THIRD EDITION

essentials of
Emergency
Care

REFRESHER FOR EMT-B

CD-ROM INCLUDED

Limmer Elling O'Keefe

Medical Editor Edward T. Dickinson, MD, FACEP

Prentice Hall
Upper Saddle River, New Jersey 07458

Library of Congress Cataloging-in-Publication Data
Limmer, Daniel
    Essentials of emergency care / Daniel Limmer, Bob Elling,
Michael O'Keefe.–3rd ed.
        p. cm.
    Includes index.
    ISBN 0-13-094559-5
    1. Medical emergencies. 2. Emergency medical technicians. I. At head of
title: Brady. II. Elling, Bob. III. O'Keefe, Michael F. IV. Dickinson, Edward
T. V. Title.

RC86.7 .L56 2002
616.02′5–dc21

2001045941

Publisher: Julie Levin Alexander
Executive Editor: Greg Vis
Managing Development Editor: Lois Berlowitz
Development Editors: Dan Zinkus, Deborah Parks
Senior Marketing Manager: Tiffany Price
Product Information Manager: Rachele Triano
Director of Manufacturing and Production: Bruce Johnson
Managing Production Editor: Patrick Walsh
Production Liaison: Cathy O'Connell
Production Editor: Navta Associates
Manufacturing Buyer: Pat Brown
Design Director: Cheryl Asherman
Senior Design Coordinator: Maria Guglielmo Walsh
Interior Design: Navta Associates
Cover Design: Blair Brown
Cover Photo: Blair Brown
Managing Photography Editor: Michal Heron
Photographers: George Dodson, Michael Gallitelli, Michal Heron,
    Richard Logan
Composition: Navta Associates
Printer/Binder: Banta Company, Menasha

PEARSON EDUCATION LTD.
PEARSON EDUCATION AUSTRALIA PTY, LIMITED
PEARSON EDUCATION SINGAPORE, PTE. LTD
PEARSON EDUCATION NORTH ASIA LTD
PEARSON EDUCATION CANADA, LTD.
PEARSON EDUCACIÓN DE MEXICO, S.A. DE C.V.
PEARSON EDUCATION—JAPAN
PEARSON EDUCATION MALAYSIA, PTE. LTD

WITH APPRECIATION
To Stephanie and Sarah Katherine
D.L.

To my future marathoners, Laura and Caitlin: Always keep chasing your dreams!
B.E.

To my parents, Mike and Noreen, my first and best teachers.
M.O'K.

NOTICE ON CARE PROCEDURES
It is the intent of the authors and publishers that this textbook be used as part of a normal EMT-Basic refresher program taught by qualified instructors and supervised by a licensed physician. The procedures described in this textbook are based upon consultation with EMT and medical authorities. The authors and publisher have taken care to make certain that these procedures reflect currently accepted clinical practice; however, they cannot be considered absolute recommendations.

The material in this textbook contains the most current information available at the time of publication. However, federal, state, and local guidelines concerning clinical practices, including without limitation, those governing infection control and universal precautions, change rapidly. The reader should note, therefore, that the new regulations may require changes in some procedures.

It is the responsibility of the reader to familiarize himself or herself with the policies and procedures set by federal, state, and local agencies as well as the institution or agency where the reader is employed. The authors and the publisher of this textbook and the supplements written to accompany it disclaim any liability, loss or risk resulting directly or indirectly from the suggested procedures and theory, from any undetected errors, or from the reader's misunderstanding of the text. It is the reader's responsibility to stay informed of any new changes or recommendations made by any federal, state, and local agency as well as by his or her employing institution or agency.

NOTICE ON GENDER USAGE
The English language has historically given preference to the male gender. Among many words, the pronouns "he" and "his" are commonly used to describe both genders. Society evolves faster than language, and the male pronouns still predominate in our speech. The authors have made great effort to treat the two genders equally, recognizing that a significant percentage of EMTs are female. However, in some instances, male pronouns may be used to describe both males and females solely for the purpose of brevity. This is not intended to offend any readers of the female gender.

NOTICE RE "Case Study"
The names used and situations depicted in "Case Study" scenarios throughout this text are fictitious.

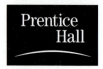

10 9 8 7 6 5 4 3 2 1

ISBN 0-13-094559-5

Dedication

This book is dedicated to the EMS, fire, and law enforcement personnel who have made the ultimate sacrifice for their communities and our nation.

May they never be forgotten.

TO OUR READERS IN THE EMS COMMUNITY

As this book goes to press, our nation is in the process of recovering from a series of terrorist attacks. These attacks, which have been unlike anything ever experienced in this country, affect all of us as individuals and as EMS providers.

In completing our work on the revision of *Essentials of Emergency Care,* we were faced with a dilemma—what to include within our text chapters regarding the challenges presented to us by terrorism. We know that the events of September 11, 2001, changed the way we look at mass casualty incidents. In fact, our thoughts on the scope and nature of what mass casualty and scene safety means have changed forever. We also realized that it is still too soon, that we may need distance and perspective on these events before we can write about how we may have to adapt our approaches to mass casualty care.

As EMS providers and educators, we will continue to study and learn from incidents big and small and bring the most recent information to you on all topics related to your study and recertification as an EMT.

As of this writing, there are still hundreds of rescuers and thousands of civilians whose bodies have not been recovered or identified as a result of the September 11th tragedy. Our thoughts, prayers, and respect are with our fallen brothers, the families and friends left behind, and those who continue to provide emergency services in any situation.

Daniel Limmer
Bob Elling
Michael F. O'Keefe

September 2001

BRIEF CONTENTS

DETAILED CONTENTS

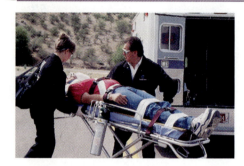
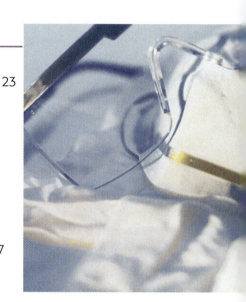
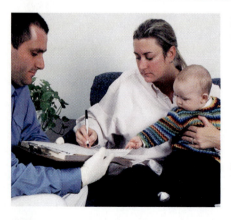

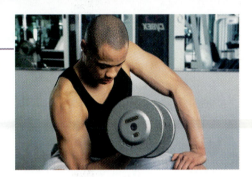
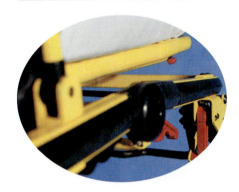
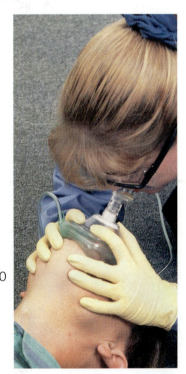

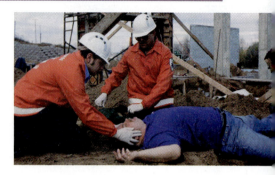

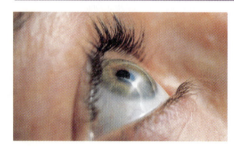

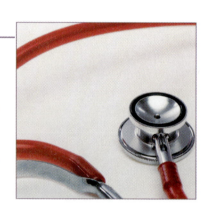

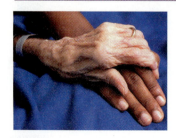

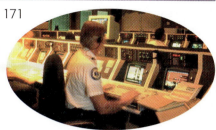
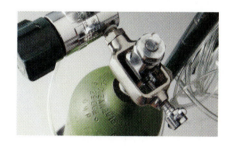
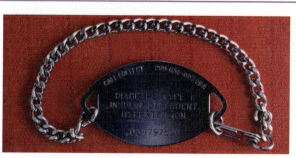

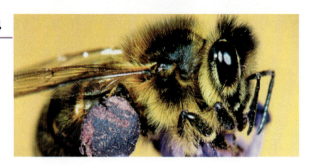

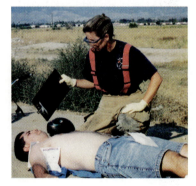

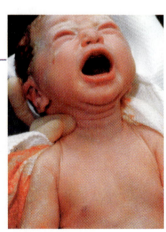

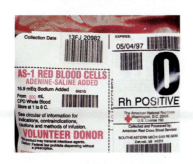

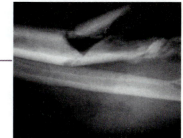

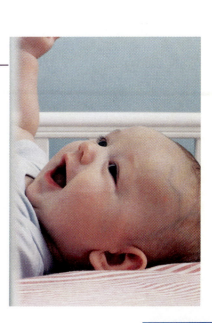

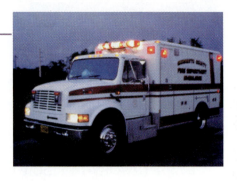

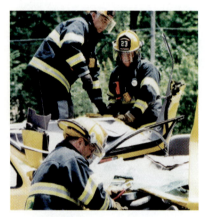

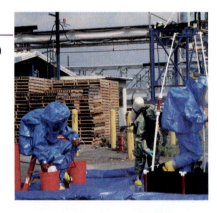

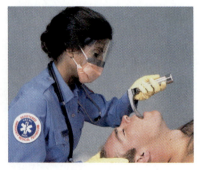

PREFACE

Essentials of Emergency Care, Third Edition, is designed for experienced EMT-Bs who are beginning, or are about to begin, an EMT-B refresher program. Traditionally, to complete such a program, EMT-Bs used their original EMT-B textbook or a subsequent edition. Such textbooks are designed to present information to a person who has no experience or training in EMS. However, the authors of this text recognize that the refresher student is different.

The authors acknowledge and respect the fact that you, an experienced EMT-B, have regularly applied the skills and knowledge learned in your original course to your work in the field. Because of your experience, expansive coverage of those skills and knowledge is not needed in a refresher text. For example, since you probably have had much field experience in bleeding control, this text does not cover it in as much detail as your original text does.

The skills and knowledge that you use less frequently, however, do require some brushing up before you take a recertification exam. Such topics are covered in *Essentials of Emergency Care* thoroughly but concisely.

National Curricula for the EMT-B

In 1994, the U.S. Department of Transportation released the "EMT-Basic: National Standard Curriculum," which has been widely accepted as the standard for instructing new EMT-Bs throughout the country. A year after its publication, the National Registry of EMTs was asked by the National Council of State EMS Training Coordinators and the National Association of State EMS Directors to develop a refresher curriculum based on the National Standard. In 1997, after consensus was achieved by the committee and the states, the U.S. Department of Transportation released the "EMT-Basic: Refresher Curriculum."

Written to help you meet all national objectives, *Essentials of Emergency Care,* Third Edition, covers both the "EMT-Basic: National Standard Curriculum" and the "EMT-Basic: Refresher Curriculum."

In addition, to make it easy for you and your instructor to be sure you are able to meet all Refresher objectives, they are listed verbatim at the beginning of every chapter and include page references that correlate related textbook material.

Correlation of Essentials of Emergency Care, Third Edition with DOT's Refresher and National Standard Curricula

Refresher Curriculum	Essentials of Emergency Care	EMT-B National Standard Curriculum
Module 1: Preparatory	Chapters 1–5	Module 1: Preparatory
Module 2: Airway	Chapter 6	Module 2: Airway
Module 3: Patient Assessment	Chapters 7–11	Module 3: Patient Assessment
Module 4: Medical/Behavioral	Chapters 12–19	Module 4: Medical/Behavioral Emergencies and Obstetrics/Gynecology
Module 5: Trauma	Chapters 21–24	Module 5: Trauma
Module 6: Obstetrics, Infants, and Children	Chapters 20, 25	Module 6: Infants and Children
	Chapters 26–28	Module 7: Operations
	Chapters 29	Module 8: Advanced Airway (Elective)

Correlations with the National Standard Curriculum may be found in a special box located next to each chapter title. This information correlates content with one or more National Standard "Lessons."

Features of the Book

In revising *Essentials of Emergency Care,* we kept our eye on the primary goal: to develop a book that provides concise yet complete coverage of the EMT-B curriculum for refresher students and people with past experience. We know you do not want to spend time preparing for your next exam by reading a book meant for beginning students. If you need to review a skill or other information, you want that information presented in a way that best meets your needs. Welcome to *Essentials of Emergency Care,* Third Edition!

This edition has kept the same successful presentation as the previous edition in addition to including new features. This edition contains:

NEW! *Essential Electronic Extras CD-ROM*

This CD-ROM contains two 150-question diagnostic examinations to help you prepare for examinations as well as identify areas where you should concentrate your study as you refresh or recertify your EMT-B credentials. The CD-ROM also contains 450 questions in chapter quizzes.

NEW! *Web Essentials*

Visit **www.prenhall.com/limmer,** a valuable online resource that includes interactive quizzes and case studies as well as links to important EMS websites.

NEW! *Case Studies*

Twelve new case studies relate chapter content to street experiences. For experienced EMT-Bs, case-based presentations make study and learning more pertinent and interesting. The case studies include critical background information and details of pathophysiology, assessment, and patient medications to provide the "big picture" of patient assessment and care.

NEW! *Core Concepts*

Each chapter begins with a list of the core concepts important to know in the topic area.

NEW! *Lifespan Development*

This new feature highlights important pediatric and geriatric issues within each chapter.

Skill Summaries

Illustrated step-by-step summaries enhance your understanding of skill procedures, summarize information, and maximize coverage.

Preceptor Pearls

Acknowledging the experienced EMT-B's role as a preceptor, mentor, and trainer, this feature highlights important topics you may wish to share with new EMT-Bs and emphasizes ways to get your points across.

Chapter Review

Each chapter ends with a summary of chapter material, multiple-choice questions to test your knowledge of chapter content, and a list of topics for which weblinks have been provided on our website.

National Registry Practical Examination

All the skills tested by the National Registry in its performance-based skills exam are included for convenient reference at the back of the book.

Comments and Suggestions

We encourage you to send your suggestions and comments about the text. They will help us improve future editions of *Essentials of Emergency Care.* Send them to the Marketing Manager at BRADY, Prentice Hall, One Lake Street, Upper Saddle River, NJ 07458. You can also reach us via e-mail:

 Daniel Limmer: danlimmer@earthlink.net
 Bob Elling: bobelling@usa.net
 Mike O'Keefe: mikeokvt@aol.com

We wish you the best of luck in your continued endeavors in EMS!

Visit Brady's Web Site
http://www.bradybooks.com

ACKNOWLEDGMENTS

The authors wish to acknowledge the many people and organizations who provided assistance to make this third edition possible. There are many reviewers and people who participated in photo shoots in this and previous editions whose time, knowledge, and dedication have been vital in creating the edition you now have before you.

The people at Brady have been dedicated and supportive as always. We would like to thank publisher Julie Alexander and our acquisitions editor, Greg Vis, for their insights and guidance in this revision. Monica Silva worked behind the scenes to keep information and material flowing, which is greatly appreciated. Dan Zinkus and Deborah Parks edited this edition skillfully. Editors make authors look good, and we always appreciate that. The production and art teams at Brady, including Pat Walsh, Cathy O'Connell, Cheryl Asherman, and Maria Guglielmo, have done a fantastic job getting the words, photos, and art to paper. Tiffany Price has been a friend and an advocate for our books. Thank you very much. Our continued gratitude goes to the Brady sales representatives who get this book from us to you.

For anyone who has read these acknowledgements over the past ten years, there have been two people whose names have been seen consistently. Those are Lois Berlowitz, Managing Development Editor, and Michal Heron, Managing Photography Editor. In every book we write we say the same things about both Lois and Michal—that the book would be impossible without them, that their dedication, organization, and talent are both amazing and critical to the book you see here. Well, it's true. And we've said it again. We have sincerely enjoyed working with you both and hope to have the pleasure of publishing successful books together for many years in the future.

And finally we would like to acknowledge our families who have stood by us and encouraged us to engage in the writing of this and other books. Some family members have even provided future case study ideas during the writing of this book. Thank you all for everything.

Reviewers

A textbook relies on reviewers for shaping the content as well as checking its accuracy. We thank our reviewers for their hard work and detailed comments.

For the Third Edition:

Edna Deacon
EMT Coordinator
Sussex County Community College
Newton, NJ

Donald Graesser
EMT Instructor, AHA Instructor Trainer
Bergen County EMS Training Center
Paramus, NJ

Jon F. Levine, EMT-P, I/C
Deputy Superintendent
Boston EMS
Boston, MA

Dennis J. O'Rourke
Bergen County EMS Training Center
Paramus, NJ

Georgia Pace
EMS Training Center
Paramus, NJ

Rose Marie Tiernan
EMS Training Center Lead Instructor
Law and Public Safety Institute EMS Liaison
Bergen County EMS Training Center
Paramus, NJ

For the Second Edition:

Bobby Baker, Paramedic Program Chair
Ivy Tech State College
Evansville, IN

James M. Courtney, NREMT-P
Vermont Department of Health
Office of Emergency Medical Services
Burlington, VT

Lynette McCullough
Program Coordinator, EMS Programs
Clayton College & State University
Fayetteville, GA

Lisa A. Shelanskas, EMT-I
Suffield Ambulance Association
Suffield, CT

Scott W. Trethaway II, EMT-P
EMS Coordinator
Chester County Emergency Services
Lansdale, PA

For the First Edition:

Beth Lothrop Adams, M.A., R.N., NREMT-P
ALS Coordinator, EMS Degree Program
Adjunct Assistant Professor of Emergency
  Medicine
The George Washington University
Washington, DC

Ralph Backenstoes
Emergency Health Services Federation
New Cumberland, PA

Marianne J. Barry, M.A., EMT-P
Allied Health/EMMT
Lee College
Baytown, TX

John L. Beckman, FF/PM Instructor
Lincolnwood Fire Department
Lincolnwood, IL

Kerry Campbell, NREMT-P
Lakeshore Technical College
Cleveland, WI

Robert Glover
Virginia Beach Fire Department
Virginia Beach, VA

Sgt. John Hannon
EMS Coordinator
Foxborough Police Department
Foxborough, MA

Debby Hassel, NREMT-P, B.S.
Denver Fire EMS Division
EMS Educator
Denver, CO

J. Kevin Henson
State EMS Training Coordinator
New Mexico EMS Bureau
Santa Fe, NM

Sgt. David M. Johnson, MICP
Emergency Services Unit
Montville Township Police
Montville, NJ

Jackie McNally, MICP
MICU Clinical Coordinator
Chilton Memorial Hospital
Pompton Plains, NJ

Greg Mullen
Director of EMS Education
HealthONE EMS
Littleton, CO

Ed Scheidel
Davenport College
Center for the Study of EMS
Grand Rapids, MI

Douglas Stevenson
EMS Department Head/Northwest College
Houston Community College System
Houston, TX

Brian J. Wilson, NREMT-P
Education Coordinator
Department of Emergency Medicine
El Paso, TX

Rhoda R. Woodard, R.N., NREMT
Chairperson, EMT 1 + 1 Paramedic
Nursing Allied Health Center
Hinds Community College
Jackson, MS

Photo Acknowledgments

All photographs not otherwise credited were photographed on assignment for Brady/Prentice Hall Health Pearson Education. Photos are credited as follows:

Photos Sources: Comstock Klips CO-2; Custom Medical Corporation/SIU 20-3f; Edward T. Dickinson, MD 6-14, 6-19, 21-4; © David Handschuh 3-3; © Michal Heron CO-1, CO-9, CO-12, CO-14, CO-25, CO-26, Table 10-1 a,b,c,d,e; Mark C. Ide CO-27; Index Stock Imagery Table 10-1f; © Craig Jackson In the Dark Photography 3-4, CS-6, 7-2, 7-4b, CS-13, CS-17, Skill Summary 19-1, 1-5, CS-22, 28-16, 10-4; Laerdal Medical Corporation 14-3; © Tracy Mack In the Dark Photography CS-16, CS-19, CS-21; Charly Miller 26-5; Omni-photo Communications CS-24; Photo Researchers 25-5; © Charles Stewart MD & Associates 23-9a, 23-9b, 24-4; Stone/Getty CO-16

Companies We wish to thank the following companies for their cooperation in providing us with photos: Ambu, Inc.; Ferno, Inc., Wilmington, OH; Laerdal Medical Corporation, Armonk, NY; Marquette Electronics, Inc., Milwaukee, WI; Nellcor Puritan Bennett, Pleasanton, CA; Nonin Medical, Inc., Plymouth, MN; PhysioControl Corporation, Redmond, WA; RMC Medical, Philadelphia, PA; Road Rescue, Inc., St. Paul, MN; SpaceLabs Medical, Inc., Redmond, WA: Wehr Engineering, Fairland, IN: and Westech Information Systems, Inc., Vancouver, BC.

Organizations We also wish to thank the following organizations for their assistance in creating the photo program for *Essentials*: Colonie Department of EMS, Colonie, NY; Fire Department New York, Bureau of Training, Bayside, NY; Hudson Valley Community College, Troy, NY; Montgomery County Public Service Training Academy, Rockville, MD; North Bethlehem Fire Department, North Bethlehem, NY; Pinellas County EMS, Largo, FL; Riverdale Fire Department, Riverdale, MD; Rockville Fire Station #3, Rockville, MD; Sandy Spring Volunteer Fire Department, Sandy Spring, MD; Sarasota County Fire Department, Sarasota, FL; Suburban Hospital, Bethesda, MD; Shady Grove Adventist Hospital, Shady Grove, MD; Town of Colonie Police Department, Colonie, NY; Town of Guilderland EMS, Guilderland, NY; Western Turnpike Rescue Squad, Albany, NY; and Wheaton Volunteer Rescue Squad, Wheaton, MD.

Technical Advisors Thanks to the following people for providing technical support during the photo shoots:

Mark T. Beall
EMT-P Instructor, Career Firefighter, Paramedic
Maryland State EMS Instructor.

Richard W.O. Beebe, B.S., R.N.

Gloria Bizjak
EMT-A, Curriculum Specialist
Maryland Fire and Rescue Institute.

Steve Carter
Manager, Special Programs
Maryland Fire and Rescue Institute.

Gail Collins, NR-EMT, EMT Instructor.

Michael Collins, EMT-P.

Ann Marie Davies, EMT-P.

Paul Dezzi
Captain, Sarasota County Fire Department
Sarasota, FL.

Bob Elling
MPA, REMT-P, Program Coordinator
Hudson Valley Community College.

Brian Gorski
Chief, Sarasota County Fire Department
Sarasota, FL.

Conrad T. Kearns
Pinellas County EMS
Largo, FL.

Lt. Willa K. Little
EMS Training Officer
Montgomery County Public Service Training
 Academy.

George Morgan
Industrial Training Specialist
Maryland Fire and Rescue Institute.

Bruce Olsen
B.S., RRT, EMT-P.

Jonathan Politis
B.A., REMT-P, Director of Emergency Medical Services
Town of Colonie, NY.

Jay Smith
EMT Class Coordinator
Montgomery County Public Service Training
 Academy.

Christine Uhlhorn
EMT-A, EMT Instructor
Maryland Fire and Rescue Institute.

Linda Zimmerman
EMT-A, EMT Instructor
Maryland Fire and Rescue Institute.

ABOUT THE AUTHORS

Daniel Limmer, EMT-P, is a faculty member at the George Washington University Health Services program in Washington, DC. He has been involved in emergency services for more than twenty years as a paramedic, police officer, and educator. He is a co-author of *Emergency Care*, Ninth Edition, *First Responder: A Skills Approach, Fire Service First Responder,* and *Advanced Medical Life Support.*

Bob Elling, MPA, REMT-P, is currently a full-time faculty member at the Institute of Prehospital Emergency Medicine at Hudson Valley Community College in Troy, NY. He is also a Professor of Management with the American College of Prehospital Medicine, and works part-time as a paramedic with the Colonie EMS Department (NY). His publications include: *Pocket Reference for the EMT-B and First Responder, First Responder: Exam Preparation and Review, Emergency Care Student Workbook,* and *Paramedic Care: Principles & Practice Volume 5 Student Workbook.* Bob has written hundreds of articles for magazines and internet websites as well as video scripts.

Michael F. O'Keefe, REMT-P, is Training Coordinator for the Vermont Department of Health's EMS division. He has been active as chairperson of the National Council of State EMS Training Coordinators and with the development of various national EMS curricula. He was a member of the curriculum development group for the "First Responder: National Standard Curriculum." He also is a co-author of *Emergency Care,* Ninth Edition.

Medical Editor

Edward T. Dickinson, M.D., NREMT-P, FACEP, is currently an Assistant Professor in the Department of Emergency Medicine, University of Pennsylvania, School of Medicine in Philadelphia where he is Director of EMS Field Operations. He is Medical Director of the Town of Colonic EMS Department (NY) and the Malvern Fire Company (PA). Dr. Dickinson is active in prehospital research and the medical editor of numerous Brady EMT-B and First Responder texts. He is also the author of *Fire Service Emergency Care* and co-author of *Emergency Incident Rehabilitation.*

Essentials of Emergency Care

In today's fast-paced learning environment, training takes place beyond the printed page. Brady has done it again and leads the field with a rich multimedia package for *Essentials of Emergency Care* that provides multiple interactive learning opportunities for students.

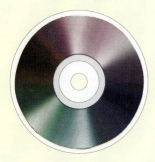

Student CD-ROM The first of its kind in EMS! Includes a 150-question **pretest** with diagnostic scoring that indicates areas of strength and weakness. Students know where they need to focus their energies when studying so they can be successful in the course and on their exams. The CD-ROM also contains chapter-specific **quizzes** with more than 400 questions that provide additional practice, and a 150-question **posttest** to help students prepare for National Registry or state-certifying exams.

Companion Web Site *(www.prenhall.com/limmer)* Contains chapter-by-chapter interactive review quizzes with immediate scoring and instant feedback, case studies, annotated links to appropriate EMS resources, and a Syllabus Manager for instructors.

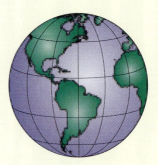

Setting the Standard for Instructor's Resources!

Essentials of Emergency Care has a comprehensive **"Instructor's Success Kit"** containing everything an instructor needs to successfully teach a refresher course. The kit includes an **Instructor's Resource Manual, Test Manager,** and **PowerPoint Slides.**

Technology at Its Best

When it comes to EMT-B refresher training, nothing beats *Essentials of Emergency Care*'s full range of multimedia support materials.

 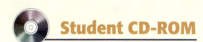 **Student CD-ROM**

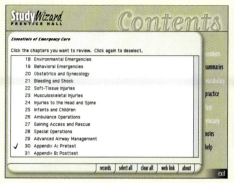 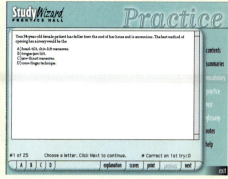

Diagnostic pretest and posttest *create a study path for students and helps students prepare for National Registry or state qualifying exams.*

Chapter-specific quizzes *provide students with extra practice.*

Companion Web Site www.prenhall.com/limmer

Syllabus Manager Online aid for instructors who wish to post course syllabi and assignments on the web for easy student access.

Case Studies Help students practice critical thinking skills in lifelike situations with these learning activities.

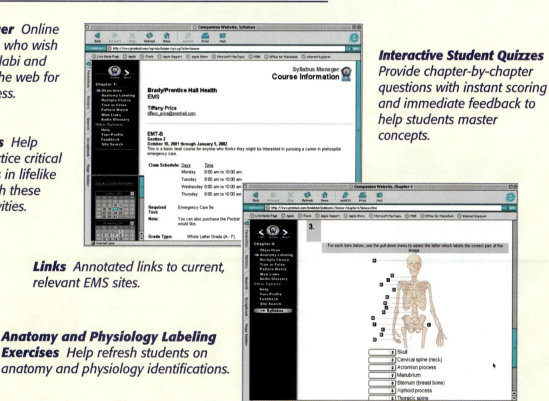

Interactive Student Quizzes Provide chapter-by-chapter questions with instant scoring and immediate feedback to help students master concepts.

Links Annotated links to current, relevant EMS sites.

Anatomy and Physiology Labeling Exercises Help refresh students on anatomy and physiology identifications.

✳ **Pocket Reference for the EMT-Basic and First Responder, 2e** *available as a PDA download.* This handy pocket-sized field reference includes skills checklists, common medications, abbreviations and acronyms, and anatomy charts. It is available for both PalmPilots and Windows CE.

Brady's Course Compass. Harness the power of the web with Brady's Course Compass to accompany *Essentials of Emergency Care*! This online course provides you with:

- Lecture notes
- Student activities and exercises
- Online testing
- Electronic gradebook
- Communications tools such as email and chat
- A whole host of course management tools for instructors.

Also available: Blackboard

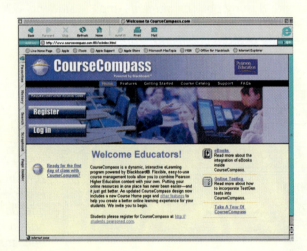

Medical Emergency Response Simulator (MERS)

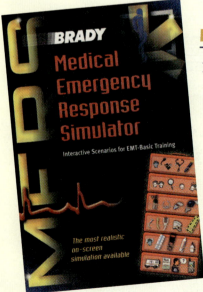

Brady's **MERS-Victor (Medical Emergency Response Simulator)** (ISBN 0-13-089857-0) contains over a dozen different "calls," providing you with truly interactive scenarios. Students and professionals can practice the decision-making skills they need to master to become and remain top-notch EMTs. Students can now also purchase **MERS Victor-Student,** which contains 2 brand-new scenarios to provide students with additional case-based practice.

Case Studies don't get any more realistic than this.

Check *www.bradybooks.com* for the latest information on our products as well as additional content to reinforce learning.

A Rich Blend of Traditional Features

Hallmark Features

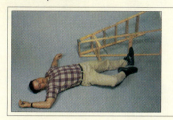

Skill Summary 8-1
Focused History and Physical Exam—Trauma Patient

FIRST take BSI precautions.

Mechanism of Injury

Reassess the MOI. If there is no significant MOI (e.g., patient has a cut finger), focus the physical exam only on the injured part. If the MOI is significant:
- Continue manual stabilization of the head and neck
- Consider requesting ALS personnel
- Reconsider transport decision
- Reassess mental status and ABCs
- Perform a rapid trauma assessment

Rapid Trauma Assessment

Rapidly assess each part of the body for the following problems (say "Dee-cap-?-LS" memor

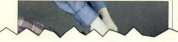

Skill Summary *Step-by-step skill procedures are presented for easy reference in illustrated scans.*

Preceptor Pearls *These special features acknowledge the experienced EMT-B's role as a mentor by pointing out important topics to share with new EMT-Bs. They emphasize ways to share information and highlight when and how to mentor new EMT-Bs.*

PRECEPTOR PEARL

Many EMT-Bs, especially at the beginning of their careers, are reluctant to apply a painful stimulus. Instead, perhaps out of a sense of shyness or a reluctance to harm the patient, they apply only a mild stimulus that is not sufficient to rouse the patient. The EMT then notifies the hospital that the patient is unresponsive to verbal and painful stimuli; but on arrival at the emergency department, the staff is easily able to elicit a response with a brisk sternal rub or a pinch of the trapezius. Watch for this tendency with new or inexperienced EMT-Bs, and give them the benefit of your experience.

A true mental status check includes more than just applying a verbal or painful stimulus. However, during the initial assessment you do not need any more information th

ment)
out a

If
faster
conce
may a
respir
tient's
of bre
ventila
spons
breath
this c

Circu
Evalua
simul
W
and l
feel th
wrist.
caroti
brach

Patient Assessment
Poisoning and Overdose Emergencies

A rapid, organized approach to patient assessment is essential in cases of possible ingested poisoning. Before you contact medical direction, you should perform an initial assessment. Look fo altered mental status. Assess ABCs. If a life-th ening condition exists, treat immediately. The your patient is responsive:

- Perform a focused history and physical exa When you gather the history, be sure to ask What substance was ingested? When was the substance ingested? How much was ingested Over what time period did the ingestion occur? What interventions have the patient, family, or bystanders taken? How much does the patient weigh? Has the patient vomited?
- Assess vital signs.
- Provide emergency care. Be sure to check with medical direction.

Or if your patient is unresponsive, perform focused history and physical exam, including a rapid trauma assessment. Gather a SAMPLE history from bystanders or family. Assess vital signs, and provide emergency care.

The following signs and symptoms are frequently associated with a poisoning or overdose emergency:

- Nausea
- Vomiting
- Diarrhea

Patient Care
Poisoning and Overdose Emergencies

Emergency care of a patient with a poisoning emergency includes the following:

1. **Perform an initial assessment.** Immediately treat life-threatening problems. Request advanced life support when appropriate.

2. **Perform a focused history and physical exam.** Be sure to remove any pills, tablets, or fragments from patient's mouth.

3. **Assess baseline vital signs.**

4. **Consult medical direction about the administration of activated charcoal** (Skill Summary 17-1). If directed by medical direction, dilute the poison with water or milk.

5. **Bring all poison containers, bottles, and labels to receiving facility.**

6. **Conduct an ongoing assessment en route to the emergency department.** ✱

Be sure to include in your prehospital care report (PCR) a thorough documentation of observations at the scene, changes in the patient's mental status, and treatment given.

For the other types of poison exposures (inhaled, absorbed, or injected poisons), apply the assessment techniques learned in this chapter. Treatment for these poison exposures remains the same (Skill Summaries 17-2 and 17-3 on the following pages).

Patient Assessment and Patient Care *Patient Assessment and Patient Care segments describe the assessment and treatment you should provide for particular types of illnesses, disorders, or injuries. Patient Assessment typically lists important signs and symptoms. Patient Care lists key steps of emergency care.*

New to this Edition

Updated coverage of the 2000 AHA Guidelines.

More Advanced Content *New coverage of advanced topics such as pathophysiology, medications, diagnosis, and infectious diseases have been added to help providers keep up-to-date with the most current information and techniques available.*

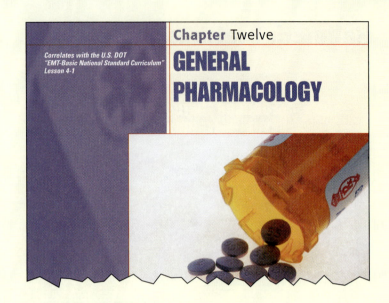

Correlates with the U.S. DOT "EMT-Basic National Standard Curriculum" Lesson 4-1

Chapter Twelve
GENERAL PHARMACOLOGY

LIFESPAN DEVELOPMENT

In children under 6 years of age, also evaluate capillary refill by pressing on the end of the nail, the back of the hand, or the top of the foot. After you release the pressure of your finger, the color should change from white to pink in less than 2 seconds. More than 2 seconds is abnormal and may be a sign of shock (hypoperfusion) or exposure to cold.

Lifespan Development *This special feature focuses on pediatric and geriatric patients, helping providers deal with the full span of emergencies.*

Identification of Priority Patients

The "sixth sense" you may have developed with experience probably alerts you to the fact that certain patients need to be transported promptly. In fact,

Case Studies *Case studies in a journal article format help providers make a connection between material in the text and real-world applications.*

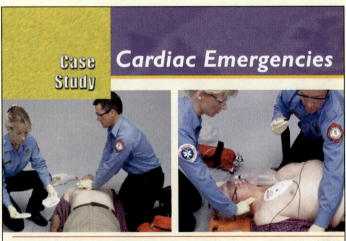

Case Study

Cardiac Emergencies

Dispatch Information 1452 Lowell Street, Apartment 2C   Chest pain   1934 hr

Your ambulance is dispatched to a 58-year-old man complaining of chest pain. When you are 2 minutes away from the scene, dispatch advises that the patient's wife has called again. The patient is now unresponsive, and the dispatcher is giving her instructions in CPR. This is a BLS system, so ALS is not available.

Mr. Tate is now secured to the backboard so he will not slide off when you carry him down the stairs. A quick carotid pulse check before you leave the apartment verifies that Mr. Tate still has a carotid pulse. The patient is not breathing spontaneously, however, so your partner continues to ventilate him with high

Instructor's Success Kit

The Most Complete Package Available

Essentials of Emergency Care has a comprehensive **"Instructor's Success Kit"** containing everything an instructor needs to successfully teach a refresher course. The kit includes an **Instructor's Resource Manual, Test Manager,** and **PowerPoint Slides.**

■ **Instructor's Resource Manual** (0-13-098332-2) Available both on disk and in print, this valuable resource contains lesson plans, lecture outlines, student activities and handouts, lists of additional resources, answers to student handouts, and more.

■ **Essentials of Emergency Care, 3e PowerPoint Slides** (0-13-091302-2) This CD-ROM contains PowerPoint slides with integrated text and images. The slides can be customized to suit individual classroom needs.

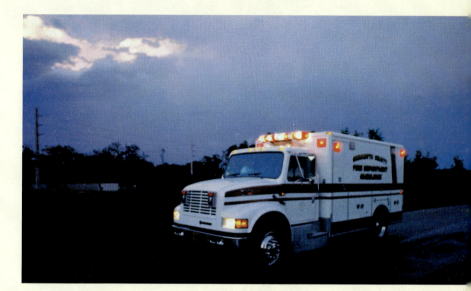

■ **Test Manager** (Win 0-13-031940-6) (MAC 0-13-032422-1) The test manager to accompany **Emergency Care, 9e** contains 1200 questions on disk in a customizable format that allows instructors to construct and administer online tests. An electronic gradebook is also included.

■ **EMT-B 35mm Slides** (0-13-091303-0) Approximately 2000 slides in traditional 35mm format.

■ **Anatomy & Physiology Color Acetates** (0-8359-5203-7) This set contains 41 acetates with 88 overlays to form multiple transparent layers that allow anatomical systems to be viewed at various depths and levels.

Correlates with the U.S. DOT "EMT-Basic National Standard Curriculum" Lesson 1-1

Chapter One

INTRODUCTION TO EMS SYSTEMS

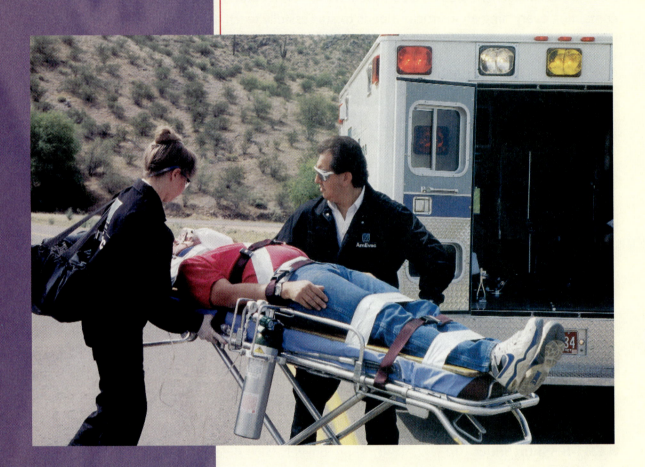

ESSENTIAL ELECTRONIC EXTRAS

CD ESSENTIALS

For preview and review of chapter material, see the student CD-ROM for

- Pretest
- Chapter quizzes
- Posttest

WEB ESSENTIALS

For additional review and enrichment, visit www.prenhall.com/limmer for

- Interactive student quizzes
- Links to online EMS resources
- Online case studies
- Audio glossary

The U.S. Department of Transportation's 1994 "EMT-Basic National Standard Curriculum," combined with state and local protocols, defines the scope of your EMT refresher training. This section discusses the Emergency Medical Services (EMS) system, the role of the experienced EMT-B as a preceptor, quality improvement (QI), and a topic that will be used frequently in the field—medical direction. Your instructor will review the related state and local policies, including the implications of the Americans with Disabilities Act (ADA).

THE EMERGENCY MEDICAL SERVICES SYSTEM

As an emergency medical technician going through an update or refresher course, you have undoubtedly experienced most if not all of the components of the Emergency Medical Services (EMS) system (Figure 1-1). The EMS system includes the following components:

- **Bystanders.** Bystanders or other persons on scene are responsible for activation of the EMS system. Bystanders also may initiate CPR or other emergency care measures prior to the arrival of the EMS units.
- **Emergency Medical Dispatchers.** EMS dispatchers take incoming emergency calls, obtain important information from callers, assign response priorities, and provide pre-arrival instructions to lay people at the scene.
- **First Responders.** Most likely the first to respond to an emergency scene, these EMS-trained rescuers may be firefighters, police, or other public, private, or industrial personnel. They provide emergency medical care until the arrival of an ambulance and more highly trained EMS personnel.
- **Emergency Medical Technicians.** The EMT-B may function in many areas, the most common of which is on an ambulance. EMT-Bs continue care started by First Responders and provide transportation of the patient. Additional training is available above the EMT-B level. EMT-Intermediates and EMT-Paramedics are considered to be advanced EMTs.
- **Emergency Department Staff.** The emergency department staff receives the patient and continues care using hospital resources. Serious trauma cases may pass quickly through the emergency department to the operating room where surgical correction of life-threatening injuries may be performed.

- **Specialty Centers.** Many hospitals are designated as specialty centers. They care for all patients but have special resources available. These include trauma centers, burn centers, pediatric centers, and poison centers.
- **Allied Health Personnel.** During the course of treatment, a patient may be seen by allied health personnel such as therapists, technicians, and other specialists.

System Access

When many EMTs began their initial training, 911 (always pronounced as "nine-one-one") communication was simply a vision. Now, many communities have **911 access** to a centralized communication center for emergency police, fire, and EMS calls. This number, made public through advertising and television, is important because it is easily remembered and it allows quick and easy access to the EMS system. In the future, it will be the only number required nationwide to get help in an emergency.

However, presently, not all areas use this number. These areas are called **non-911 systems.**

CORE CONCEPTS

In this chapter, you will learn about the following topics:

- Components of the EMS system

- Roles and responsibilities of the EMT-B

- Quality improvement and the role of the EMT-B in the process

- Medical direction (on-line, off-line, and standing orders)

✔ **Knowledge**

☐ **1.** Provide for safety of self, patient, and fellow workers. (pp. 5–6)

☐ **2.** Participate in the quality improvement process. (pp. 8–9)

  • Define "quality improvement" and discuss the EMT-Basic's role in the process. (pp. 8–9)

☐ **3.** Use physician medical direction for authorization to provide care. (pp. 9–10)

  • Define "medical direction" and discuss the EMT-Basic's role in the process. (p. 9)

✔ **Attitude**

☐ **4.** Assess areas of personal attitude and conduct of the EMT-Basic. (pp. 6–8)

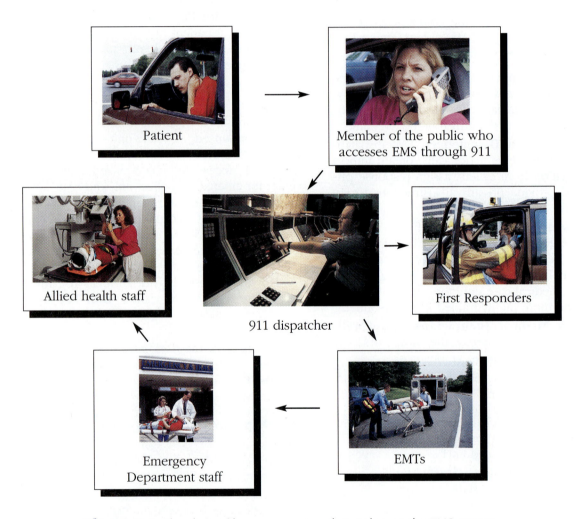

Figure 1-1 The chain of human resources that makes up the EMS system.

Dialing 911 in these areas may not be ideal. Calls are routed to operators who, while trained, may not even be in the same city or region as the patient and thus may cause delays in EMS response.

Enhanced 911 (sometimes called "E-911") is a system set up so that the caller's number and location are displayed on the screen for the emergency dispatcher. This is especially helpful in cases in which the patient loses consciousness or is unable to speak or when the caller is a small child. It has benefits in police emergencies as well.

Levels of Training

The training of EMS personnel in the U.S. differs from state to state. In the early 1990s EMS professionals representing many national organizations convened to discuss this matter. As a result, they developed the "National Emergency Medical Services Education and Practice Blueprint," which outlines the skills that should be performed at each level of EMS training. This attempt at standardization was adopted by the U.S. DOT National Highway Traffic Safety Administration and incorporated in the new official curricula.

While there will always be some differences in training among the states and regions, the following are levels of EMS training defined by the "Blueprint" and the NHTSA:

- First Responder
- Emergency Medical Technician–Basic
- Emergency Medical Technician–Intermediate
- Emergency Medical Technician–Paramedic

The **National Registry of Emergency Medical Technicians** is an organization that provides a means of nationally registering First Responders and all three types of Emergency Medical Technician. It uses a written and practical examination to qualify candidates for registration. It also is active in many EMS issues such as curriculum development, standardization, and research. Many states use the National Registry for their final examinations and for license reciprocity. Having this certification may make it easier to relocate to other states or regions. (See Figure 1-2 for the National Registry's EMT-B patch.)

Roles and Responsibilities of the EMT-Basic

After performing the job of an EMT-B for a period of time, one might think that the roles and responsibilities you are bound by would be relatively obvious. You may, in fact, practice without thinking about them. However, the roles and responsibilities are important to know, both for your practice as an

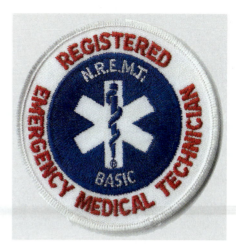

Figure 1-2 The National Registry's EMT-Basic patch.

EMT-B and for your recertification exam. They are (Figure 1-3):

- **Personal safety.** The EMT-B curriculum stresses safety in several areas, most notably in scene size-up. Safety issues include hazards from chemicals, violence, traffic, and natural forces.
- **Safety of the crew, patient, and bystanders.** Continuing the emphasis on safety, the EMT-B must also look out for the safety of others. Emergency scenes are dynamic events. Untrained personnel may act in unusual ways when in emergency situations.
- **Patient assessment.** You will perform a patient assessment throughout a call on every patient you encounter. This will help you to make appropriate treatment and transport decisions.
- **Patient care.** Patient care is based on patient assessment.
- **Lifting and moving patients.** Since EMS treatment almost always results in transportation to a hospital, lifting and moving the patient safely and effectively is very important. Improper lifting and moving not only can injure the patient, but it also can worsen the patient's condition and injure the EMT-B.
- **Transport and transfer of care.** Once moved to the ambulance, the patient must be safely delivered to the hospital. At the hospital, the patient and the patient information you have gathered must be turned over to hospital personnel.
- **Record keeping and data collection.** While some may not consider filling out a run report as record keeping, this report is a legal document and must be completed neatly and accurately. As

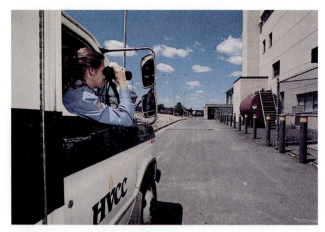

A Personal and crew safety

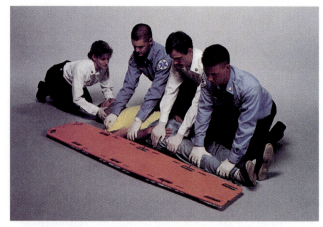

C Lifting and moving, transport, and transfer of care

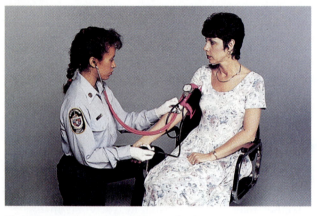

B Patient assessment, care, and advocacy

Figure 1-3A, B, C Some roles and responsibilities of the EMT-B.

EMS grows, research will be needed to determine trends and information that will help improve EMS care. Thus, accurate and thorough record keeping and data collection can contribute to improving patient care. (See Appendix A, "Research in EMS" for more on this topic.)

- **Patient advocacy.** Remember, an advocate does more for a patient than provide textbook emergency care. In the time you spend with your patient, you can learn a great deal about his or her condition and needs. For example, you may find that the patient has a special concern that you can bring to the attention of hospital personnel in order to comfort him or her. Or you might submit a social service referral for the geriatric patient who may require additional home care. Performing such a significant task can make a tremendous positive difference to a patient.

Professional Attributes of an EMT-Basic

Several professional attributes that are desirable for an EMT-B include a neat, clean appearance, positive image, maintaining up-to-date knowledge, and safely placing the patient's needs above your own. For example, a patient who is experiencing chills on a hot day would not want the ambulance air conditioner running full force. You should turn the air conditioner off because it is in the best interest of the patient.

An EMT-B must maintain a positive attitude when dealing with patients and coworkers. Personal conduct also must be beyond reproach.

The EMT-Basic as a Preceptor

Since you (or your instructor) chose this book, you most likely have some experience as an EMT-B. You will notice that this book takes a slightly different look at the EMT-B curriculum. Most notably, it covers the curriculum objectives in an abbreviated way since you have been taught much of the material earlier in a full course.

The second way this text differs is it takes into account the fact that you will be an example for new EMT-Bs as they finish their training. In the past, being a trainer has not been considered a major part of the roles and responsibilities of an EMT. But try to recall your first few months or years as an EMT. You most likely had some good and bad experiences. Some experienced EMTs were extremely helpful and supportive. Others may have actually helped you learn the wrong information.

The receipt of an EMT-B card is not the end of EMS learning. It is the beginning. As an experienced EMT, you will be called upon to teach new EMT-Bs, both formally when giving orientation sessions and informally by example. This section discusses ways you can help teach the new EMT-B through your everyday role as a **preceptor,** or mentor.

Webster's Dictionary defines "mentor" as "a wise and trusted counselor and teacher" and "preceptor" as "tutor." These definitions capture the essence of what you are called to do when working with new EMT-Bs. Remember that the EMT-B course is primarily classroom and lab work with minimal field experience. Students emerge from the course with a considerable amount of new knowledge but with little experience applying that knowledge in the field. The transition from classroom to field is not smooth or easy. A new EMT-B's first calls are critical for developing the confidence that will form the basis of a successful EMS career.

Even before you begin to teach skills such as assessment or splinting, you can provide some important, practical insight into EMS:

- Let new EMT-Bs know that their EMS education is a life-long commitment. It does not stop with their EMT-B training. Show them that you mean it by participating in continuing medical education (CME) and other available training. Stimulate the newcomer by quizzing or offering challenging situations for him or her to solve.

- Since EMS is not all excitement, help the new EMT-B understand this. People who are led to believe that EMS is all emergencies are disillusioned when they learn the truth. Cultivate a life-long provider rather than a flash in the pan!

- Encourage the qualities of loyalty, reliability, compassion, and good judgment in a new EMT-B.

While it is important to recognize that not all people are cut out for EMS, it is equally important to recognize that we lose talented people because they are never "broken in" properly. They never see good examples or work with those who can act as mentors.

The following "Preceptor Pearl" is one of many that will be offered throughout this text. It is designed to remind you of your role as a preceptor and to provide "pearls of wisdom" that are important to pass along to students.

PRECEPTOR PEARL

A disservice is done to new EMT-Bs when they are told "forget what you learned in the classroom. You're on the street now." This is damaging and confusing. Even shortcuts in assessment and care can confuse new EMT-Bs. Help integrate classroom knowledge into the field experience. Allow the newcomer to cement a foundation of knowledge and skills before you provide new "tricks."

It is very difficult to determine just how much freedom to give a new EMT-B. While many agree that it is improper to allow the newly trained person to be crew chief, there are more subtle issues that are very important. Some experienced people never allow the newcomer to participate, while others allow the new EMT-B to perform tasks that are above his or her current capabilities. The resultant failures erode the confidence of the student.

How you choose to lead an EMT-B will depend on his or her capabilities. An EMT-B may have excellent assessment skills, but may never have applied a traction splint. The preceptor must recognize that a different approach must be taken when supervising each skill:

- **Direct.** The direct approach may be needed when the EMT-B is highly motivated but has no experience. If a new EMT-B is allowed to "get in over his head," he will lose (or never initially gain) confidence. The new EMT-B also may believe that he or she knows it all. This may cause problems when helping the newcomer.

- **Coach**. Use this approach when students have motivation or confidence problems. Coaching provides support and encouragement at a crucial time. Give them a gentle nudge to get involved in a new experience while letting them know they have you there as a safety net.

- **Support.** Support newcomers who are unmotivated but who have good skills and experience. This approach is often useful when students have reached a plateau in learning. Provide challenging case studies or review sessions to challenge these EMT-Bs.
- **Delegate.** Use this approach when EMT-Bs are self-motivated and have developed a high level of experience and proficiency. This person essentially can do it on his or her own.

It is easy to imagine what could happen when an EMT-B who lacks confidence or motivation is assigned to a task for which he or she is not ready. New EMT-Bs will reach different levels of confidence and expertise for different skills and experiences. An EMT-B who was able to assess and treat a patient with a single broken bone in an extremity may not be ready to manage a multiple-trauma patient. This means that you may be able to delegate the EMT-B to perform alone in some situations while coaching, supporting, or even directing the EMT-B in others.

Remember, a person is not a failure because he or she lacks confidence and motivation. These are qualities that must be cultivated by organizations and individuals. If you direct, coach, support, and delegate in the appropriate situations, the end result will be a high quality, life-long EMS provider.

Feedback is essential to any EMS provider, because it leads to growth. Provide feedback often. But remember to "praise in public, reprimand in private."

Remember the EMTs who made positive impressions on you. Stay alert to the impressions you make with new EMT-Bs. Avoid influencing them negatively.

Finally, participate in training or instructor workshops offered in your area. Your role as a teacher, mentor, and preceptor is valuable in and out of the classroom.

QUALITY IMPROVEMENT AND MEDICAL DIRECTION

Quality Improvement (QI)

Quality improvement (QI) is a system of internal and external reviews and audits of all aspects of an EMS system. It is meant to identify aspects that need improvement in order to make sure the public receives the highest quality prehospital care. Most EMS systems have some type of QI program in place. In some systems it may be called QA (quality assurance) or it may be a part of a TQM (total quality management) or PI (process improvement) program. The end result is basically the same.

A group of people is usually assigned the function of quality improvement. A QI review session may proceed this way: The group decides to review traumatic cardiac-arrest calls for a given period. The run reports are then pulled for all calls meeting that criterion in the set time period. The calls will be reviewed for specific, objective criteria such as scene time, spinal immobilization, other skills, and documentation.

If calls are found in which the crew did not appear to meet the standards set by the organization, those crews are notified of the results. A plan of action is then put in place to assure that the standards are met in the future. If calls are found to meet the standards, letters of commendation may be issued documenting the work done by crews who have provided superior patient care and have met or exceeded the desired standards.

Quality improvement is not a once-a-month proposition. As an EMT-B, you must strive to provide quality care at all times. Your agency's medical director also must be actively involved in the QI process. There are several ways that you can work toward quality patient care and improvement every day:

- **Documentation.** Since committees that review prior calls rely on your documentation, this is a critical aspect of the QI process. If a report is incomplete or improperly completed, a QI committee would be forced to assume that substandard care was given. Furthermore, incomplete documentation may result in, or worsen, lawsuits filed against you and your organization. A run report should honestly "tell the story" of your patient so that others reading the report can get a clear picture of the patient's condition, your assessment, and treatment given.
- **Review and audit run reports.** As an EMT-B, you may volunteer to be a member of your agency's QI committee. Even when not functioning as part of a committee, review your run reports before submission to be sure they are complete. Have another person on your crew review your reports for accuracy and completeness.
- **Gathering feedback from patients and hospital staff.** If you never receive feedback or comments, you may never improve. Many people can offer comments that will help improve your patient care. In addition, questionnaires sent to patients after a call may be returned with just such valuable information.

- **Conduct preventive maintenance.** Extremes in temperature, the weight of repeated patients, and the nature of emergency scenes take a great toll on your equipment and your emergency vehicle. Preventive maintenance (PM) and regular equipment checks will extend the life of your equipment. It also can ensure that it will be in good working order for use with the next patient.

- **Continuing education.** If not used every day, the knowledge and skills you learned in your original EMT class may be forgotten. Also, new techniques and procedures have undoubtedly come about since your certification. Continuing education is an important part of quality improvement. Reading journals, attending seminars or classes, and completing other continuing education endeavors is a necessary part of EMS quality today.

- **Maintain skills.** Skills that are not practiced frequently usually deteriorate. If you have not performed a traction-splint application in some time, you may require additional practice *before* you perform this procedure on a patient. To provide quality patient care, you must maintain proficiency in all skills.

A true quality improvement program transcends agency politics and personalities. It focuses on the true issue: *quality.* Members of any profession must continually strive for quality to gain community and peer respect.

Medical Direction

A **medical director** is a physician who is responsible for the clinical and patient-care aspects of an EMS system. All ambulance services and rescue squads must have one. The medical director will be actively involved with the QI committee. Medical direction is also important due to the various EMT-administered or patient-assisted medications available in the field.

Medical direction can be **on-line** or **off-line.** Physicians authorized by regional or local agencies may provide medical direction on a call-by-call basis. On-line medical direction may be contacted by telephone, cellular phone, or radio (Figure 1-4). A brief report on the patient is presented, followed by "orders" from the on-line physician.

Off-line medical direction is done through **standing orders,** or **protocols.** These are written orders issued by the medical director that may be used any time a certain situation is encountered. The standing order may be issued as shown in Figure 1-5. Your system may have standing orders such as this. Other drugs—such as oral glucose, activated charcoal, and prescribed inhalers—may have similar orders. *Always follow local protocols.*

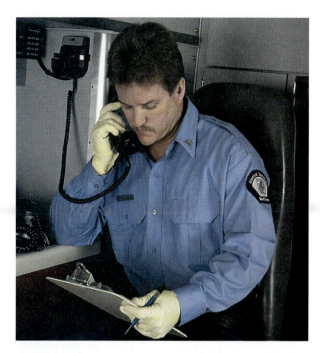

Figure 1-4 On-line medical direction may be obtained by way of phone or radio.

The practice of medicine and the ability to prescribe and administer drugs are rights primarily given to physicians. If you, as an EMT-B, administer a medication, it is generally considered an extension of the medical director's authority or license. When you carry out an on-line or off-line order, you are the **designated agent** of the physician. This is a tremendous responsibility. You would not be able to perform these tasks without your medical director. *Performing advanced skills and medication administration without approval from the medical director is the equivalent of practicing medicine without a license.*

LIFESPAN DEVELOPMENT

Though you receive training in calls involving infants and children, such calls may be infrequent. If so, medical direction may be a valuable resource. Remember to take advantage of the guidance that medical direction can give for general issues, medications, and problems that you encounter.

MORGANVILLE AMBULANCE CORPS

Standing Order: Nitroglycerin

An EMT-B is authorized to assist the patient in administering nitroglycerin tablets or spray if the following circumstances exist:

1. The nitroglycerin medication has been prescribed to the patient. No other person's nitro may be administered in this situation.

2. The patient must have suspected cardiac chest pain, which may include substernal pain with radiation to the neck, arm, or jaw; or a patient must have a previous cardiac history and be experiencing pain similar to a prior cardiac event.

3. At no point will more than two nitroglycerin tablets be administered in the field without contacting on-line medical direction. The doses are to be administered 5 minutes apart with an evaluation of chest pain and vital signs prior to each dose being administered. This 5-minute wait between administrations includes nitro that may have been taken by the patient before your arrival.

4. Nitroglycerin will be administered only to patients with a systolic blood pressure above 110 mmHg.

5. EMT-Bs will follow directions on the prescription for administration of the drug.

6. Nitroglycerin is a potentially beneficial drug for patients with chest pain. It is a *drug,* however, and must be treated with respect. Monitor the patient carefully before and after administration of this or any drug. **If you have any doubts or questions, contact your on-line physician immediately!**

Joe Otz

Joe Otz, MD
Medical Director

Figure 1-5 A sample protocol.

Most states have enacted legislation that creates and authorizes the EMS systems in your area. Authority may be given to state, regional, or local agencies to set policies and procedures that affect you as an EMT-B. Become familiar with those regulations and the agencies that set them.

Minimum Data Set

In order to improve the way EMS cares for patients, research is ongoing. This research includes EMS response, care, and other responsibilities. To be effective and accurate, researchers must be able to collect similar data from many different systems. If each system's data differed from the next, the data and, most importantly, the research would be meaningless.

For example, if a study were to focus on EMS response time as it relates to a patient's survival from cardiac arrest, the researchers may find that there was a problem with the times received from certain systems. One system may use the time the ambulance arrived "on scene." This may or may not reflect the time that the EMT-Bs reached the patient. In some high-rise buildings, for example, it could take another five minutes to actually get to the patient's side.

A **minimum data set** was developed to standardize arrival time at patient location and other pieces of information (Table 1-1). This means that all the data elements should be present in each prehospital care report (PCR). It also means that the definition of each data element should be standardized from region to region and state to state. Note that there are two types of information: patient information and administrative information.

Table 1-1 The Minimum Data Set

Patient Information at initial contact, following all interventions, and upon arrival at medical facility

- Chief complaint
- Level of consciousness (AVPU), mental status
- Systolic blood pressure for patients more than 3 years old
- Skin perfusion (capillary refill) for patients less than 6 years old
- Skin color and temperature
- Pulse rate
- Respiratory rate and effort

Administrative Information

- Time of incident report
- Time unit notified
- Time of arrival at patient
- Time unit left scene
- Time of arrival at destination
- Time of transfer of care

SUMMARY

- The EMS system has been developed to provide prehospital as well as hospital emergency care.
- The Emergency Medical Services System is made up of bystanders, EMS dispatchers, First Responders, Emergency Medical Technicians, emergency department staffs, specialty centers, and allied health personnel who work together to provide emergency care.
- The "National Emergency Medical Services Education and Practice Blueprint" outlines the skills expected at each level of EMS training— First Responder, EMT-Basic, EMT-Intermediate, and EMT-Paramedic.

- Your responsibilities as an EMT-B include safety; patient assessment and care; lifting, moving, and transporting patients; transfer of care; record keeping and data collection; and patient advocacy.
- As an EMT-Basic, you are also expected to pass information about health and emergency care on to patients and others in the EMS system.
- Education (including refresher training and continuing education), quality improvement procedures, and medical direction are all essential to maintaining high standards of EMS care.

REVIEW QUESTIONS

1. Which of the following are responsible for activation of the EMS system?
   a. bystanders
   b. EMT-Paramedics
   c. First Responders
   d. Emergency Medical Dispatchers

2. A community with access to a centralized communication center for emergency police, fire, and EMS calls has a(n) _____ system
   a. access number
   b. non-911
   c. computer
   d. 911

3. As an EMT-B, your role in quality improvement involves all of the following EXCEPT:
   a. documenting your assessment and treatment of patients.
   b. gathering feedback from patients and hospital staff.
   c. issuing standing orders and medical protocols.
   d. completing continuing education courses.

4. The _____ is responsible for the clinical and patient-care aspects of an EMS system.

   a. EMT-Basic

   b. medical director

   c. designated agent

   d. emergency department staff

5. Which of the following would NOT be considered off-line medical direction?

   a. radio contact with a physician

   b. quality control process

   c. standing orders

   d. locol protocols

WEB MEDIC

Visit Brady's *Essentials of Emergency Care* web site for direct web links. At **www.prenhall.com/limmer,** you will find information related to the following Chapter 1 topics:

- National Registry of EMTs
- National Association of EMTs
- National Highway Traffic Safety Administration
- Quality Improvement for EMS Systems
- Continuing education for EMS

Chapter Two

WELL-BEING OF THE EMT-BASIC

Correlates with the U.S. DOT "EMT-Basic National Standard Curriculum" Lesson 1-2

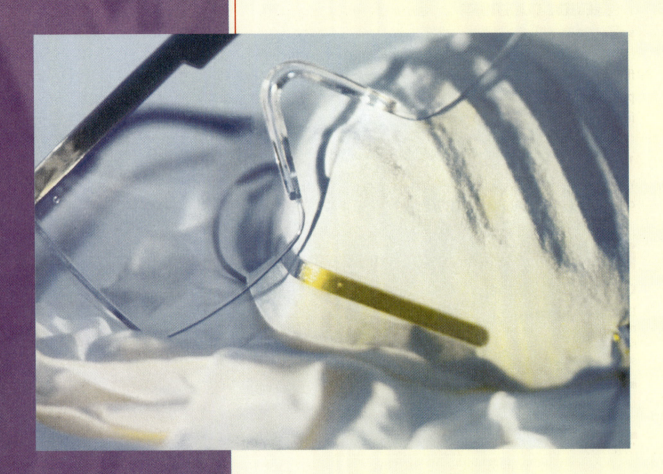

ESSENTIAL ELECTRONIC EXTRAS

CD ESSENTIALS

For preview and review of chapter material, see the student CD-ROM for

- Pretest
- Chapter quizzes
- Posttest

WEB ESSENTIALS

For additional review and enrichment, visit www.prenhall.com/limmer for

- Interactive student quizzes
- Links to online EMS resources
- Online case studies
- Audio glossary

Learning how to safeguard your well-being as an EMT-Basic is critical. During your EMS service you may be exposed to all kinds of stress, including that which accompanies death and dying and dangerous situations. This section will help you to learn strategies that can help you stay emotionally well as well as physically safe.

Scene safety is perhaps the most important part of any call. Without assuring your safety and the safety of others at the scene, the remainder of the call is destined to fail. This section deals with the concept of well-being, with an emphasis on scene safety. As a practicing EMT-B, you have experience in managing emergency scenes. With this experience, you will find it easier than a first-time student to integrate and understand the value of scene-safety methods on every call.

Attitudes and practices have changed over the past several years regarding exposure to blood and other body fluids and therefore to potentially infectious disease. This increased awareness has extended beyond the EMS provider's well-being to patients. An EMT-B must be acutely aware of the cleanliness of patient-care equipment in order to decrease any potential for passing on an infectious disease from patient to patient.

This section outlines the Occupational Safety and Health Administration (OSHA) standard 29 CFR Part 1910.1030 for an exposure control plan and annual refresher training regarding bloodborne pathogens. It also reviews the Ryan White CARE Act reporting requirements and BSI precautions for EMT-Bs during an ambulance call, as well as decontamination procedures for emergency equipment and vehicles.

EMOTION AND STRESS

Causes of Stress

Emergencies are stressful. That is their nature. While most emergencies are considered "routine," some seem to have a higher potential for causing excess stress in EMS providers. High-stress calls include:

- *Multiple-casualty incident (MCI).* This is an emergency in which there are three or more patients.
- *Infants and children.* Calls involving the injury or illness of an infant or child are known to be particularly stressful to all health-care providers.
- *Amputations* and other types of severe injuries
- *Abuse and neglect* of children, adults, and the elderly
- *Death or injury of a coworker* or other public safety personnel

Stress may be caused by a single event or it may be the cumulative result of several incidents. Remember, any incident may affect you and coworkers differently. Two EMT-Bs on the same call may have opposite responses. Do not make negative judgments about another person's reaction.

Stress also may stem from a combination of factors, including problems in your personal life. One common cause of stress is people who "just don't

CORE CONCEPTS

In this chapter, you will learn about the following topics:

- The effects of emotion and stress on the EMT-B

- Death and dying and the reactions of the patient, the family, and the EMT-B

- Safety at the scene

- Exposure control

- Body substance isolation throughout the call

✔ **Knowledge**

☐ 1. Provide for safety of self, patient, and fellow workers. (pp. 18–27, 33)

- Discuss the importance of body substance isolation. (BSI). (pp. 20–23)
- Describe the steps the EMT-Basic should take for personal protection from airborne and bloodborne pathogens. (pp. 20–24)

☐ 2. Identify the presence of hazardous materials. (pp. 19–20)

- Break down the steps to approaching a hazardous situation. (pp. 18–20)

☐ 3. Use methods to reduce stress in self, patients, bystanders, and coworkers. (pp. 15–17)

- Recognize the signs and symptoms of critical incident stress. (pp. 15–17)

- State possible steps that the EMT-Basic may take to help reduce/alleviate stress. (pp. 16–17)

✔ **Attitude**

1. Explain the rationale for serving as an advocate for the use of appropriate protective equipment. (pp. 21–24)

understand" the job. For example, your EMS organization may require you to work on weekends and holidays. Time spent on call may be frustrating to friends and family members. They may not understand why you can't participate in certain social activities or why you can't leave a certain area. You, too, might get frustrated because you can't plan around the unpredictable nature of emergencies. In fact, after a very trying or exciting call, you may wish to share your feelings with a friend or someone you love. You find instead that the person does not understand your emotions. This can lead to feelings of separation and rejection, which are highly stressful.

Signs and Symptoms of Stress

The signs and symptoms of excess stress include irritability with family, friends, and coworkers; inability to concentrate; changes in daily activities, such as difficulty sleeping or nightmares, loss of appetite, and loss of interest in sexual activity; anxiety; indecisiveness; guilt; isolation; and loss of interest in work (Figure 2-1).

Dealing with Stress

Life-Style Changes

There are several ways to deal with stress. They are called "life-style changes," and they include the following:

- **Develop more healthful and positive dietary habits.** Avoid fatty foods, reduce sugar, and eat more carbohydrates. Also reduce your consumption of alcohol and caffeine, which can have negative effects, including an increase in stress and disturbances of sleep patterns.
- **Exercise.** When performed safely and properly, this life-style change helps to "burn off" stress. It

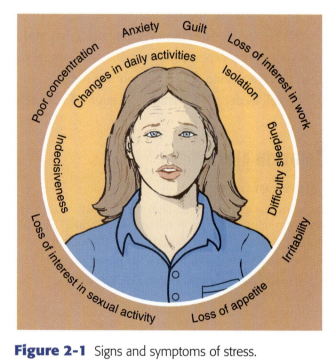

Figure 2-1 Signs and symptoms of stress.

also helps you deal with the physical aspects of your responsibilities, such as carrying equipment and performing physically demanding emergency procedures. Experts recommend aerobic exercise for at least 20-30 minutes, three times each week.

- **Devote time to relaxing.** Try relaxation techniques, too. These techniques are valuable stress reducers. They include deep-breathing exercises, meditation, and visualization of peaceful or relaxing places and events.

In addition to changing your personal life, you can also make changes in your professional life that help reduce and prevent stress. For example, if you are in an organization with varied shifts and locations, consider asking for a location that offers a lighter call volume or different types of calls. You also may want to change your shift to one that allows more time with family and friends.

There are many types of help available for EMT-Bs and others who are experiencing stress. Seek them out. It is not a sign of weakness. There are many professionals who can help you deal with the stress you feel, and much of their care may be covered by health insurance policies.

Critical Incident Stress Debriefing (CISD)

A **critical incident stress debriefing (CISD)** is a process in which a team of trained peer counselors and mental health professionals meet with rescuers who have been involved in a major incident (Figure 2-2). The meetings are generally held within 24 to 72 hours after the incident. The goal is to assist rescuers in dealing with the related stress. Only those involved in the incident may attend. No media are allowed.

A CISD is an open discussion of the feelings experienced during and after the call. Participants are encouraged to talk about any fears or reactions they have had. It is critical that the CISD does not become a method of investigation of the events of the call, so everything discussed at the meetings is confidential. All participants are asked not to disclose information once the meeting is over. Any breach in confidentiality prevents others from sharing information that can help them. After an open discussion, the CISD team offers suggestions on how to deal with and overcome the stress. It is important once again to state that stress after a major incident is normal and should be expected. The CISD process is meant to help accelerate the recovery process.

Sometimes a "defusing" session is held within the first few hours after a critical incident. While CISD includes all personnel involved in the incident, a defusing session is usually limited to a small group, often the people who were most directly involved with the most stressful aspects of the incident. A defusing gives them an opportunity to vent their feelings and receive information about stress before the larger group meets.

After a CISD, follow-up is essential. A member of the peer team should contact all CISD attendees within 24 hours to offer support and referrals. No two emergency care workers will perceive, experience, or recover from critical incident stress in the same way. The process of overcoming the stress will be different from person to person. Resources must be available immediately as well as long after the incident, including the "anniversaries" of stressful events.

Comprehensive critical incident stress management goes beyond the CISD session to include pre-incident stress education, on-scene peer support,

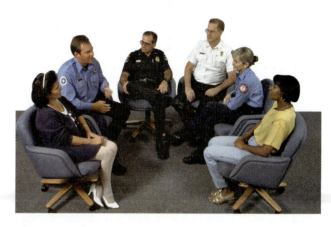

Figure 2-2 Critical incident stress management usually includes a debriefing 24 to 72 hours after an incident.

one-on-one support, disaster support services, spouse and family support, community outreach programs, and other health and welfare programs such as wellness programs.

You may have read that there has been debate over whether or not critical incident stress debriefing works. The science of medicine constantly looks for research to determine if procedures actually benefit medical and stress-related conditions. There are many EMT-Bs who have gone through the debriefing process and feel they have been helped. Others dispute the process. Regardless of the method you choose to deal with stress, remember that it is a normal and perhaps inevitable response to a critical incident. Learn to recognize the signs and symptoms, and find out where to turn for help in your area.

Understanding Reactions to Death and Dying

As an EMT-B, you will undoubtedly be called to patients who are in various stages of a terminal illness. Understanding what the families and the patients go through can help you deal with their stress, as well as your own.

When a patient finds out that death is near, he or she goes through emotional stages. The stages vary in duration and magnitude, sometimes overlap, and all affect both the patient and the family. They are:

- **Denial or "not me."** The patient denies that he or she is dying. This puts off dealing with the inevitable end of the process.
- **Anger or "why me?"** The patient becomes angry at the situation. This anger is commonly vented at family members and EMS personnel.
- **Bargaining or "okay, but first let me . . ."** In the mind of the patient, bargaining seems to postpone death, even if only for a short time.
- **Depression or "okay, but I haven't . . ."** The patient is sad, depressed, and despairing, often

mourning things not accomplished, dreams that won't come true. He or she retreats into a private world, unwilling to communicate with others.

- **Acceptance or "okay, I'm not afraid."** The patient may come to accept death, although does not welcome it. Often, the patient may accept the situation before family members do. At this stage, the family may need more support than the patient.

The patient and family are on an emotional roller coaster after a terminal condition has been diagnosed. They may actually seem to be in more than one stage at one time, or their attitudes may reflect thoughts that do not fit easily into any of the stages. However, a general understanding of the process can help you to communicate with them effectively.

As an EMT-B, you also will encounter sudden, unexpected death (as a result of a collision, for example). In these cases, family members are likely to react with a wide range of emotions.

There are steps or approaches that you can take in dealing with the patient and family members confronted with death or dying. They are:

- **Recognize the patient's needs.** Treat the patient with respect. Do everything you can to preserve his or her dignity and sense of control. For example, talk directly to the patient. Avoid talking about the patient to family members in the patient's presence, as if he or she were incompetent or no longer living. Be sensitive to how the patient seems to want to handle the situation. For example, allow or encourage the patient to share feelings and needs. Don't cut off such communications because of your own embarrassment or discomfort. Respect the patient's privacy if he or she does not want to communicate personal feelings.

- **Be tolerant of angry reactions.** They can come from the patient or family members who have feelings of helpless rage about the death or prospect of dying. The anger is not personal. It would be directed at anyone in your position.

- **Listen empathetically.** You can't "fix" the situation, but just listening with understanding and patience will be very helpful.

- **Do not falsely reassure.** Avoid saying things like "everything will be all right," which you, the patient, and the family all know are not true. Offering false reassurance will only be irritating or convey the impression that you don't really understand.

- **Offer as much comfort as you realistically can.** Comfort both the patient and the family. Let them know that you will do everything you can to help or to get them whatever help is available. Use a gentle tone of voice and a reassuring touch, if appropriate.

SCENE SAFETY

Observe the Scene

The best way to avoid danger is to prevent it. It is very easy to get caught up in an emergency and feel the need to rush in. Don't do it! It is during the approach to the scene that information vital to your safety may be obtained.

Since you have been an EMT-B for some time, you may find that you have developed "gut feelings" about calls. It is important to listen to these feelings since they are often correct. The feelings may be in reference to a patient who you feel may be worse than he appears to be or about a scene that may be more dangerous than it appears. While "gut feelings" may be correct, it is also important to develop concrete information about a call. Always check for these indicators of danger at a scene:

- **Fighting or loud voices.** Fighting is a relatively obvious sign of trouble, but one that is often ignored. Loud voices, posturing, or other signs of imminent fighting indicate danger. While you might not be involved in the fight, you can still be injured. Since you may be seen as a symbol of authority, you could be attacked. Fighting may take place on the street or in the home. Domestic violence is alarmingly common and a source of many EMS calls.

- **Intoxicants or illegal drugs.** When people abuse alcohol or other drugs, their behavior becomes unpredictable. Many of us have seen intoxicated persons acting anywhere from sleepy to combative. When drugs are abused or they are observed on scene, it is likely that criminals associated with the drugs are close by.

- **Weapons.** Weapons are a clear indicator of potential danger. When weapons are visible or in use, or their use is threatened, retreat! Remember that almost anything may be used as a weapon. It takes careful observation of the people and surroundings at a scene to prevent the use of a weapon against you.

- **Crime scenes.** Danger exists when the crime is in progress, as well as after the crime has been committed. Perpetrators may be hiding on scene. They also may return to the scene during your time there. There even have been calls where the "victim" assaults police and EMT-Bs. Even if the police have secured the crime scene, consider it potentially dangerous at all times.

- **Pets.** Almost any dog can be dangerous if it or its owners are threatened. There are many breeds of dogs that are trained to protect and attack. Exotic animals (snakes, reptiles, etc.) may also pose a threat to the EMT-B.

Use Your Senses

Use your senses to observe and prevent danger. While it is sometimes difficult to remember to observe constantly, practicing your observational techniques daily will make this task second nature. When it comes to safety, however, some senses are obviously better than others.

Sight is the sense most EMT-Bs think of when it comes to safety. You are able to see a weapon, an unstable vehicle, or a hazmat situation and respond to it appropriately. But do not underestimate the remaining senses. Hearing is vital for detecting scene danger. You can hear sounds from other rooms, from behind doors, or from some distance away. Smell is valuable for identifying dangerous chemicals, leaking gasoline, and other situations that may pose a hazard. (Touch and taste are not practical to use, since they bring you too close to the danger.)

Some people claim to have a "sixth sense." If you do, heed it. Your gut feeling may not require immediate action, but may simply create a reason for you to act more slowly and observe more carefully until you can gain additional information. Many crime victims have told police that they "had a feeling" that something was about to happen but ignored it. Act cautiously until the feeling is resolved, but avoid overreacting.

Respond to Danger

When you observe danger, these tactics can help keep you safe until the police or other appropriate agencies arrive to secure the scene:

- **Use cover and concealment** (Figures 2-3 and 2-4). No doubt you have heard of the term "take cover." Cover is taking a position behind some sturdy barricade that will hide your body and offer ballistic protection. Examples of cover include brick walls, the engine of your ambulance, and large trees. Surprisingly, some common items offer little coverage. The box of an ambulance offers little or no protection. Most doors and walls are also poor cover.

    Concealment is hiding your body, but it does not offer protection from projectiles and should be used only when solid cover cannot be found safely. Doors, walls, smaller trees, and shrubs can be used for concealment.

- **Retreat.** If danger is observed, the most appropriate action is to immediately move a safe distance away. Retreat when you confront hazardous materials, unstable vehicles and terrain, and violence.

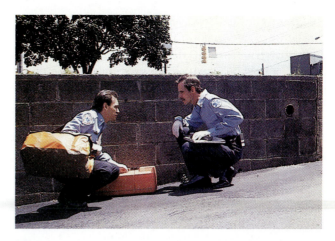

Figure 2-3 To take cover, find a position that both hides you and protects your body from projectiles.

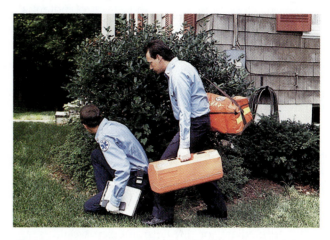

Figure 2-4 To conceal yourself, place your body behind an object that can hide you. Choose this option only when solid cover cannot be found.

When you retreat from danger, get far enough away. It is best to have a clear idea of exactly how far is far enough before you find yourself in a potentially life-threatening situation.

Retreat to a position where there are two major obstacles between you and the violence. If a dangerous person is able to get through one of the obstacles, one remains there as a buffer. One or both of the obstacles should be cover. One of the obstacles may be distance, as much as moving several hundred yards away. However, distance alone will not provide protection from gunfire.

Ideally, you should be able to get away from the danger and find a position of cover. This way, if someone tries to move toward you, you have time to retreat further and find another position of cover. When possible, return to the rescue vehicle and drive away. However, this should be done only when it is safe to go to your vehicle.

- **Use distractions if necessary.** If you must retreat, it may help you to put something in the path of the danger. If you are fleeing through a doorway, wedging the stretcher there will slow down a potential aggressor. Throwing a medical kit at someone's feet will have a similar effect.
- **Carry a portable radio.** If you do observe danger, report it. Provide as much information as possible, such as the location of the problem, the nature of the problem (fighting, gunshots, dangerous drugs), your response to the problem (retreat, etc.), and details about the incident.

Many EMT-Bs are concerned about preventing liability when retreating from a scene. The key to any liability prevention is adequate and objective documentation. Document all the indicators of potential danger and your response to them. When you retreat from the scene, do not return to service. Stand by at a safe location until the scene is declared safe by law enforcement and emergency care can be provided safely. Document the time you retreated from and returned to the scene. Notify a supervisor if necessary.

Carrying weapons can be cause for significant danger. Carrying a weapon may give you a false sense of security that might allow you to enter a scene from which you should and would normally retreat. It also is dangerous to carry any weapon you are not trained to use. You wouldn't think of using advanced life support equipment unless you were an EMT-Intermediate or EMT-Paramedic, would you? Remember, too, that weapons may be taken from you and used against you or your partners. Using a weapon also may result in considerable liability. Observation and proper response before the danger strikes are much safer and more practical methods of dealing with danger than the use of weapons.

Plan for Safety

It is always best to plan for safety. Planning begins with having a base of safety knowledge, such as the information presented earlier in this section. To be safe, there are certain things that can be done in advance:

- **Work together.** The sum of a team's efforts is greater than its individual parts. This is especially true when it comes to safety. Crews can work together to observe and use predetermined signals to communicate dangers to other members of the crew.

  Split up the carrying of equipment between crew members so no one person is bogged down. Having a hand free helps you to hold railings, open doors, stabilize yourself on uneven surfaces, and retreat more easily.

- **Make your equipment work for you.** Make sure your equipment is easily carried and not burdensome. Carry the equipment that you will realistically need in kits of a reasonable size and shape.
- **Dress for safety.** Wear clothing or protective equipment that is appropriate for the task you are performing. Hazardous material incidents and rescue scenes require specific safety equipment (see Chapter 28). Everyday EMS work requires safe shoes and outerwear that are reflective and appropriate for the weather and time of day or night.
- **Use body armor, if necessary.** Some EMT-Bs wear body armor, or bulletproof vests (Figure 2-5). Many urban EMS agencies are providing body armor for employees or contributing sums toward its purchase. Even if body armor isn't for you at this time, the following information can help you make an informed decision about its purchase and possible use.
  - Body armor is *not* totally bulletproof. It will stop most handgun bullets, but not rifle bullets. Body armor is not a guarantee. It is only an added safety measure you may choose to take.
  - Body armor may stop knife penetration and prevent trauma from steering wheel impact in motor vehicle collisions.
  - To be effective, equipment must be worn! A vest will not afford any protection when it is in your locker or behind the seat of the ambulance. So choose comfortable body armor and a practical way to wear it.
  - Body armor is flexible. It is not truly "armor." The panels are made of soft Kevlar™ or other fibers that are woven together to give ballistic protection.

Scene safety techniques are not designed to instill paranoia. In your chosen career as an EMT-B, it would be unrealistic to believe that you will never face danger. Emergencies are dynamic events during which emotions run high. If the skill of observation is necessary, then that skill will be part of EMT-B activities on every call, just like the skills of patient assessment and care.

THE EXPOSURE CONTROL PLAN

The Occupational Safety and Health Administration (OSHA) developed and enforces standards for EMT-Bs to use when dealing with bloodborne pathogens. This standard—called Title 29 CFR 1910.1030—will be reviewed in this section and may be used by EMT-Bs as a basis for annual refresher training requirements.

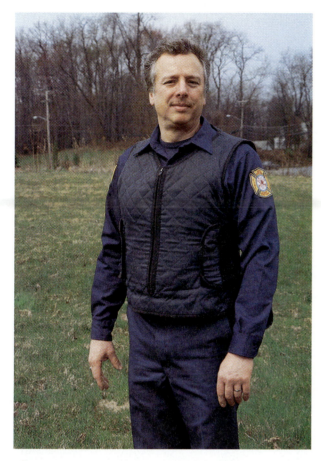

Figure 2-5 Body armor, or bulletproof vest.

The OSHA standard requires an EMS service or employer to establish an exposure control plan. The exposure control plan must include:

- General hazards associated with exposures to blood or body fluids
- Specific tasks considered to present a potential exposure to these hazards
- Job classifications or descriptions of the employees/personnel expected to perform the above tasks
- Personal protective equipment (PPE) and safe work practices designed to prevent exposures
- Vaccination (hepatitis B) requirements
- Training requirements under the exposure control plan
- Exposure determination and follow-up medical care including record keeping

As you know, bacteria and viruses are pathogens, or organisms that may cause infections or diseases. The spread of pathogens may be through the air or through contact with blood or other body fluids. Direct contact with blood or other body fluids through an open wound or break in the skin, mucous membrane of the mouth, nose or eyes, or parenteral contact (stick by a needle or other sharp object) increases the risk for contracting a bloodborne disease such as human immunodeficiency virus (HIV) or hepatitis B virus (HBV). Airborne pathogens, such as those of tuberculosis (TB), are spread through tiny droplets released by breathing, sneezing, or coughing. These pathogens may be absorbed through the EMT-B's eyes or inhaled into the respiratory system. Airborne pathogens will be covered in more detail under the Ryan White Act later in this section.

HIV/AIDS, HBV, and TB are communicable diseases of greatest concern because they are life-threatening. However, there are many communicable diseases health-care personnel may be exposed to. See Table 2-1, which lists common ones, their modes of transmission, and incubation periods (the time between contact and first symptoms).

Occupational Exposure

Since it is impossible to determine which body fluids are infectious, *all* blood and body fluids must be considered infectious and appropriate safeguards must be taken whenever they are present. When an EMT-B has contact with blood or body fluids through a break in the skin, eyes, mucous membranes, or parenteral contact resulting from the performance of his or her duties, it is referred to as **occupational exposure.**

Duties in which EMS providers are considered "at risk" include CPR, managing the airway, bleeding control for trauma patients, other medical emergencies such as childbirth, and cleaning and decontamination of equipment used during patient care.

Body Substance Isolation (BSI)

Exposure control plans outline procedures to use when the potential for contact with blood or other body fluids exists. **Body substance isolation (BSI) precautions** are infection-control procedures designed to reduce the risk for exposure to potentially infectious blood and body fluids. Because each situation you encounter is slightly different, it is important that you take the appropriate BSI precautions for a specific situation.

Both the employer and the employee are responsible for ensuring that proper BSI precautions are taken. The employer is responsible for implementing the exposure control plan, as well as providing appropriate training, immunizations, and the proper **personal protective equipment (PPE).** The employee has the responsibility to take the training and to follow the exposure control plan.

Table 2-1 Communicable Diseases

Disease	Mode of Transmission	Incubation
AIDS (acquired immune deficiency syndrome)	AIDS- or HIV-infected blood via intravenous drug use, semen and vaginal fluids, unprotected sexual contact, blood transfusions, or (rarely) accidental needle sticks. Mothers also may pass HIV to their unborn children.	Several months or years
Chicken pox (varicella)	Airborne droplets, which also can be spread by contact with open sores.	11 to 21 days
German measles (rubella)	Airborne droplets. Mothers may pass it to unborn children.	10 to 12 days
Meningitis, bacterial	Oral and nasal secretions.	2 to 10 days
Mumps	Droplets of saliva or objects contaminated by saliva.	14 to 24 days
Pneumonia, bacterial and viral	Oral and nasal droplets and secretions.	Several days
Staphylococcal skin infections	Direct contact with infected wounds or sores or with contaminated objects.	Several days
Tuberculosis (TB)	Respiratory secretions, airborne or on contaminated objects.	2 to 6 weeks
Hepatitis (B, C)	Blood, saliva, sexual contact, or contaminated objects.	Weeks or months
Whooping cough (pertussis)	Respiratory secretions or airborne droplets.	6 to 20 days

The employee also is to use the proper PPE except in the most extraordinary circumstances, such as when an off-duty EMT-B encounters a patient who must be given CPR. Extraordinary situations are reserved for those instances when, in the EMT-B's professional judgment, the specific PPE will prevent the delivery of appropriate emergency medical care or will pose an increased hazard to the safety of the employee. Documentation of these extraordinary situations is required and must be followed up by the employer.

Engineering Controls

The exposure control plan must include **engineering controls** that outline specific equipment to use when dealing with blood or body fluid specimens, contaminated equipment, contaminated needles, sharps containers, and disposal of contaminated disposable items. Blood and body fluid specimens should be labeled with the appropriate "biohazard" identification and placed in a leak-proof container (Figure 2-6).

Nondisposable equipment that is contaminated with blood or body fluids should be examined for any contaminants and cleaned with disinfectant prior

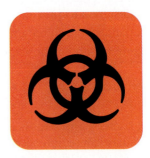

Figure 2-6 This biohazard symbol must be on containers used for disposal of contaminated items.

to returning it to service. If equipment cannot be adequately decontaminated, then it must be labeled with a "biohazard" identification.

Contaminated needles or other "sharps" should not be recapped, bent, or otherwise altered. They should be placed immediately into a puncture- and leak-proof container appropriately labeled with a "biohazard" identification. Such containers should not be allowed to overflow and should be replaced routinely and disposed of properly.

Following a call, contaminated disposable items—such as dressings, bandages, and gloves—should be disposed of immediately in an appropriately marked "biohazard" waste container. This action usually takes place while you are at the receiving facility but in some cases may occur at the ambulance station or base. Detailed procedures for cleaning and disinfecting equipment are presented later in this section.

Work Practice Controls

Work practice controls are the part of the exposure control plan used to complement the engineering controls. This section of the plan includes promotion of handwashing, usually the best defense against contracting an infectious disease. It also outlines procedures for dealing with contaminated needles or other sharps; procedures for personnel to follow regarding eating, drinking, or applying cosmetics in the patient compartment of the vehicle; and procedures to minimize the splashing or spattering of blood and body fluids.

Personal Protective Equipment (PPE)

To prevent transmission of any diseases, OSHA standards require that personal protective equipment (PPE) must be used any time there is a potential for contact with blood or body fluids. Always follow BSI guidelines and wear appropriate PPE on every call. Personal protective equipment is considered "appropriate" only if it prevents blood and body fluids from passing through the skin or from reaching the eyes, mouth, or other mucous membranes. Personal protective equipment includes:

- Disposable vinyl or latex gloves
- Impervious gowns
- Eye shields or protection
- Surgical masks
- Resuscitation bags such as BVM
- Pocket masks with one-way valves

All PPE used during patient care should be disposed of or cleaned according to procedures out-

lined in your agency's exposure control plan. Protective gloves may be either latex, vinyl, or other similar synthetic material and should be worn if there is any possibility of contact with blood or body fluids, such as during bleeding control, suctioning, CPR, or any situation in which handling or touching contaminated items or surfaces is anticipated. Gloves should not be washed. Instead, they should be replaced between patients or if punctured, ripped, or torn.

When you anticipate blood or body fluid splash or spatter, wear eye protection and masks because the mucous membranes of the eyes are capable of absorbing fluids. Eyewear should provide protection from both the front and the sides. EMS services must provide protective eyewear for employees to use. In the case of prescription glasses, protective side shields, or clip-on barriers, should be available.

Wear impervious gowns to protect clothing from spilled or splashed blood or body fluids that occur during childbirth or other bleeding. In cases of suspected tuberculosis (TB), an N-95 or a high-efficiency particulate air (HEPA) respirator is required (Figure 2-7).

> ## PRECEPTOR PEARL
>
> Be sure to explain to new EMT-Bs—and serve as an example for—the use of personal protective equipment both for BSI and for protection during rescue.

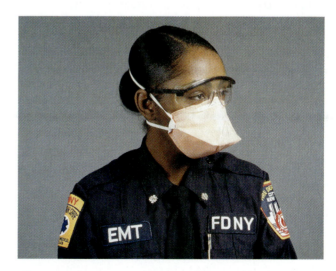

Figure 2-7 Wear a NIOSH-approved respirator when you suspect a patient may have tuberculosis.

Housekeeping Procedures

Housekeeping procedures are outlined in an exposure control plan to establish and maintain sanitary conditions of the workplace and vehicle. All employees are responsible for ensuring that vehicles and work areas are kept clean and sanitary. This portion of an exposure control plan establishes a schedule for cleaning as well as methods of decontaminating work areas and vehicles. These procedures are presented later in this chapter.

Vaccinations

All employers are required to make available to all identified employees the hepatitis B (HBV) vaccination series free of charge. Hepatitis B is one of several types of infections that can affect the liver. HBV infections can occur in two phases—the acute phase and the chronic phase. The acute phase occurs just after a person becomes infected and lasts from a few weeks to several months. Most people will recover after the acute phase and will no longer be infectious. However, some people are infected for the remainder of their lives and are chronic carriers of the HBV.

Acute hepatitis B begins with symptoms such as loss of appetite, generalized weakness, nausea, vomiting, a jaundice or yellow appearance, and dark-colored urine. However, over half the people infected with HBV never become sick or ill. HBV is passed by blood or other body fluids through direct contact with nonintact skin, mucous membranes, unprotected sexual intercourse, or parenteral contact (needle stick).

As an EMS provider, you are at risk for exposure to blood or other body fluids. For this reason, if possible, you should be immunized with the HBV vaccine. The vaccinations are given in three shots: the first shot within 10 days of the initial job functions, the second shot one month after the first, and the third shot five months after the second.

An EMS employee may elect to decline the series of shots but will then need to sign a hepatitis vaccination declination form. The signing of the form, however, does not preclude the employee from deciding that he or she wishes to be vaccinated at a later date. In this case, the employer is still required to make the vaccination available. All vaccination records should be stored in the medical records of the employee's personnel files.

As an EMT-B, you also should have all the up-to-date immunizations, including tetanus prophylaxis, recommended by your personal physician and medical direction.

Post-Exposure Procedures

By definition, an **exposure** is any occurrence of blood or body fluids coming in contact with nonintact skin, the eyes or other mucous membranes, or parenteral contact (needle stick). In general, post-exposure procedures require immediate washing of the affected area with soap and water, immediate medical evaluation, notification of the agency's infection-control liaison, and follow-up reporting to document the circumstances surrounding the exposure. If feasible and applicable to state law, the source individual's and employee's blood should be tested for the presence of HBV and HIV. The exposed employee may also be required to attend post-exposure counseling. All information obtained through post-exposure follow-up is confidential and becomes part of the employee's medical record.

PRECEPTOR PEARL

Since an exposure incident may be anxiety provoking to new EMT-Bs, discuss with them your state laws and local policies regarding post-exposure procedures.

Other Plan Requirements

Other parts of the exposure control plan include hazard requirements, training requirements, and record keeping. The "biohazard" label is required to be affixed to all containers used to store, transport, or ship blood or other body fluids. EMT-Bs must be provided with training that includes information about the employer's exposure control plan, general disease transmission, uses and limitations of PPE, workplace practices that reduce or prevent exposures, exposure incident procedures, and labeling requirements. OSHA also requires that records be kept for medical and training purposes. Medical records are confidential and kept for the duration of employment plus 30 years. Training records are kept for three years.

RYAN WHITE CARE ACT

In 1994, the Centers for Disease Control (CDC) issued the final notice for the Ryan White Comprehensive AIDS Resources Emergency (CARE) Act. This federal mandate applies to all 50 states and all emergency response employees, which includes all EMS, firefighting, and police personnel who provide emergency medical care. The Ryan White Act establishes procedures by which all emergency response employees (EREs) can determine if they have been exposed to a potentially infectious disease while providing patient care. It identifies a list of potentially life-threatening, infectious, and communicable diseases to which EREs may be exposed. This list includes infectious pulmonary tuberculosis, HIV/AIDS, hepatitis B, hemorrhagic fevers, plague, diphtheria, meningococcal disease, and rabies.

The Ryan White Act requires that "every State public health officer must designate an official of every employer of EREs in the State who will be responsible for notifying EREs of exposure." This person is called the **designated officer,** or D.O. The D.O. is responsible for gathering all information regarding an exposure to an airborne or bloodborne infectious disease and reporting to the receiving medical facility to request a determination of exposure. There are two separate notification procedures—one for airborne exposures and another for bloodborne exposures (Figure 2-8).

The reason for the two distinct reporting requirements is that exposure to airborne diseases, such as infectious pulmonary tuberculosis, may not be evident until well after the patient is transferred to the medical facility. Tuberculosis is usually diagnosed during hospitalization. However, you will know immediately if you had significant contact with blood or body fluids and can request immediate follow-up.

Several states have laws regarding patient testing after an exposure that are not covered under the

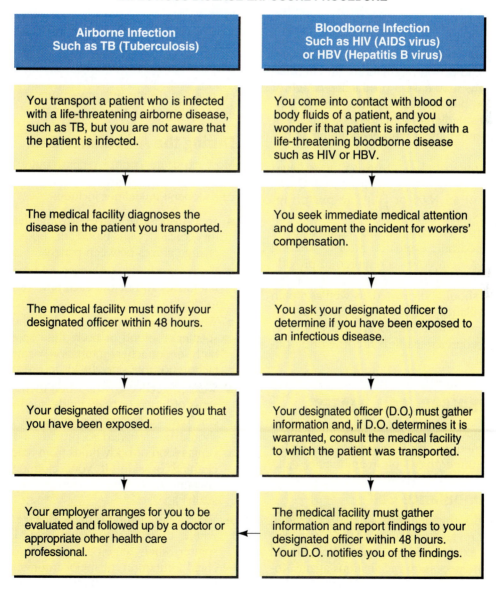

INFECTIOUS DISEASE EXPOSURE PROCEDURE

Airborne Infection Such as TB (Tuberculosis)	Bloodborne Infection Such as HIV (AIDS virus) or HBV (Hepatitis B virus)
You transport a patient who is infected with a life-threatening airborne disease, such as TB, but you are not aware that the patient is infected.	You come into contact with blood or body fluids of a patient, and you wonder if that patient is infected with a life-threatening bloodborne disease such as HIV or HBV.
The medical facility diagnoses the disease in the patient you transported.	You seek immediate medical attention and document the incident for workers' compensation.
The medical facility must notify your designated officer within 48 hours.	You ask your designated officer to determine if you have been exposed to an infectious disease.
Your designated officer notifies you that you have been exposed.	Your designated officer (D.O.) must gather information and, if D.O. determines it is warranted, consult the medical facility to which the patient was transported.
Your employer arranges for you to be evaluated and followed up by a doctor or appropriate other health care professional.	The medical facility must gather information and report findings to your designated officer within 48 hours. Your D.O. notifies you of the findings.

Figure 2-8 Under the Ryan White CARE Act, there is a procedure for finding out and following up if you have been exposed to an infectious disease.

Ryan White Act. Review all applicable laws in your area regarding your rights to request patient testing after an exposure incident.

TUBERCULOSIS REQUIREMENTS

Based upon the 1990 Centers for Disease Control (CDC) recommendations, OSHA in 1993 issued policies and procedures for providing care for patients with suspected or confirmed TB. They are called "Guidelines for Preventing the Transmission in Health Care Settings with Special Focus on HIV-Related Issues." They outline those situations in which there is a risk for contracting and transmitting TB, procedures for prevention of transmission, and the training required for use of personal protective equipment such as an N-95 or high-efficiency particulate air (HEPA) respirator.

As an EMT-B, you should suspect TB in patients who have a suppressed immune system such as occurs in HIV/AIDS, in prison populations, and in nursing homes. Patients may have a productive cough of either sputum or blood, night sweats, loss of appetite, weight loss, lethargy or weakness, and fever. Always consider any patient who is coughing as potentially infectious.

In cases of anticipated exposure to the exhaled air of a patient with potential or confirmed TB, OSHA requires the use of an N-95 or HEPA respirator approved by the National Institute for Occupational Safety and Health (NIOSH). You are required to be "fit tested" and medically evaluated prior to wearing any HEPA mask. An employer is required to provide a written procedure for training in the use of the mask and how it should be cleaned, as well as a plan for medical surveillance, including TB skin tests.

Always review your state, local, and employer policies and procedures regarding airborne or bloodborne pathogens.

BSI AND AMBULANCE CALL PHASES

Various BSI techniques and other infection control procedures outlined in the exposure control plan take place in the three phases of an ambulance call.

Before the Ambulance Call

Before performing any duties as an EMS provider, make sure you review and understand your employer's specific exposure control plan. You should also have all of the necessary vaccinations against infectious diseases, such as HBV, as well as the TB skin test or purified protein derivative (PPD) test for tuberculosis.

As you begin each shift, inspect your vehicle for cleanliness as you complete other equipment checklists. All equipment, especially airway, oxygen, and suction equipment, should be in good working order and free of any blood or body fluids from previous patient-care activities. If any equipment is found to be contaminated, it should be immediately cleaned and checked for proper functioning. Some EMS services have a daily or weekly infection-control cleaning schedule that should be followed.

In general, all surfaces should be checked and cleaned of any blood or body fluids. Any contaminated items in waste receptacles should be emptied, and the receptacles should be cleaned. Sharps containers should be checked to ensure they are not overflowing or leaking. Never try to empty sharps containers. When they are full, seal and dispose of them properly. Check to make sure you have adequate supplies of infection-control equipment such as gloves, masks, eye protection, biohazard waste bags, and intermediate- and low-level disinfectants for cleaning up spills of blood or body fluids. Also remember to wash your hands after cleaning or disinfecting any equipment or vehicle surfaces and prior to going on any calls.

During the Ambulance Call

Most exposure control plans require the use of PPE based upon the degree of risk associated with each call. General guidelines include:

- Wear disposable gloves anytime there is a potential for contact with blood or body fluids. Always change gloves between patients.
- Wash your hands with soap and water after removing gloves and before each time you eat or use cosmetics.
- Wear protective eyewear when there is a risk for splatter of blood or body fluid spatter, as in childbirth, endotracheal intubation, or major trauma. Attach removable side shields to prescription glasses.
- Wear protective gowns when there are large splash areas of blood or body fluids, such as in emergency childbirth or with major trauma victims. The gowns should be designed to provide a barrier that prevents blood or body fluids from reaching your inner clothing or skin. If your clothing does become contaminated, have a change of uniform readily available.
- Wear a surgical-type mask or face shield in cases where there is anticipated blood or body fluid spatter, such as emergency childbirth, endotracheal intubation, or major trauma. In cases of potential infectious respiratory tuberculosis, an N-95 or high-efficiency particulate air (HEPA) respirator is required. A surgical-type mask also should be

worn by the patient in cases of airborne disease. Monitor the patient's airway carefully while the mask is in place.

In addition to PPE, use other protective barrier equipment, such as face shields and pocket masks with one-way valves, to decrease the possibility of any disease transmission. The key to prevention of disease transmission is to always have PPE available when and where you need it.

Termination of the Ambulance Call

Even after you have transferred care of the patient to the receiving facility, your call has not ended. As an EMT-B, you are responsible for preparing for the next call by decontaminating and cleaning the ambulance and all equipment used for patient-care activities.

Always wash your hands after transferring care at the receiving facility. The practice of good handwashing techniques is the best defense against the transmission of disease. Wash your hands with soap and water or other disinfectant as soon as possible upon removing gloves after patient contact.

Follow engineering controls and housekeeping procedures to ready yourself, your crew, and the ambulance for the next response. While still at the receiving facility, take the following steps (Skill Summary 2-1):

1. **Prepare the ambulance for service.** While wearing heavy duty, dishwashing-style gloves, quickly clean the patient compartment. Follow biohazard disposal procedures according to your agency's exposure control plan. Clean up blood, vomitus, and other body fluids that may have soiled the floor. Wipe down any equipment that has been splashed. Place disposable towels used to clean up blood or body fluids directly in a red bag. Remove and dispose of trash such as bandage wrappings and opened but unused dressings. Sweep away caked dirt that may have been tracked into the patient compartment. Sponge up water and mud from the floor that may have been tracked in due to inclement weather. Bag dirty linens or blankets to be appropriately laundered. Use a deodorizer to neutralize odors of vomit, urine, and feces.

2. **Prepare respiratory equipment for service.** Clean and disinfect nondisposable, used BVMs and other used reusable parts of respiratory-assist devices. This will keep them from becoming reservoirs of infectious agents that can easily contaminate the next patient. Disinfect the suction unit, and place used disposable items in a plastic bag and seal it. Replace the items with the spare ones carried in the ambulance.

3. **Replace expendable items.** If you have a supply replacement agreement with the hospital, replace expendable items from the hospital storerooms on a one-for-one basis. However, do not abuse this exchange program. Keep in mind that the constant abuse of a supplies replacement program usually leads to its discontinuation.

4. **Exchange equipment according to your local policy.** Exchange items such as splints and spine boards. Benefits associated with an equipment exchange program include: there is no need to subject patients to injury-aggravating movements just to recover equipment, crews are not delayed at the hospital, and ambulances can return to quarters fully equipped for the next response. When equipment is available for exchange, quickly inspect it for completeness and operability. Parts are sometimes lost or broken when an immobilizing device is removed from a patient. If so, notify someone in authority so the device can be repaired or replaced.

5. **Make up the ambulance stretcher.** Each service has its own favorite way to make up a stretcher. It is a good practice to clean the mattress and flip it over prior to making the stretcher. Learn the procedure for your service and always make up the stretcher so it is neat and clean.

> ## PRECEPTOR PEARL
>
> Remember if patients see stained sheets or other examples of failure to prepare a vehicle, they also may question the quality of care they receive. Remind new EMT-Bs that they can make a good first impression on a patient and the patient's family by making the stretcher presentation a matter of personal and professional pride.

Specific cleaning and decontamination solutions will vary according to local procedures. In general, three levels of disinfectants are used: a high-level disinfectant (strong enough to destroy mycobacterium tuberculosis), an intermediate-level disinfectant such as 1:100 solution of bleach (1 part bleach to 100 parts water), and a low-level disinfectant such as Lysol®, (Skill Summary 2-2). Sterilization—another process used to clean and disinfect equipment—is generally used in a hospital and is not practical in the out-of-hospital setting.

You may elect to wait until you are back in quarters to disinfect and clean equipment (Skill Summary 2-3). However, always remember to bag

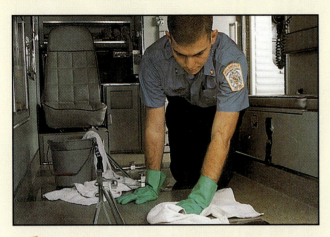

▲ **1.** Clean the ambulance interior as required.

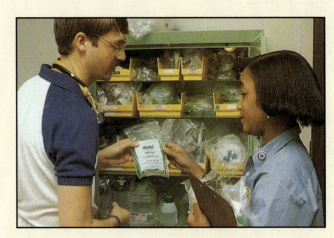

▲ **2.** Replace respiratory equipment as required.

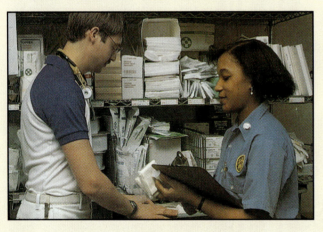

▲ **3.** Replace expendable items per local policies.

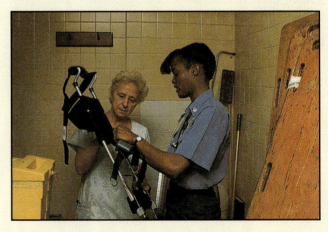

▲ **4.** Exchange equipment per local policies.

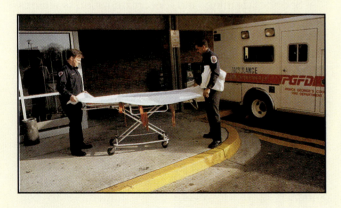

▲ **5.** Make up the wheeled stretcher.

Cleaning and Disinfecting Equipment

There are four levels of cleaning and disinfecting.

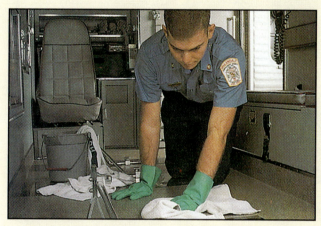

▲ **1.** A *low-level disinfectant* approved by the U.S. Environmental Protection Agency—for example, a commercial product like Lysol®—will clean and kill germs on ambulance floors and walls.

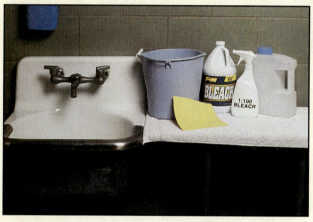

▲ **2.** An *intermediate-level disinfectant*—such as a 1:100 bleach-to-water mixture—can be used to clean and kill germs on equipment surfaces.

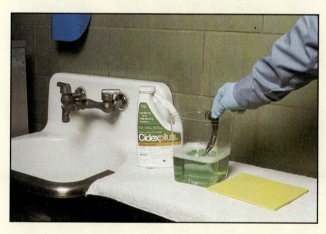

▲ **3.** A *high-level disinfectant*—such as Cidex Plus®—will destroy all forms of microbial life except high numbers of bacterial spores.

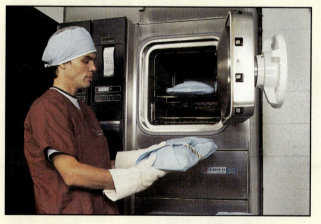

▲ **4.** *Sterilization* is required to destroy all possible sources of infection on equipment that will be used invasively.

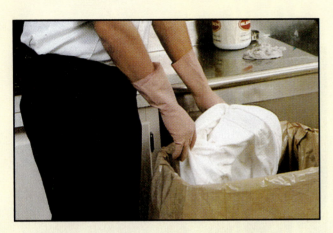

▲ **1.** Place contaminated linens in a biohazard container. Place noncontaminated linens in a regular hamper.

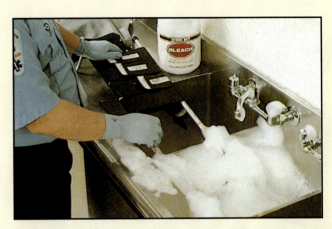

▲ **2.** Remove and clean patient-care equipment as required.

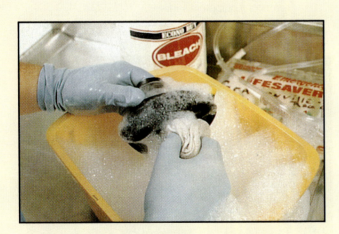

▲ **3.** Clean and sanitize respiratory equipment as required.

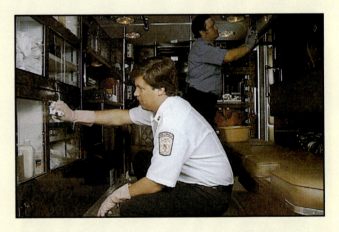

▲ **4.** Clean and sanitize the ambulance interior as required. Use germicide to clean any devices or surfaces that have come in contact with a patient's blood or body fluids.

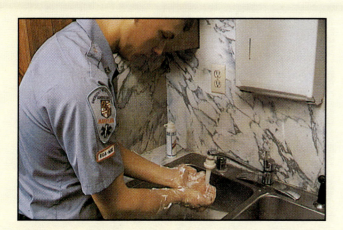

▲ **5.** Wash thoroughly. Change soiled clothing. If you were exposed to a communicable disease, you should wash and change first.

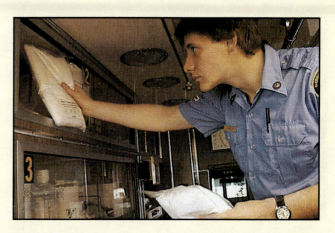

▲ **6.** Replace expendable items as required.

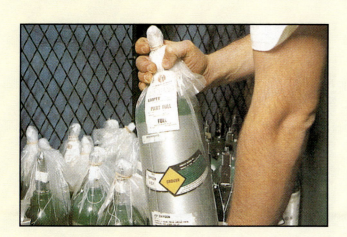

▲ **7.** Always be sure to replace oxygen cylinders as necessary.

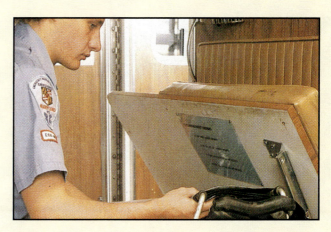

▲ **8.** Replace patient-care equipment as needed.

(continued)

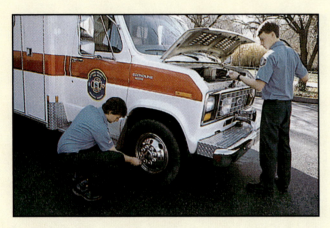

▲ **9.** Maintain the ambulance as required. Report problems that may take the vehicle out of service.

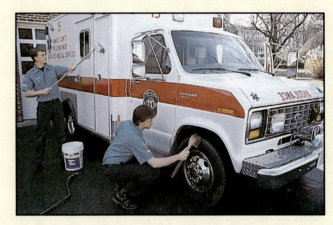

▲ **10.** Clean the ambulance exterior as needed.

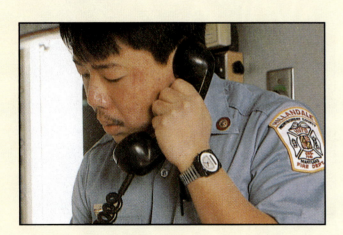

▲ **11.** Report the unit ready for service.

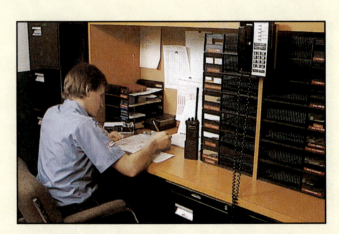

▲ **12.** Complete any unfinished report forms as soon as possible.

this equipment properly to isolate and separate it from clean equipment while returning to quarters. This prevents the possibility that you will use "dirty" equipment if you receive a call prior to disinfecting and cleaning. If the floor, cots, or walls of the vehicle are blood-covered, then the ambulance may need to be placed out of service until cleaning can occur.

At the station, place all contaminated equipment in the proper solution for disinfecting and cleaning. Check the ambulance for any surfaces that may have come in contact with blood or body fluids. After the equipment and vehicle have been cleaned, allow surfaces to air dry. Wash your hands thoroughly, and check to see if your uniform has become soiled with blood or body fluids. Prepare yourself for service by washing your hands and changing your uniform if it was soiled with a body substance on the call. Replace expendable items with items from the unit's storeroom. Refill oxygen cylinders even if only a small volume of gas was used. Replace patient care equipment. Check vehicle fluid levels, tire pressures, warning devices, and lights. Clean the vehicle (a clean exterior lends a professional appearance to an ambulance), and check it for broken lights, glass and body damage, door operation, and other parts that may need repair or replacement. Complete any unfinished report forms and report the unit ready for service.

SUMMARY

- Stressful calls include MCIs, calls involving children, grotesques injuries, and injury or death of a coworker.

- Signs of stress include irritability, inability to concentrate, difficulty sleeping, and loss of interest in pleasurable activities.

- To deal with stress, exercise, rotate your duty assignment (by changing location or shift) if possible, and relax.

- The stages of the death and dying process include denial, anger, bargaining, depression, and acceptance.

- Scene safety is the first priority on every call.

- Be alert for signs of danger, including violence, unstable vehicles or surfaces, and hazardous materials.

- Use tactics such as cover, concealment, and retreat in response to violence.

- Personal protective equipment should be used any time that the potential exists for coming in contact with the blood or body fluids of another person.

- Personal protective equipment (PPE) includes disposable gloves, eye shields, masks, gowns, N-95 or HEPA respirators, BVMs, and pocket masks.

- EMS agencies are required to have exposure control plans.

- The Ryan White CARE Act specifies procedures to follow in the event that exposures (airborne or bloodborne) to a potentially infectious disease occur.

REVIEW QUESTIONS

1. Signs and symptoms of critical incident stress include all of the following EXCEPT:
   a. delusional thoughts.
   b. general irritability.
   c. inability to concentrate.
   d. nightmares and difficulty sleeping.

2. A critical incident stress debriefing is usually:
   a. an investigation of conduct during an incident.
   b. held within the first hour or so after an incident.
   c. arranged for EMS workers who breach confidentiality.
   d. to assist emergency personnel in dealing with stress.

3. Which of the following actions is most appropriate for an EMT-B at a violent scene?
   a. Attempt to stop the violence.
   b. Put on body armor and then enter.
   c. Wait for more EMT-Bs before entering the scene.
   d. Retreat to a safe place and then call police.

4. When an EMT-B has contact with blood or body fluids through a break in the skin, eyes, mucous membranes, or parenteral contact resulting from the performance of his or her duties, it is referred to as a(n):
   a. occupational exposure.
   b. body substance isolation.
   c. passive or accidental infection.
   d. perquistice infection.

5. Usually the best defense against contracting an infectious disease from a patient is to:

    a. disinfect all your equipment.

    b. wear a face shield on every call.

    c. wash your hands after every patient.

    d. wear protective gloves with all patients.

W**EB MEDIC**

Visit Brady's *Essentials of Emergency Care* web site for direct web links. At **www.prenhall.com/limmer,** you will find information related to the following Chapter 2 topics:

- the Centers for Disease Control
- the Ryan White CARE Act
- OSHA exposure control standards
- Critical incident stress
- Stages of grief associated with death and dying

Chapter Three

MEDICAL/LEGAL AND ETHICAL ISSUES

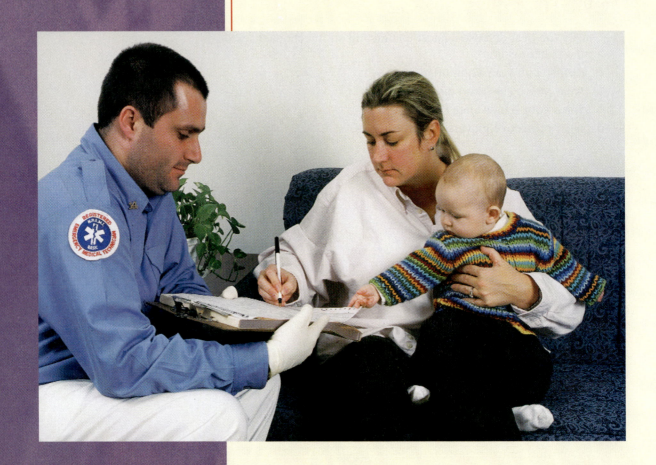

ESSENTIAL ELECTRONIC EXTRAS

CD ESSENTIALS

For preview and review of chapter material, see the student CD-ROM for

- Pretest
- Chapter quizzes
- Posttest

WEB ESSENTIALS

For additional review and enrichment, visit www.prenhall.com/limmer for

- Interactive student quizzes
- Links to online EMS resources
- Online case studies
- Audio glossary

This section covers the legal obligations and moral considerations you will encounter as you continue your practice as an EMT-B. These considerations include scope of practice, patient consent and refusal, abandonment and negligence, battery, the duty to act, confidentiality, and issues related to organ donation. In addition, the EMT-B's responsibilities at a crime scene are reviewed.

SCOPE OF PRACTICE

Simply stated, the **scope of practice** defines medical/legal boundaries and expectations for the care you provide as an EMT-B. The scope of practice for any medical professional is usually defined by state legislation. Just as physicians, nurses, technicians, and others have definitions of what they are allowed to do, EMT-Bs are also bound by legislative guidelines. The scope of practice of an EMT-B may be enhanced by medical direction through the use of standing orders and protocols.

PATIENT CONSENT AND REFUSAL

Do Not Resuscitate (DNR) Orders

In general, mentally competent patients have the right to refuse care, including resuscitation efforts. This situation is most commonly encountered in a patient with a terminal disease. Generally, refusal of resuscitation requires a written order from a physician before care may be withheld. This written order is called a **Do Not Resuscitate (DNR) order** (Figure 3-1). A DNR order is a type of "advance directive" because it is signed in advance of an emergency situation.

DNR orders may be issued in varying degrees. That is, some orders are issued to prevent all resuscitative measures including CPR. Others are issued to prevent only long-term care such as feeding tubes. When in doubt or when written orders are not present, you should begin resuscitation efforts.

Be sure to review your protocols regarding DNR orders before you must make these decisions. A scene in which the patient or family does not want emergency care for a critical illness is not the time to look up the protocol.

Expressed Consent

In order to provide care for any patient, you must obtain consent. To be able to give consent, a patient must be of legal age, able to make a rational decision, mentally competent, and informed about the care that will be given, the procedures involved, and all related risks. Consent must be obtained from every adult patient before rendering treatment.

Implied Consent

If a patient is unconscious and therefore unable to give consent, it is assumed or implied that the patient, if conscious, would consent to your care. If an unconscious patient regains consciousness and is able to give expressed consent, you must obtain it in order to continue care.

Consent of Minors

Because of their age, minors are unable to give consent. This also applies to individuals who are mentally incompetent. Consent for care of these patients must be obtained from a parent or legal guardian. Each state has its own laws that determine the age at which a minor can legally give consent. The ages for consent may vary depending on whether the child is

CORE CONCEPTS

In this chapter, you will learn about the following topics:

- Scope of practice

- Patient consent and refusal issues

- Advance directives

- Performing assessment and care at crime scenes

emancipated (living on his or her own) or married. If a child is critically ill or injured and a parent or guardian is not present, begin care based on implied consent.

Patient Refusal

A patient who is competent and of legal age may refuse your care and/or transportation. The patient also may withdraw consent at any time. Most agencies have a "release" form that the patient signs to indicate refusal of care (Figure 3-2). It should be witnessed. The purpose of this form is to release the EMT-B and ambulance service from liability should the patient suffer ill effects from the refusal.

A patient must be fully informed of the risks involved with refusing care or transportation. A patient who refuses care and whose condition then deteriorates can be a significant source of liability for EMT-Bs, even though the patient signed the release form. Always make every effort to convince the patient to accept your care and transportation. In the event the patient still refuses, always tell the patient that you can be called again at any time. Furthermore, try to convince the patient to call a doctor for follow-up care. Having a family member or other concerned person stay with the patient may also be helpful should problems develop after you leave. Carefully document attempts you have made to convince the patient to accept your care and the provisions you made for the patient when care was refused.

Consent is not always clear cut. It is not always easy to determine if a patient is rational and capable of making informed decisions. In your experience as an EMT-B, you may have responded to calls in which

a patient was intoxicated, suffered from head injury, or incurred another medical problem that may have clouded his or her judgment. If patients such as these are allowed to "sign off" and refuse care, you could be held responsible if they suffer a worsening of their condition as a result of not being transported.

There are several steps that may be taken to provide quality care while still respecting the patient's rights. If you question whether or not a patient is competent to refuse, or if you feel that not caring for the patient may result in a worsening of the patient's condition, you must take action. Consider the following steps:

■ **Contact medical direction for advice.** The medical control physician may be able to provide advice and input on the patient's condition and ways, such as talking to the patient, to convince him or her to accept care and transportation.

■ **Utilize family members to help the patient accept your care.** Often family members can help convince the patient that care is actually needed. Family members can also provide insight into the patient's reasoning for refusing care (denial, fear of hospitals, etc.).

■ **Notify the police if necessary.** In many states, police have the authority to order patients to be transported against their will. If you have a supervisor, notify him or her as well.

Remember to document all your actions. It is usually considered best to err on the side of caution and seek input from medical control, the police, or other appropriate parties before accepting refusal.

Department of Health

Nonhospital Order Not to Resuscitate (DNR order)

Person's Name (Print) _____

Date of Birth ____/____/____

Do not resuscitate the person named above.

Person's Signature_____

Date____/____/____

Physician's Signature_____

Print Name_____

License Number _____

Date____/____/____

It is the responsibility of the physician to determine, at least every 90 days, whether this order continues to be appropriate, and to indicate this by a note in the person's medical chart. The issuance of a new form is **NOT** required, and under the law this order should be considered valid unless it is known that it has been revoked. This order remains valid and must be followed, even if it has not been reviewed within the 90 day period.

Figure 3-1   A sample Do Not Resuscitate (DNR) order.

EMS PATIENT REFUSAL CHECKLIST

PATIENT's NAME: _____ AGE: _____

LOCATION OF CALL: _____ DATE: _____

AGENCY INCIDENT #: _____ AGENCY CODE: _____

NAME OF PERSON FILLING OUT FORM: _____

I.   ASSESSMENT OF PATIENT (Check appropriate response for each item)

1.   Oriented to: Person?   ☐ Yes ☐ No
                    Place?   ☐ Yes ☐ No
                    Time?   ☐ Yes ☐ No
                    Situation? ☐ Yes ☐ No

2.   Altered level of consciousness?   ☐ Yes ☐ No

3.   Head injury?   ☐ Yes ☐ No

4.   Alcohol or drug ingestion by exam or history?   ☐ Yes ☐ No

II. PATIENT INFORMED (Check appropriate response for each item)

☐ Yes ☐ No   Medical treatment/evaluation needed

☐ Yes ☐ No   Ambulance transport needed

☐ Yes ☐ No   Further harm could result without medical treatment/evaluation

☐ Yes ☐ No   Transport by means other than ambulance could be hazardous in light of patient's illness/injury

☐ Yes ☐ No   Patient provided with Refusal Information Sheet

☐ Yes ☐ No   Patient accepted Refusal Information Sheet

III. DISPOSITION

☐ Refused all EMS assistance

☐ Refused field treatment, but accepted transport

☐ Refused transport, but accepted field treatment

☐ Refused transport to recommended facility

☐ Patient transported by private vehicle to_____

☐ Released in care or custody of self

☐ Released in care or custody of relative or friend

   Name: _____ Relationship: _____

☐ Released in custody of law enforcement agency

   Agency: _____ Officer: _____

☐ Released in custody of other agency

   Agency: _____ Officer: _____

IV. COMMENTS: _____

_____

_____

_____

Figure 3-2   A sample patient refusal checklist (from Spokane County Emergency Medical Services, Washington State

OTHER LEGAL ASPECTS OF EMERGENCY CARE

Abandonment and Negligence

Terminating care of a patient without making sure the patient is in the hands of a provider at the same or higher level of training is considered abandonment.

Negligence is deviation from the accepted standard of care that results in injury to a patient. There are four components to a successful negligence action or lawsuit:

- The EMT-B had a **duty to act.** This means that the EMT-B was in a situation through employment, position in a volunteer squad, or other position in which the EMT-B is required to provide care and . . .
- The EMT-B breached, or failed to perform, that duty and . . .
- Injuries, which may be physical or psychological, or damages were inflicted and . . .
- The actions or lack of action caused the injury or damage.

PRECEPTOR PEARL

When someone new to the profession is completing a prehospital care report (PCR), remember your role as an experienced provider. Coach the new EMT-B to "paint a word picture" of the patient. Someone who has never seen the patient should be able to clearly "picture" the patient by reading the PCR. Remind the newcomer that when it comes to interventions: "If it's not written down, it wasn't performed." Proper documentation is important for liability prevention.

Battery

Battery is subjecting a person to contact against his or her will. If a patient who is legally able to refuse care is treated anyway, the patient has grounds for criminal charges or civil suit or action against the EMT-B for battery.

Duty to Act

In some situations, EMT-Bs have a duty to act. Often this duty is very clear, such as when you are riding an ambulance dispatched to a call. Other times— such as when you are off-duty in another ambulance district—you may not have a legal duty to act, but you may be morally obligated to provide care or take action until EMS arrives. In most cases, for both legal and moral reasons, it is better to provide care than not to.

Confidentiality

When you treat a patient, the details of your assessment and care are confidential. They may not be told to others, with some exceptions. The information may be given to other health-care providers who need the information to provide care, under judicial subpoena, when law requires (child abuse, gunshot wounds, etc.), and for some insurance purposes. Releasing information for other reasons requires a signed release form from the patient.

Organ Donors/Organ Retrieval

In general, organs may be donated only if there is a signed document giving permission to harvest them. A signed donor card is a legal document. So is the sticker on the reverse side of some driver licenses.

There are many people who are waiting to receive donated organs to save or prolong life. While the EMS care you give to organ donor patients must not differ from that for other patients, there are some things that may be done to assist in the harvesting of organs from a donor. If you find yourself caring for a patient who is an organ donor and that patient is in cardiac arrest, continue to treat the patient as you would any other. Advise medical direction that the patient may be an organ donor. The physician may direct you to continue CPR when it normally would be stopped in order to maintain organs in a viable condition. You may confront this situation in a trauma incident in which a patient has mortal wounds. Mortal head injuries are the most common scenario for organ donations. CPR may be initiated solely for the purpose of organ harvesting.

Special Reporting Situations

As an EMT-B, you will be called upon to treat patients who have been assaulted or abused. There will be times when these acts are committed by strangers and other times when they are committed by family members. Emergency care is the same for all injuries, regardless of the causes. However, the patient who has received injuries through abuse or neglect may require additional emotional care and reassurance.

There will be times when you suspect abuse, although the patient denies it. Conflicting stories, injuries in various stages of healing, or an unusual fear of a parent or spouse are just a few of the possible indicators. These suspicions should be reported to hospital personnel or other agencies as required by law. Document your observations objectively (injury patterns, unusual behavior, etc.), but avoid conclusions or opinions.

You may be required to notify local law enforcement officials of domestic violence, sexual assault, and gunshot wounds, as well as child and elder abuse and neglect. Become familiar with the laws in your area.

EMS AT CRIME SCENES

Crime scenes are very dynamic situations. Providing emergency medical care at crime scenes can be very challenging. Remember that your safety is always the most important concern. Crime scenes should always be secured by the police before you enter and begin

care. Even then, the perpetrator may return or even be well hidden at the scene.

Once your safety is reasonably assured, there are still some very major issues: patient care, preservation of evidence, and working with the police. This section will give an overview of EMS actions at the crime scene. Just as there are many types of patients, there are many types of crime scenes and evidence. Use your local resources to set up additional training in conjunction with police agencies in your area.

Scene Safety

Obviously, scene safety is the most important part of any call. Danger at a crime scene may come from things other than human beings. While physical violence is an obvious danger, remember that downed wires, hazardous materials, controlled substances, booby traps, and other materials may pose a danger to you. Even if the danger is not directed at you as an EMS provider, you may still be affected by it.

The police have the training, authority, and responsibility to secure the scene for violent or potentially violent persons. Failing to let police perform this task, or unreasonably attempting it yourself, may cause you to fall victim to the same violence that harmed your patient. Fight the urge to rush in without doing a thorough scene size-up. Remember that scenes change rapidly. A scene that was not violent initially may become violent when the perpetrator returns or emerges from hiding. Patients themselves can become violent. You can never be too careful (Figure 3-4).

Cooperating with the Police

While some may feel that public service agencies automatically cooperate, as an experienced provider you will realize that this is not always the case. Agencies and personnel may fail to cooperate, not out of malicious intent but because emergency scenes are very stressful.

There is one fundamental difference between the responsibilities of police and EMS. EMS must get a trauma patient off the scene in 10 minutes or less. The police may have hours to examine a crime scene carefully.

Even the most experienced and well-meaning EMT-B can disturb a crime scene. It is inevitable. One fundamental disturbance is caused by taking the patient to the hospital. This action removes a key piece of evidence (the patient) from the scene.

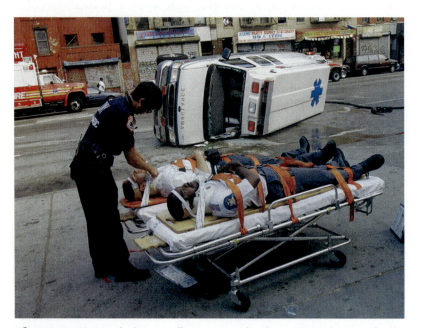

Figure 3-3 Ambulance collisions are a leading cause of injury, death, and legal liability to EMTs.

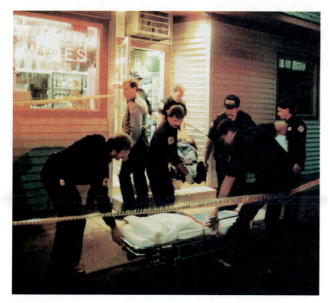

Figure 3-4 Example of a crime scence

The combination of the stress felt by members of both agencies plus their conflicting roles is often the cause of less than ideal EMS/police interaction. The following steps may help prevent these negative interactions:

- **Learn to identify and preserve evidence.** While you must always put patient care first (after your own safety), learn how to recognize evidence on scene and preserve it. Knowledge of types of evidence can help you carry out your patient-care tasks as well as keep from disturbing important evidence.

- **Be observant.** Small things may be the key to a criminal case. Remembering the condition of the area when you arrive is very important. Whether or not the door was locked, whether the lights were on or off, and statements made by the patient can be extremely useful to police.

- **Remember what you touch.** You may find it necessary to move a patient from a couch to the floor to provide treatments such as CPR. You may also need to move furniture to perform this task. Remembering these actions and reporting them to the police is very important. If you do not, a police officer at the scene may see furniture moved and blood in two locations. The officer may improperly conclude that a struggle took place because of changes you made.

- **Minimize your impact on the scene.** While you may have to move items at the scene, do so carefully and minimally. A good rule of thumb would be to do what you must to provide proper patient care and no more. Remember what changes have been made and report them to the police. If you have moved an item, leave it where you moved it. Do not try to replace items to their original locations. Do not use a telephone on the scene because the police may be interested in the redial function.

Learn more about communicating with police. It may not be possible to provide a thorough report to the police and still keep your time at the scene to an acceptable level. Many police agencies will request a statement about your actions and observations at the crime scene. Do this according to your agency's policies. There is a good chance that you will be required to testify about the conditions at the crime scene and the actions you took while there and en route to the hospital. When the call is over, critique the scene from a patient-care as well as an evidence-preservation standpoint. Invite police officers to speak at your training sessions to learn more about crime scenes.

You may also be sent to calls that appear to be routine medical or trauma calls and which later are determined to be crime scenes. Many experienced EMT-Bs have received calls days, weeks, or months later from a police officer indicating that a call they had been to some time ago was actually a crime scene. EMT-Bs may also uncover situations that are suspicious and be the first to alert the police to a crime. In either case, being observant will help you to remain safe, to uncover the mechanism of injury or medical history, and to document important facts about the patient.

Crime scenes are challenging situations. Your first priority is always patient care, with attention to aspects of the crime scene that may be preserved as you go. Remember that you are under a certain amount of stress at a crime scene. So are the police. Any interpersonal relationship will suffer when stress is added. Crime scenes are no different. Understanding, training, and cooperation will make the next crime scene you respond to successful for both yourself and the police.

SUMMARY

- As an EMT-B, you have legal obligations, including a duty to act.
- If you do not act or if you act in a way that deviates from the accepted standard of care, you may be liable to a charge of abandonment or negligence.
- You must stay within your scope of practice and provide emergency care only with the informed consent of your patient or your patient's legal guardian.
- If the patient is not able to give consent, you may be able to provide emergency care under the law of implied consent.
- If a competent, informed patient refuses your help either before or during patient care, you must stop. If you do not stop, you may be charged with the crime of battery.
- When a patient does refuse care, you must make sure he or she is informed of the risks involved, obtain a signed and witnessed release form, and document all your actions.
- Remember that you are obliged to keep all patient information confidential.
- You also have an obligation to assure your own safety. Do not enter a violent scene or a crime scene until the police have given you the okay.

REVIEW QUESTIONS

1. The medical and legal boundaries for the care the EMT-B may provide are referred to as:
   a. professional guidelines.
   b. the scope of practice.
   c. local protocols.
   d. the area of responsibility.

2. A written order limiting care that can be provided to a patient by an EMT-B must be signed by the:
   a. witnessing policeman.
   b. patient's physician.
   c. patient.
   d. EMS system's director.

3. Patients who are _____ and of legal age have the right to refuse emergency medical care.
   a. concious
   b. competent
   c. unresponsive
   d. terminally ill

4. An EMT-B may be charged with _____ if care of a patient is terminated without making sure the patient is in the hands of a provider at the same or higher level training.
   a. battery
   b. negligence
   c. abandonment
   d. breach of contract

5. When an EMT-B is in a situation in which he or she is required to provide emergency medical care, he or she is said to have a(n):

   a. duty to act.

   b. standard of care.

   c. order to respond.

   d. judicial subpoena.

6. If you have to move a piece of furniture at a crime scene, you should:

   a. try to put it back in its original location.

   b. leave it where you moved it and forget it.

   c. remember and report it to the police.

   d. allow the police to figure it out.

WEB MEDIC

Visit Brady's *Essentials of Emergency Care* web site for direct web links. At **www.prenhall.com/limmer,** you will find information related to the following Chapter 3 topics:

- DNR orders
- Organ sharing
- Legal actions involving paramedics
- Confidentiality
- Crime scene evidence

Chapter Four

THE HUMAN BODY

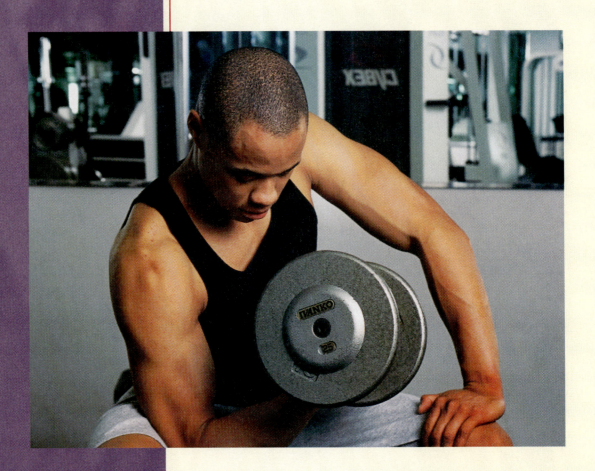

ESSENTIAL ELECTRONIC EXTRAS

CD ESSENTIALS

For preview and review of chapter material, see the student CD-ROM for

- Pretest
- Chapter quizzes
- Posttest

WEB ESSENTIALS

For additional review and enrichment, visit www.prenhall.com/limmer for

- Interactive student quizzes
- Links to online EMS resources
- Online case studies
- Audio glossary

The human body is the organism we are called upon to treat when illness or injury strikes. It should go without saying that it is important to be knowledgeable about the structure and function of the body. This chapter will briefly review basic anatomy, or structure of the body, regions of the body, and some of the major organ systems. Other systems are covered as appropriate throughout this textbook.

ANATOMICAL TERMS AND DIRECTION

On prehospital care reports it is not possible to describe injuries, signs, or symptoms without having a common point of medical reference and without having common terms that other medical professionals recognize and understand. The following terms are used to describe body parts and locations:

- **Anatomical position.** In this position a person is standing, facing forward, with palms facing forward.
- **Midline.** The midline of the body is created by dividing the body in half. An imaginary line is drawn from the top of the head between the eyes, extending through the umbilicus. This divides the body into right and left halves. It also allows us to use the terms **medial** (closer to the midline) and **lateral** (farther away from the midline).
- **Mid-axillary line.** The mid-axillary line extends vertically from the armpit to the ankle. This line divides the body into front and back halves. From this division we may determine **anterior** (front) and **posterior** (back).
- **Mid-clavicular.** This line is drawn from the center of the collarbone (clavicle) through the nipple below. Since there are two clavicles, there are two mid-clavicular lines. This "landmark" is important when listening for breath sounds.
- **Bilateral.** This term refers to both sides of anything. "Lungs sounds present bilaterally" means that there are lung sounds in both lungs.
- **Superior and inferior.** Superior means "above," while inferior means "below."
- **Proximal and distal.** These are terms of relative direction. Proximal refers to a position closer to the body or midline. Distal is a position farther away. For example, the elbow is proximal to the wrist, but distal to the shoulder.
- **Right and left.** In the health-care setting, these terms are no different from anywhere else. It is, however, important to use the patient's right and left, rather than yours, when documenting signs of illness or injury.

See Figures 4-1 through 4-4, pp. 47–49, for illustrations of body regions, directional terms, abdominal quadrants, and anatomical postures.

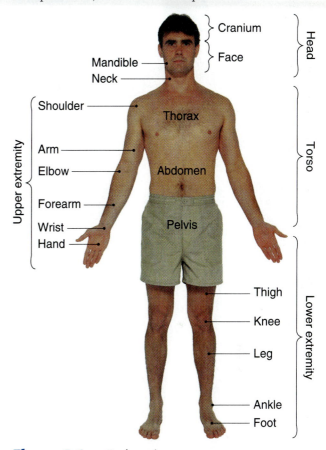

Figure 4-1 Body regions.

CORE CONCEPTS

In this chapter, you will learn about the following topics:

- Terms used to refer to regions and directions of the body

- Structure and function of the respiratory, cardiovascular, musculoskeletal, nervous, and endocrine systems

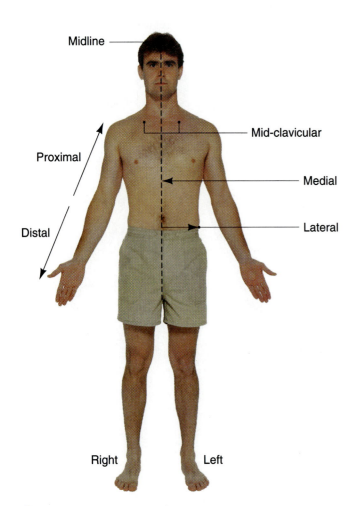

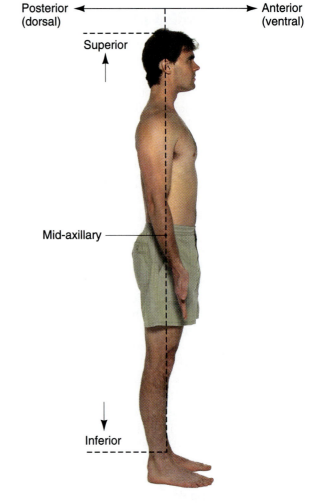

Figure 4-2   Directional terms.

BODY SYSTEMS

The following text and illustrations offer brief descriptions of the basic structures and functions, or physiology, of the human body for your review.

Respiratory System

The respiratory system is responsible for bringing oxygenated blood into the body and turning it over to the circulatory system for distribution to the body. It also excretes carbon dioxide through exhalation.

The respiratory system functions by inhaling air through the mouth and nose, through the **oropharynx** and **nasopharynx**, through the **larynx**—which contains the vocal cords—past the **cricoid cartilage** and through the **trachea**, through the mainstem **bronchi**, and gradually to the **alveoli** where the oxygen is turned over to the circulatory system (Figure 4-5, p. 49).

The **epiglottis** is a leaf-shaped structure which prevents food and foreign objects from entering the trachea during swallowing.

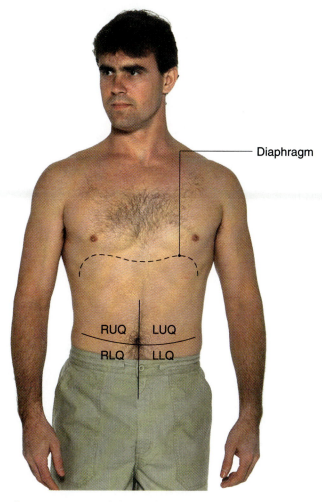

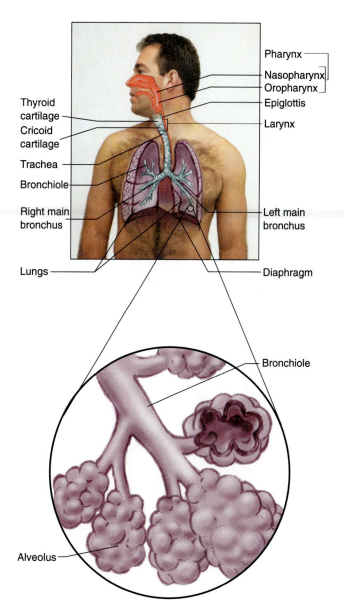

Figure 4-3   Abdominal quadrants.

Figure 4-5   The respiratory system.

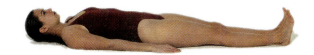

Supine

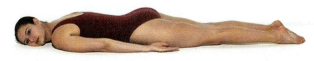

Prone

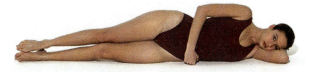

Recovery (lateral recumbent) position

Figure 4-4   Anatomical postures.

Cardiovascular System

Also known as the circulatory system, the cardiovascular system consists of the heart and blood vessels (Figure 4-6, p. 50). The heart consists of four chambers (Figure 4-7, p. 51). The two upper chambers are called **atria,** and the two lower chambers are called **ventricles.** Both atria contract at the same time. Both ventricles contract at the same time. One-way valves between the chambers of the heart—and at the blood vessels that leave the heart—prevent blood from traveling backward through the system.

Review the path of blood through the heart. Blood enters the right atria from the **vena cava.** It is next pumped through the right atria to the right ventricle into the pulmonary artery. Then, the blood travels through the lungs, where it receives oxygen.

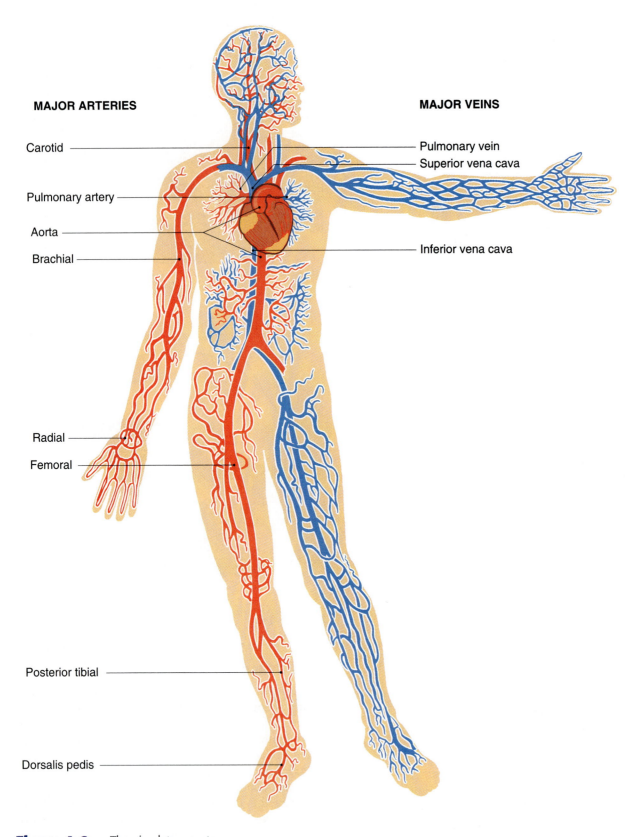

MAJOR ARTERIES

Carotid

Pulmonary artery

Aorta

Brachial

Radial

Femoral

Posterior tibial

Dorsalis pedis

MAJOR VEINS

Pulmonary vein

Superior vena cava

Inferior vena cava

Figure 4-6   The circulatory system.

THE HEART

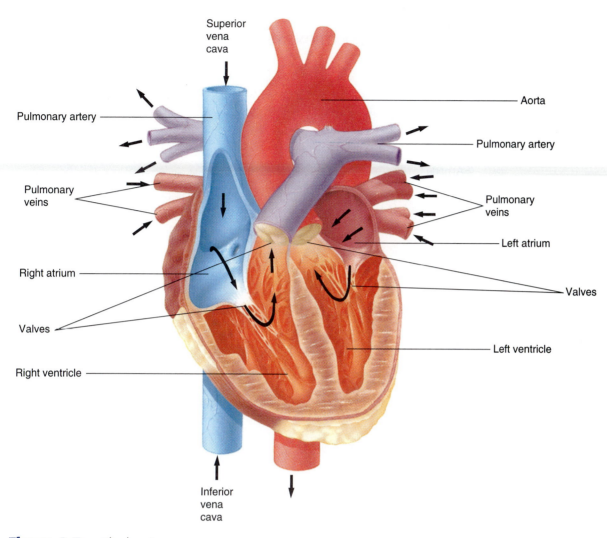

Superior vena cava

Pulmonary artery

Pulmonary veins

Right atrium

Valves

Right ventricle

Aorta

Pulmonary artery

Pulmonary veins

Left atrium

Valves

Left ventricle

Inferior vena cava

Figure 4-7   The heart.

The pulmonary veins return oxygenated blood to the left atrium of the heart. Blood is pumped down into the left ventricle, the most muscular chamber, where a contraction sends blood into the **aorta** for distribution to all parts of the body. Remember that **veins** carry blood toward the heart and **arteries** carry blood away from the heart.

The heart also has a specialized **cardiac conduction system** which sends electrical impulses through the heart (Figure 4-8, p. 52). It is these impulses that give heart muscle direction to beat. Irregularities in the conduction system can cause serious illness and death.

The sinoatrial (SA) node in the right atrium is the normal pacemaker of the heart. Impulses spread throughout the atria to the atrioventricular (AV) node. Here the impulses are transmitted through to the ventricles. The ventricular conduction system causes the ventricles to contract.

You have most likely learned to use the term "ventricular fibrillation." This condition occurs when the conduction system of the ventricles fibrillate, or fire randomly rather than in the normal organized pattern. Fibrillation does not cause contraction of the ventricles. Fortunately, the condition is often reversible through automated external defibrillation by EMTs.

Although the heart is constantly filled with blood, it obtains the blood supply needed to contract from the coronary arteries. These arteries branch off of the aorta. When they narrow, the pain known as "angina pectoris" is caused. If the arteries are occluded, heart muscle dies and the result is a myocardial infarction, or heart attack.

A. THE CARDIAC CONDUCTION SYSTEM

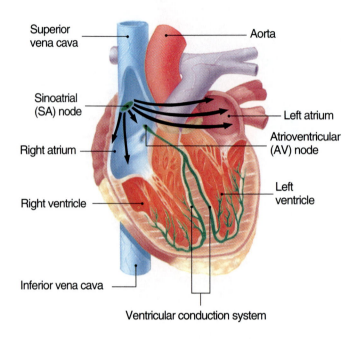

Superior vena cava

Aorta

Sinoatrial (SA) node

Left atrium

Atrioventricular (AV) node

Right atrium

Left ventricle

Right ventricle

Inferior vena cava

Ventricular conduction system

B. THE CORONARY ARTERIES

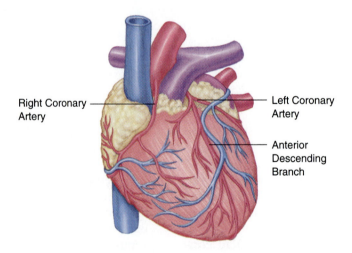

Right Coronary Artery

Left Coronary Artery

Anterior Descending Branch

Figure 4-8   (A) The cardiac conduction system and (B) the coronary arteries.

Musculoskeletal System

The musculoskeletal system is a system of muscles and bones which extend to every part of the body. The main functions of the musculoskeletal system are to give the body shape, to protect internal organs, and to provide for movement of the body. Figures 4-9 through 4-11 and Table 4-1 present the major bone structures of the body (see pp. 53–54).

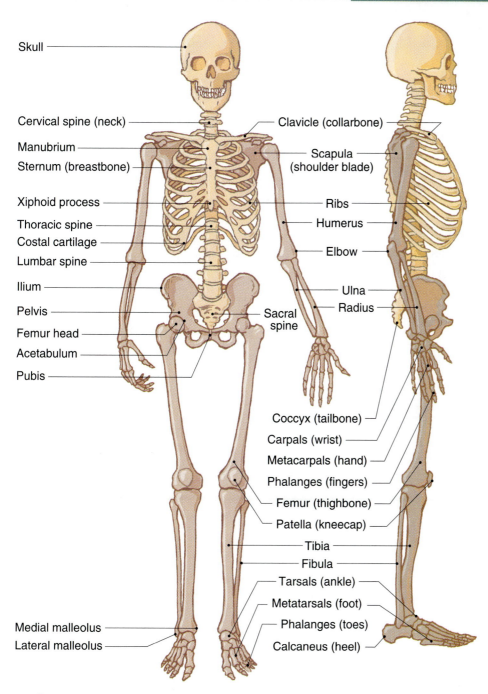

Skull

Cervical spine (neck)

Clavicle (collarbone)

Manubrium

Scapula (shoulder blade)

Sternum (breastbone)

Xiphoid process

Ribs

Thoracic spine

Humerus

Costal cartilage

Elbow

Lumbar spine

Ilium

Ulna

Pelvis

Radius

Femur head

Sacral spine

Acetabulum

Pubis

Coccyx (tailbone)

Carpals (wrist)

Metacarpals (hand)

Phalanges (fingers)

Femur (thighbone)

Patella (kneecap)

Tibia

Fibula

Tarsals (ankle)

Metatarsals (foot)

Medial malleolus

Phalanges (toes)

Lateral malleolus

Calcaneus (heel)

Figure 4-9   The skeleton.

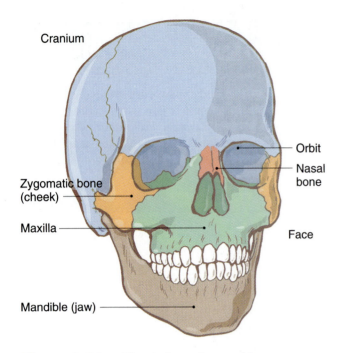

Cranium

Orbit

Nasal bone

Zygomatic bone (cheek)

Maxilla

Face

Mandible (jaw)

Figure 4-10   The skull: cranium and face.

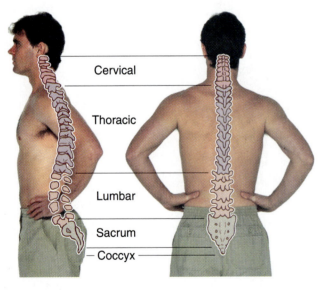

Cervical

Thoracic

Lumbar

Sacrum

Coccyx

Figure 4-11   The divisions of the spine.

Table 4-1   **Body Regions**

Region	Bones
Skull	Cranium
	Orbits
	Zygomatic (cheek) bones
	Maxilla (upper jaw)
	Mandible (lower jaw)
Spine	Consists of 33 vertebrae in the following regions:
	Cervical (neck), 7
	Thoracic (chest), 12
	Lumbar (lower back), 5
	Sacral (back wall of pelvis), 5
	Coccyx (tailbone), 4
Torso	Sternum (breastbone)
	Clavicle (collarbone)
	Scapula (shoulder blade)
	Ribs—12 pair (two of these pair are "floating" ribs)
Pelvis	Ilium (bony "wings")
	Ischium (base)
	Pubis (anterior)
Upper extremity	Humerus (upper arm)
	Radius
	Ulna
	Carpals (wrist)
	Metacarpals (hand)
	Phalanges (fingers)
Lower extremity	Femur (thigh)
	Tibia
	Fibula
	Tarsals (ankle)
	Metatarsals (foot)
	Phalanges (toes)

There are three types of muscle in the human body. **Involuntary muscle** is contained in our internal organs and responds directly to orders from the brain. **Voluntary muscle** is found in our extremities and is under our conscious control. **Cardiac muscle** is found in the heart. A unique feature of cardiac muscle is automaticity, or the ability to generate electrical impulses.

Nervous System

The nervous system consists of the brain, spinal cord, and nerves (Figure 4-12). The nervous system is necessary to transmit messages from the brain to all parts of the body. Without it, we could not move, react to pain, or communicate. The **central nervous system** consists of the brain and spinal cord. The **peripheral nervous system** consists of the nerves, which travel from the spine to all parts of the body.

The nervous system also assures we respond to stresses. You have undoubtedly heard of the "fight or flight" responses of the **sympathetic nervous system,** which allows us to respond to stressful situations. The opposite of the sympathetic nervous system is the **parasympathetic nervous system,** which slows the body and controls vegetative functions such as digestion and reproduction.

Endocrine System

The endocrine system produces chemicals called **hormones,** which help to regulate body activities and functions. The most notable hormone is insulin. This hormone, created in the pancreas, is critical to allowing glucose in the blood to be used in the body's cells.

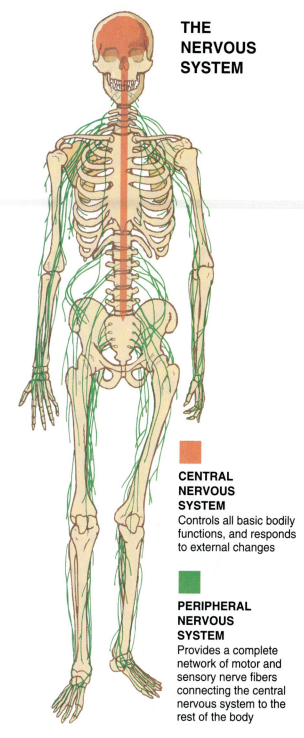

THE NERVOUS SYSTEM

CENTRAL NERVOUS SYSTEM
Controls all basic bodily functions, and responds to external changes

PERIPHERAL NERVOUS SYSTEM
Provides a complete network of motor and sensory nerve fibers connecting the central nervous system to the rest of the body

Figure 4-12   The nervous system.

SUMMARY

- Anatomical terms such as superior, inferior, proximal, and distal are used frequently.
- The respiratory system includes the upper and lower airways.
- The cardiovascular system includes the arteries, veins, capillaries, atria, ventricles, and cardiac conduction system.
- The musculoskeletal system includes voluntary, involuntary and cardiac muscle, bones, ligaments, and tendons.
- The nervous system includes the central (brain and spinal cord) and peripheral portions.
- The endocrine system functions through hormones, particularly insulin.

REVIEW QUESTIONS

1. The functions of the body are called its:
   a. kinesiology.
   b. physiology.
   c. pathology.
   d. anatomy.

2. The term "anterior" refers to:
   a. both sides of anything.
   b. the front side of the body.
   c. one side of a two-sided object.
   d. a position closer to the midline.

3. Blood vessels that carry blood away from the heart are called:
   a. veins.
   b. systolic.
   c. arteries.
   d. platelets.

4. The divisions of the spine in order from top to bottom are:
   a. thoracic, lumbar, sacrum, coccyx, cervical.
   b. cervical, thoracic, lumbar, sacrum, coccyx.
   c. cervical, lumbar, sacrum, thoracic, coccyx.
   d. coccyx, sacrum, thoracic, cervical, lumbar.

REVIEW QUESTIONS *continued*

5. The components of the ______ system are the brain, spinal cord, and nerves.

a. nervous
b. endocrine
c. respiratory
d. circulatory

6. The endocrine system produces chemicals called:.

a. antibodies.
b. antigens.
c. hormones.
d. toxins.

WEB MEDIC

Visit Brady's *Essentials of Emergency Care* web site for direct web links. At **www.prenhall.com/limmer,** you will find information related to the following Chapter 4 topics:

- the cardiovascular system
- the respiratory system
- the musculoskeletal system
- the nervous system
- the endocrine system

Chapter Five

LIFTING AND MOVING PATIENTS

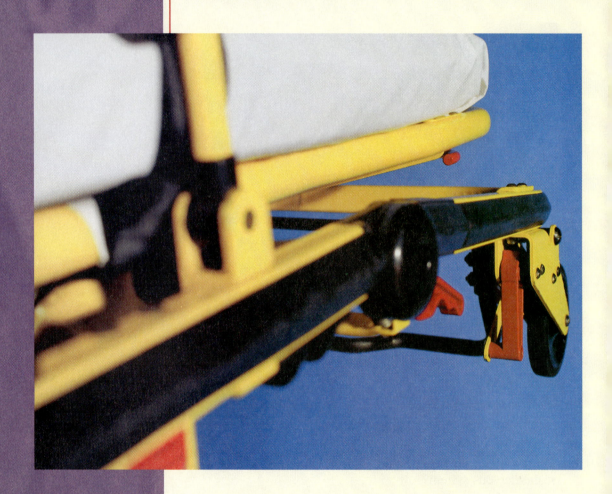

Lifting and moving patients is an important part of emergency care. The methods chosen to transport a patient depend on a number of factors including location, terrain, and patient condition. A wide variety of patient-carrying devices are available, each with a specific purpose. This chapter reviews the options available in lifting and moving patients. It also describes methods of safe lifting, as well as classifying emergency, urgent, and non-urgent moves.

BODY MECHANICS

The term "body mechanics" refers to how to best use the body during the process of lifting and moving. In EMS personnel, improper lifting is a significant cause of musculoskeletal injuries, some of which result in permanent disability and shattered careers.

Even if you have been successfully lifting and moving patients for many years, it never hurts to review the proper procedures. The actual process of lifting and moving can be broken down into two steps. The first step is decision making and planning. The second is lifting and moving.

Decision Making and Planning

Decision making and planning are essential for any successful move of a patient. They set crucial groundwork that makes the actual move more efficient. Consider these points:

- **What are the needs of the patient?** The condition of the patient will be an important part of transportation planning. Many patients with respiratory complaints are clearly more comfortable sitting up. That same position is improper for patients with spinal injuries.
- **What is the terrain like?** Elevators, stairs, narrow hallways, and other difficult places will affect transportation decisions. When possible, use wheeled devices such as the ambulance stretcher or stair chair to reduce the amount of carrying.
- **What is the weight of the patient?** What are the physical abilities and limitations of your crew and equipment? Can you handle the weight? These questions must be answered as part of the decision-making process.
- **What communication is necessary?** When planning or physically preparing to lift a patient, communication is essential. The communication process should include readiness, problems encountered during the move, and planning for

the next phase. This becomes especially important when coordinating a move and administering treatments such as CPR.

Lifting and Moving

Follow these guidelines to lift or move a patient:

- Position your feet properly.
- Use your legs, not your back, when lifting.
- Keep the weight you are lifting as close to your body as possible.
- Never twist your body while lifting. Attempting to turn or twist during a lift is a major cause of injury.
- For a one-handed carrying technique, pick up and carry the object with your back in the locked-in position. Avoid leaning to either side to compensate for the imbalance.
- When the weight requires more than one person, make sure an even number of people perform the lift. Uneven numbers may cause the lifting device to go off balance and result in injury to the EMT-Bs and patient. Partners also should have similar strength and height.

Whenever you have to lift a weight, use the squat lift or **power lift** (Figure 5-1a). (The squat lift is also called the "power lift" because it is used by

DOT OBJECTIVES

✔ **Knowledge**

☐ **1.** Use body mechanics when lifting and moving a patient. (pp. 59–61)

- Relate body mechanics associated with patient care to its impact on the EMT-Basic. (pp. 59–61)

✔ **Attitude**

☐ **2.** Explain the rationale for properly lifting and moving patients. (pp. 59–61)

✔ **Skills**

☐ **3.** Working with a partner, move a simulated patient from the ground to a stretcher and properly position the patient on the stretcher. (pp. 66–67)

☐ **4.** Working with a partner, demonstrate the technique for moving a patient secured to a stretcher to the ambulance and loading the patient into the ambulance. (p. 71)

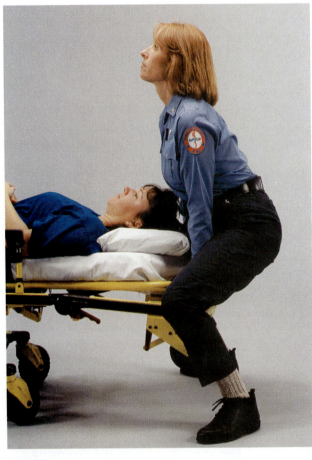

Figure 5-1a   The power lift, or squat lift.

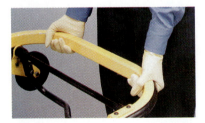

Figure 5-1b   The power grip.

weightlifters.) Squatting, instead of bending at the waist, allows the muscles of the legs rather than the back to do the work. It also is useful for individuals with weak knees or thighs. To perform a power lift, straddle the object. Then place your feet a comfortable distance apart. Let your abdominal muscles lock your back in a slight inward curve. Keep your feet flat, and distribute weight to the balls of your feet or just behind. Stand, lifting your upper body before your hips.

The **power grip** also is important to get the most force from your hands. To perform a power grip, position your hands about 10 inches apart. Your palms and fingers should be in complete contact with the object, and all fingers should be bent at the same angle (Figure 5-1b).

Reaching, Pushing, and Pulling

Simple lifting is not the only strenuous task performed by an EMT-B. Reaching, pushing, and pulling can cause injury as easily as lifting. These movements put the body at an unusual angle, which may cause injury. Follow these guidelines when you must reach at an emergency scene:

- Keep your back in a locked-in position.
- Use caution when reaching overhead. Avoid hyperextended positions.
- Avoid twisting while reaching.
- Avoid reaching more than 15 to 20 inches in front of the body.
- Avoid situations where prolonged reaching combined with lifting or other strenuous effort is required.

Reaching is commonly required when assisting in log rolling a patient onto a backboard. When performing a log roll, remember to keep the back straight, lean from the hips, and use your shoulder muscles to help with the roll (Figure 5-2). Follow the guidelines below whenever you must push or pull:

- Push, rather than pull, whenever possible.
- Keep your back locked in. Then push from the area between the waist and shoulder.
- If the weight is below the level of your waist, use a kneeling position.
- Keep your elbows bent with your arms close to your sides.
- Avoid pushing or pulling from an overhead position when possible.

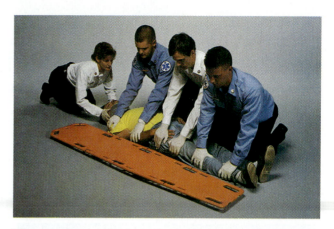

Figure 5-2 When performing a log roll, keep your back straight, lean from the hips, and use your shoulder muscles.

TYPES OF MOVES

There are three types of moves you will make as an EMT-B: emergency moves, urgent moves, and non-urgent moves.

Emergency Moves

Emergency moves are those which must be made immediately but only when definite life threats exist, such as:

- Fire, explosives, or other hazardous materials threaten the lives of the patient and the EMT-B.
- A patient who requires immediate care cannot be accessed because another patient is in the way.
- The patient requires positioning in order to immediately administer life-saving care (for example, turning a cardiac-arrest patient from a prone to a supine position).

The obvious problem with emergency moves is that they provide minimal protection for patients with spinal injuries. (See emergency moves illustrated in Skill Summaries 5-1 through 5-3.) However, since these moves are used in life-threatening situations only, you may have no other choice but to use them. In order to minimize aggravation of a spine injury, move the patient along the long axis of the body.

Urgent Moves

Urgent moves are used when the patient must be moved quickly but with precautions for spinal injury. An example would be a trauma patient who needs treatment for inadequate breathing. Rapid extrication is another example of an urgent move. It takes into account the need for spinal precautions but is quicker than standard extrication procedures. A collision patient who is breathing but who is in critical condition is a candidate for this type of move. The delay caused by taking the time to fully immobilize the patient could actually cause harm. (Rapid extrication is reviewed in more detail in Chapter 24.)

Non-Urgent Moves

Non-urgent moves are performed when no harm will come to the patient due to the delay or to the external environment. The patient will generally receive complete emergency medical care prior to being moved in a non-urgent manner.

A patient with neck pain who does not have a serious mechanism of injury and is in no danger of further injury from an unstable vehicle, fire, or so on would receive a full assessment, short-board immobilization, and transfer to a long spine board. Non-urgent moves are shown in Skill Summary 5-4.

PATIENT-CARRYING DEVICES

Many experienced EMT-Bs will be familiar with most patient-carrying devices (Figures 5-3 through 5-8). Your choice of a patient-carrying device will depend on terrain. Stairs, elevators, hills, and other situations each may require a different device. Patient condition also affects your choice. For example, patients with cardiac and respiratory complaints often feel more comfortable sitting up. If they are stable enough, a stair chair is usually *(continued on page 68)*

Caution: Always pull in the direction of the long axis of the patient's body. Do not pull the patient sideways. Avoid bending or twisting the trunk.

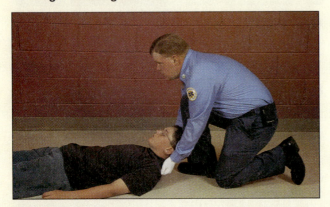

The Clothes Drag

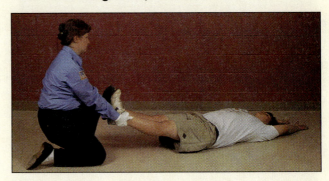

The Incline Drag Always head first.

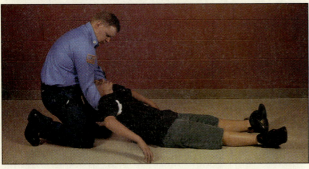

The Shoulder Drag Be careful not to bump the patient's head.

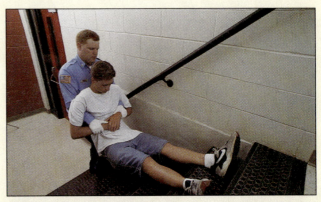

The Foot Drag Be careful not to bump the patient's head.

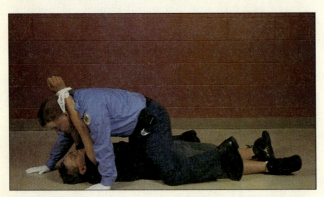

The Firefighter Drag Place the patient on his back and tie his hands together. Straddle the patient, facing his head. Crouch and pass your head through his trussed arms and raise your body. Crawl on your hands and knees. Keep the patient's head as low as possible.

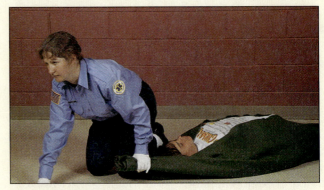

The Blanket Drag Gather half of the blanket material up against the patient's side. Roll the patient toward your knees so that you can place the blanket under him. Gently roll the patient back onto the blanket. During the drag, keep the patient's head as low as possible.

Emergency Moves— One-Rescuer Carries

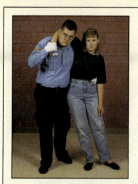

The One-Rescuer Assist   Place patient's arm around your neck, grasping her hand in yours. Place your other arm around patient's waist. Help her walk to safety. Be prepared to change your technique if level of danger increases. Be sure to communicate with patient about obstacles, uneven terrain, and so on.

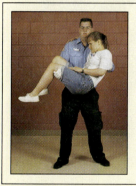

The Cradle Carry   Place one arm across patient's back with your hand under her arm. Place your other arm under her knees and lift. If patient is conscious, have her place her near arm over your shoulder. Note: This carry places a lot of weight on the carrier's back. It is usually appropriate only for very light patients.

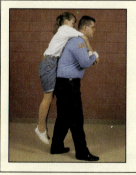

The Pack Strap Carry   Have patient stand. Turn your back on her, bringing her arms over your shoulders to cross your chest. Keep her arms as straight as possible, and her armpits over your shoulders. Hold patient's wrists, bend, and pull her onto your back.

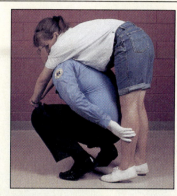

The Piggy Back Carry   Assist the patient to stand. Place her arms over your shoulders so they cross your chest. Bend over and lift patient. While she holds on with her arms, crouch and grasp each leg. Use a lifting motion to move her onto your back. Pass your forearms under her knees and grasp her wrists.

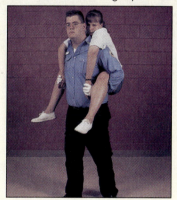

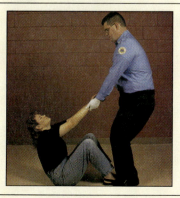

The Firefighter's Carry   Place your feet against her feet and pull patient toward you. Bend at waist and flex knees. Duck and pull her across your shoulder, keeping hold of one of her wrists. Use your free arm to reach between her legs and grasp her thigh. When weight of patient falls onto your shoulders, stand up. Transfer your grip on thigh to patient's wrist.

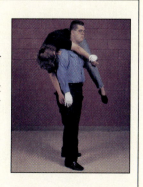

Emergency Moves— Two-Rescuers

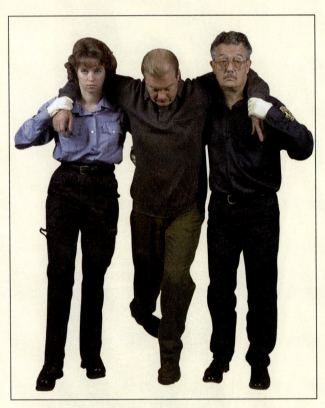

Two-Rescuer Assist Patient's arms are placed around shoulders of both rescuers. They each grip a hand, place their free arms around patient's waist, then help him walk to safety.

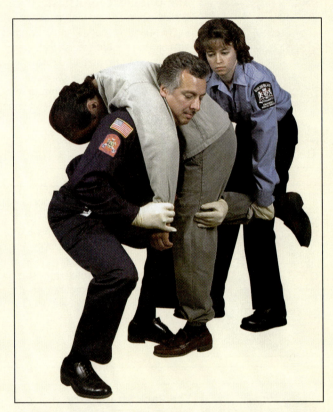

Firefighter's Carry with Assist Have a second rescuer help to lift and position the patient.

Non-urgent Moves, No Suspected Spine Injury

Extremity Carry

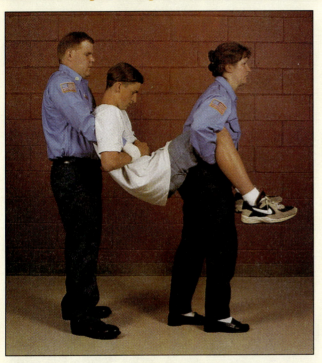

The extremity carry may be an emergency move or a non-urgent move for a patient with no suspected spine injury. To perform it, place patient on his back with knees flexed. Kneel at his head, and place your hands under his shoulders. Helper kneels at patient's feet and grasps patient's wrists. Helper lifts patient forward while you slip your arms under patient's armpits and grasp his wrists. Helper can grasp patient's knees while facing patient or turn and grasp patient's knees while facing away from patient. Direct helper so you both move to a crouch. Stand at the same time, and move as a unit when carrying the patient.

If patient is found sitting, crouch and slip your arms under patient's armpits and grasp his wrists. Helper crouches, and then grasps patient's knees. Lift patient as a unit.

Draw Sheet Method

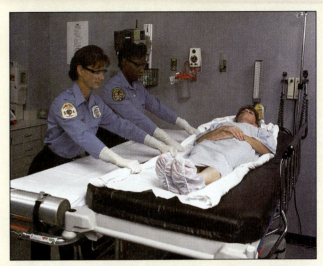

▲ **1.** Loosen bottom sheet of bed and roll it from both sides toward patient. Rails lowered, the stretcher is placed parallel to and touching side of bed. Use your bodies and feet to lock the stretcher against the bed.

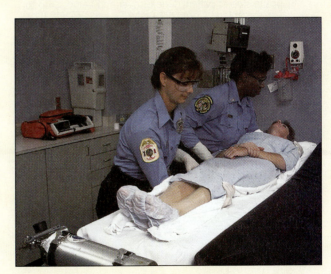

▲ **2.** Pull on draw sheet to move patient to side of bed. You and helper each use one hand to support patient while you both reach under him to grasp draw sheet. Then both you and helper simultaneously draw patient onto stretcher.

(continued)

Direct Ground Lift

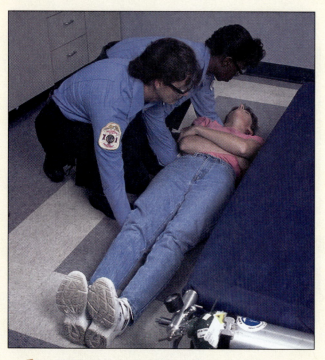

▲ **1.** Stretcher is set in its lowest position and placed on opposite side of patient. One rescuer and helper drop to one knee, facing patient. Patient's arms are placed on chest if possible. Rescuer at the head cradles patient's head and neck by sliding one arm under the neck to grasp shoulder, and the other arm under the lower back. The foot-end rescuer slides one arm under the patient's knees and the other under the patient above the buttocks.

    Note: If a third rescuer is available, he or she should place both arms under patient's waist while the other two slide their arms up to the mid back or down to the buttocks as appropriate.

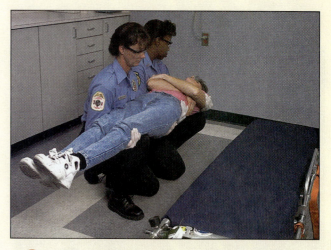

▲ **2.** On a signal, both rescuers lift the patient to their knees.

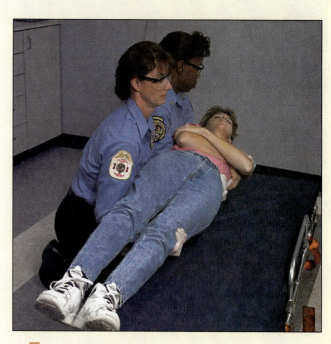

▲ **3.** On a signal, both rescuers stand and carry patient to stretcher, drop to one knee, and roll forward to place patient onto mattress.

Direct Carry

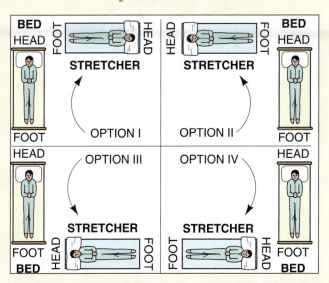

Stretcher is placed at 90° angle to bed, depending on room configuration. Rescuers prepare stretcher by lowering rails, unbuckling straps, and removing other items. They then stand between stretcher and bed, facing patient.

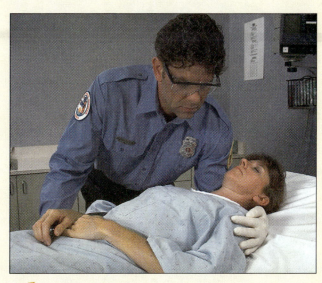

▲ **1.** The head-end rescuer cradles patient's head and neck by sliding one arm under her neck to grasp shoulder.

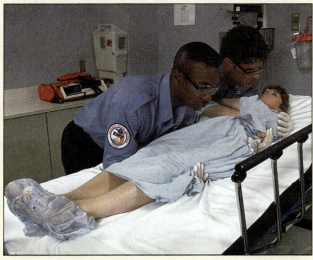

▲ **2.** The foot-end rescuer slides hands under patient's hip and lifts slightly. The head-end rescuer slides arms under her back. Foot-end rescuer then places arms under patient's hips and calves.

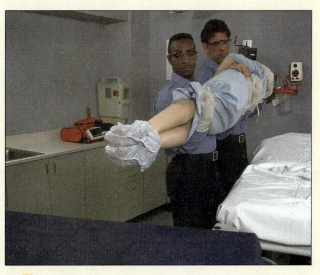

▲ **3.** Both rescuers slide patient to edge of bed and bend toward her with their knees slightly bent. They lift and curl patient to their chests and return to a standing position. They rotate, then slide patient gently onto stretcher.

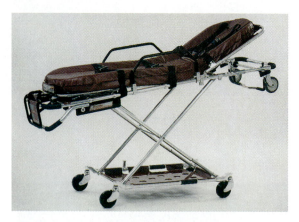

Figure 5-3　Wheeled ambulance stretcher.

appropriate. A spine-injured patient, however, must be immobilized and supine for transport.

Use these general guidelines for selecting a patient-carrying device:

- Use the wheeled ambulance stretcher when there is an unrestricted pathway to the ambulance or a large elevator to an upper story.
- Use the portable ambulance stretcher, flexible stretcher, stair chair, Reeves stretcher, scoop stretcher, or long spine board when a patient must be removed from a confined space or carried through a narrow opening or narrow hallway.
- Use a stair chair when it is impossible to carry a patient down stairs on a stretcher and when an elevator is too small for a stretcher.
- Use a basket (Stokes) stretcher to move a patient from one elevation to another by rope or ladder or when the patient must be carried over debris, rough terrain, or uphill. Some Stokes stretchers can be fitted with a detachable wheel to facilitate movement over rough terrain.

When a person has a possible spine injury, the patient-carrying device must provide straight-line neck and back immobilization. Selection of the device will be influenced by the location of the person and how the person must be moved, as described below:

- Use a long spine board when a spine-injured patient is on the ground or on the floor of a structure. Once immobilized on the board, the patient may be carried directly to the ambulance or secured to the cot and wheeled there.
- Use a long spine board to immobilize a patient who has already been immobilized with a short spine board or flexible, vest-type extrication device. Once a seated patient has been immobilized on a short spine board or vest, he or she can be pivoted onto a long spine board.
- Use a long spine board to immobilize the patient. Secure the board and patient in a basket (Stokes)

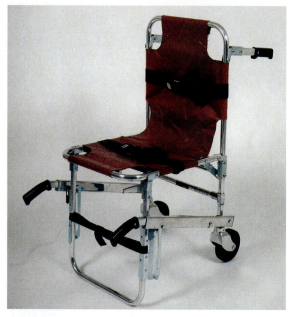

Figure 5-4　Stair chair.

stretcher when the patient must be moved from one level to another and there are no stairs or elevators. Then, if you have been appropriately trained, use a rope to lower the stretcher or to slide it down the beams of a ladder.

LIFESPAN DEVELOPMENT

Always be careful how you package a patient whose extremities may be paralyzed, as in the case of a patient who may have sustained a spinal injury or a stroke. Make sure the patient's weight is not crushing the paralyzed extremity and that the extremity is properly secured in the blankets and bedding. This will prevent the paralyzed extremity from suddenly flopping off the side of the stretcher as you travel through a doorway, which could easily cause additional injury to the patient.

Normally a patient with a spinal injury will be immobilized on a long backboard, so just make sure the patient's extremities are strapped in. The patient who has experienced a stroke is usually transferred on a wheeled ambulance stretcher, so be careful to strap in all of his or her extremities. It is also a good idea, if you are strapping an oxygen cylinder in by the patient's legs, to place the cylinder next to the leg that is not paralyzed. This way, should the patient have any discomfort from the cylinder squeezing up against the leg, he or she can feel the pain and, if able to speak, let you know.

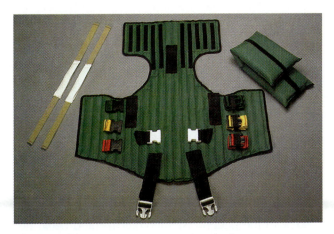

Figure 5-5 Vest-type extraction device.

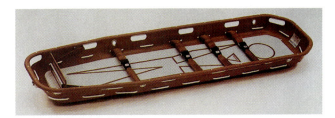

Figure 5-6 Plastic Stokes basket stretcher.

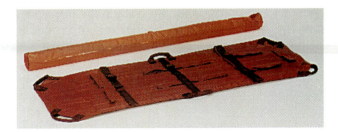

Figure 5-7 Reeves flexible stretcher.

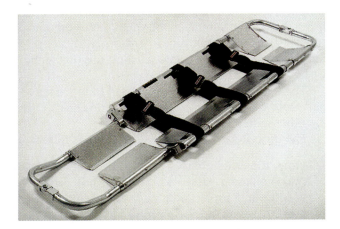

Figure 5-8 Scoop (orthopedic) stretcher.

Ambulance Stretcher

The ambulance stretcher is the most commonly used patient-carrying device. However, if used improperly, it can be a source of injury to the EMT-B as well as a potential liability risk. In general, the principles of transfer for this device also apply to all other patient-carrying devices.

The patient on an ambulance stretcher should be covered by a top sheet and blankets, as required by weather. The side rails should be locked in the up position and the body straps fastened. Whenever you move a conscious patient, explain what you are doing and what obstacles you are maneuvering around, which will help to comfort him or her.

The transfer of a bed-level or ground-level patient may require special lifting techniques such as the draw-sheet or direct-carry method. Regardless of the method used, protect yourself from back injury and hernia. Do not position yourself too far from the patient and do not strain to lift the patient. Keep your balance to avoid possible injury to yourself, your partner, and the patient.

Regardless of the method used to move a patient, you and your partner should walk naturally at a smooth, fairly slow pace. Use two hands on the bed of the stretcher—rather than just pulling on the handles—to roll and maneuver the stretcher at a safe, constant speed. Turn corners slowly and squarely to keep the stretcher level and to minimize discomfort to the patient. Lift the stretcher over thresholds and rugs. Use caution when maneuvering the stretcher to avoid bumping into and damaging walls and furniture.

The stretcher may be carried by the end-carry method or by the side-carry method. The end-carry is most widely used when moving the stretcher to the ambulance. The side-carry is usually used to load the patient into the ambulance (Skill Summary 5-5).

Often a stretcher is wheeled in the raised position by two EMT-Bs, one at the head end and one at the foot. The stretcher is guided by the EMT-B at the head. Never leave a patient unattended on a wheeled stretcher in the raised position for even a few seconds. The patient may shift position and the stretcher can easily topple over. Some services have policies that restrict moving the stretcher in the raised position. Other services simply require four hands on a raised stretcher at all times.

Many services now have stretchers with which the patient is loaded into the ambulance with minimal lifting. The wheels and suspension fold underneath the stretcher as it is wheeled into the ambulance. However, this must be done very carefully. The stretchers must be used and maintained properly or they can malfunction, causing serious injury to the patient and EMT-B.

After loading the stretcher, make sure that the cot and the patient are secure before moving. When you arrive at the hospital, you will move the patient from the ambulance stretcher to the hospital stretcher. See Skill Summary 5-6 for procedures.

Folding Stair Chair

The folding stair chair is useful in narrow corridors, doorways, small elevators, and stairways. Since the device has wheels, it can be rolled on landings and other surfaces, thereby reducing strain on the EMT-Bs. A stair chair is not recommended for use with an unconscious or disoriented patient or with a patient who has a possible spine injury or possible fracture of the lower extremities.

Unfold and secure the stair chair in the open position by the positive locking devices (not on all chairs). Unfasten and position the safety straps so they do not become tripping hazards. Do not use a patient's wheelchair when carrying the patient because it may collapse in your hands.

The direct-carry method may be modified when a bed-level or ground-level patient must be moved into a stair chair. The first part of the technique is the same as for transfer of a patient to a wheeled stretcher. However, the foot-end EMT slides his arm under the patient's thighs rather than under the mid-calf. This maneuver allows the lower part of the patient's legs to drop down into a sitting position as he or she is eased into the chair.

The extremity transfer can be used to move a patient from the floor or ground to a stair chair or to any other patient-carrying device.

The procedure for using a stair chair is as follows:

1. Drape the stair chair with a sheet or blanket, which will be used to protect the patient's modesty and protect him from the elements. Be sure the sheet or blanket does not dangle and trip the EMTs on stairs.
2. Assume a head-end position. Have your partner take the foot-end position.
3. Your partner then assists the patient to a sitting position.
4. You should reach under the patient's armpits and grasp the patient's wrists, holding the arms to his chest.
5. Your partner flexes the patient's knees, and slides his hands into position under the knees.
6. Simultaneously, on your command, both you and your partner move to a standing position, lifting the patient.
7. Carry the patient to the chair, and lower him onto it.
8. Drape the patient with a sheet, and place a blanket over his body and shoulders.
9. Secure the patient to the chair with two straps. Fasten one around the chest and the back of the chair. Place the second strap across the thighs and around the seat of the chair.

A loaded stair chair is fairly easy to carry and maneuver, especially if the chair is on wheels. As with the ambulance stretcher, stair chairs should be rolled whenever possible. Rolling reduces your risk of back strain and injury to the patient. However, the following procedure is suggested when a stair chair must be carried over level ground:

1. When the stair chair and patient are to be moved, get behind the chair to tilt the chair back. Always warn the patient that you are going to tilt the chair.
2. If the chair has wheels, tilt it carefully. Your partner should stand at the patient's feet with his back to the patient. As the chair is tilted back, he should crouch and grasp the chair by its legs.
3. Both you and your partner should lift the chair simultaneously, and carry the patient to the wheeled stretcher. Be sure the patient's feet are on the bar, not below it, so you don't set the chair on the patient's feet when you rest it on the ground.
4. Transfer the patient to the wheeled stretcher as soon as possible and before he is loaded onto the ambulance.

If a patient must be carried down stairs on a stair chair, the EMT-B at the foot-end should face the patient. A third person should spot the foot-end EMT-B while moving down steps. If the chair has wheels, do not allow them to touch the steps.

> ### PRECEPTOR PEARL
>
> New EMT-Bs may feel awkward when walking down stairs, especially if they are facing backwards. Tell them: if you begin to lose your balance while carrying a patient down stairs, sit down if you are at the head end. If you are at the foot end, lean into the stairs to regain your balance.

Scoop-Style (Orthopedic) Stretchers

A scoop-style stretcher is given its name because it splits in two. When the two pieces are brought together again, they cause a scooping action to occur. A Scoop comes in either steel or hard plastic. Note that a scoop-style stretcher should not be used to transport a patient with a possible spine injury.

Always adjust the length of a scoop-style stretcher to the patient's height. Separate the stretcher halves, and place one half on each side of the patient. If the stretcher is the folding type, make sure the pins are properly set.

Loading the Wheeled Stretcher into the Ambulance

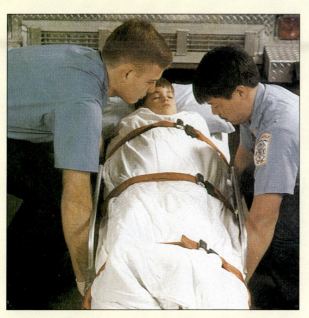

▲ **1.** Clear interior of ambulance and lift rear step if necessary. Move stretcher as close to ambulance as possible. Lock stretcher in its lowest level before lifting. Rescuers get in position on opposite sides of stretcher, bend at knees, and grasp lower bar of stretcher frame.

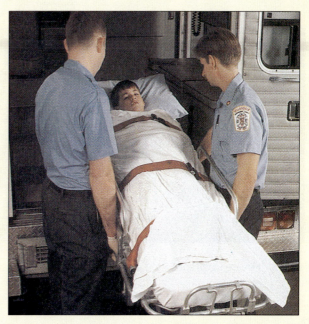

▲ **2.** Both rescuers come to a full standing position with their backs straight. Small sideways steps are used to move stretcher onto ambulance.

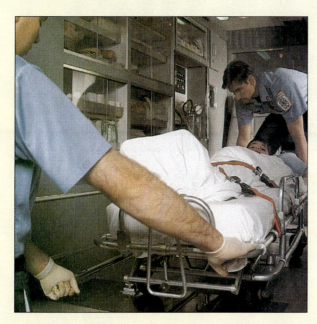

▲ **3.** Stretcher is moved into securing device.

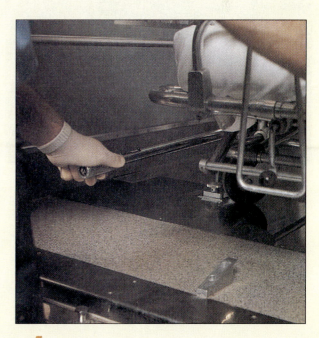

▲ **4.** Both forward and rear catches are engaged.

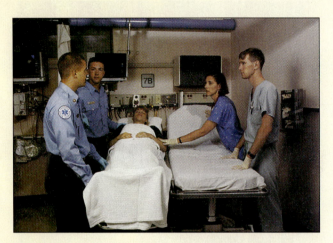

▲ **1.** Rescuers position raised ambulance cot next to hospital stretcher. Hospital personnel adjust stretcher (raise or lower head) to receive patient from ambulance cot.

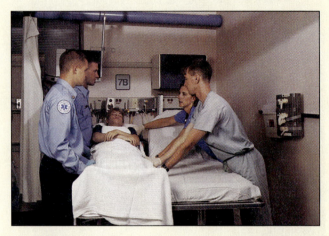

▲ **2.** Rescuers and hospital personnel gather sheet on either side of patient and pull taut in order to transfer patient securely.

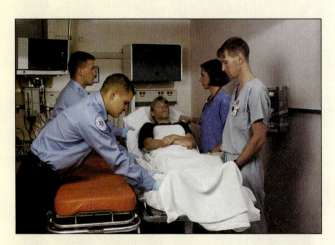

▲ **3.** Holding gathered sheet at support points near shoulders, mid-torso, hips, and knees, rescuers and hospital personnel slide patient in one motion to hospital stretcher.

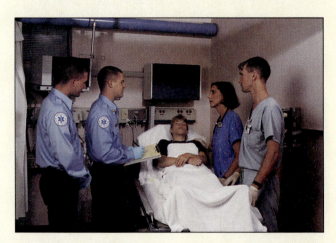

▲ **4.** Assure patient is centered on stretcher. Make sure stretcher rails are raised before turning patient over to emergency department staff.

Slide the stretcher halves under the patient one at a time. This may be difficult since the stretcher may snag on clothing, grass, or debris. If necessary, roll the patient as a unit to either side to allow for proper positioning of the stretcher's parts. Mate the latch parts and ensure stretcher halves are locked together. Latching should be done from head to feet. Be careful not to pinch the patient when latching the two halves together. Adjust the head support and secure the patient.

Then lift the scoop by the end-carry method. Move the patient to a long spine board as soon as possible. Secure the patient and long spine board as a unit to the wheeled ambulance stretcher by using three straps.

Special Transfer Devices

Additional stretchers used in the field today include:

- **Basket-style (Stokes) stretcher.** Use the basket-style stretcher to move patients from one level to another or over rough terrain. Do not move a patient in a basket stretcher by rope or ladder unless you have been specifically trained in the techniques used for such moves.
- **Reeves sleeve.** This sleeve has an envelope configuration into which a regular long spine board can be inserted. Tabs with quick-hitch straps encapsulate the patient, providing security in almost any carrying position.
- **SKED®.** The SKED® stretcher comes rolled in a package. When opened, it can be quickly assembled and used to rescue someone from a confined space, height, or snow or water emergency.
- **Air mattress.** Some services use an air mattress to transport the patient with multiple fractures or a spine injury. The mattress is placed under the patient and air is evacuated using a pump. A bead-like material hardens, forming a rigid stretcher that conforms to the patient's body position.

Always follow manufacturer's recommendations for inspection, cleaning, repair, and upkeep on all patient-carrying devices.

The selection and use of patient-carrying devices are important factors in the safety and condition of your patient. If transportation is not performed properly and taken seriously, you may harm your patient and incur liability for improper actions.

Packaging the Patient

The term "packaging" refers to combining the patient and the patient-carrying device into a unit ready for transfer. A patient must be packaged so that his or her condition is not aggravated. Before a low-priority patient is placed on the patient-carrying device, complete necessary care for injuries, stabilize impaled objects, and check all dressings and splints.

PRECEPTOR PEARL

Do not waste time with extensive packaging of a badly traumatized patient. New EMT-Bs may not realize that critical or unstable patients should not receive the same detailed packaging that a stable patient would receive. Critical patients obviously must have safe packaging, but priorities are resuscitative measures, immobilization, and prompt transport to an appropriate facility. To convey the message, you might explain: "A neatly packaged corpse has not received optimal care!"

Cover and secure the properly packaged patient to the patient-carrying device. Covering a patient helps to maintain body temperature, prevents exposure to the elements, and helps assure privacy. A single blanket or sheet may be all that is required in warm weather. A sheet and blankets should be used in cold weather. When practical, cuff the blankets under the patient's chin with the top sheet outside. Do not leave sheets and blankets hanging loose. Tuck them under the mattress at the foot and sides of the stretcher. In wet weather, a plastic cover should be placed over the blankets during transfer. Once the stretcher is in the ambulance, the cover may be removed to prevent the patient from overheating.

If a scoop-style stretcher or long spine board is used, fold a blanket once or twice lengthwise and carefully tuck the blanket under the patient. Cover the patient as best you can, place the patient and scoop-style stretcher on a wheeled ambulance stretcher, and then apply full covering. When using a basket (Stokes) stretcher, line the basket with a blanket prior to positioning the patient. If you are unable to do so, cover the patient as you would when using a scoop-style stretcher.

Before seating a patient in a stair chair, place a sheet or blanket on the chair. This will facilitate transfer of the nonambulatory patient later. Once seated on the chair, the patient should be covered. Have the patient sit upright with legs together and with hands folded over the lap. Drape a sheet and then a blanket over the patient's body and shoulders. Carefully tuck in the sheet and blanket all around. In cold or wet weather, cover the patient's head, leaving the face exposed.

Today's devices for the transfer and transport of patients should have a minimum of three straps to secure a patient to the device. The first strap is at the chest level. The second is at the hip or waist level. The third is on the lower extremities. Secure all patients—including those receiving CPR—to the patient-carrying device before transfer to the ambulance.

SUMMARY

- Moving patients is an important part of emergency care that is done on almost every call.
- Whenever lifting, reaching, pulling or pushing, you should practice proper body mechanics in order to avoid injury.
- Emergency moves are used when a patient must be moved immediately.
- Urgent moves are used when a patient must be moved quickly but with precautions for the spine.
- Non-urgent moves are used when no harm will come to the patient due to the delay or to the external environment.
- The EMT-B has at his or her disposal various patient-carrying devices, and should be familiar with the operation of each, such as the wheeled ambulance stretcher, scoop, flexible stretcher, specialty stretchers, and the stair chair.

REVIEW QUESTIONS

1. Which of the following is NOT one of the basic guidelines an EMT-B should follow for safely lifting and moving a patient?:
   a. Position your feet properly.
   b. Use your back, not your legs, when lifting.
   c. Keep the weight as close to the body as possible.
   d. Do not twist your body when lifting.

2. To perform the power grip, the EMT-B should position his or hands about _____ inches apart.
   a. 5
   b. 10
   c. 12
   d. 18

3. It is best to use a kneeling position if you must push or pull a weight that is below the level of your:
   a. chin.
   b. shoulders.
   c. chest.
   d. waist.

4. When the patient must be moved quickly, but with precautions for spinal injury, the EMT-B should use a(n):
   a. emergency move
   b. rapid move
   c. urgent move
   d. firefighter's move

5. Which patient-carrying device would be used if the EMT-B must move a patient from one elevation to another by rope?
   a. stair chair
   b. flexible stretcher
   c. scoop stretcher
   d. Stokes stretcher

WEB MEDIC

Visit Brady's *Essentials of Emergency Care* web site for direct web links. At **www.prenhall.com/limmer,** you will find information related to the following Chapter 5 topics:
- Back injuries in EMS
- Body mechanics
- Patient-carrying devices

CHAPTER Six

AIRWAY MANAGEMENT

*Correlates with the U.S. DOT
"EMT-Basic National Standard Curriculum"
Lesson 2-1*

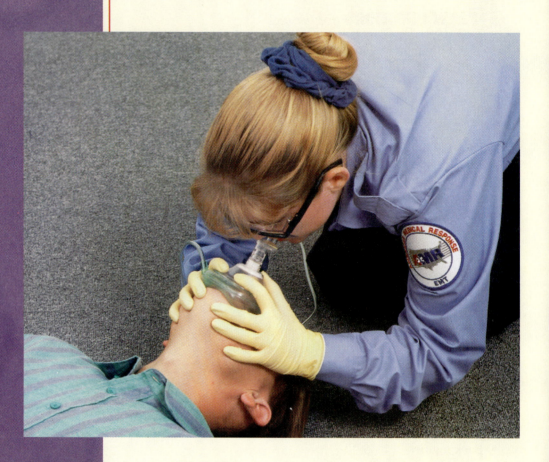

ESSENTIAL ELECTRONIC EXTRAS

CD ESSENTIALS

For preview and review of chapter material, see the student CD-ROM for

- Pretest
- Chapter quizzes
- Posttest

WEB ESSENTIALS

For additional review and enrichment, visit www.prenhall.com/limmer for

- Interactive student quizzes
- Links to online EMS resources
- Online case studies
- Audio glossary

Airway maintenance and ventilation take priority over almost anything else you will do for a patient. It is critical to maintain proficiency in airway skills. If skills are not used on a regular basis, they must be practiced. Improperly performed procedures can harm your patient. Simply stated, if the patient does not have a patent airway and adequate respirations he or she will surely die.

AIRWAY ANATOMY AND PHYSIOLOGY REVIEW

Another word for breathing is **respiration.** The body system that allows breathing to occur is the respiratory system. As an experienced EMT-B, you should be able to label the following major structures on a diagram (Figure 6-1):

- **Nose.** Allows air to enter, warms inhaled air, and filters out impurities with the help of nose hairs and mucus.
- **Mouth.** One of the openings to the airway and respiratory system that allows the taking in of air.
- **Oropharynx.** The inside of the mouth posterior to the tongue and leading to the throat.
- **Nasopharynx.** The area between the nasal passages and the oropharynx.
- **Epiglottis.** A flap of tissue that covers the glottic opening of the trachea when swallowing or gagging takes place.
- **Larynx.** The voice box, which holds the vocal cords and the glottic opening to the trachea.
- **Trachea.** The windpipe, which is a tube in the front of the throat that carries air from the oropharynx to the bronchii.
- **Cricoid cartilage.** A ring of cartilage that completely surrounds the trachea at the lower edge of the larynx.
- **Bronchi.** The right and left mainstem tubes leading into the lungs.
- **Lungs.** The organs where oxygen is exchanged for carbon dioxide.
- **Alveoli.** Grape-like sacs within the lungs that are surrounded by capillaries whose red blood cells pick up inhaled oxygen and drop off carbon dioxide.
- **Diaphragm.** A large primary muscle of breathing that separates the thorax from the abdomen.

The respiratory system enables the body to inhale oxygen and exhale carbon dioxide. Oxygen is used by all the body's cells and organs. Carbon dioxide is the major waste product of respiration. If anything obstructs or disrupts the breathing process, the patient is likely to develop the sensation of **dyspnea** (shortness of breath) and be at risk for respiratory failure.

When the diaphragm contracts, it moves downward as the intercostal muscles pull the ribs up and out to create a larger cavity into which air can rush. This is called **inhalation.** The lungs are wrapped in two membranes: the *visceral pleura,* which is found directly around the lung tissue, and the *parietal pleura,* which is found directly around the inside of the chest wall. These membranes have a small amount of fluid between them that causes them to stick together, much like a drop of water between two glass slides under a microscope. Due to this "surface tension," when the intercostal muscles move the rib cage, the lungs also enlarge in size.

CORE CONCEPTS

In this chapter, you will learn about the following topics:

- Identifying and using body substance isolation procedures for airway techniques
- Providing artificial ventilation and assisted ventilations
- Using airway adjunct devices
- Identifying the need for and providing suctioning to patients
- Identifying the need for and administering oxygen to patients

✔ **Knowledge**

☐ **1.** Perform techniques to assure a patent airway. (pp. 80–82, 84–91, 93–98)

- Describe the steps in performing the head-tilt chin-lift. (pp. 80–81)
- Describe the steps in performing the jaw thrust. (pp. 81–82)
- Describe the techniques of suctioning. (pp. 82, 84–85)

- Describe how to measure and insert an oropharyngeal (oral) airway. (pp. 90–91)
- Describe how to measure and insert a nasopharyngeal (nasal) airway. (pp. 91, 93)

☐ **2.** Provide ventilatory support for a patient. (pp. 85–90)

- Describe the steps in performing the skill of artificially ventilating a patient with a bag-valve-mask for one and two rescuers. (pp. 87–89, 90)

- Describe the steps in artificially ventilating a patient with a flow-restricted, oxygen-powered ventilation device. (pp. 85, 89–90)

☐ **3.** Use oxygen delivery system components (nasal cannula, face mask, etc.). (pp. 93–97)

- Identify a nonrebreather mask and state the oxygen flow requirements needed for its use. (p. 96)

When the diaphragm relaxes, it moves upward as the intercostal muscles allow the ribs to fall back in and down. This action decreases the space inside the chest cavity and forces air out of the lungs (Figure 6-2). This process is referred to as **exhalation**.

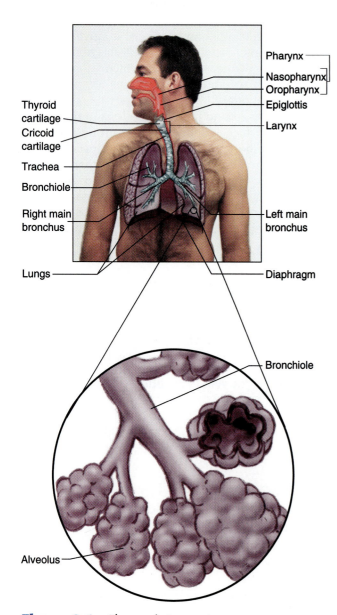

Figure 6-1   The respiratory system.

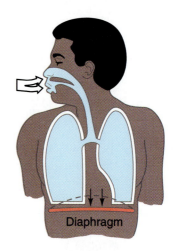

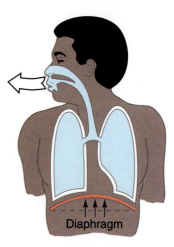

Figure 6-2   The lungs and diaphragm.

- Identify a nasal cannula and state the flow requirements needed for its use. (pp. 96–97)

✔ **Attitude**

☐ **4.** Explain the rationale for basic life support artificial ventilation and airway protection skills taking priority over most other life support skills. (p. 77)

☐ **5.** Explain the rationale for providing oxygenation through high inspired oxygen concentrations to

patients who in the past may have received low concentrations. (pp. 93–94)

✔ **Skills**

☐ **6.** Demonstrate the steps in performing the skill of artificially ventilating a patient with a bag-valve-mask for one and two rescuers. (pp. 88–90)

☐ **7.** Demonstrate how to insert an oropharyngeal and nasopharyngeal airway. (pp. 90–93)

☐ **8.** Demonstrate the use of a nonrebreather face mask and a nasal cannula. (pp. 96–97)

☐ **9.** Demonstrate artificial ventilation of a patient with a flow-restricted, oxygen-powered ventilation device. (pp. 89–90)

☐ **10.** Demonstrate the techniques of suctioning. (pp. 82, 84–85)

Patient Assessment

Adequate Breathing

When examining a patient for adequate breathing:

- Look for adequate and equal expansion of both sides of the chest with inhalation.
- Listen for air entering and leaving the nose, mouth, and chest. The breath sounds should be present and equal on both sides of the chest. Any sounds heard from the mouth should be free of gurgling, gasping, crowing, snoring, and wheezing. Feel for air moving out of the nose or mouth.
- Check for typical skin coloration. There should be no blue (cyanotic) or gray discoloration.
- Take note of the rate, rhythm, quality, and depth of breathing.

Adequate breathing consists of a normal rate of 12 to 20 per minute for an adult, 15 to 30 for a child, and 25 to 50 for an infant. A patient with adequate breathing should exhibit equal and present breath sounds and have visible and symmetric chest expansion with minimal effort. ✳

PRECEPTOR PEARL

Breathing is not an all-or-nothing proposition. New EMT-Bs may believe that they will find a patient who is breathing—or not. Perhaps the most important airway intervention that can be made is assisting the ventilations of a person who is breathing inadequately. It may seem odd for the new EMT to do this. Be sure to coach him or her to bag while the patient attempts a breath and to fill in the spaces between the patient's ventilations with additional BVM ventilations.

Patient Assessment

Inadequate Breathing

When evaluating patients with inadequate breathing, you may observe any of the following signs:

- Chest movements are absent, minimal, or uneven.
- Movements associated with breathing are limited to the abdomen (diaphragmatic or abdominal breathing).
- Breath sounds are diminished or absent.
- Noises such as wheezing, snoring, gurgling, or gasping (and in children, grunting) are heard during breathing.
- The rate of breathing is too rapid or too slow.
- Breathing is very shallow, very deep, or labored.
- The patient's skin, lips, tongue, ear lobes, or nail beds are **cyanotic** (blue or gray). On dark-skinned patients, check the lips and tongue.
- Inspirations are prolonged, indicating a possible upper airway obstruction.
- Expirations are prolonged, indicating a possible lower airway obstruction.
- Inability to speak or cannot speak in full sentences due to shortness of breath.
- Tripod position (leaning forward with hands on knees or another surface).
- In children, there may be retractions (pulling in) of the skin and tissues above the sternum and clavicles and of the muscles between and below the ribs.
- Nasal flaring, or widening of the nostrils during respirations, may be present especially in infants and children. ✳

OPENING THE AIRWAY

The airway is the passageway by which air enters or leaves the body. The structures of the upper airway include the nose, mouth, pharynx, and larynx. The larynx contains the epiglottis, which separates the upper airway from the lower airway. The lower airway contains the trachea, lungs, bronchi, and alveoli.

You will need to open and maintain the airway in any patient who cannot do so for him- or herself. This includes patients without a gag reflex, patients with an altered mental status, or patients in respiratory or cardiac arrest.

Airway assessment for patients who are unresponsive or have an altered mental status is usually done on a patient in the supine position. If a patient is found in a sitting position or slumped over the wheel of a car, take spinal precautions and carefully move him or her to a supine position. Then assess airway status.

Moving a trauma patient before immobilizing the head and spine could cause serious injury. However, in certain situations an "emergency move" of this type would be needed (see Chapter 5). If you suspect injury to the spine, protect the patient's head and neck as you position him. As you know, airway and breathing have priority over spine protection and must be assured as quickly as possible. If the trauma patient must be moved in order to open the airway or to provide ventilations, you will probably not have time to provide immobilization with a cervical collar, head immobilizer, and long backboard. In this case, manually stabilize the head and spine while a partner or two help you reposition the patient into a supine position. Then you can stabilize the patient's head and do a jaw-thrust maneuver to open the airway.

Most airway obstructions are anatomical obstructions caused by the tongue flopping back into the patient's airway when the head is flexed. When a patient is unconscious, the tongue frequently loses muscle tone and muscles of the lower jaw relax. Since the tongue is attached to the mandible (lower jaw), the risk of airway obstruction is even greater during unconsciousness.

PRECEPTOR PEARL

Don't forget to inform new EMT-Bs that a common sign of a partial airway obstruction is a snoring noise. As an experiment, if you can do so without waking up a snoring person, you should simply hyperextend the person's neck and listen as the snoring noise disappears!

Head-Tilt Chin-Lift Maneuver

The basic procedure for opening the airway to correct the position of the tongue is called the **head-tilt chin-lift maneuver.** Use this maneuver for a patient who has no suspected spine injuries. As you can see in Figure 6-3, when the jaw is pulled or lifted, the tongue moves away from the back of the throat. This procedure provides the maximum opening of the airway. Follow these steps to perform a head-tilt chin-lift (Figure 6-4):

1. **Position the patient.** The patient should be in a supine position.
2. **Position your hands.** Place one hand on the forehead. Place the fingertips of the other hand under the bony area at the center of the patient's lower jaw.
3. **Lift the patient's chin.** Use your fingertips to lift the chin and to support the lower jaw. Move the jaw forward to a point where the lower teeth are almost touching the upper teeth.

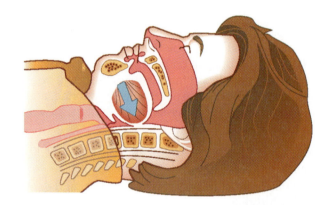

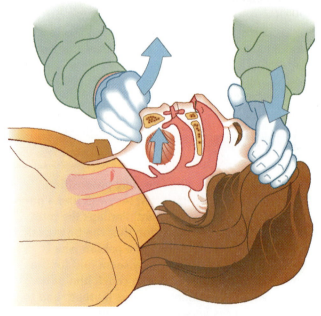

Figure 6-3 When you open the airway, you help to position the tongue.

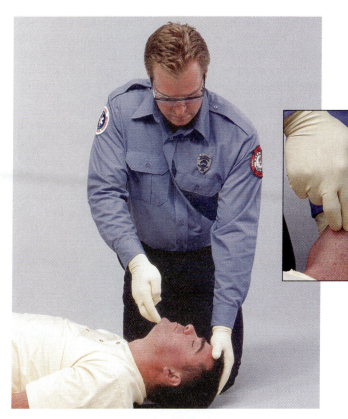

Figure 6-4 Head-tilt, chin-lift maneuver, side view. Inset shows EMT's fingertips under bony area at center of patient's lower jaw.

If a patient has no gag reflex, use an oropharyngeal airway (OPA) to keep the tongue from occluding the airway. In some situations it may be helpful to use the thumb of the hand supporting the chin to pull back the patient's lower lip. To avoid being bitten, do not insert your thumb into the patient's mouth.

LIFESPAN DEVELOPMENT

When performing the head-tilt chin-lift on a child, be careful to avoid pushing in on the fleshy tissue under the chin, as it may actually cause the tongue to partially occlude the airway. Your fingers should be placed so that they hold by the lower jaw only. Also, do not hyperextend an infant's neck; simply place it into an extended position. Hyperextension could occlude the soft trachea and larynx.

Jaw-Thrust Maneuver

If you suspect that the patient has a spine injury, the head-tilt chin-lift is *not* indicated since it can harm the patient's spine further. The *jaw-thrust maneuver* is the only recommended procedure for use on patients when trauma is suspected. To perform the jaw-thrust, follow these steps (Figure 6-5):

1. **Position the patient.** As you place the patient in a supine position, move him or her as a unit. Be sure to keep the head, neck, and spine aligned. Note that it will take more than one rescuer to move the patient into this position, and the rescuer holding the head and neck should direct all movement of the patient.
2. **Get in position yourself.** Kneel at the top of the patient's head, resting your elbows on the same surface on which the patient is lying.
3. **Position your hands.** Carefully reach forward and place one hand on each side of the patient's lower jaw at the angle of the jaw below the ears.
4. **Push the patient's jaw forward.** Stabilize the patient's head with your wrists while you use your index fingers to "jut the jaw," or push the lower jaw forward.

It is essential that you have your fingers behind the angle of the jaw, not just on the bottom; otherwise you will just shut the patient's mouth. You may

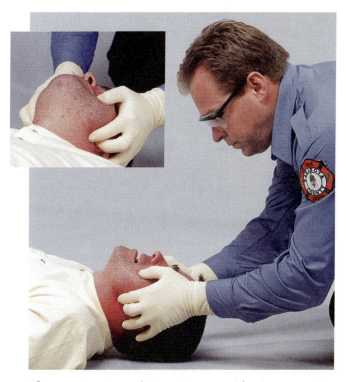

Figure 6-5 Jaw-thrust maneuver, side view. Inset shows EMT's finger position at angle of the jaw just below the ears.

need to retract the patient's lower lip with your thumb to keep the mouth open. Do not tilt or rotate the patient's head since any movement may cause an injury to the cervical spine.

SUCTIONING

As you know, keeping the patient's airway clear of vomitus, secretions, blood, and foreign materials is one of the most important jobs of the EMT-B. If a patient aspirates foreign material into the lungs, complications ranging from severe pneumonia to complete airway obstruction could occur.

The esophagus and stomach are lined with a tough coating that can tolerate anything from spicy sauces to peanuts and beer. In fact, the stomach contains hydrochloric acid, which helps break down food. The trachea and lungs, however, are made up of very delicate tissue that is easily damaged. When a patient is unconscious and regurgitates or vomits stomach contents into the pharynx, there is a danger that some of this "toxic" material may be aspirated into the lower airway. It only takes about an ounce of stomach acid to cause a potentially lethal pneumonia. So make clearing the patient's airway your first priority!

> ### PRECEPTOR PEARL
>
> Be sure to stress the importance of suctioning to new EMT-Bs. In patients who survive cardiac arrest, the most common preventable cause of death is aspiration pneumonia. It is tragic to think that patients who are saved with defibrillation may ultimately die from pneumonia as a result of aspirated vomitus.

Suction Devices

There are basically three types of suction units: electric, oxygen-powered (or gas-powered), and manual (Figure 6-6). There are "on-board," or portable, versions of each. Typical on-board units are mounted near the head end of the stretcher and are powered by the suction vacuum produced by the engine's manifold or the vehicle's battery. To be effective, a suction unit should furnish an air intake of at least 30 liters per minute at the open end of the collection tube. This will occur if the system can generate a vacuum of no less than 300 mmHg when the collecting tube is clamped. Your suction device should be inspected each shift before it is needed.

Since patients can vomit or have fluid in their airways at any time, always carry a portable suction unit to the patient's side. Some EMT-Bs carry a "turkey baster" as a manual unit until the larger unit is at the patient's side.

> ### LIFESPAN DEVELOPMENT
>
> Carry a bulb syringe in your pediatric kit to use as a manual suction unit for infants. Use a turkey baster for toddlers and older children.

There are pros and cons to each type of portable suction unit. Use the one that works best for your service area. Things to consider when choosing a portable suction unit include:

- **How easy is it to clean?** Material in the suction unit tubing and reservoir is a biohazard. Many units now have self-contained disposable parts that limit your potential exposure to the infectious materials you collect.
- **Does it deplete too much oxygen?** If you rely on an oxygen-powered suction unit, you may find that it runs down smaller tanks of oxygen quickly, consuming oxygen that should be administered to the patient.
- **Is the collection container large enough?** If you will be away from the ambulance for a long time and there is a great amount of suctioning to be done, you may have a problem if the collection container is too small.
- **How reliable is the unit?** Manual units work well when there is someone to pump them. Many EMT-Bs carry a manual hand-operated suction unit such as the V-Vac™ in their first-in bag to cover them until they return to the ambulance. Electric units work well, but the batteries should be checked every shift.

In addition to the suction unit, you need tubing, tips, and catheters. The tubing should be thick-walled, non-kinking, and wide-bored. It must allow "chunks" of suctioned material to pass through it. A tube that kinks or collapses decreases the amount of suction. The tubing must also be long enough to reach from the wall of the ambulance to the patient's head when the patient is on the stretcher. If it is necessary to suction a large volume of thick material, the tubing can be used without a tip as long as the steps for suctioning are followed.

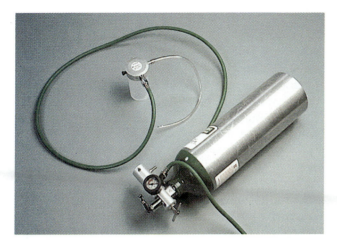

A

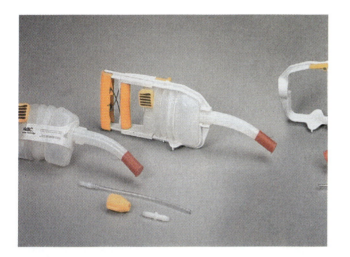

B

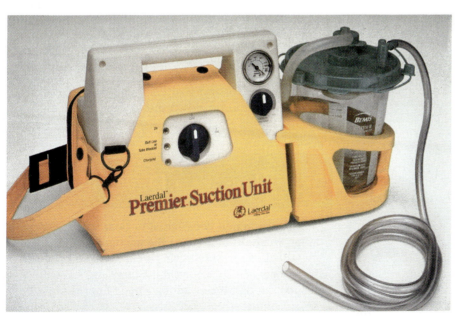

C

D

Figure 6-6 (A) An oxygen-powered portable suction unit. (B) Portable manual suction units (V-Vac™ Manual Suction Units from Laerdal). (C) An on-board suction unit. (D) An electric battery-powered portable suction unit (Laerdal™ Premier™ Suction Unit).

The most popular type of suction tip is the rigid pharyngeal tip, also called a "Yankauer" or "tonsil-tip." Basically, this is a disposable straight version of the suction tip a dentist places in the corner of your mouth. The Yankauer offers excellent control over the distal end of the device as you suction a patient's mouth and throat. It also has a larger bore than a catheter. However, be sure the Yankauer has a port to use as an on-off control. This way, with one hand you can open the mouth using the crossed-finger technique, while the other hand controls the Yankauer as well as the on-off control.

If the patient has a gag reflex, be careful not to cause gagging or to stimulate the vagus nerve by tickling the back of the throat. The vagus nerve, when stimulated, will cause the heart rate to slow down—a dangerous occurrence in critical situations. Always suction a few seconds at a time with a maximum of 15 seconds before oxygenating an adult patient. Always keep the end of the tip in sight, inserting no deeper than the base of the tongue to avoid damaging any soft tissue.

Suction catheters are flexible plastic tubes that come in various sizes identified by a number French. The larger the number, the larger the catheter. For example, a "14 French" catheter is larger than an "8 French." Actually, catheters are designed to be passed down a tube, such as an endotracheal tube or a nasopharyngeal airway (NPA). Some catheters have an on-off control port. For those that do not, it is necessary to kink the tubing to turn the suction on and off.

When using a suction catheter, use the largest diameter that fits. Measure the catheter from the center of the patient's mouth to the angle of the jaw or from the corner of the mouth to the ear-lobe. The length measured should be the maximum placed into the mouth at one time. Three hands are needed to properly position a catheter that is not being placed down a tube. One hand is used to open the mouth, another is used to control movement of the catheter tip, and the "third hand" is needed to turn the vacuum on and off.

Suctioning Procedure

Follow these steps for suctioning:

1. **Always take BSI precautions.** Most EMT-Bs routinely wear gloves when suctioning but fail to wear masks and eyeshields. Yet, the potential for being sprayed with oral secretions or other infectious material is great when suctioning a patient. You should use eye protection that you feel comfortable wearing with a mask, or wear a combination mask and eyeshield.

2. **Position yourself at the patient's head, and turn the patient to the side, if he or she is not at risk of a cervical-spine injury.** Positioning the patient in this way allows secretions to drain from the mouth. If the patient has a potential cervical-spine injury, one EMT-B should maintain manual stabilization of the patient's neck while another quickly suctions. If you are unable to adequately suction a supine patient, it will be necessary for at least two rescuers to carefully log roll the patient to the side. Remember that the airway is the highest treatment priority. If the patient is immobilized on a long spine board, then the entire spine board should be rolled on its side.

3. **Measure the catheter.** It is not necessary to measure a rigid-tip (Yankauer) catheter as long as you do not lose sight of the tip. Insert it no deeper than the base of the tongue. If using a flexible catheter, measure the same way you measure for an oropharyngeal airway (OPA).

4. **Open the patient's mouth using a crossed-finger technique.** Then clear the mouth of large pieces of material by using a finger sweep as necessary. If the patient has an OPA inserted, remove it while you are suctioning.

5. **Place the Yankauer so the convex (bulging-out) side is against the roof of the patient's mouth. Insert the tip to the base of the tongue.** Follow the pharyngeal curvature (Figure 6-7). Do not push the tip down into the throat or into the larynx.

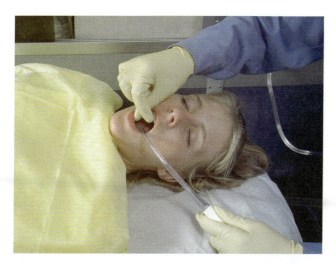

Figure 6-7 Placing a rigid-tip Yankauer following the pharyngeal curvature.

6. Apply suction only after the Yankauer or catheter tip is in place. Suction on the way out, moving the catheter from side to side for a maximum of 15 seconds. Then reoxygenate the patient. Remember that as long as the suction unit is on, it is removing oxygen from the patient's respiratory system. In infants and children a shorter suction time is suggested: 10 seconds for toddlers and 5 seconds for infants.

If the patient produces frothy secretions as rapidly as suctioning can remove them, suction for 15 seconds and then artificially ventilate for two minutes. Suction for 15 seconds and again artificially ventilate. Continue in this manner until secretions are resolved or you arrive at the hospital. It is a good idea to consult medical direction en route to the hospital if this situation exists.

If necessary, you may need to quickly rinse the catheter and tubing with water to prevent obstruction of the tubing from dried material.

PRECEPTOR PEARL

Rather than counting out 15 seconds as the maximum amount of time for suctioning, just take a breath and hold it before beginning to suction. When you need a breath, so does the patient. So stop suctioning and ventilate. In the excitement of a serious call, you will need to breathe more often than four times a minute!

ARTIFICIAL VENTILATION

If you determine that a patient is either not breathing or respiratory effort is inadequate, immediately provide artificial ventilation. **Artificial ventilation** is the forcing of air, or oxygen, into the lungs when a patient has either stopped breathing or has inadequate breathing. Of the techniques used to perform artificial ventilation, the American Heart Association (AHA) recommends the following in order of preference:

■ **Mouth-to-mask ventilation with high-flow supplemental oxygen at 15 liters or more per minute.** This procedure allows for delivery of a large volume of oxygen and provides an excellent mask seal that is created by the use of both hands on the mask.

■ **Two-rescuer bag-valve-mask ventilation with high-flow supplemental oxygen at 15 liters or more per minute.** When using the BVM, one rescuer uses two hands to seal the mask with the "double-OK hand position," as the second rescuer squeezes the bag. This also gives the EMT-B a good sense of the patient's lung compliance.

■ **Flow-restricted, oxygen-powered ventilation device (FROPVD).** This procedure provides excellent volume. In fact, you need to watch closely to prevent over-inflation, which would fill the patient's stomach with gas. In the field, this device is not recommended for use on infants and children.

■ **One-rescuer bag-valve-mask ventilation with supplemental oxygen at 15 liters or more per minute.** The one-handed mask seal necessary for this technique is difficult to maintain over a long time period.

NOTE: When you are using the mouth-to-mask or BVM with supplemental oxygen, the American Heart Association recommends smaller ventilatory volumes (400-600 mL). Since it is difficult to determine exact volumes while ventilating, deliver slow ventilations which cause the chest to rise visibly without overinflating and causing gastric distention.

First choice is always mouth-to-mask ventilation with high-flow supplemental oxygen. However, if the patient has been endotracheally intubated by a Paramedic, for example, or a specially trained EMT-B, the first choice would be ET ventilation with a bag-valve-mask, which is discussed later in this section.

Mouth-to-Mask with Supplemental Oxygen

Although DOT's "EMT-Basic National Standard Curriculum" identifies mouth-to-mouth or mouth-to-stoma as objectives, you know as an experienced

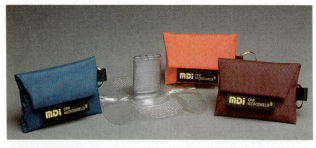

A

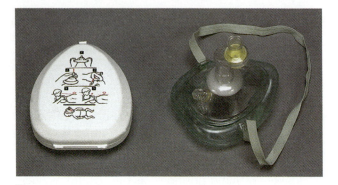

B

Figure 6-8 Examples of (A) barrier devices and (B) a pocket face mask.

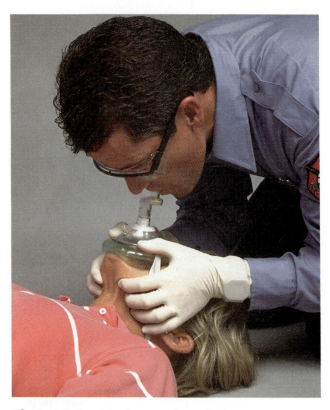

Figure 6-9 Mouth-to-mask ventilation.

EMT-B that these procedures are rarely if ever performed in the field. As a citizen who finds a family member in need of resuscitation, you might do mouth-to-mouth until either barrier protection or a pocket face mask becomes available. However, for EMS responses due to the potential for spreading infection, you should make it a practice to bring a pocket face mask to the patient's side on each call.

Mouth-to-mask ventilation is performed using a pocket face mask. The pocket face mask, or barrier protection device, is made of soft, collapsible material that can be easily carried in your pocket, jacket, glove compartment, or purse (Figure 6-8).

Pocket face masks have an important infection-control purpose. To prevent direct contact with the patient's mouth, ventilations are given into a valve in the mask. Most pocket face masks have one-way valves that allow ventilations to enter but prevent the patient's exhaled air from exiting through the ventilation port into the rescuer. The pocket face mask must be made of see-through plastic so you can observe the color of the patient's face and immediately respond if the patient regurgitates.

Follow these steps to apply a pocket face mask for artificial ventilation (Figure 6-9):

1. **Take BSI precautions.** Wear gloves and eye protection. You will not be able to wear a disposable mask.

2. **Position yourself at the patient's head and open the airway.** It may be necessary to quickly suction and clear obstructions in the patient's mouth. If available, insert an OPA to help keep the patient's airway open. Note that if your patient is an infant, do not hyperextend the neck as this may close the airway.

3. **Apply oxygen.** Connect oxygen to the inlet on the face mask. Run oxygen at 15 liters or more per minute.

4. **Position the mask on the patient's face.** Make sure the apex is over the bridge of the nose and the base is between the lower lip and prominence of the chin.

5. **Hold the mask firmly in place while maintaining the proper head tilt.** To lift the jaw forward, place both thumbs on the sides of the mask and the index, third, and fourth fingers on each side of the patient's face between the angle of the jaw and the earlobe. Jut the jaw up to the mask; avoid squeezing the mask down onto the face since this squeezing closes the mouth and airway.

6. **Ventilate.** Take a deep breath and exhale into the mask's one-way valve at the top of the mask port. Each ventilation should be delivered over 2 seconds in adults and 1 to 1½ seconds in infants and children. Watch closely for the patient's chest to rise. Remember this is your primary goal.

7. Remove your mouth from the port and allow for passive exhalation. Continue the procedure for ventilating following the AHA's rescue breathing or CPR guidelines.

Two-Rescuer Bag-Valve-Mask Ventilation

The bag-valve mask is a hand-held ventilation device which may be referred to as a bag-valve-mask unit, system, or device; resuscitator; Ambu-bag™; or BVM. It is used to ventilate a nonbreathing patient, as well as to assist the respirations of a patient who is not adequately ventilating on his or her own. The parts of the BVM include the clear face mask with air cushion, the nonrebreather valve, the squeezable bag, the oxygen reservoir, and the oxygen inlet. When you are ventilating a patient, the BVM provides an excellent barrier to infection but must be properly disposed of or sterilized after its use.

BVMs come in various sizes. Ambulances should carry the adult, pediatric, and neonatal (newborn) sizes. The bag must be a self-refilling shell. The system must have a non-jam valve that allows an oxygen inlet flow of 30 liters per minute. The valve should be nonrebreathing to prevent the patient from rebreathing his or her own exhalation and not subject to freezing in the cold temperatures experienced in the field. Most systems have the standard 15/22 mm respiratory fitting to ensure a proper fit with other respiratory equipment, face masks, and endotracheal tubes. The BVM should not have a pop-off or pressure relief valve.

The BVM's squeezable bag is designed to hold anywhere from 1,200 to 1,600 milliliters of air, depending on the brand. According to AHA guidelines, 700–1000 milliliters of air must be delivered to the adult patient with each squeeze of the bag (less when supplemental oxygen is used). The BVM should always be used with an oxygen reservoir system attached. To operate the BVM, the oxygen should flow at 15 liters or more per minute.

There are two types of reservoir systems—open and closed. In the open system, the BVM usually has a long open tube, or "elephant's trunk," which backfills with oxygen between ventilations. When the bag is squeezed, the oxygen in it goes into the patient; then the bag immediately fills with the oxygen that has collected in the reservoir. Since the end of the tube is open to the outside environment, there is a possibility that some room air will mix with the oxygen in the bag. Therefore, oxygen concentration is usually expressed as 90% oxygen.

In the closed system, a collapsible bag acts as the reservoir (Figure 6-10). Since this bag is not open to the outside environment, it contains 100% oxygen. The closed system operates the same way as the open system, but since there is no outside air mixed with the contents of the reservoir, the patient receives 100% oxygen.

The most difficult part of delivering BVM ventilations is obtaining an adequate mask seal so that air meant for the patient's respiratory system does not leak in or out around the mask's edges. It is difficult to maintain the seal with one hand while

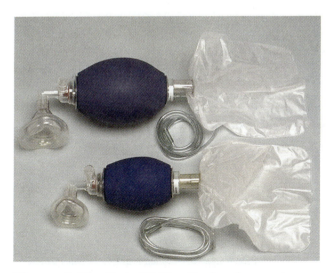

Figure 6-10 Typical BVMs with closed reservoir systems in adult and child sizes.

squeezing the bag with the other hand. For this reason, the one-rescuer bag-valve-mask technique is often inadequate. It is strongly recommended that BVM ventilation be performed by two rescuers. The two-rescuer technique can be used when no trauma is suspected, or it can be modified by using a jaw-thrust maneuver if trauma to the spine is suspected.

Signs of adequate BVM ventilation would include those listed for adequate breathing on page 79. Inadequate BVM ventilation would include a rapidly swelling stomach and/or any of the signs listed on page 79 for inadequate breathing.

BVM Ventilation for a Patient with No Suspected Trauma

The procedure for using a BVM with a patient who has no suspected trauma is as follows (Figure 6-11):

1. **Take BSI precautions.**
2. **Open the patient's airway.** Use the head-tilt chin-lift maneuver, suction as needed, and insert an oral or nasal airway.
3. **Select the proper size BVM for the patient** (infant, child, or adult).
4. **Get in position.** Kneel at the patient's head. Place your thumbs over the top half of the mask, and your index and middle fingers over the bottom half.
5. **Position the mask on the patient's face.** Make sure the apex is over the bridge of the nose and the base is between the lower lip and prominence of the chin. Note: If the mask you use has a large, round cuff—the "blob" type—surrounding a ventilation port, center the port over the patient's mouth.

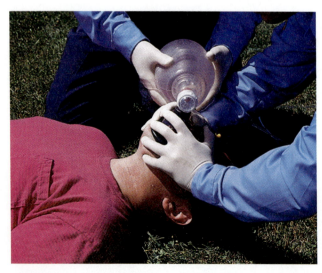

Figure 6-11 Providing BVM ventilation when *no* trauma is suspected.

6. **The second rescuer should kneel at the patient's side and connect the bag to mask,** if this has not already been done.
7. **Maintain seal while the bag is squeezed.** The second rescuer should squeeze the bag with two hands until the patient's chest rises. The rate should be once every 5 seconds for an adult or once every 3 seconds for infants and children.

If the chest does not rise or fall, you should re-evaluate the situation. It is probably necessary to reposition the head. If any air is escaping from under the mask, it will be necessary to reposition your fingers and the mask. Check to see if there are any obstructions that you did not notice previously. If after trying these adjustments the chest still does not rise and fall, try using an alternative method of artificial ventilation such as a pocket mask or manually triggered device.

BVM Ventilation for a Patient with Suspected Spinal Trauma

The procedure for using a BVM with a patient who you suspect may have a spine injury is as follows (Figure 6-12):

1. **Take BSI precautions.**
2. **Open the patient's airway.** Position yourself at the patient's head about 12 to 18 inches above the supine patient. Use the jaw-thrust maneuver, suction as needed, and insert an OPA or NPA.
3. **Select the proper size BVM for the patient** (infant, child, or adult).
4. **Position the mask on the patient.** Place the apex of the triangular mask over the bridge of the patient's nose. Then lower the mask over the mouth and upper chin. Place your thumbs over the nose portion of the mask and your index and middle fingers over the portion of the mask that covers the mouth, reaching to grasp the angle of the jaw. Use the ring and little fingers to jut the patient's jaw, bringing the jaw up to the mask without tilting the head or neck. Your palms will help to manually stabilize the patient's head and neck.
5. **The second rescuer should kneel at the patient's side.** Consider applying a rapid extrication collar.
6. **Maintain seal while the bag is squeezed.** The second rescuer should squeeze the bag with two hands until the patient's chest rises. The rate should be once every 5 seconds for an adult or once every 3 seconds for infants and children.

If the chest does not rise or fall, you should re-evaluate the situation. If the abdomen rises, it may be

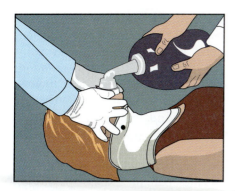

Figure 6-12 Providing BVM ventilation when trauma is suspected.

necessary to reposition the jaw. If any air is escaping from under the mask, it will be necessary to reposition your fingers and the mask. Check to see if there are any obstructions that you did not notice previously. If after trying these adjustments you find the chest still does not rise and fall, try using an alternative method of artificial ventilation such as a pocket mask or manually triggered device.

PRECEPTOR PEARL

It is impossible to do a one-handed jaw-thrust maneuver. Therefore, it is impossible to use a BVM on an unconscious trauma patient unless the patient has an endotracheal tube inserted or unless a second rescuer can assist.

BVM Ventilation for a Patient with a Stoma

The BVM can be used to artificially ventilate patients with a stoma who are found to be in severe respiratory distress or respiratory arrest. These patients often have thick secretions blocking the stoma, which will first need to be suctioned with a catheter. Due to the high potential for spread of infection from secretions in a stoma, mouth-to-stoma ventilation is not done in the field by EMT-Bs. Use this procedure:

1. **Take BSI precautions.**
2. **Clear the stoma.** Suction any mucous plugs or secretions from the stoma using a sterile suction catheter.
3. **Keep the patient's head and neck in a neutral position.** It is not necessary to position a stoma breather's airway prior to ventilating.
4. **Establish a seal around the stoma.** Use a pediatric-sized mask to do so.
5. **Ventilate at the appropriate rate.**

If you are unable to ventilate through the stoma, consider sealing the stoma and attempting artificial ventilations through the mouth and nose. (This technique may work if the patient is a partial neck breather. It will not work in a patient whose trachea has been permanently connected to the neck opening, since there is no remaining connection to the mouth, nose, or pharynx.)

Flow-Restricted, Oxygen-Powered Ventilation Device (FROPVD)

A flow-restricted, oxygen-powered ventilation device (FROPVD) uses pressurized oxygen delivered through a mask to provide artificial ventilation. This device is similar to the traditional positive-pressure ventilator, multifunction regulator, or "demand-valve resuscitator." However, the FROPVD includes a redesigned valve that optimizes ventilations and safeguards the patient (Figure 6-13). In the past, the FROPVD was referred to as a manual transport ventilator (MTV). A ventilator called an automatic transport ventilator (ATV) (Figure 6-14) is commonly used by ALS providers for inter-facility transport.

LIFESPAN DEVELOPMENT

The FROPVD is designed to be used only on adults, unless members of your service have been specially trained in its use for children and a very sophisticated unit in which the ventilation volume can be adjusted is available.

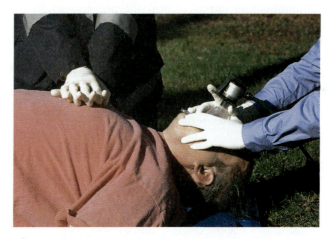

Figure 6-13 Providing ventilation with a flow-restricted, oxygen-powered ventilation device (FROPVD).

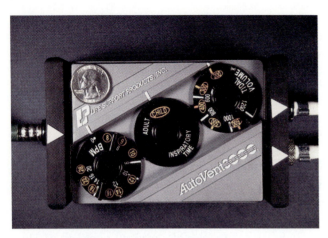

Figure 6-14 An automatic transport ventilator (ATV).

The procedure for using the FROPVD for a patient is the same as the BVM procedures described already. When purchasing a FROPVD, look for the following features:

■ A peak flow rate of 100% oxygen at up to 40 liters per minute.

■ An inspiratory pressure relief valve that opens at approximately 60 cm of water pressure and vents any remaining volume to the atmosphere or ceases gas flow.

■ An audible alarm that sounds when the relief valve pressure is exceeded.

■ A rugged design and construction that produces satisfactory operation under ordinary environmental conditions and extremes of temperature.

■ A trigger that enables the EMT-B to use both hands to maintain a mask seal while pressing the trigger.

One-Rescuer Bag-Valve-Mask Ventilation

As noted earlier in this section, the one-rescuer BVM procedure is the last choice for artificial ventilation. It is not designed for trauma patients since it is not possible to do a one-handed jaw-thrust maneuver. If it must be performed because of the lack of helpers or the lack of an available flow-restricted, oxygen-powered ventilation device (FROPVD) or pocket face mask, follow these steps:

1. **Take BSI precautions.**
2. **Get in position, and establish an airway.** Position yourself at the patient's head about 12 to 18 inches above the supine patient. Use the head-tilt chin-lift maneuver, suction as needed, and insert an OPA or NPA.
3. **Select the proper size BVM for the patient** (infant, child, or adult).

4. **Position the mask on the patient, and create a seal with one hand.** To create a seal, use the "OK hand position." That is, form a "C" with your thumb and index finger around the ventilation port. Place your middle, ring, and little fingers under the patient's jaw to pull it up to the mask.

5. **With your other hand, squeeze the bag against the side of the patient's face.** The squeeze should be a full one, causing the patient's chest to rise. Then release pressure on the bag, letting the patient exhale passively. While this takes place, the bag will refill with oxygen from the reservoir. The rate should be once every 5 seconds for an adult or once every 3 seconds for infants and children.

If the chest does not rise or fall, you should re-evaluate the situation. If the chest does not rise, reposition the head. If any air is escaping from under the mask, reposition your fingers and the mask. Check to see if there are any obstructions that you did not notice previously. If after trying these adjustments you find the chest still does not rise and fall, try using an alternative method of artificial ventilation such as a pocket mask or manually triggered device.

PRECEPTOR PEARL

Teach your crews that if any leaks are heard during BVM ventilation, immediately reopen the airway and reposition the mask seal to correct the mask leak. If the chest does not rise and fall, check for airway obstruction or obstruction in the BVM system. Consider inserting an OPA if one is not yet in place. If these steps are unsuccessful, do not continue to ventilate the patient inadequately. Instead, quickly switch to the two-rescuer BVM technique, pocket-face-mask technique, or flow-restricted, oxygen-powered ventilation device.

AIRWAY ADJUNCTS

Devices that aid in maintaining an open airway are referred to as **airway adjuncts.** In addition to performing either the head-tilt chin-lift maneuver or, if you suspect trauma, the jaw-thrust maneuver, two common airway adjuncts are used: the **oropharyngeal airway (OPA)** and the **nasopharyngeal airway (NPA).** (The prefix "oro" refers to the mouth, and "naso" refers to the nose. "Pharyngeal" refers to the throat or pharynx.)

Use these general guidelines for OPAs and NPAs:

- Always take BSI precautions when working in or around a patient's airway. This includes gloves, mask, and an eyeshield.
- Use OPAs only on patients who do not have a gag reflex. The gag reflex causes vomiting or retching when something is placed in the back of the throat. When a patient is unconscious, the gag reflex usually disappears but may reappear as consciousness is regained. A patient with a gag reflex may tolerate the NPA because it contacts the tongue only at its base.
- Open the patient's airway manually before using an airway adjunct.
- Do not continue to insert the OPA if the patient starts to gag. Continue manual maneuvers and, if the patient remains unconscious, try insertion again in a few minutes.
- While the OPA or NPA is in place, continue to provide either the head-tilt chin-lift or the jaw-thrust maneuver.
- While the OPA or NPA is in place, always have a rigid-tipped suction device readily available.
- If the patient regains consciousness or develops a gag reflex, remove the airway adjunct immediately and prepare to suction.

Oropharyngeal Airway (OPA)

Since you are an experienced prehospital care provider, you have most likely used an OPA, or oral airway, frequently. To review: The OPA cannot be used effectively unless you select the correct airway size for the patient. Always measure for the proper size before using an OPA. If the wrong size is inserted, you could actually occlude the patient's airway. The proper size will extend either from the center of the patient's mouth to the angle of the jaw *or* from the corner of the patient's mouth (lips) to the earlobe.

To insert an OPA, follow these guidelines (Figure 6-15):

1. **Take BSI precautions.**
2. **Position the patient.** First place the patient in a supine position. Then open the airway using either the head-tilt chin-lift maneuver or, if you suspect trauma, the jaw-thrust maneuver.
3. **Open the patient's mouth and jaws using the crossed-finger technique.** Cross the thumb and forefinger of one hand and place them on the patient's upper and lower teeth at the corner of the mouth. Then spread your fingers apart.
4. **Insert the OPA.** First position the correct size airway so that its tip is pointing toward the roof

of the patient's mouth. Then insert it by sliding it along the roof of the patient's mouth, past the soft tissue hanging down from the back (the uvula), or until you encounter resistance against the soft palate. Be certain not to push the patient's tongue back into the throat.

Now flip the airway 180 degrees over the tongue so the tip is pointing down into the patient's throat and the flange is resting on the patient's teeth. This prevents pushing the tongue back.

5. **Reposition the patient.** Once the OPA has been inserted, place the non-trauma patient in a maximum head-tilt position (hyperextension). If the airway is too long or short, replace it with the proper size.

An alternative insertion method for adults is: start with the airway pointing "down" the patient's throat (normal anatomical position) and then using a tongue depressor, press the tongue down and forward to avoid obstructing the airway.

LIFESPAN DEVELOPMENT

The preferred method for inserting an OPA in infants and children is to use a tongue depressor and insert the airway straight in. This method prevents damage to the soft palate or uvula. Note that an OPA is used in children only when prolonged ventilation is necessary.

Nasopharyngeal Airway (NPA)

The nasopharyngeal airway (NPA), or nasal airway, is not as widely used as an OPA. However, those who do use it often prefer it because it is less likely to stimulate a gag reflex.

NPAs may be used on patients who are responsive but need assistance keeping the tongue from obstructing the airway. Remember that even though the tube is lubricated, it still is a painful stimulus. The NPA is also useful on patients with clenched teeth or oral injuries. When a patient has clenched teeth and the airway is filled with secretions, the NPA and a suction catheter provide access to the secretions without ever opening the patient's mouth.

Because the hard plastic NPAs tend to cause nasal bleeding, soft flexible latex or silicone ones are used in the field. The sizes used for adults range from 28, 30, 32, to 34 "French." A small adult female would probably take a 28. A large male would probably take a 34.

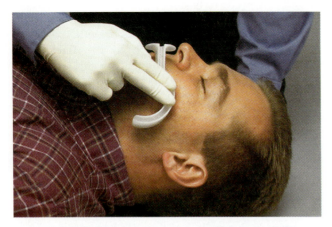

A The proper size OPA will extend either from the center of the patient's mouth to the angle of the jaw.

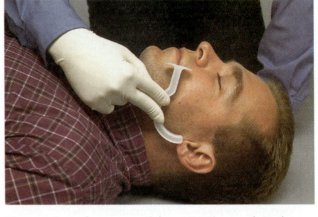

B . . . or from the corner of the patient's mouth to the earlobe.

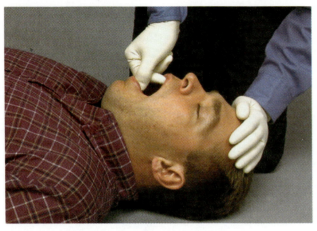

C After the patient is in position, use the crossed-finger technique to open the patient's mouth.

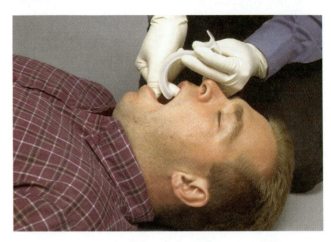

D Insert the OPA by sliding it along the roof of the patient's mouth until you meet resistance against the soft palate. Then rotate it into position.

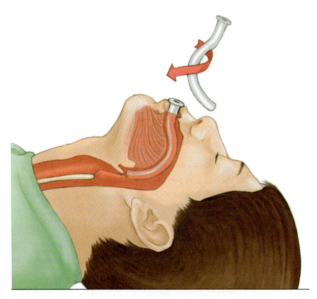

E Rotate it 180 degrees into position. When the airway is properly positioned, the flange rests against the patient's mouth.

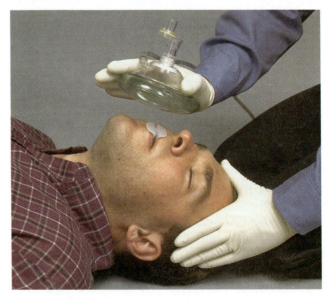

F After proper insertion, the patient is ready for ventilation.

Figure 6-15   Inserting an oropharyngeal airway.

There are two ways to size NPAs. Either use an NPA that is the diameter of the patient's smallest finger, or use one that extends from the tip of the patient's nose to the earlobe. Your goal is to insert the largest diameter that will fit into the nostril.

To insert an NPA follow these guidelines (Figure 6-16):

1. **Take BSI precautions.**
2. **Position the patient.** First place the patient in a supine position. Then open the airway using either the head-tilt chin-lift maneuver or, if you suspect trauma, the jaw-thrust maneuver.
3. **Lubricate the NPA.** Use a water-based lubricant such as KY Jelly®, Lubifax®, or Surgilube®. Do not use an oil-based lubricant, such as Vaseline®. It could damage the tissue that lines the nasal cavity and, if aspirated, can cause pneumonia.
4. **Insert the NPA.** Most NPAs are designed to be placed in the right nostril. The beveled, or angled, portion at the tip of the airway should point toward the nasal septum, the wall that separates the nostrils. Then gently push the tip of the nose upward while keeping the patient's head in a neutral position. Advance the NPA until the flange rests firmly against the patient's nostril.

Never force an NPA. If you experience any difficulty advancing it, pull it out, rotate 180 degrees, and try to insert it in the other nostril. Also, do not attempt to use an NPA if there is evidence of clear or blood-tinged (cerebrospinal) fluid coming from the nose or ears. This may indicate a skull fracture in the base of the cranium, which could potentially create an opening for the NPA to enter the brain.

There are a number of advanced airway adjuncts that fall under the elective sections of the EMT-B curriculum. In this textbook, Chapter 29 introduces the use of advanced airway adjuncts, such as the endotracheal tube, Combitube®, and LMA . Your state and local Medical Directors decide which, if any, of these devices are taught in your region.

OXYGEN ADMINISTRATION

One of the most beneficial treatments an EMT-B can provide is oxygen. **Hypoxia** is an insufficient supply of oxygen to the body's tissues. If a patient develops hypoxia while breathing atmospheric air (which contains only 21% oxygen), it is essential that the patient receive aggressive oxygen therapy. Clinically, the hypoxic patient may present with cyanosis or with restlessness and confusion if the brain is not receiving adequate oxygen.

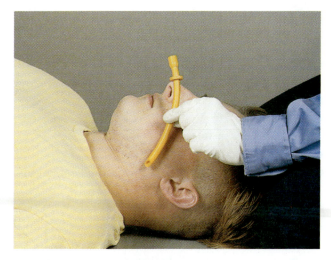

A Find the correct size NPA.

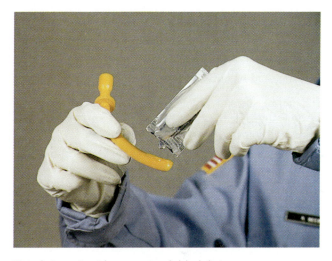

B Lubricate it with a water-soluble lubricant.

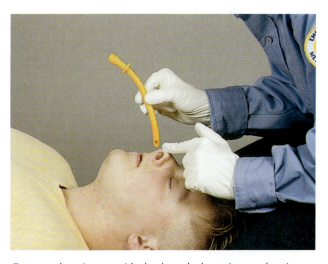

C Insert the airway, with the beveled portion at the tip pointing toward the nasal septum.

Figure 6-16 Inserting a nasopharyngeal airway.

Indications for Oxygen Therapy

Indications for oxygen therapy include:

- Shock or hypoperfusion
- Respiratory distress or arrest
- Cardiac abnormality or arrest
- Patients with chronic lung disorders who present in respiratory distress
- Smoke or toxic fume inhalation
- Poisoning or drug overdose causing ventilations that are too shallow or too slow
- Multiple-system trauma
- Head trauma resulting in brain tissue swelling and hypoxia
- Stroke, seizure, or a diabetic emergency

Hazards of Oxygen Therapy

The use of oxygen can involve non-medical and medical hazards.

Non-medical hazards include:

- If a pressurized oxygen cylinder is dropped and the valve breaks off, the cylinder can become a missile injuring everyone in its path.
- Oxygen supports combustion, causing fire to burn more rapidly.
- Pressurized oxygen and oil do not mix. When they come in contact, an explosion can occur. Never lubricate an oxygen cylinder.

Medical hazards include:

- Oxygen toxicity or air-sac collapse can occur in an environment where high-concentration oxygen has been administered to a patient for an extended period, such as in hospitals and long-term care facilities.
- If premature infants are given too much oxygen over an extended period of time, eye damage may occur. Excessive oxygen, along with other factors, can cause scar tissue to develop on the retinas. However, in the field, if you suspect that an infant or premature infant is in respiratory distress, never withhold oxygen for fear of injuring the patient's eyes.
- Patients with chronic lung diseases—such as asbestosis, black lung, emphysema, and chronic bronchitis—as well as elderly asthmatics, may be in the last stage of these diseases. In such cases, administering high-concentration oxygen could cause breathing to stop. Although this is rare, always evaluate a patient's oxygen needs. If a patient is in respiratory distress, administer high-concentration oxygen. If a patient has a minor problem,

such as a twisted ankle, and normally is on a long nasal cannula at home, then continue the liter flow and device the patient has been using at home.

The normal stimulus to breathe is the level of carbon dioxide in the blood. In chronic lung diseases, gas (mostly carbon dioxide) is trapped in the lungs due to chronic lower airway obstruction. When this occurs, the **chronic obstructive pulmonary disease (COPD)** patient switches over to a secondary stimulus to breathe, which is a low level of oxygen in the blood. This condition is called "hypoxic drive." A patient who is in hypoxic drive and who is administered high-concentration oxygen may stop breathing because his blood level of oxygen would be so high that the brain thinks no more oxygen is needed.

PRECEPTOR PEARL

Be sure to remind your crew that in the field, you may never see oxygen toxicity or other adverse conditions that result from oxygen administration since the time required for such conditions to develop is lengthy. Therefore, if the patient requires oxygen and is adequately ventilating him- or herself, use a nonrebreather mask at 15 liters per minute; otherwise ventilate the patient. The bottom line is never withhold high-concentration oxygen from a patient who needs it!

Oxygen Delivery Systems

Oxygen equipment used in the field must be safe, lightweight, portable, and dependable (Figure 6-17).

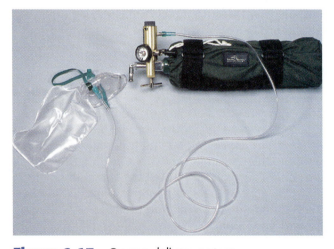

Figure 6-17 Oxygen delivery system.

Oxygen Cylinders

The standard source of oxygen is the oxygen cylinder, which is made of seamless steel or alloy and is filled with oxygen under pressure, usually 2,000 to 2,200 psi when full. A cylinder, or tank, is 75% full when it reads 1,500 psi. It is 50% full when it reads 1,000 psi, and 25% full at 500 psi. Change the tank when it is at 500 or less, but never allow it to empty completely since this can damage its insides.

Cylinders come in various sizes. The higher the letter in the alphabet, the larger the cylinder. For example, a "D" tank holds 350 liters of oxygen, and an "E" tank holds 625 liters. The larger tanks—such as a "G" tank, which holds 5,300 liters, or an "H" tank, which holds 6,900 liters—are used on board the ambulance.

The *U.S. Pharmacopoeia* has assigned a color code to distinguish compressed gases. Green and white cylinders have been assigned to all grades of oxygen. Also, unpainted stainless steel or aluminum cylinders are frequently used for oxygen.

Safety is a prime concern when working with oxygen cylinders. When using an oxygen tank,

ALWAYS:

- Use pressure gauges, regulators, and tubing that are intended for use with oxygen.
- Use nonferrous metal oxygen wrenches for changing gauges and regulators or for adjusting flow rates to avoid sparks.
- Ensure that valve seal inserts and gaskets are in good condition to prevent dangerous leaks.
- Use medical-grade oxygen. Industrial oxygen contains impurities. The cylinders should be labeled "OXYGEN U.S.P." and should not be more than five years old.
- Open the valve of an oxygen cylinder fully. Then close it half a turn. This prevents someone else from thinking the valve is closed and attempting to force it open. Remember: "Right is Tight and Left is Loose."
- Store reserve oxygen cylinders in a cool, vented room, properly secured in place.
- Have oxygen cylinders hydrostatically tested every 5 years. Some tanks only need testing every 10 years, if they have a star after the date of test (e.g., 4M92*). The date a cylinder was last tested is stamped on the cylinder.

When using an oxygen tank:

NEVER:

- Drop a tank or let it fall against any object. When transporting a patient with an oxygen cylinder, make sure it is strapped or secured to the stretcher.

- Leave an oxygen tank standing in an upright position without securing it.
- Allow smoking around oxygen equipment in use. Clearly mark the area of use with signs that read "OXYGEN—NO SMOKING."
- Use grease, oil, or fat-based soaps on devices that will be attached to an oxygen cylinder. Do not handle these devices when your hands are greasy. Use greaseless tools when making connections.
- Use adhesive tape to protect an oxygen tank outlet or to mark or label any oxygen tank or delivery apparatus. The oxygen can react with the adhesive and debris and cause a fire.
- Try to move an oxygen cylinder by dragging it or rolling it on its side or bottom.

Regulators

A pressure regulator must be attached to the oxygen cylinder. It measures the amount of pressure in the tank and the liters you wish to flow. Regulators are either screw-in types for the larger tanks or pin-yoke assembly types. The pin system is designed to assure the regulator is used only on an oxygen tank. The procedure for changing a regulator on a tank is as follows:

1. Select the desired cylinder. Check the label for "Oxygen U.S.P."
2. Place the cylinder in an upright position and stand to one side.
3. Remove the plastic wrapper or cap protecting the cylinder outlet.
4. Keep the plastic washer and change if necessary.
5. "Crack" the main valve for a second.
6. Select the correct pressure regulator and flowmeter (either pin-yoke or threaded).
7. Place the cylinder valve gasket on the regulator oxygen port.
8. Make certain that the pressure regulator is closed.
9. Align pins or thread by hand.
10. Tighten the T-screw for the pin yoke by hand or tighten the threaded outlet with a wrench.
11. Attach tubing and appropriate oxygen delivery device.

Flowmeters

The flowmeter allows control of the flow of oxygen in liters per minute. It is connected to the regulator but may be a separate unit as in the on-board oxygen system. The three types of flowmeters commonly used in the field are:

- **Bourdon Gauge Flowmeter™.** This flowmeter operates at almost any angle and is fairly rugged, but the gauge is inaccurate. When the tubing is kinked, the flowmeter does not compensate for the back pressure, and the gauge will give a falsely high reading.
- **Pressure-compensated flowmeter (Thorpe™ tube-type).** This unit is gravity dependent so it must be in an upright position. It has a ball float in an upright glass tube and indicates very accurately the flow at all times. It is often used in the on-board system.
- **Constant-flow selector valve.** This type of flowmeter is gaining popularity for use with portable tanks. It allows for adjustment in stepped increments (2, 4, 6, 8, . . . 15 liters per minute).

Humidifiers

A humidifier can be connected to the flowmeter to provide moisture to the dry oxygen coming from the supply cylinder. Dry oxygen can dehydrate the mucous membranes of a patient's airway and lungs. When used for a short time, oxygen dryness is not a problem. However certain patients (infants, children, and those with COPD or respiratory burns) are better off if offered humidified oxygen, especially on long ambulance trips. Sterile, single-use humidifiers are available for use.

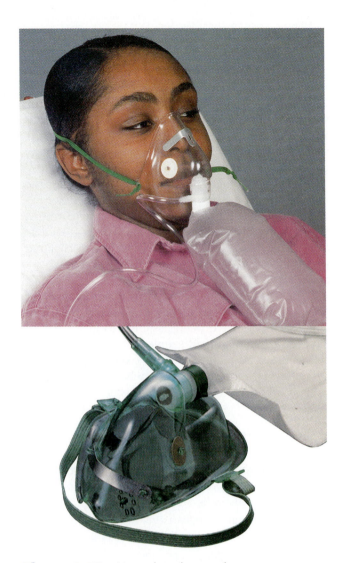

Figure 6-18 Non-rebreather mask

> ## PRECEPTOR PEARL
>
> **Remind your crew that some EMT-Bs like to keep Betadyne® in their on-board suction container to keep it clean. However, putting Betadyne® in the humidifier could kill an asthmatic patient. Never use any substance other than sterile water in the humidifier unless directed to do so by a physician!**

Delivering Oxygen to the Breathing Patient

Two devices are used in the field to treat both adult and pediatric patients who are breathing and have adequate ventilation—the **nonrebreather mask** and the **nasal cannula.** If patients need oxygen, give them a high flow of 15 liters per minute with a nonrebreather mask, which produces an oxygen concentration of 80% to 90%.

The nonrebreather mask is the preferred method for an EMT-B to deliver high concentrations of oxygen to a patient who is breathing adequately (Figure 6-18).

The mask must be properly placed on the patient's face to provide the necessary seal, which ensures that a high concentration is delivered. The reservoir bag must be inflated before the mask is placed on the patient's face. To inflate the reservoir bag, use your finger to cover the connection between the mask and the reservoir. The reservoir must always contain enough oxygen so that it does not deflate by more than one third when the patient takes his or her deepest inspiration. Oxygen supply can be maintained by flowing at least 15 liters per minute. Air exhaled by the patient does not return to the reservoir; instead it escapes through a flutter valve in the face piece.

New design features allow for one emergency port in the mask, so that the patient can still receive atmospheric air should the oxygen supply fail. This feature keeps the mask from delivering 100% oxygen but it is necessary for safety. Nonrebreather masks come in infant, child, and adult sizes.

Some patients will not tolerate a mask-type delivery device because they feel "suffocated" by it. If they need a higher concentration of oxygen, try to convince them to use the nonrebreather mask. For the patient who refuses to wear it, the nasal cannula is better than no oxygen at all.

A nasal cannula provides low oxygen concentrations between 24% and 44%. Oxygen is delivered to the patient by the two prongs that rest in the patient's nostrils. The device is usually held to the patient's face by placing the tubing over the patient's ears and securing the slip-loop under the patient's chin. When a cannula is used, deliver no more than 6 liters of oxygen per minute. At higher flow rates, the cannula begins to feel like a windstorm in the nose and dries out the nasal mucous membranes.

The Complicated Airway

Not all patients needing oxygen are as simple as "apply a nonrebreather mask and set the liter flow to 15 lpm." Some of the most complicated airway problems involve a traumatized patient. One example, which has become too common, is the following case:

As the elderly male pulls into his driveway, he's thinking of the activities he has planned for the day. Distracted, he begins to get out of the car without placing it in "park." Due to the slight incline of the driveway, the car begins to roll before he has his feet firmly on the ground. Rather than simply jumping back in, the man grabs the door to stop the car. As the car picks up speed, he falls and is caught by the undercarriage of the vehicle. Fortunately, he is not run over. But as you arrive on scene, his problems give you grave concern. Aside from abrasions and contusions and potential for serious burns from the hot spots on the undercarriage of the vehicle, the patient's most serious problem is facial trauma. (See Figure 6-19 for an example of this type of injury.)

After the vehicle is stabilized and the patient is removed from beneath the vehicle, you expose a grotesquely disfigured face. You find it difficult to make out the mouth and nose without first noticing the blood bubbles that appear as the patient attempts to breathe.

This is a complicated airway. It will require all of your attention to oxygenate the patient and make sure he does not aspirate blood or vomitus. A BVM device may not work well due to the inability to get an adequate seal, and a nonrebreather will most likely not be appropriate. Suctioning, however, is absolutely essential. This is one time where more personnel can be helpful in treating the patient.

Advanced life support is available in your community, so you call for them to respond

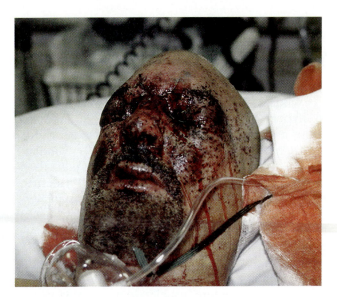

Figure 6-19 Facial injuries often involve airway complications.

immediately, as endotracheal or nasotracheal intubation may be life-saving in this patient's care. The complicated airway will most likely need surgical intervention and possibly a surgical airway. So you get the patient immobilized, deal with the ABCs (suction and attempt to assist ventilations with high-concentration oxygen), and get rolling to the most appropriate emergency department. (Depending on your local EMS system and how fast they can be accessed, an aeromedical evacuation may be more appropriate.)

Fortunately, cases such as this are not everyday occurrences. They are very stressful and use 100% of an EMT-B's abilities just to keep the patient alive. In order to be ready, you must be expert at all the skills presented in this chapter. You also must have a thorough knowledge of the capabilities of your EMS system so you can make quick, life-saving decisions for these patients.

ASSISTING WITH ENDOTRACHEAL TUBE PLACEMENT

Endotracheal intubation involves placing a tube directly into the trachea of a patient. This creates a direct route into the trachea for ventilations and medication administration. The endotracheal tube for adults is "cuffed," which means that a balloon at the end of the tube can be inflated to prevent aspiration.

Its combination of features makes the endotracheal, or ET, tube the best way to secure the airway of a person who is not breathing or has severe respiratory distress. In a vast majority of EMS systems, intubation is performed only by EMT-Paramedics and EMT-Intermediates, although intubation is an optional skill for the EMT-B and is covered in Chapter 29 of this text. You may, however, be called upon to assist in this procedure.

When assisting in intubation, you may be asked to hyperventilate the patient with the BVM for about a minute or so before the Paramedic inserts the ET tube. This can be accomplished by ventilating once every 2 seconds. The Paramedic then places the non-traumatic patient in the **sniffing position** (neck elevated approximately 2 inches, chin and nose thrust forward, and head tilted back) to align the mouth, throat, and trachea. The Paramedic then removes the OPA and passes the ET tube through the mouth (sometimes the nose), into the throat through the vocal cords, and into the trachea. This procedure usually requires a laryngoscope to illuminate the airway and to move the tongue and other obstructions out of the way.

In order to maneuver the ET tube past the vocal cords correctly, the Paramedic needs to see them. You may be asked to push the vocal cords into view by gently and carefully pressing your thumb and index finger just to either side of the medial throat over the cricoid cartilage. This procedure is known as "cricoid pressure" or Sellick's maneuver (Figure 6-20).

Once the ET tube is properly placed, the cuff is inflated with air from a 10 cc syringe. To assure proper placement of the ET tube, the Paramedic, while holding the tube, uses a stethoscope to listen for lung sounds on both sides and over the epigastrium (the area of the upper abdomen just under the xiphoid process). If the tube is incorrectly placed, the Paramedic immediately repositions or removes the tube, asks you to reoxygenate the patient, and repeats the intubation procedure.

The correctly positioned tube is anchored in place with tape or a commercial tube-securing device. The entire procedure, including the last ventilation, passing the tube, and the next ventilation, should take less than 30 seconds.

Complications of Intubation

When asked to ventilate the intubated, or "tubed," patient, keep in mind that it takes very little movement to displace the ET tube. Look at the graduations on the side of the tube. In the typical adult male, for example, the 22 cm mark will be at the teeth when the tube is properly placed. If the tube moves, report this to the Paramedic immediately.

Be especially careful not to disturb the ET tube. If the tube is pushed in, it will most likely enter the right mainstem bronchus, preventing oxygen from

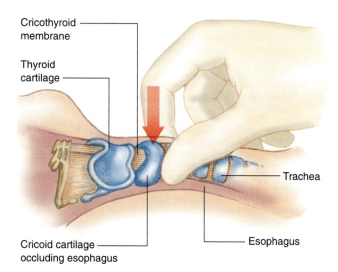

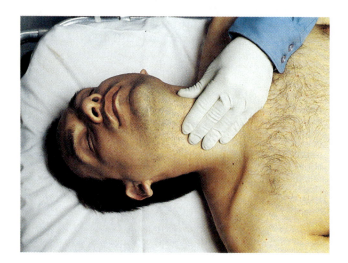

Figure 6-20 Sellick's manuver

entering the patient's left lung. If the tube is pulled out, it can easily slip into the esophagus and send ventilations directly to the stomach. This is a fatal complication if it goes unnoticed.

When holding the tube, place the tube with two fingers of one hand against the patient's teeth (Figure 6-21). If you are ventilating a breathing patient, be sure to time your breaths with the respiratory efforts of the patient. You want to enlarge the patient's breaths, not fight them. Pay close attention to how the ventilations feel. Report any change in resistance, since increased resistance when ventilating with the BVM is one of the first signs of air escaping through a hole in the lungs and filling the space around the lungs (pneumothorax). A change

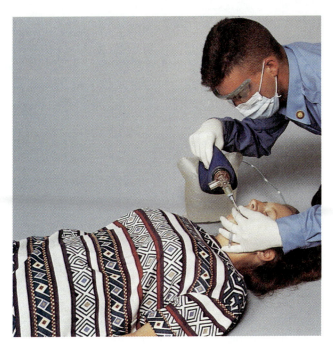

Figure 6-21 Make sure the endotracheal tube does not move. Hold it with two fingers against the patient's teeth.

in resistance can also indicate that the tube has slipped into the esophagus.

Whenever a patient is to be defibrillated, carefully remove the BVM from the tube, because the weight of the unsupported bag may accidentally dislodge the tube. Watch for any changes in the patient's mental status. As the patient becomes more alert, he or she may need to be restrained from pulling the tube out.

Assisting with a Trauma Intubation

Occasionally you will be asked to assist in the endotracheal intubation of a patient with a suspected cervical-spine injury. Since using the sniffing position increases the risk of further injuring the neck, you may be required to provide manual in-line stabilization during the entire procedure.

To accomplish this, the Paramedic holds manual stabilization while you apply a rigid cervical collar to the patient. (In some systems the patient

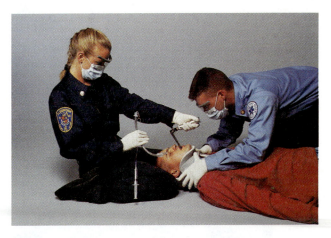

Figure 6-22 To assist in the intubation of a patient with suspected cervical-spine injury, maintain manual stabilization throughout the procedure. The EMT-B may straddle the patient, if necessary, to maintain stabilization.

may be intubated without the collar.) Since the Paramedic must stay at the patient's head, it is necessary for you to stabilize the head and neck from the patient's side (Figure 6-22). Once you are in position, the Paramedic leans back and uses the straight laryngoscope blade to bring the patient's vocal cords into view.

After intubation, hold the ET tube against the patient's teeth until placement is confirmed and the tube is anchored. At that time, you can change your position to a more comfortable one. However, until the patient is immobilized on a long backboard, it is necessary to assign another rescuer to maintain manual stabilization while you ventilate the patient.

> ### PRECEPTOR PEARL
>
> Never assume that a collar alone provides adequate immobilization. In addition to a collar, manual stabilization must be used until the patient's head is secured in place on the backboard.

Airway Emergencies

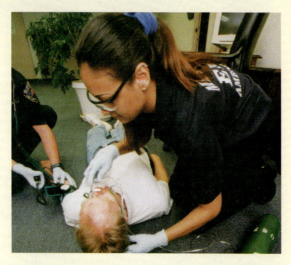

A call comes in for a "sick person" at 24662 East Densmore Road. You and your crew climb into the ambulance to respond to the call. You are in charge. You have a driver and a new EMT-B riding on her first call with you. Upon arrival at what turns out to be a single-family home, you judge the scene safe and move toward the residence. You are greeted by a concerned, well-kept woman in her 60s who tells you, "My husband, my husband! He is very sick!"

Entering the living room, you find a man, also in his 60s slumped over in a chair. He does not respond to loud verbal stimulus and has snoring respirations. You work with your crew to bring him gently to the floor. You assign Jane, the new EMT-B on your crew, to the airway. After a few seconds, Jane tells you that the patient is breathing. "Adequately?" you ask. Jane does a reassessment and notes that the respirations are deep, there is chest expansion, and the patient's color is good. Jane continues the initial assessment, while the driver suctions the patient. Once Jane is set with the initial assessment, the driver gets the stretcher. You now obtain a quick history. Speaking with the patient's wife, you find that the patient's name is Howard Engel. He is 64, has high blood pressure, and was released from the hospital 2 weeks ago after having a "mini-stroke." He had no complaints or precipitating events such as falls or injuries. Mrs. Engel last saw her husband in a

chair about 2 hours earlier. He was sitting in front of the TV, so she had originally assumed that he had fallen asleep while watching a baseball game. Mr. Engel, you learn, takes a high blood pressure medication, a multi-vitamin, and an aspirin daily. He has no known allergies and ate a sandwich for lunch.

Jane has placed an oral airway in the patient, and he tolerates it. She administers 15 liters of oxygen via nonrebreather mask. You explain your history findings to Jane, and ask her to form an initial impression. "Critical patient," she says. "Priority transport."

A rapid survey of the patient's body has revealed no signs of injury. Vital signs are pulse 94 strong and regular, respirations 12 and adequate, blood pressure 154/94. The patient's skin is cool and dry and his pupils equal and reactive to light.

Bob, the experienced EMT driver, appears with the stretcher. Jane smiles and is happy to be working with an experienced crew. The patient is loaded onto the stretcher, with Jane still stationed at the airway. You ask the patient's wife a few more questions. "Has Howard ever had seizures? Diabetes?" The wife shakes her head no. "How about heart problems?" Still "No." "Has he been drinking at all today or taken anything other than his medications that you know of?" "No, he hasn't," his wife replies. "One more question. Has he been depressed or have any history of psychiatric problems?" "Goodness no," she replies. You thank Mrs. Engel for her help and arrange for her to get a ride to the hospital with a neighbor. Jane nods her head to you after you finish asking questions, indicating she realizes why you were asking the questions you did.

On the way to the hospital, you talk more about the patient, including the need to monitor his airway for signs of inadequate breathing. Jane identifies inadequate breathing a short time later by noting that the bag on the NRB mask deflates only minimally. The chest is not rising, and the respiratory rate is now 10. Jane attaches supplemental oxygen to the BVM and squeezes the bag while you hold the seal on the patient's face. Jane squeezes the bag with the patient's own breaths and in-between when the breaths are slow. You report all patient information to the emergency department. The medical direction phycian confirms your suspicion of a stroke and requests your ETA.

CASE DISCUSSION

Your patient presented with an altered mental status. He needed airway maintenance with an oral airway, suction, and eventually BVM-assisted ventilations. Scene time was kept to a minimum while maintaining priorities and obtaining an adequate history.

Patients who have transient ischemic attacks (TIAs or "mini-strokes") are at a high risk for subsequent TIAs or strokes (cerebrovascular accidents or CVAs). This was probably the reason the patient took aspirin as a preventative measure.

Jane, the new EMT-B, learned two important lessons on this call. First, she obtained some good airway experience, while still having the support of a seasoned EMS crew. She inserted an oral airway, suctioned, and eventually identified inadequate ventilations and assisted with a BVM.

Second, Jane saw the reasons an EMT-B asks the standard questions for an altered mental status patient. While Howard may have suffered a stroke, there are other potentially treatable causes which may have been the cause of his unresponsiveness.

Name: Howard Engel
Age: 64
Chief Complaint: Sick person/unresponsive male

ASSESSMENT INFORMATION	RELEVANCE TO THIS PATIENT
History of "mini stroke" (TIA?)	• Patients who have had one TIA or CVA are at a greater risk for another in the weeks after the first one.
Patient history	• Since the patient was unable to communicate and there did not appear to be trauma, the history is a key part of the assessment process. • The EMT looked for potential causes of altered mental status other than the obvious potential for stroke. These included seizure, diabetic conditions, alcohol or drug overdose, psychiatric causes, and cardiac problems.
Medications	• The patient most likely took aspirin to prevent further strokes. Aspirin can help prevent a blood clot (also known as a thrombus), which is the cause of a majority of strokes. • The high blood pressure history and medications were important to note because of the patient's elevated blood pressure. Had elevated blood pressure been present with a low pulse, intracranial bleeding might have been suspected.
Other considerations	• This patient should be transported to a facility that would be able to provide aggressive care for patients with possible stroke. • Several opportunities existed for you to act as a preceptor and positive influence for Jane, the new EMT on the crew. Being able to perform critical airway skills and your observations will help promote confidence when she has to do it by herself at a later date. You also provided a good example of how to take the history of a patient with altered mental status.

SUMMARY

- Body substance isolation must be used when performing airway techniques.
- Patients who are breathing adequately will have adequate and equal expansion of both sides of their chest, normal skin color, and adequate rate and depth of breathing.
- Patients who are breathing inadequately will have inadequate respiratory rate and/or depth, unequal or inadequate chest expansion, and poor skin color.
- The airway may be opened with the head-tilt chin lift or, in patients with spine injuries, the jaw-thrust maneuver.
- Suction should be used any time that a patient's airway has vomitus, secretions, blood or other foreign materials and the patient is unable to maintain his or her own airway.

- Suction should not be performed for more than 15 seconds.
- Mouth-to-mask with supplemental oxygen is the preferred method of providing artificial ventilation. The next methods, in order of preference, include: two-rescuer BVM ventilation with supplemental oxygen, FROPVD, and one-rescuer BVM with supplemental oxygen.
- Airway adjuncts include oropharyngeal and nasophgeal airways. They should be used when patients cannot maintain the airway on his or her own.
- Oxygen should be administered at high concentration (10–15 lpm) to all patients who need oxygen. Some of these patients include those with hypoperfusion, respiratory or cardiac distress, or trauma.

REVIEW QUESTIONS

1. When examining a patient for adequate breathing, you should do all of the following EXCEPT:
   a. listen for sounds such as gurgling or gagging.
   b. assess the carotid pulse for at least 5 seconds.
   c. look for equal expansion of both sides of the chest.
   d. note the rate, rhythm, and quality of the breathing.

2. Suspect an upper airway obstruction when the patient has:
   a. an asthmatic disorder.
   b. prolonged expirations.
   c. prolonged inspirations.
   d. a chronic pulmonary disase.

3. Another name for an Yankauer is:
   a. gag reflex.
   b. rubber bulb syringe.
   c. nasopharyngeal airway.
   d. rigid-tip suction device.

4. If you don see the patient's chest rise or fall when you are performing BVM ventilation, you should first try to:
   a. squeeze harder on the bag.
   b. switch to a different bag.
   c. perform CPR or defibrillate.
   d. reposition the patient's head.

5. When a bag-valve-mask device is used on an adult, each ventilation should deliver at least _____ milliliters of air.

a. 400   c. 800

b. 600   d. 1000

6. To select the proper size oral airway, you should measure from the patient's:

a. tip of the nose to the earlobe.

b. corner of the mouth to the earlobe.

c. one side of the mouth to the other.

d. bridge of the nose to tip of the chin.

7. A large male would most likely take a size _____ French nasopharyngeal airway.

a. 28   c. 32

b. 30   d. 34

8. When an end-stage COPD patient is given too much oxygen, he or she may:

a. stop breathing.

b. lower his or her pulse rate.

c. itch and turn red.

d. become sensitive to light.

9. When using an oxygen cylinder, you should NOT:

a. store it in a cool, dry place.

b. ensure that the valve seal inserts are in good condition.

c. leave it in an upright position without securing it.

d. use industrial grade oxygen with your patients.

10. The best way for an EMT-B to deliver high-concentration oxygen to a breathing, conscious patient is to use a(n):

a. nasal cannula.

b. N-95 or HEPA mask.

c. constant-flow valve.

d. nonrebreather mask.

WEB MEDIC

Visit Brady's *Essentials of Emergency Care* web site for direct web links. At **www.prenhall.com/limmer,** you will find information related to the following Chapter 6 topics:

- Controlled ventilations
- Automatic transport ventilators
- Oxygen cylinders
- Suction-tip catheters
- Bag-valve masks

Chapter Seven

SCENE SIZE-UP, INITIAL ASSESSMENT, BASELINE VITALS, AND SAMPLE HISTORY

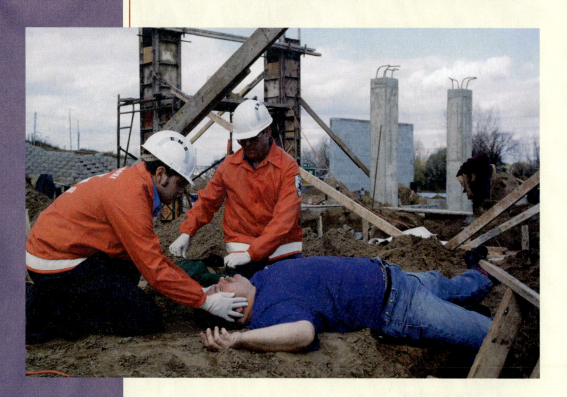

ESSENTIAL ELECTRONIC EXTRAS

CD ESSENTIALS

For preview and review of chapter material, see the student CD-ROM for

- Pretest
- Chapter quizzes
- Posttest

WEB ESSENTIALS

For additional review and enrichment, visit www.prenhall.com/limmer for

- Interactive student quizzes
- Links to online EMS resources
- Online case studies
- Audio glossary

The beginning stages of patient assessment are the same for all patients. Each scene will be sized-up for dangers, needed resources, and pertinent patient information such as mechanism of injury. Then each patient will receive an initial assessment that will identify and correct life threats and help determine which assessment steps to follow. At some point in the care of your patient, depending on whether the patient is a medical patient or trauma patient and whether the patient is conscious or not, you will perform a SAMPLE history.

SCENE SIZE-UP

The scene size-up is the first step of the patient assessment process, and it begins the assessment with a logical theme: It will not be possible to act as an EMT-B if you are injured. The size-up also focuses on several other factors that must be determined early on, such as the **mechanism of injury (MOI)** or **nature of illness (NOI)** and the resources needed to adequately handle the call (Table 7-1).

Components

The parts of the scene size-up are:

- **Scene safety.** The first and foremost part of the scene size-up is safety. This process begins before you approach the scene or exit the ambulance. Observe the scene as you drive up and before you exit the vehicle (Figure 7-1). This process continues throughout the call since hazards can change and violence can escalate at any time.

- **BSI review.** One of the initial determinations that must be made during the size-up is the amount of BSI equipment that will be required for the call (Figure 7-2). Make this determination as soon as possible. Getting to the patient without appropriate equipment can be awkward and potentially dangerous.

- **Mechanism of injury/nature of illness.** Even before you touch the patient, you should have some idea about the patient's chief complaint. Before emergency care can begin, determine the mechanism of injury (the physical force that caused the injuries) or nature of illness.

If the patient is injured, it is your responsibility to determine the force that caused the injuries (the mechanism of injury, or MOI), how it applies to the patient's condition, and the emergency care you will provide. (Does the patient require cervical-spine stabilization? Is there a potential for hidden injuries?) In the case of a motor-vehicle collision, there are different impacts (Figure 7-3). Specific types of motor-vehicle collisions have specific injury patterns (Table 7-2 and Figures 7-4 through 7-11). The amount of deformity in the passenger compartment is also significant in determining the MOI. Injury from falls depends on the height, the surface landed on, and the part of the body that struck the ground. Penetrating injuries always have a high index of suspicion since the path of damage under the skin cannot be seen.

CORE CONCEPTS

In this chapter, you will learn about the following topics:

- Components of the scene size-up and how they relate to your personal safety as well as to other parts of the call

- The initial assessment, including identification and correction of life threats and priority determination

- The SAMPLE history and vital signs

☐ **1.** Assess scene safety.
(pp. 105–107, 109–112)

- Recognize hazards/potential hazards. (pp. 105–107, 109–112)

- Describe common hazards found at the scene of a trauma and medical patient. (pp. 105–112)

- Determine if the scene is safe to enter. (pp. 105–112)

☐ **2.** Assess the need for additional resources at the scene. (pp. 106–107)

- Explain the reason for identifying the need for additional help or assistance. (pp. 106–107)

☐ **3.** Assess mechanism of injury. (pp. 105–109)

☐ **4.** Assess nature of illness. (pp. 105–107, 112–113, 116–122)

- Discuss common mechanisms of injury/nature of illness. (pp. 105, 108)

☐ **5.** Perform an initial patient assessment and provide care based on initial assessment findings. (pp. 112–123)

- Summarize the reasons for forming a general impression of the patient. (pp. 112–113)

- Discuss methods of assessing the airway on the adult, child, and infant patient. (pp. 116–118)

- Describe methods used for assessing if a patient is breathing. (pp. 116–118)

Table 7-1 **Components of the Scene Size-up**

Size-up Components	Actions
Scene Safety	Make sure that the scene is safe from all potential hazards (violence, hazmats, fire, explosion, unstable vehicles or surfaces, etc.)
BSI Review	Make sure your BSI precautions are adequate for the patient and situation.
Mechanism of Injury (trauma) or Nature of illness (medical)	Determine whether the call is trauma or medical in nature. Observe for physical forces in injury.
Number of Patients and Needed Resources	Determine number of patients and if resources will be needed. Call for additional help before beginning patient care.

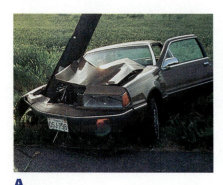

A

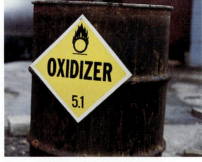

B

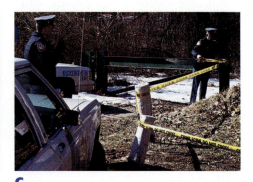

C

Figure 7-1 Hazards you may encounter include (A) unstable vehicles and downed power lines, (B) hazardous materials, (C) and crime scenes.

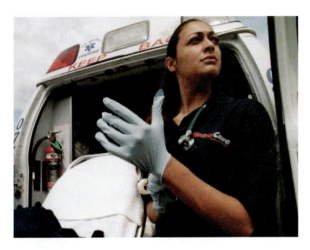

FIGURE 7-2 Take BSI precautions before you approach the patient.

If trauma is ruled out, it is necessary to determine what type of medical problem the patient is experiencing. This is called "nature of illness." Determine from the patient, family, or bystanders why EMS was activated.

■ **Number of patients and needed resources.** You must determine the number of patients and needed resources early in the call, since you are less likely to call for help once you become involved with patient care. You may simply call for an additional ambulance in smaller incidents to activation of a multiple-casualty incident (MCI) plan. Do not forget to request any special teams (hazmat, power company, etc.).

There are various sections in this text that deal with specific components of the scene size-up. Chapter 2 deals with BSI precautions. Chapter 28 addresses hazardous material incidents and multiple-casualty incidents.

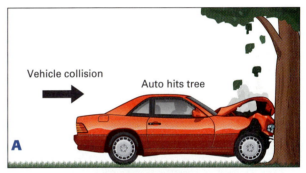

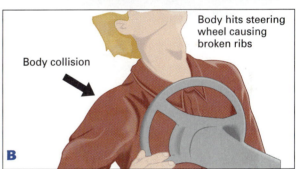

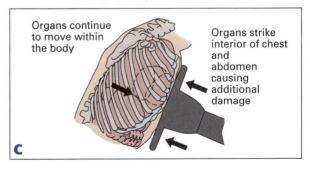

Figure 7-3 Three types of impact are possible in an auto collision. (A) The vehicle impacts an object. (B) The occupant continues to move forward and impacts the steering wheel. (C) Internal organs continue to move forward and impact the inside of the chest and other organs.

Table 7-2 Mechanisms of Injury—Motor-Vehicle Collisions

Type of Collision	Possible Injury Patterns
Head-on Impact	*Up-and-over pathway*—the body may be thrown over the steering wheel, head and neck may sustain injuries from the windshield, chest and abdomen may strike the steering wheel. *Down-and-under pathway*—the body slides under steering wheel, resulting in chest and abdominal injuries with pelvis, femur, knee, and lower leg injuries.
Rear Impact	Injuries to cervical spine, especially when a head rest is not used; other injury types are possible.
Side Impact	Patient on the side of impact absorbs more energy than patient on opposite side. The body and head may be pushed in opposite directions laterally. Suspect all injury patterns, especially if patients may have struck door post, etc. Determine extent (in inches) of intrusion into passenger compartment.
Rotational Impact	Occurs when vehicle is struck, then spins, often resulting in collisions with other vehicles or objects; multiple injury patterns.
Rollover	Causes multiple injury patterns; items inside vehicle become projectiles causing further injury.

Note: Attempt to determine if occupant restraints (safety belts) were in use at the time of the collision and what type was used (lap belt, lap and shoulder belt, etc.). Also determine if an airbag was deployed and "lift and look" under the airbag after the patient has been removed since the driver may have hit the steering wheel after the bag was deployed.

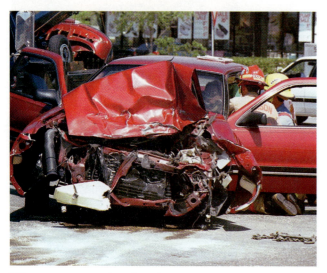

Figure 7-4 A head-on impact.

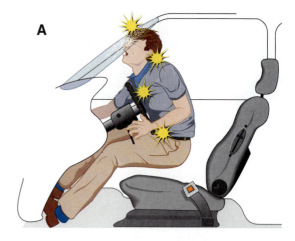

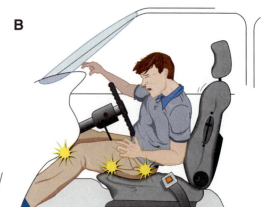

Figure 7-5 In a head-on collision, an unrestrained person is likely to travel in (A) an up-and-over pathway causing head, neck, chest and abdominal injuries or in (B) a down-and-under pathway causing hip, knee and leg injuries.

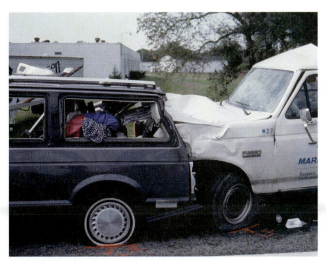

Figure 7-6 Rear imapact

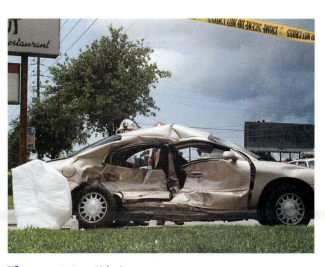

Figure 7-8 Side impact.

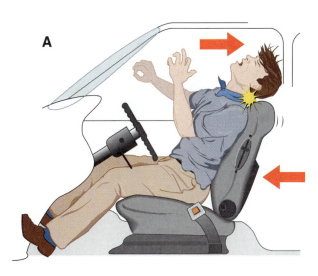

A

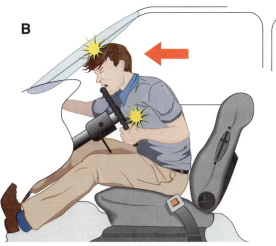

B

Figure 7-7 In a rear-end collision, the unrestrained person's head is jerked violently (A) backward and then (B) forward, causing neck, head, and chest injuries.

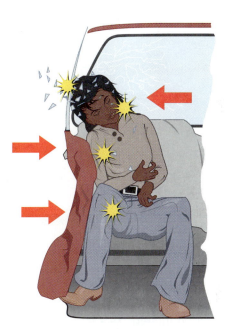

Figure 7-9 A side-impact collision may cause head and neck injuries as well as injuries to the chest, abdomen, pelvis, and thighs.

Scene-Safety Techniques

Observation

The best way to avoid danger is to prevent it. In order to do so, you must observe it early. Always check for these common indicators of danger at a scene:

- **Fighting or loud voices.** Fighting is a relatively obvious sign of trouble, but it is one that is often ignored. Loud voices, posturing, or other signs of imminent fighting are also indicators. While you might not be the one who is involved in the fight,

Figure 7-10 Rollover collision.

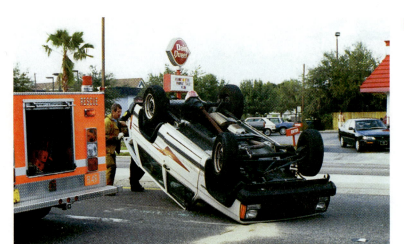

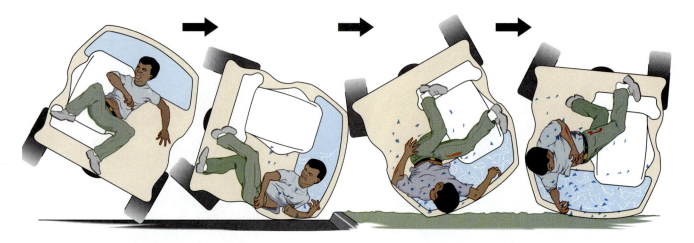

Figure 7-11 In a rollover collision, the unrestrained person wil suffer multiple impacts and possible multiple injuries.

you can still be injured. As a symbol of authority, you could be attacked. Fighting may take place on the street or in the home. Domestic violence is alarmingly common and a source of many EMS calls.

- **Intoxicants or illegal drugs.** When people abuse alcohol or other drugs, their behavior becomes unpredictable. Many of us have seen intoxicated persons acting anywhere from sleepy to combative. When drugs are abused or when they are observed on the scene, it is likely that the criminal element associated with the drugs is close by.

- **Weapons.** Weapons are a clear indicator of potential danger. When weapons are visible, being used, or are threatened to be used, retreat! Remember that almost anything may be used as a weapon. It takes careful observation of the people and their surroundings to prevent the use of a weapon against you.

- **Crime scenes.** Danger exists both during and after a crime. It is not unusual for the perpetrators to be in hiding at the scene. They also may return to the scene during your time there. There have been calls where the "victim" assaults police and EMT-Bs too! Even if the police have secured the crime scene, consider it potentially dangerous at all times.

- **Pets.** Almost any dog can be dangerous if it or its owners are threatened. Many breeds of dogs are trained to protect and attack. Exotic animals, such as snakes, also may pose a threat to the EMT-B.

Use of Your Senses

Use your senses to observe and prevent danger. While it is sometimes difficult to remember to observe constantly, practicing observational techniques every day will make this task second nature.

When it comes to safety, some senses are obviously better than others. Sight is the sense most EMT-Bs think of when it comes to safety; you are able to see a weapon, an unstable vehicle, or hazmat situation and respond appropriately. But do not underestimate the remaining senses. You do not need to see a danger directly in order to detect it. You can listen from other rooms, from behind doors, or from some distance away. Smell is valuable for identifying dangerous chemicals, leaking gasoline, and other situations that may pose a hazard. The senses of touch and taste are not practical to use since they bring you too close to the danger.

Some people claim to have a "sixth sense." If you do, heed it. Your gut feeling may not require immediate action, but it may give you a reason to react more slowly and to observe carefully until you can gather more information. Many crime victims have told police that they "had a feeling" that something was about to happen but they ignored it. Act cautiously until the feeling is resolved. Avoid overreacting.

Responses to Danger

When you observe danger, the following tactics can help keep you safe until the police or other appropriate agencies arrive to secure the scene:

- **Use cover and concealment** (Figure 7-12). No doubt you have heard of the term "take cover." Cover is taking a position behind some sturdy barricade that will hide your body and offer ballistic protection. Examples of cover include brick walls, the engine of your ambulance, and large trees. Surprisingly, some common items offer little coverage. The box of an ambulance offers little or no protection. Most doors and walls are also poor cover.

  Concealment is hiding your body, but it does not offer protection from projectiles and should be used only when solid cover cannot be found safely. Doors, walls, smaller trees, and shrubs may be used for concealment.

- **Retreat.** If danger is observed, the most appropriate action is to immediately move a safe distance away. Retreat when you confront hazardous materials, unstable vehicles and terrain, and violence. When you are retreating from danger, a common mistake is not getting far enough away. It is best to have a clear idea exactly how far is far enough before a potentially life-threatening situation develops.

  Move to a position where there are two major obstacles between you and the violence. If a dangerous person is able to get through one of the obstacles, one remains there as a buffer. One or both of the obstacles should be cover. One of the

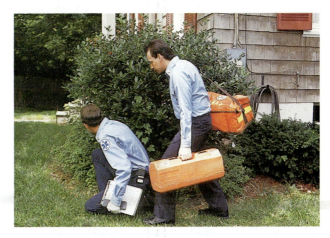

(A) Concealing yourself is placing your body behind an object that can hide you from view.

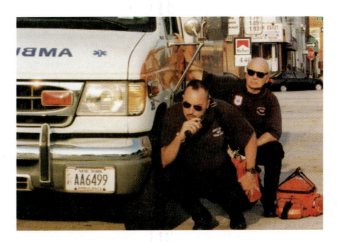

Figure 7-12 (B) Taking cover is finding a position that both hides you and protects you from projectiles.

obstacles can be distance, as in moving several hundred yards away. However, distance alone will not provide protection from gunfire.

Ideally, you should be able to get away from the danger and find a position of cover. This way, if someone tries to move toward you, you have time to retreat further and find another position of cover. When possible, return to the rescue vehicle and drive away. However, this should be done only when it is safe to do so.

- **Use distractions if necessary.** If you must retreat, it may help you to put something in the path of the danger. If you are fleeing through a doorway, wedging the stretcher there will slow down a potential aggressor. Throwing a medical kit at someone's feet will have a similar effect.

- **Carry a portable radio.** If you do confront danger, it must be reported. Carry a portable radio, especially if you are unable to return to the ambulance. When you report the danger, provide as much information as possible, such as:

- The location of the problem.
- The nature of the problem (fighting, gunshots, dangerous drugs).
- Your response to the problem (retreat, etc.).
- Details about the incident.

Many EMT-Bs are concerned about preventing liability when retreating from a scene. The key to liability prevention is adequate, objective documentation. Document all the indicators of potential danger and your responses to them. When you retreat from the scene, do not return to service. Stand by until the police secure the scene and emergency care can be performed safely. Document the time you left and returned to the scene. Notify a supervisor if necessary.

Carrying a weapon may be cause for liability and danger. A weapon can give you a false sense of security, causing you to enter scenes from which you would normally retreat. It is also dangerous to carry any weapon you are not trained to use (you wouldn't think of using advanced life support equipment unless you were an EMT with advanced training). Also remember that weapons may be taken from you and used against you or your partners. The use of a weapon also may result in considerable liability.

Observation and proper response before the danger strikes are much safer and more practical methods of dealing with danger than is the use of weapons.

Planning for Safety

It is always best to plan for safety. Planning begins with having a base of safety knowledge, such as the information presented earlier in this section. In addition, there are certain things that can be done in advance:

- **Work together.** The sum of a team's efforts is greater than its individual parts. This is especially true when it comes to safety. Crews can work together to observe and then use predetermined signals to communicate dangers to other members of the crew. Split up the carrying of equipment between crew members so no one person is bogged down. Having a hand free helps you to hold railings, open doors, stabilize yourself on uneven surfaces, and retreat more easily.
- **Make your equipment work for you.** Make sure your equipment is easily carried and not burdensome. Carry the equipment that you will realistically need in kits of a reasonable size and shape.
- **Dress for safety.** Wear clothing or protective equipment that is appropriate for the task you are

performing. Hazardous material incidents and rescue scenes require specific safety equipment. Everyday EMS work requires safe shoes and outerwear that is reflective and appropriate for the weather.

- **Use body armor, if necessary.** Some EMT-Bs wear body armor, or bulletproof vests. Many metropolitan EMS agencies are providing body armor for employees or contributing a sum toward purchase. Even if body armor is not for you at this time, the following information can help you make an informed decision about its purchase and possible use:
  - Body armor is not totally bulletproof. It will stop most handgun bullets, but not rifle bullets. Body armor is not a guarantee; it is an added safety measure that you may choose to take.
  - Body armor may stop knife penetration and prevent trauma from steering-wheel impact in motor-vehicle collisions.
  - To be effective, it must be worn! Choose comfortable body armor and a practical way to wear it. A quilted cover designed for outerwear will be very hot in the summer. A vest will not afford any protection when it is in your locker or behind the seat of the ambulance.
  - Body armor is flexible. It is not truly "armor." The panels are made of soft Kevlar™ or other fibers that are woven together to give ballistic protection.

Scene safety techniques are not designed to instill paranoia. In our chosen careers as EMT-Bs, it would be unrealistic to believe that we will never face danger. Emergencies are dynamic events at which emotions run high. If we accept that the skill of observation is necessary, then that skill will be part of our activities on every call, just as are patient assessment or splinting skills.

INITIAL ASSESSMENT

Elements of the Initial Assessment

The six elements of the **initial assessment** are: general impression, mental status, airway, breathing, circulation, and identification of priority patients (Skill Summary 7-1). In performing an initial assessment, you will quickly find and correct immediate threats to life and also discover information that determines the kind and extent of assessment you will perform next (e.g., your patient is responsive or unresponsive).

General Impression

After you completed your EMT course and gained some experience, you probably developed a "sixth sense" that alerted you when there was something wrong with a patient. There is now a name for this. It's called the **general impression.** Forming a general impression helps you to determine the priority of care. You do this by evaluating the environment, the patient's appearance, and the patient's chief complaint, among other things. As part of your general impression, you also should determine the patient's age and sex. In addition, if you have not already done so, determine whether the patient is injured, ill, or both. If the patient has sustained an injury, identify the mechanism of injury (MOI). If the patient is ill, determine the nature of illness.

If you see an immediate threat to life, such as a heavily bleeding wound, treat it before proceeding further.

Mental Status

Begin your evaluation of **mental status** as you approach the patient and introduce yourself. Tell the patient your name, that you are an emergency medical technician, and that you are there to help.

The response you get will vary. Most of the time, the patient is awake, with eyes open, and is able to answer questions. At other times, a patient's eyes may be closed, but he or she will respond to the sound of your voice. Another possibility is that the patient does not respond to your voice but moves or speaks after you apply a painful stimulus. A painful stimulus may be rubbing your knuckles on the patient's sternum, squeezing the trapezius muscle (though not in a patient who may have a cervical-spine injury), or pinching the muscle between the thumb and index finger. This last method has the advantage of allowing you to compare the response to a painful stimulus on each side of the body. The worst possibility is that the patient does not respond to either your voice or to a painful stimulus. This is the **AVPU** scale of assessing mental status (Figure 7-13).

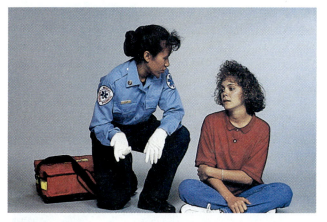

Figure 7-13 (A) In the AVPU system, the patient is Alert, or . . .

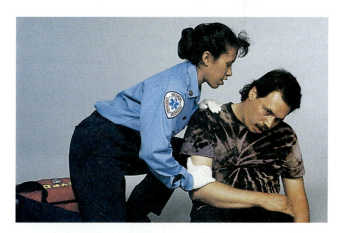

(B) responsive to Verbal stimulus, or . . .

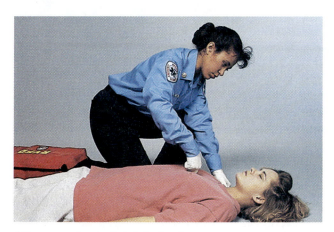

(C) responsive to Painful stimulus, or . . .

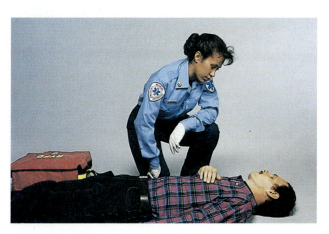

(D) Unresponsive.

Note: A trauma patient has been used to summarize the steps in the initial assessment.
Always take BSI precautions first.

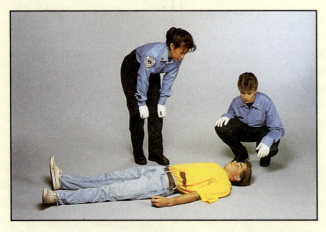

▲ **1.** Form a general impression of the patient and patient's environment.

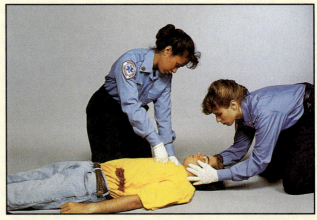

▲ **2.** Assess the patient's mental status using the AVPU scale.

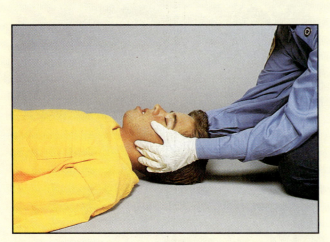

▲ **3.** Assess the airway. (Interventions: Perform appropriate maneuver to open and maintain the airway. If necessary, suction and insert an oro- or nasopharyngeal airway).

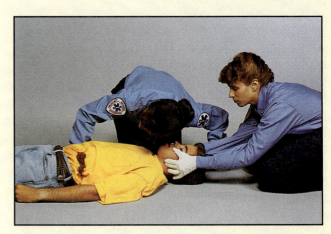

▲ **4.** Assess breathing. (Interventions: If there is respiratory arrest or inadequate breathing, ventilate with 100% oxygen. If breathing is above 24, give high-concentration oxygen).

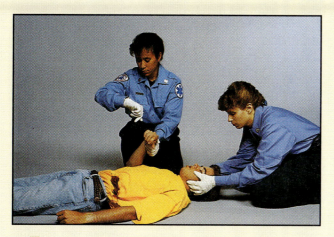

▲ **5.** Assess circulation by taking the patient's pulse and evaluating skin color, temperature, and condition, and . . .

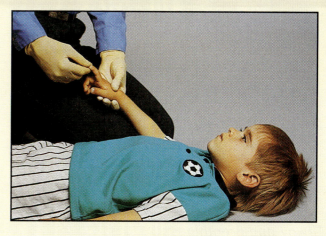

. . . in infants and children, also assess circulation by testing capillary refill. (Interventions: For indications of poor circulation, treat for shock).

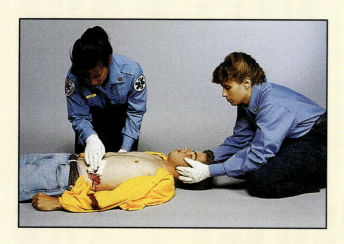

Assess and control severe bleeding.

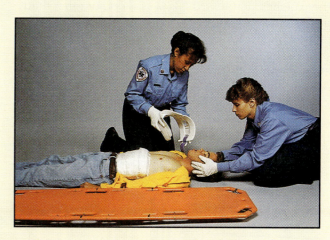

▲ **6.** Make a decision about patient priority for further assessment, interventions, or immediate transport.

A true mental status check includes more than just applying a verbal or painful stimulus. However, during the initial assessment you do not need any more information than this to determine your next steps. There is usually time later to gather more detailed information on the patient's mental status.

Airway and Breathing

In the responsive patient, there is rarely difficulty in confirming that the airway is patent. You can determine this by the absence of any trauma to the airway, the patient's alertness, the lack of blood or other fluid in the mouth, and the ability to speak without difficulty. You also can note that the respiratory rate appears to be in the normal range (although you do not stop to count respirations during the initial assessment) and that breathing is of adequate depth without any signs of difficulty.

If the patient's respiratory rate appears to be faster than 24 breaths per minute, administer high-concentration oxygen by nonrebreather mask. You may also wish to apply oxygen early to patients with respirations in the normal range, based on the patient's chief complaint (e.g., chest pain or shortness of breath). If the patient's breathing is inadequate, ventilate with supplemental oxygen. Although responsive patients sometimes do have inadequate breathing, it is much more likely that you will find this condition in unresponsive patients.

Circulation

Evaluating circulation involves checking three things simultaneously: pulse, bleeding, and perfusion.

When assessing a responsive patient, the easiest and least intrusive way of checking the pulse is to feel the radial pulse on the thumb side of the anterior wrist. If you do not feel a radial pulse, palpate the carotid pulse. In children less than a year old, the brachial pulse inside the upper arm is more reliable.

Palpating the pulse provides valuable information about the status of the patient's circulation. A rapid, weak pulse leads you to suspect shock (hypoperfusion). A slow pulse (less than 60) in an infant is an indication of the need for you to begin chest compressions. The most common finding on checking the pulse is a full (neither weak nor bounding) pulse in the normal range for the age of the patient (Table 7-3).

At the same time that you are palpating the pulse, look around the patient for blood and bleeding. If you see bleeding, control it now to minimize blood loss.

Table 7-3 Pulse, Normal Ranges

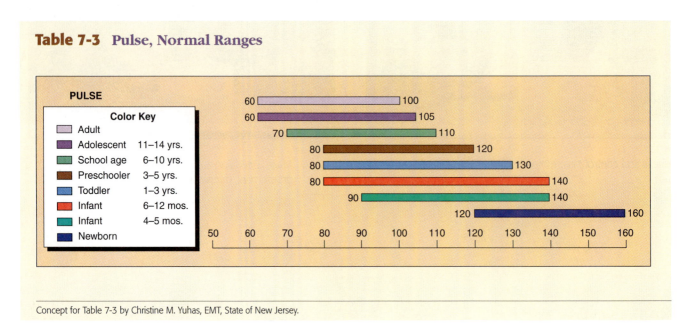

PULSE	Color Key	Range
Adult		60–100
Adolescent	11–14 yrs.	60–105
School age	6–10 yrs.	70–110
Preschooler	3–5 yrs.	80–120
Toddler	1–3 yrs.	80–130
Infant	6–12 mos.	80–140
Infant	4–5 mos.	90–140
Newborn		120–160

Concept for Table 7-3 by Christine M. Yuhas, EMT, State of New Jersey.

To evaluate perfusion, check skin color, temperature, and condition. Under normal conditions, lightly pigmented skin is pink. In skin that is darkly pigmented, the nail beds, lips, and inner surface of the eyelids should be pink. Abnormal skin conditions in any patient include:

- **Pallor.** Paleness from blood loss, shock, fright.
- **Cyanosis.** Blue or blue-gray color from hypoxia.
- **Flushing.** Redness from exertion or exposure to heat.
- **Jaundice.** A yellowish cast from liver disease.

When you feel a patient's skin temperature, you will frequently find it to be *warm*—the way it should be. It also can be *hot* (from fever or exposure to heat), cool (from hypoperfusion), or *cold* (from exposure to cold temperatures).

Skin condition refers to the amount of moisture on the skin. Normally, skin is *dry*. You also may find it *moist* or *wet*. If the skin is both cool and moist, it is called clammy, a condition that can result from hypoperfusion.

LIFESPAN DEVELOPMENT

In children under 6 years of age, also evaluate capillary refill by pressing on the end of the nail, the back of the hand, or the top of the foot. After you release the pressure of your finger, the color should change from white to pink in less than 2 seconds. More than 2 seconds is abnormal and may be a sign of shock (hypoperfusion) or exposure to cold.

Identification of Priority Patients

The "sixth sense" you may have developed with experience probably alerts you to the fact that certain patients need to be transported promptly. In fact, some patients need additional treatment and stabilization that only can be provided in an emergency department or hospital operating room. Conditions that fit in this category include:

- Poor general impression.
- Unresponsiveness.
- Responsive, but not following commands.
- Difficulty breathing.
- Shock (hypoperfusion).

- Complicated childbirth.
- Chest pain with systolic blood pressure less than 100.
- Uncontrolled bleeding.
- Severe pain anywhere.

The initial assessment is a critical part of the patient assessment process. In it, you will identify and correct life-threatening problems such as respiratory or cardiac arrest, inadequate ventilations, the need for suctioning, etc., but you will also use this assessment to set the tone and identify a patient's priority and plan for the remainder of your patient care.

BASELINE VITAL SIGNS

Vital signs reflect a patient's condition over time. The EMT-B should take them early, often, and accurately.

An EMT-Basic must be able to accurately assess and record a patient's vital signs. This is important not only for the first assessment (baseline vital signs), but also for repeated assessments, which can identify trends in a patient's condition. Such trends may alert the emergency department staff to the need to prepare certain equipment or a certain area of the emergency department. In order to detect such trends, you must record the time each set of vital signs was taken. Be sure your watch or clock has the same time as your dispatcher's clock. This will assist the health-care providers who take over the care of your patient.

There are five vital signs that must be measured: respiration, pulse, skin, pupils, and blood pressure. In the hospital, temperature is another vital sign that is frequently obtained, but in the field it has little value under ordinary circumstances and can be difficult to obtain accurately.

PRECEPTOR PEARL

New EMT-Bs, in their desire to explain to the patient everything that is going on, may say something like, "I'm going to count your breaths right now, so just relax." Of course, the patient who knows someone is counting his or her breathing rate will think about it and probably breathe either faster or slower as a result. If you hear new EMT-Bs using this approach, remind them that counting a respiratory rate should be done without bringing the patient's attention to it.

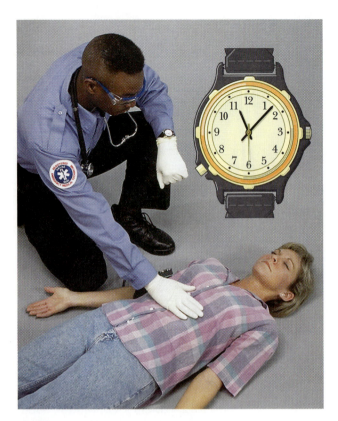

Figure 7-14 Assess respiration rate and quality. Count for 30 seconds and multiply by 2.

Table 7-4 Respirations—Rates and Sounds

Normal Respiration Rates (breaths per minute, at rest)	
Adult	12 to 20 (Above 24 or below 10 is serious.)
Adolescent, 12–18 years	12 to 20
School age, 6–12 years	15 to 30
Preschooler, 3–6 years	20 to 30
Toddler, 1–3 years	20 to 30
Infant, 6–12 months	20 to 30
Infant, birth–6 months	25 to 50

Respiratory Sounds	Possible Causes/Interventions
Snoring	Airway blocked. Open patient's airway, provide prompt transport.
Wheezing	Medical problem such as asthma. Assist patient in taking prescribed medications, provide prompt transport.
Gurgling	Fluids in airway. Suction airway, provide prompt transport.
Crowing	Medical problem that cannot be treated on scene. Provide prompt transport.

Respirations

Respirations, one of the most frequently forgotten vital signs, are easily assessed by observing the patient's chest rise and fall. You determine the rate by counting the number of breaths in a 30-second period and multiplying by 2 (Figure 7-14).

The quality of respirations is easy to determine while assessing the rate. Quality falls into one of four categories—normal, shallow, labored, or noisy:

- **Normal respirations.** The patient shows average chest wall motion and does not use accessory muscles to breathe.
- **Shallow respirations.** The patient shows only slight chest or abdominal wall motion.
- **Labored breathing.** This is usually easy to recognize by an increase in the effort of breathing, grunting, and stridor; the use of accessory muscles; and sometimes outright gasping. In children, you may also see nasal flaring and retractions in the supra-clavicular (above the clavicles) and intercostal (between the ribs) areas.
- **Noisy breathing.** Noisy respirations are just that—easy to hear because of the noise they make (Table 7-4).

Pulse

The radial pulse is the pulse you should assess first in all breathing patients one year or older. In infants less than one year old, assess the brachial pulse instead. When assessing a patient's pulse, feel for rate and quality. Determine the rate by counting the number of beats you feel in 30 seconds and multiplying that number by 2 (Figure 7-15). The quality of the pulse is classified as strong or weak and regular or irregular (Table 7-5).

Use only gentle pressure when palpating the pulse. This is especially true if you cannot feel a radial pulse and try the carotid pulse instead. Too much pressure can actually "shut off" the pulse by

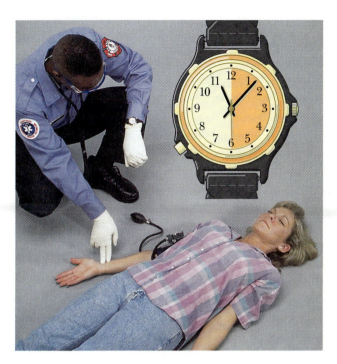

Figure 7-15 Assess pulse rate and quality. Count for 30 seconds and multiply by 2.

Table 7-5 Pulse

Normal Pulse Rates (beats per minute, at rest)

Adult	60 to 100
Adolescent, 12–18 years	60 to 105
School age, 6–12 years	70 to 110
Preschooler, 3–6 years	80 to 120
Toddler, 1–3 years	80 to 130
Infant, 6–12 months	80 to 140
Infant, birth–6 months	100 to 160

Pulse	Significance/Possible Causes
Rapid, regular, and full	Exertion, fright, fever, high blood pressure, first stage of blood loss
Rapid, regular, and thready	Shock, later stages of blood loss
Slow	Head injury, drugs, some poisons, some heart problems
No pulse	Cardiac arrest (clinical death)

not allowing any blood through the artery past where you are pressing it. When palpating a carotid pulse, especially in elderly patients, you may also slow the pulse by inadvertently putting pressure on an area called the "carotid sinus." Naturally, you should refrain from assessing carotid pulses on both sides of a patient at the same time.

Skin

Assess the color, temperature, and condition of the skin, looking for abnormalities like cyanosis or clamminess (Table 7-6).

Pupils

The pupils have been called the windows to the brain, and for good reason. They can give a very quick indication of serious problems in the brain, such as hypoxia or swelling inside the skull.

Assess the pupils by briefly shining a light into the patient's eyes one at a time. When you do this, cover the eye that you are not assessing. This will prevent light in that eye from affecting the size of the pupil in the other one.

When you assess pupils, look for size, reactivity, and equality (Table 7-7). Dilated pupils are very big, so big that it is difficult to tell what color eyes the patient has. Constricted pupils are very small. Normal pupils are in between these two extremes. A normal pupil constricts when you shine a light into it and returns to its normal size after you remove the light. Normal pupils also are the same size when you first look at them and both constrict at about the same rate when you shine a light into them (Figure 7-16).

Blood Pressure

The arterial blood pressure may be obtained with a BP cuff (or sphygmomanometer). It consists of two types of pressure, the systolic and diastolic. These are the pressures against the walls of the arteries when the heart is contracting and relaxing.

There are two methods of obtaining a blood pressure, **auscultation** and **palpation** (Figure 7-17). To auscultate the blood pressure, place a cuff of the appropriate size on the upper arm of the sitting or supine patient. The cuff should fit snugly. Find the location of the brachial artery by palpating just medial to the center of the crease of the elbow. Put a stethoscope in your ears so that the ear pieces face forward, and place the diaphragm over the brachial artery. Inflate the cuff until you can no longer hear the pulse. Slowly deflate the cuff until you hear the first return of the sound of the artery. This is the **systolic pressure,** or the pressure exerted against the walls of the arteries during

Table 7-6 Skin Color, Temperature, and Condition

Skin Color	Significance/Possible Causes
Pink	Normal in light-skinned patients, or at inner eyelids, lips, and nail beds of dark-skinned patients
Pale	Constricted blood vessels possibly resulting from blood loss, shock, heart attack, emotional distress
Cyanotic (blue)	Lack of oxygen in blood cells and tissues, resulting from inadequate breathing or heart function
Flushed (red)	Exposure to heat, high blood pressure, emotional excitement
Jaundiced (yellow)	Liver abnormalities
Mottling (blotchiness)	Occasionally in patients with shock

Skin Temperature/Condition	Significance/Possible Causes
Cool, clammy	Usual sign of shock, anxiety
Cold, moist	Body is losing heat
Cold, dry	Exposure to cold
Hot, dry	High fever, heat exposure
Hot, moist	High fever, heat exposure
"Goose pimples," shivering, blueness, paleness	Chills, communicable disease, exposure to cold, pain, or fear

contraction of the heart. Continue to deflate slowly until you no longer hear the sound. This is the **diastolic pressure.** Allow the cuff to deflate the rest of the way quickly. When listening for the diastolic

Table 7-7 Pupils

Pupil Appearance	Significance/ Possible Causes
Dilated (larger than normal)	Fright, blood loss, drugs, treatment with eye drops
Unequal	Stroke, head injury, eye injury, artificial eye
Lack of reactivity	Drugs, lack of oxygen to brain

pressure, be careful not to put any more pressure than necessary on the diaphragm. Too much pressure will give you a falsely low diastolic pressure.

To palpate the blood pressure, position the cuff in the same way as before. Instead of putting the stethoscope diaphragm over the brachial artery, palpate the radial pulse. Inflate the cuff until you can no longer feel the pulse. Slowly deflate the cuff until you feel the return of the pulse. This is the systolic pressure. Allow the cuff to deflate the rest of the way, since there is no way to get an accurate diastolic pressure by palpation.

When obtaining a blood pressure, be sure to use the proper cuff size. A cuff that is the right width should take up about two-thirds of the distance between the shoulder and the elbow. It should also have a bladder that does not overlap when the cuff is wrapped around the arm. The center of the bladder should be over the brachial artery when it is positioned properly.

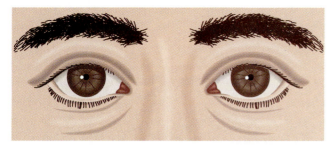

Constricted pupils

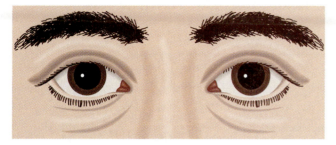

Dilated pupils

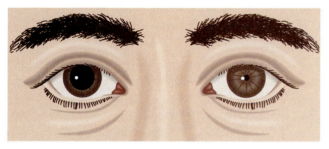

Unequal pupils

Figure 7-16 Constricted, dilated, and unequal pupils.

Hypertension (high blood pressure) has many definitions, but most authorities would agree that it is present when the diastolic is greater than 90 millimeters of mercury (mmHg) (Table 7-8). Hypertension is important because it indicates that the heart is working harder than it should to pump blood to the body. When the heart pumps, no blood leaves the left ventricle until the ventricle generates a pressure greater than the diastolic pressure (the diastolic is the lowest pressure in the arteries). If the diastolic pressure is higher than it should be, then the heart has to pump extra hard in order to do its job. Left untreated, this additional workload on the heart has the effect of weakening the heart and worsening other cardiovascular diseases such as angina.

LIFESPAN DEVELOPMENT

Cuff size is especially important when assessing children. You should determine a blood pressure in all patients older than 3 years. Below this age, the blood pressure is difficult to obtain and has very limited value. Instead, the general appearance of the patient, e.g., weak, in respiratory distress, or unresponsive, is more valuable than the numbers obtained from a blood pressure measurement.

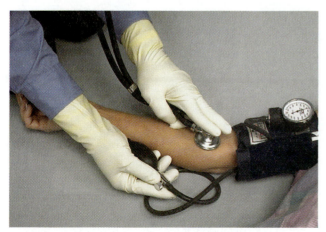

Figure 7-17 (A) Measuring blood pressure by ausculation.

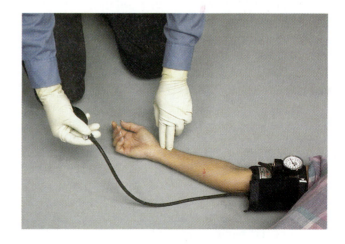

(B) Measuring blood pressure by palpation.

Table 7-8 Blood Pressure

Blood Pressure Normal Ranges

	Systolic	Diastolic
Adult	90 to 150	60 to 90
Infants and Children	approx. 80 + (2 × age)	approx. 2/3 systolic
Adolescent, 12–18 years	average 114 (88 to 140)	average 76
School age, 6–12 years	average 105 (80 to 122)	average 69
Preschooler, 3–6 years	average 99 (78 to 116)	average 65

Blood Pressure	Significance/Possible Causes
High blood pressure	Medical condition, exertion, fright, emotional distress or excitement
Low blood pressure	Athlete or other person with normally low blood pressure; blood loss; late sign of shock

Note: The systolic blood pressure usually parallels the pulse rate; that is, when the pulse rate increases, the systolic blood pressure increases, too. Also note that blood pressure usually is not taken on a child under three years of age. In cases of blood loss or shock, a child's blood pressure will remain within normal limits until near the end, then fall swiftly.

Hypertension is rarely something to be concerned about in the short term. However, document it and bring it to the attention of the hospital staff.

You should reassess the patient's vital signs as part of your ongoing assessment and also after each medical intervention.

SAMPLE HISTORY

An important part of the information you obtain on all of your patients is information about the present problem plus a relevant past medical history (Figure 7-18). The acronym *SAMPLE* can help you remember all the elements of such a history: signs and symptoms, allergies, medications, past medical history, last oral intake, and events leading to the present injury or illness.

To obtain a SAMPLE history, ask these questions:

S — Signs and symptoms. What is wrong? (A sign is any condition that can be identified by the EMT-B. A symptom is any condition that can only be described by the patient.) Be sure to ask about associated symptoms. For example, in the patient with a chief complaint of chest pain, you should ask whether the patient is having any difficulty breathing or shortness of breath.

A — Allergies. Are you allergic to medications, foods, or environmental substances?

M — Medications. What medications (prescription, over-the-counter, or herbal) are you currently taking?

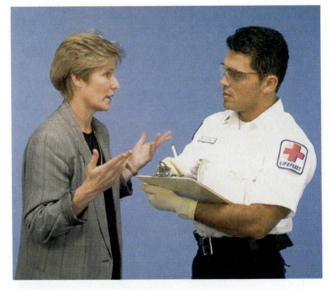

Figure 7-18 Get the SAMPLE history from family members or bystanders if the patient is unable to give information.

P — Past medical history. What medical illnesses has the patient had in the past or is the patient currently receiving treatment for? If the patient is injured, has this area been injured before?

L — Last oral intake. What did the patient last eat or drink? This information can help you prepare for potential airway problems, especially in the patient who is nauseated.

E — Events leading to the injury or illness. What, if anything, happened that led to today's problem?

This information may be very useful to the emergency department staff in determining the proper treatment for your patient. In the unresponsive patient, you may be able to gather some of this history from a medical ID tag or from family members.

LIFESPAN DEVELOPMENT

The geriatric patient often presents a challenge when the EMT-B attempts to take a history. Some complicating factors include:

- Impairments to vision or hearing that may hinder communication
- Multiple medical problems and medications
- Poor memory about past events

- Denial and/or fear of hospitalization, serious illness, and death

To overcome these problems:
- Speak slowly and clearly.
- Deal with fears and questions as you would with any patient. Offer reassurance and compassion. Explain your care and the importance of transportation to the hospital. Offer to make sure loved ones are contacted upon arrival at the hospital if this is a concern.
- Ask to see medications. Often medications are kept in one place. Use the medications as a means of identifying medical problems.
- If a family member is present, attempt to clarify information as necessary. (But do not ignore the patient and speak around him or her to another.)
- Ask a question in a number of ways. For example, ask a patient if he or she has any medical problems. Then ask if a doctor is seen for anything. Asking about hospitalizations may also uncover important history points.
- If the patient denies any history, it is beneficial to ask about certain conditions specifically. These include:
  — Cardiac (heart) problems
  — Stroke or "mini strokes"
  — Diabetes
  — Seizures
  — Blood pressure problems (high or low)

SUMMARY

- The scene size-up consists of:
—Scene safety
—BSI review
—Determination of mechanism of injury or nature of illness
—Resource determination (number of patients, need for special units or other help).
- The initial assessment consists of:
—General impression
—Mental status determination
—Checking and dealing with problems with
  Airway
  Breathing
  Circulation
—Priority determination.

- The vital signs consist of:
—Respirations
—Pulse
—Skin
—Pupils
—Blood pressure
- The SAMPLE mnemonic stands for:
—*S*igns and symptoms
—*A*llergies
—*M*edications
—*P*ast medical history
—*L*ast oral intake
—*E*vents leading up to the present injury or illness.

REVIEW QUESTIONS

1. The first and foremost part of the scene size-up is:
   a. BSI review.
   b. determining the mechanism of safety.
   c. ensuring scene safety.
   d. determining the nature of illness.

2. All of the following are elements of the initial assessment EXCEPT::
   a. mental status.
   b. breathing.
   c. identification of priority patients.
   d. vital signs.

3. The "P" in AVPU stands for:
   a. positive.
   b. pallor.
   c. perception.
   d. painful.

4. The normal pulse range for an infant 6 to 12 months old is _____ beats per minute:
   a. 60 to 100
   b. 70 to 100
   c. 80 to 140
   d. 120 to 160

5. If a patient's respiratory rate appears to be faster than _____ breaths per minute, administer high-concentration oxygen via nonrebreather mask.
   a. 15
   b. 18
   c. 20
   d. 24

6. A blue or blue-gray skin color that results from hypoxia is:
   a. cyanosis.
   b. pallor.
   c. flushing.
   d. jaundice.

7. If you press your finger to the back of the hand of a child under 6 years, an abnormal capillary refill, in which the skin regains its normal color, is longer than _____ seconds.
   a. 2
   b. 4
   c. 6
   d. 8

8. A respiratory sound caused by fluids in the airway is:
   a. snoring.
   b. wheezing.
   c. crowing.
   d. gurgling.

9. Most authorities agree that hypertension is present when diastolic pressure is greater than:
   a. 70 mmHg.
   b. 75 mmHg.
   c. 80 mmHg.
   d. 90 mmHg.

10. The "A" in SAMPLE history stands for:
    a. anemia.
    b. anaphylaxis.
    c. allergies.
    d. arthritis.

WEB MEDIC

Visit Brady's *Essentials of Emergency Care* web site for direct web links. At **www.prenhall.com/limmer,** you will find information related to the following Chapter 7 topics:
- Measuring blood pressure
- Hypertension
- Drug evaluation and research
- *Physician's Desk Reference*

Chapter Eight

ASSESSMENT OF THE TRAUMA PATIENT

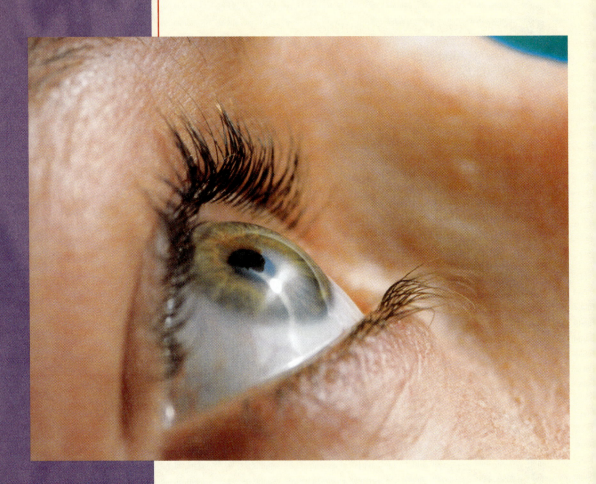

ESSENTIAL ELECTRONIC EXTRAS

CD ESSENTIALS

For preview and review of chapter material, see the student CD-ROM for

- Pretest
- Chapter quizzes
- Posttest

WEB ESSENTIALS

For additional review and enrichment, visit www.prenhall.com/limmer for

- Interactive student quizzes
- Links to online EMS resources
- Online case studies
- Audio glossary

Trauma patients make up only a small portion of EMS patients, but they are one of the most visible reasons for the existence of EMS systems. Although medical patients receive a great deal of attention today, it was the unnecessary deaths of patients on the highways in the 1960s that led to the American system of delivering EMS.

Today, the death rate from trauma on the highways is decreasing because of successful prevention measures, organized systems of trauma care, attention to the airway, control of bleeding, and prompt transport. Although EMT-Bs can and do participate in all of these components of trauma care, the last three are critical EMT-B interventions if patients are to survive potentially fatal injuries.

Trauma patients with significant internal injuries usually require interventions that are not available in the field. Rarely, if ever, can out-of-hospital providers stabilize a critical trauma patient. Such patients require interventions that are available only in an emergency department or a hospital operating room. Most trauma patients do not have critical injuries. Distinguishing between critical and non-critical patients can be difficult, but a systematic, efficient approach to assessment will make this process much easier.

Some trauma patients require significant interventions from the EMS system if they are to survive and do well. Most of the things an EMT-B can do that will make the difference between life and death are included in the initial assessment. Sometimes a rapid trauma exam will also reveal serious conditions that the EMT-B must manage. Mastering a systematic, efficient way to detect these conditions is an essential part of being an EMT-B.

SCENE SIZE-UP

Sizing up the scene is a critical part of any assessment. A trauma scene in particular can present a confusing array of information that the EMT-B must quickly evaluate and use to make decisions. For example, scene size-up includes taking BSI precautions, evaluating the scene for actual and potential dangers, identifying the mechanism of injury, and determining whether to institute multiple-casualty procedures. You reviewed the principles of BSI and scene safety earlier in this textbook. This section will concentrate on mechanism of injury.

The first step is to anticipate, based on dispatch information, what you might encounter when you arrive at the scene. This can help you to begin a plan of action. For example, if you receive a call for a motor-vehicle collision, you should anticipate blunt trauma with the possible need for extrication. On the other hand, a patient with a stab wound will have a penetrating injury with very little need for extrication under ordinary circumstances. Beware, though, of depending too much on dispatch

information. As you have no doubt discovered, the scene you arrive at sometimes bears little resemblance to the scene your dispatcher described. The patient in the motor vehicle may have gone off the road because of mental status changes due to hypoglycemia. The patient with the stab wounds may also have fallen (or been pushed) down a flight of stairs. Use dispatch information to start a plan, but be prepared to change your plan based on additional information at the scene.

CORE CONCEPTS

In this chapter, you will learn about the following topics:

- Distinguishing between patients who have and don't have significant mechanism of injury

- Performing a focused history and physical exam for a trauma patient

- Sizing and applying a cervical collar

- Ongoing assessment

DOT OBJECTIVES

✔ **Knowledge**

☐ 1. Perform an initial patient assessment and provide care based on
initial assessment findings.
(pp. 128–131, 137, 139)

- Summarize the reasons for
forming a general impression
of the patient. (p. 129)

- Discuss methods of assessing
altered mental status. (p. 129)

- Discuss methods of assessing
the airway in the adult, child,
and infant patient. (p. 129)

- Describe methods used for
assessing if a patient is
breathing. (p. 130)

- Differentiate between a patient
with adequate breathing and
inadequate breathing. (p. 130)

- Explain the reason for prioritizing a patient for care and
transport. (p. 130)

☐ 2. Perform a rapid trauma assessment
and provide care based on assessment findings. (pp. 130, 137)

- State the reasons for performing a rapid trauma assessment.
(pp. 130, 137)

- Recite examples and explain
why patients should receive a
rapid trauma assessment.
(pp. 130, 137)

The goals of patient assessment are always the same: to detect and correct conditions you can treat, to gather information for other members of the health-care team, and to identify and respond to trends in the patient's condition. How you accomplish these goals in the trauma patient will depend to a great extent on the mechanism of injury.

In all trauma patients, you perform an initial assessment, followed by a focused history and physical exam. En route to the hospital, you will conduct an ongoing assessment. In the patient with a significant mechanism of injury, after you perform the initial assessment, you will conduct a focused history and physical exam by doing a rapid trauma assessment, getting baseline vital signs, and gathering a SAMPLE history. En route to the hospital, if time allows, you will perform a detailed physical exam and ongoing assessment, re-evaluating the patient for changes and trends.

After you perform an initial assessment on the patient with no significant mechanism of injury, you will examine areas the patient tells you are injured and areas you suspect may have been injured based on your evaluation of the mechanism of injury. You will also get baseline vital signs and gather a SAMPLE history. En route, you will perform ongoing assessment.

SIGNIFICANT MECHANISM OF INJURY

Experience has shown that certain mechanisms of injury carry with them a greater risk of serious or life-threatening injury. Some are quite apparent, such as a gunshot to the chest. Others are not as obvious. (For example, how far can someone fall before it is likely that he or she will sustain serious injury?) Trauma specialists and researchers have examined

Table 8-1	Some Significant Mechanisms of Injury

Significant Mechanisms of Injury

- Ejection from a vehicle
- Death in same passenger compartment
- Fall of more than 15 feet or three times patient's height
- Rollover of vehicle
- High-speed vehicle collision
- Vehicle-pedestrian collision
- Motorcycle crash
- Unresponsiveness or altered mental status
- Penetrations of the head, chest, or abdomen; e.g., stab and gunshot wounds

Additional Significant Mechanisms of Injury for a Child

- Falls from more than 10 feet
- Bicycle collision
- Medium-speed vehicle collision

thousands of cases and drawn up a list of some of the more dangerous mechanisms (Table 8-1). However, this is only a partial list. It is important that the EMT-B have a high index of suspicion. When in doubt, assume that the patient has a significant mechanism of injury and treat him or her as such.

Initial Assessment

The components of the initial assessment are the same in medical and trauma patients, but they can take very different forms. This is due to the potential for spinal-cord injury in trauma patients. You should suspect spine injury in any patient who has sustained significant force to the upper part of the body or when there is a wound to the head, face, or neck. As you assess and treat a patient you suspect has a potential spine injury, avoid moving the neck and head as much as possible. Even a slight movement in the wrong direction can turn a potential spine injury into an actual one, which can be devastating or even life-threatening.

There are six parts of the initial assessment:

- Forming a general impression
- Assessing mental status
- Assessing the airway
- Assessing breathing
- Assessing circulation
- Determining the priority of the patient

Forming a General Impression

As with the medical patient, form your general impression by looking at the patient and getting an idea of the severity of the patient's condition. Also gather information such as the patient's sex and approximate age. It is at this point that you start to determine whether the patient is injured, ill, or both. If you see an immediate threat to life in the initial assessment, it is appropriate to treat it at this time.

Assessing Mental Status

The AVPU system of determining mental status gives you a good way of describing the type of stimulus you used and the patient's response to it. For example, a patient may moan in response to verbal stimuli or may withdraw both hands from a painful stimulus. When applying a painful stimulus, be sure not to

cause or worsen an injury. To avoid this, it is wise to avoid pinching the trapezius muscle near the neck in trauma patients. At the same time that you assess mental status, your partner should apply manual stabilization of the head and neck (Figure 8-1).

Assessing the Airway

If the patient is not talking (or not crying, if the patient is an infant or child), assume that the airway is not open and take steps to establish one. When assessing the airway of a patient with a potential spine injury, you must take care not to move the patient's head or neck any more than necessary. The jaw-thrust maneuver is the preferred way to open the airway of the patient who cannot keep his or her airway open alone. Suction the mouth and oropharynx to remove blood and other fluids as necessary.

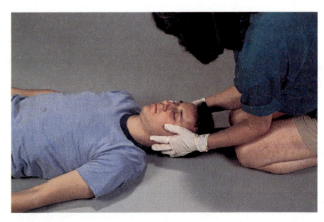

Figure 8-1 Stabilize a supine patient's head from the top.

Assessing Breathing

If the patient is unresponsive, put your ear near his or her mouth and look toward the chest. Look, listen, and feel for air movement. If the patient is responsive, look at the chest as you approach. Estimate the rate and depth of the patient's breaths. If the patient is unresponsive with breathing less than 8 per minute, ventilate with high-concentration oxygen. This is also appropriate if the patient's breathing is faster than 8 per minute but inadequate in depth.

If the depth of the patient's breathing is sufficient but the rate is faster than 24 per minute, administer high-concentration oxygen by nonrebreather mask.

Assessing Circulation

To determine how adequate the patient's circulation is, check pulse, bleeding, and perfusion. The radial pulse is easy to find and allows you not only to check the rate and strength, but also to gauge how good the circulation is in the extremities. If the radial pulse is difficult to find, palpate the carotid pulse.

Significant external bleeding is uncommon but important to identify and correct. Direct pressure on a heavily bleeding wound will stop or slow hemorrhage from all but the most serious of wounds. (See Chapter 21 for a review of bleeding and shock.)

It is easy to determine the adequacy of perfusion by checking skin color, temperature, and condition.

LIFESPAN DEVELOPMENT

In infants and children, capillary refill gives additional information about perfusion. A capillary refill time greater than 2 seconds indicates reduced perfusion from either shock or exposure to cold temperatures.

Determining the Priority of the Patient

High-priority conditions include poor general impression, unresponsiveness, inability to follow commands, difficulty breathing, uncontrolled bleeding, shock, complicated childbirth, chest pain with systolic blood pressure less than 100, and severe pain anywhere. Your local protocols may describe others. Some systems have very clearly defined conditions that require scene time to be kept to a minimum. In addition, this is the time in the initial assessment to decide whether

advanced life support (ALS) backup is needed or not. Based on the information gathered so far, you also will decide the next steps in the assessment.

Focused History and Physical Exam— Trauma

When you are treating a patient who has a significant mechanism of injury, spend as little time on scene as possible. Rather than doing a complete physical exam, you should perform a rapid trauma assessment and a detailed physical exam en route. This is why you should reconsider the mechanism of injury at this point in the assessment.

Rapid Trauma Assessment

The rapid trauma assessment, or rapid physical exam, is a quick assessment that allows you to find major problems that need to be treated quickly. The rapid trauma assessment consists of inspecting, palpating, and auscultating particular areas of the body: the head, neck, chest, abdomen, pelvis, extremities, and posterior (Skill Summary 8-1). When you assess these areas, search for DCAP-BTLS:

D — Deformities
C — Contusions
A — Abrasions
P — Punctures/penetrations
B — Burns
T — Tenderness
L — Lacerations
S — Swelling

A part of the rapid trauma assessment is not assessment at all. It is application of a cervical collar to limit motion of the patient's head and neck. Even after the collar is in place, the person applying manual stabilization must continue to do so. No collar limits motion enough for you to depend on it alone. Skill Summary 8-2 starting on page 134 describes the proper sizing and application of a cervical collar.

Sometimes as you perform a rapid trauma assessment, you will discover changes in the patient's condition that require you to act immediately. That means you may have to postpone the remainder of the exam for a short period. For example, if while you are performing a rapid trauma assessment, your patient's respiratory rate decreases to 6, you need to begin ventilations with high-concentration oxygen immediately.

Baseline Vital Signs

A complete set of baseline vital signs is essential in both determining the patient's condition now and

continued on page 137

FIRST take BSI precautions.

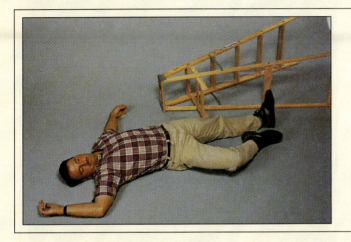

Mechanism of Injury

Reassess the MOI. If there is no significant MOI (e.g., patient has a cut finger), focus the physical exam only on the injured part. If the MOI is significant:

- Continue manual stabilization of the head and neck
- Consider requesting ALS personnel
- Reconsider transport decision
- Reassess mental status and ABCs
- Perform a rapid trauma assessment

Rapid Trauma Assessment

Rapidly assess each part of the body for the following problems (say "Dee-cap B-T-L-S") as a memory prompt for:

Deformities	**B**urns
Contusions	**T**enderness
Abrasions	**L**acerations
Punctures and	**S**welling
Penetrations	

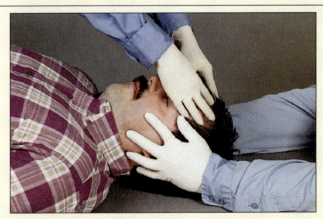

Head: DCAP-BTLS plus crepitation.

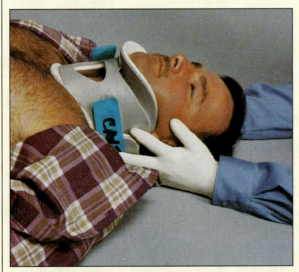

Neck: DCAP-BTLS plus jugular vein distention and crepitation (then place cervical collar).

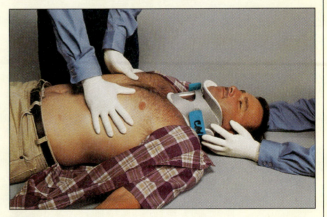

Chest: DCAP-BTLS plus crepitation and breath sounds (absent/present, equal).

(continued)

Chapter 8 • Assessment of the Trauma Patient **131**

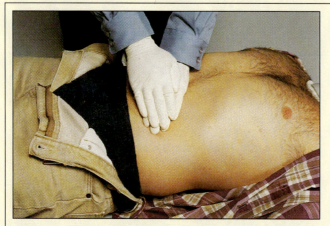

Abdomen: DCAP-BTLS plus firm, soft, distended.

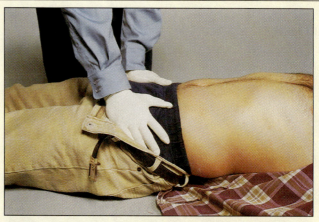

Pelvis: DCAP-BTLS, using gentle compression for tenderness.

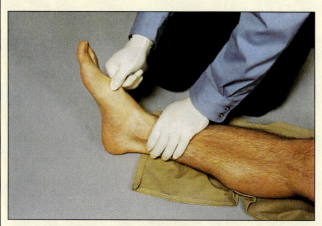

Extremities: DCAP-BTLS plus pulses, motor function, and sensation (PMS).

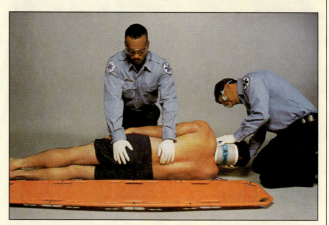

Posterior: DCAP-BTLS. (To examine posterior, roll patient using spinal precautions.)

Vital Signs

Assess the patient's vital signs:
- Respirations
- Pulse
- Skin color, temperature, conditions (and capillary refill in infants and children)
- Pupils
- Blood pressure

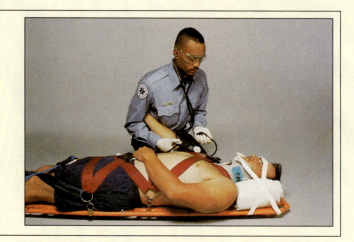

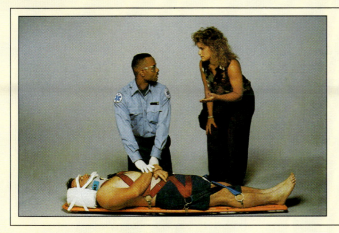

SAMPLE History

Interview patient, or if patient is unresponsive, interview family and bystanders to get as much information as possible about the patient's problem. Ask about:

Signs and symptoms
Allergies
Medications
Past medical history
Last oral intake
Events leading to injury.

Interventions and Transport

Contact on-line medical direction as needed.
Perform interventions as needed. Package and transport patient.

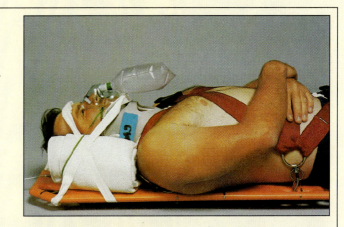

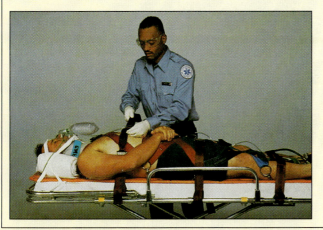

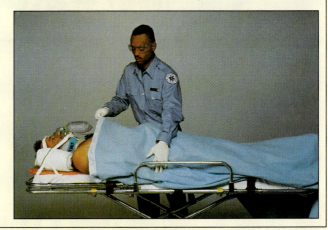

Rigid cervical collars are applied to protect the cervical spine. Do not apply a soft collar.

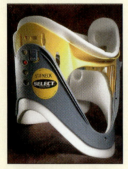

STIFNECK® SELECT™—
Rigid extrication collar
(Laerdal Medical Corporation/
John Hill Photography)

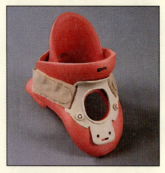

PHILADELPHIA CERVICAL COLLAR™

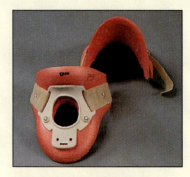

PHILADELPHIA CERVICAL COLLAR™—Open

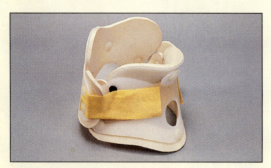

NEC-LOC™—Rigid extrication

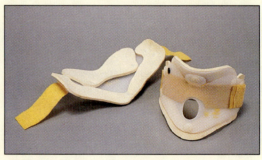

NEC-LOC™—Open

Sizing a Rigid Cervical Collar

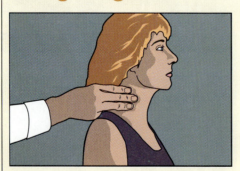

▲ **1.** Measure the patient's neck.

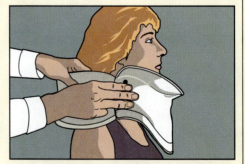

▲ **2.** Measure the collar. Make sure that the chin piece will not lift the patient's chin and hyperextend the neck. Make sure the collar is not too small and tight, which would act as a constricting band.

STIFNECK® SELECT™ Collar–Seated Patient

FIRST take BSI precautions.

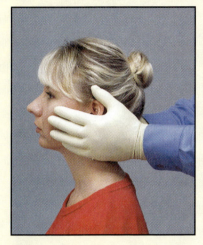

▲ **1.** Stabilize the head and neck from the rear.

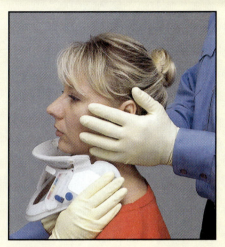

▲ **2.** Properly angle the collar for placement

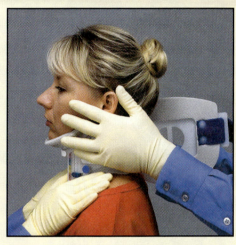

▲ **3.** Position the collar bottom.

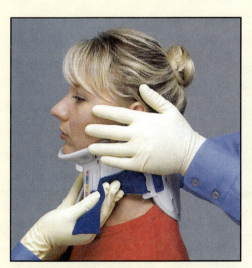

▲ **4.** Set the collar in place around the neck.

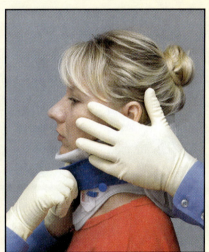

▲ **5.** Secure the collar.

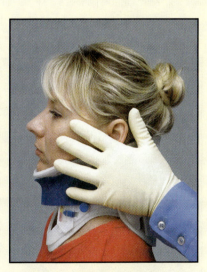

▲ **5.** Maintain manual stabilization of the head and neck

(continued)

STIFNECK® SELECT™ Collar–Supine Patient

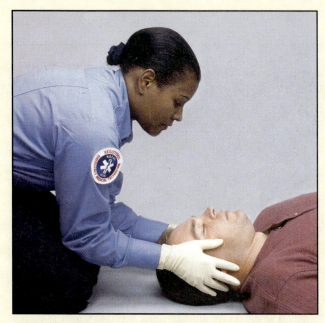

▲ **1.** Kneel at the patient's head, and stabilize the head and neck.

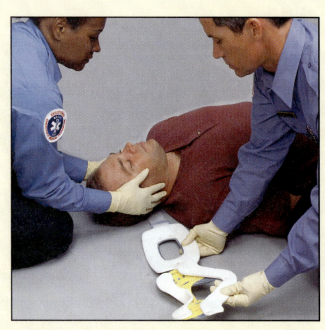

▲ **2.** Set the collar in place.

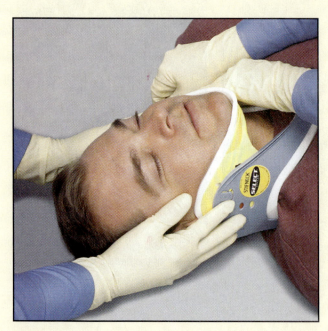

▲ **3.** Secure the collar.

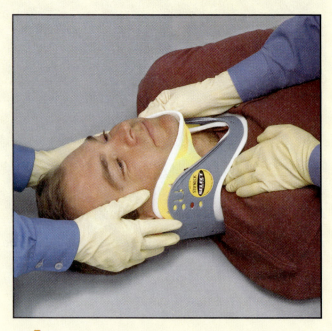

▲ **4.** Continue to manually stabilize the head and neck.

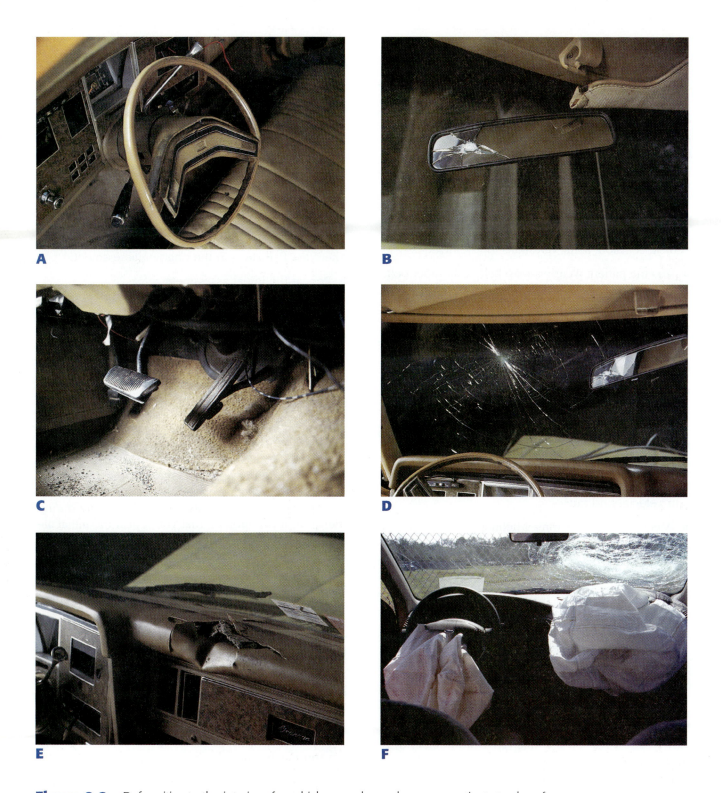

Figure 8-2 Deformities to the interior of a vehicle may show where your patient struck surfaces, revealing mechanisms of injury.

detecting changes later. Be sure to determine the patient's respirations, pulse, skin (color, temperature, and condition), and blood pressure. As appropriate, assess the pupils.

SAMPLE History

Although a trauma patient has an injury and not an illness, there is still important information you can gain by way of a SAMPLE history. Remember, the patient may have a medical condition that affects the way you or the emergency department staff manage the patient. You should also find out more about how the patient was injured. If the patient was in a motor-vehicle collision, some questions to ask include:

- Was the patient wearing a lap belt, a shoulder belt, or both?
- Was there any loss of consciousness?
- Did the patient strike the inside of the vehicle?

Examination of the vehicle will lead to answers to the following questions (Figure 8-2 on p. 138):

- Is there deformity of the steering wheel?
- Is there deformity of the pedals, mirror, gear shift, or other items inside the vehicle?
- Is the windshield cracked or spider-webbed?
- Did an airbag deploy?

If the patient was on a motorcycle, bicycle, or all-terrain vehicle, find out:

- Was the patient wearing a helmet?
- If there is a helmet but it is not on the patient when you arrive, who removed it?

Detailed Physical Exam

Generally, the best place to perform the detailed physical exam is en route to a hospital.

There are two other ways in which the detailed physical exam differs from the rapid trauma assessment. First, the detailed physical exam includes examination not only of the areas you assessed in the rapid trauma assessment, but also of the face, ears, eyes, nose, and mouth. Second, it is done more slowly, allowing you the time to be thorough and to locate injuries.

As you perform the detailed physical exam, you may come across injuries or signs that you must treat right away. For example, if you find a broken or dislodged tooth in the patient's mouth, you should remove it immediately so that it does not become a cause of airway obstruction. You might also find a reason to administer oxygen when performing this part of patient assessment. Do not wait until the detailed physical exam is complete for instituting these important measures.

Other findings will guide your treatment of the patient, but it can be delegated to others (e.g., dressing a non-bleeding wound) or carried out after you have finished the physical exam (e.g., splinting a lower-leg injury).

Whenever you examine a patient and to the extent possible, always explain to the patient what you are going to do, particularly if your actions will cause some discomfort or pain. This will help calm the patient and reassure him or her that you know what you are doing.

Ongoing Assessment

There are five steps in the ongoing assessment:

- Repeat the initial assessment.
- Re-establish the priority of the patient.
- Reassess and record vital signs.
- Reassess injuries found previously.
- Check the interventions you have instituted.

For the trauma patient with a significant mechanism of injury, an intervention check might include verifying that oxygen continues to flow into the non-rebreather mask, the straps on the backboard are snug without compromising respiration, and any splints you applied are secure without limiting circulation. For the unstable patient, ongoing assessment should be repeated every 5 minutes.

Although most patients do not deteriorate during transport, it is important that you repeat the initial assessment in order to detect signs of life-threatening changes. Be sure to continue to inform and reassure the patient. You may have been on lots of EMS calls, but the patient probably has not.

No Significant Mechanism of Injury

Most trauma patients are not critically injured. In these cases, you have a little more time to assess them and provide emergency care. However, it is important to keep a high index of suspicion. When in doubt, treat the patient as though he or she has a significant mechanism of injury.

Initial Assessment

The initial assessment consists of the same six steps as before: general impression, mental status, airway, breathing, circulation, and patient priority. When there is no significant mechanism of injury, most patients will not display life-threatening problems. However, do not be lulled into a false sense of security. Evaluate every patient for threats to life as soon as you can.

Focused History and Physical Exam—Trauma

In situations where there is no significant mechanism of injury, your focused history and physical exam are truly focused. You assess the areas the patient has injured and also areas you believe may have been injured based on your evaluation of the mechanism of injury. Since there is no significant mechanism of injury, there is no need to do a complete head-to-toe physical exam. Instead, the patient's complaints will lead you to the areas that were injured.

Search for the same wounds and signs that you looked for in the physical exam of the patient with a significant mechanism of injury (DCAP-BTLS). As part of your focused history and physical exam, also take baseline vital signs and gather a SAMPLE history.

Ongoing Assessment

If the patient is stable and does not have a significant mechanism of injury, you should perform an ongoing assessment at least every 15 minutes. This includes repeating the initial assessment, re-establishing the priority of the patient, reassessing and recording vital signs, reassessing injuries, and checking the interventions you have instituted.

CHAPTER REVIEW

SUMMARY

- To help the patient with critical injuries, you must quickly find and treat threats to life.

- Perform scene size-up first.

- When you do the initial assessment, determine whether there is a significant mechanism of injury (MOI).

- If there is no significant MOI, assess areas the patient complains about and which the MOI suggests might be injured, take vital signs, gather a SAMPLE history, and perform ongoing assessment every 15 minutes.

- If there is a significant MOI, perform a rapid trauma exam, take vital signs, gather a SAMPLE history, immobilize the patient in the supine position and transport. As time allows, perform a detailed physical exam, then ongoing assessment every 5 minutes.

REVIEW QUESTIONS

1. A significant mechanism of injury for a child would be:
   a. a skateboard fall.
   b. a fall of more than 10 feet.
   c. a low-speed vehicle collision.
   d. scissors cuts to the arm.

2. The "A" in DCAP-BTLS stands for:
   a. acne.
   b. allergies.
   c. abrasions.
   d. anaphylaxis.

3. For a trauma patient with a significant mechanism of injury, perform an ongoing assessement every _____ minutes.
   a. 2
   b. 5
   c. 10
   d. 15

REVIEW QUESTIONS *continued*

4. Provide ventilations with high-concentration oxygen for an unresponsive patient breathing less than ______ times a minute.

a. 8

b. 10

c. 12

d. 16

5. For a trauma patient with a significant mechanism of injury, the best time to perform a detailed physical exam is:

a. before the SAMPLE history.

b. before the vital signs.

c. en route to the hospital.

d. after establishing patient priority.

WEB MEDIC

Visit Brady's *Essentials of Emergency Care* web site for direct web links. At **www.prenhall.com/limmer,** you will find information related to the following Chapter 8 topics:

- Kinematics of injury
- Trauma
- Athletic injuries
- Whiplash injuries
- Injury facts

Correlates with the U.S. DOT "EMT-Basic National Standard Curriculum" Lessons 3-3 through 3-6

ASSESSMENT OF THE MEDICAL PATIENT

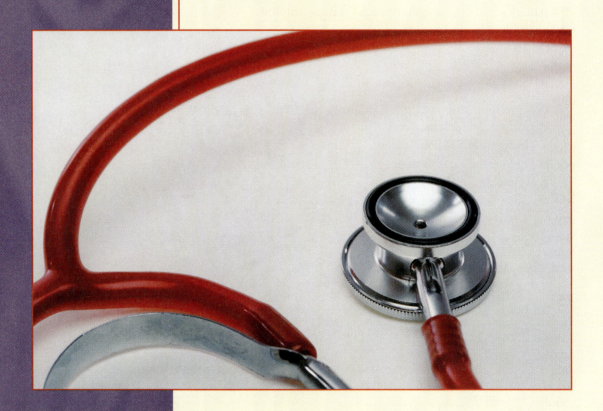

ESSENTIAL ELECTRONIC EXTRAS

CD ESSENTIALS

For preview and review of chapter material, see the student CD-ROM for

- Pretest
- Chapter quizzes
- Posttest

WEB ESSENTIALS

For additional review and enrichment, visit www.prenhall.com/limmer for

- Interactive student quizzes
- Links to online EMS resources
- Online case studies
- Audio glossary

Many of the calls you will respond to as an EMT-B will be for medical patients or patients who are not injured. After sizing up the scene and performing the initial assessment, you will assess medical patients in different ways depending upon whether they are responsive or unresponsive. The EMT-B will be able to administer medications to some and to assist others in taking their own medications. In these cases, there are specific questions to ask that will determine whether the medication is the appropriate intervention. Since many things can be going on at the same time with any particular patient, the obvious treatment may not always be the best or only treatment. Determining this accurately depends on an appropriate assessment that is done well.

ASSESSING MEDICAL PATIENTS

The elements of the scene size-up are the same for medical and trauma patients, but the application of those elements is frequently different because of the different kinds of scenes or environments they are usually associated with. How to perform the scene size-up and the initial assessment is discussed in Chapter 7. There are, however, some significant points that should be stressed.

Scene Safety

Pay special attention to the presence of fighting, loud voices, alcohol and other drugs, weapons, and household pets. Follow the instructions of working at a crime scene described in Chapter 7.

BSI Review

In an efficient EMS system with well-trained dispatchers, you may be able to predict the need (or lack of need) for donning personal protective equipment (PPE) before entering the scene. However, you should always carry sufficient PPE to protect yourself should the information you received be inaccurate or should the circumstances at the scene change.

Nature of Illness

Good dispatchers can improve your efficiency in this area as well. Use the dispatch information regarding the nature of illness to determine the equipment you bring to the scene, but keep in mind there are some calls where the caller gives the dispatcher inaccurate information. Keep the nature of illness from dispatch in mind, but stay open to the possibility that the patient's problem is not what you were told. Avoid tunnel vision and evaluate the nature of illness yourself.

Number of Patients and Needed Resources

At medical scenes, the number of patients is usually obvious, but many an experienced EMT-B has responded to a call for difficulty breathing or chest pain and found a spouse in worse shape than the person EMS was called to assist. Keep this possibility in mind, particularly with elderly patients.

THE RESPONSIVE MEDICAL PATIENT

When you assess a medical patient, you get most of your information from the patient's history and vital signs. You can usually get this information only from an individual who is able to communicate with you. For the purpose of learning to assess a medical patient, this patient is referred to as "responsive."

Since the individual who cannot communicate with you also cannot give you a history, assessing this patient will necessarily be different. The assessment

CORE CONCEPTS

In this chapter, you will learn about the following topics:

- How to perform a focused history and physical exam for a medical patient

- The differences in assessment of responsive and unresponsive medical patients

- How to perform an ongoing assessment for a medical patient

DOT OBJECTIVES

✓ **Knowledge**

☐ **1.** Assess nature of illness. (p. 143)

☐ **2.** Perform an initial patient assessment and provide care based on initial assessment findings. (pp. 144–145, 148–149)

- Summarize the reasons for forming a general impression of the patient. (pp. 144, 149)

☐ **3.** Explain the reason for prioritizing a patient for care and transport. (pp. 144, 149)

☐ **4.** Perform a history and physical examination focusing on the specific injury and provide care based on assessment findings. (pp. 144–145, 149)

- Discuss the reason for performing a focused history and physical examination. (pp. 144–145, 149)

- Differentiate between the history and physical examination that are performed for responsive patients with no known prior history and responsive patients with a known history. (pp. 144–145, 148)

- Differentiate between the assessment that is performed for a patient who is unresponsive or has an altered mental status and other medical

of the unresponsive medical patient is described later in this chapter. See Table 9-1 for a summary of the assessment of mental status, airway, breathing, and circulation in adults, children, and infants.

Initial Assessment

Follow the steps described in Chapter 7 when performing an initial assessment. Your general impression will give you a good idea of how much time you can spend at the scene. A responsive medical patient will be alert and able to answer questions. Airway and breathing are usually easy to assess in these patients. Keep in mind that a patient with a respiratory rate over 24 breaths per minute should receive high-concentration oxygen by nonrebreather mask. Checking circulation in these patients typically includes looking for external bleeding, palpating a peripheral pulse, and determining perfusion status as described in Chapter 7. Priority responsive medical patients include those with:

- A poor general impression
- Inability to follow commands
- Difficulty breathing
- Shock (hypoperfusion)
- Complicated childbirth
- Chest pain with systolic blood pressure less than 100 mm
- Uncontrolled bleeding
- Severe pain anywhere

Focused History and Physical Exam— Responsive Medical Patient

Once immediate threats to life have been detected and corrected, gather information that will determine the interventions you must provide and that will assist the emergency department staff in preparation for the patient's arrival. The four elements of the EMT-B focused history and physical exam for a responsive medical patient are OPQRST history, SAMPLE history, physical exam, and baseline vital signs (Skill Summary 9-1).

OPQRST History

The history of the present illness is also known as the **OPQRST history** because it serves as a reminder of the information that must be obtained. The OPQRST history allows you to describe the patient's chief complaint in some detail:

O — Onset. What were you doing when the episode started?

P — Provokes. Did anything bring on this episode?

Q — Quality. What kind of pain are you having?

R — Radiation. Does the pain spread anywhere?

S — Severity. How bad is the pain? How does it compare to previous episodes?

T — Time. When did the episode start? Has the pain changed since it started?

OPQRST is very useful for conditions characterized by pain but, as you may have discovered, it needs to be modified when a patient's chief complaint does not involve pain. For example, when interviewing a patient with shortness of breath, it does not make sense to ask the patient whether or not the shortness of breath radiates anywhere.

Important principles to remember when interviewing a patient include:

- **Position yourself properly.** You should be close to the patient and at about the same height without being so close that the patient feels "closed in."
- **Introduce yourself in a calm, confident, and reassuring manner.** Although emergencies may be routine to you, chances are this is not the case for the patient. Reassuring the patient and behaving

patients requiring assessment. (pp. 148–149)

☐ **5.** Perform on-going assessments and provide care based on assessment findings. (pp. 148, 149)

- Discuss the reasons for repeating the initial assessment as part of the ongoing assessment. (pp. 148, 149)

- Describe the components of the ongoing assessment. (pp. 148, 149)

✔ **Attitude**

☐ **6.** Explain the value of performing each component of the prehospital patient assessment. (pp. 143–144, 148–149)

✔ **Skills**

☐ **7.** Demonstrate the steps in performing a focused history and physical on a medical and trauma patient. (pp. 144–145, 148–149)

Table 9-1 Initial Assessment of Adults, Children, and Infants

	Adults	Children 1–6 yrs	Infants to 1 yr
Mental Status	AVPU: Is patient alert? Responsive to verbal stimulus? Unresponsive? If alert, is patient oriented to person, place, and time?	Same as for adults.	If not alert, shout as a verbal stimulus, flick feet as a painful stimulus. (Crying would be infant's response.)
Airway	Trauma: jaw-thrust. Medical: head-tilt chin-lift. Consider oro- or nasopharyngeal airway, suctioning.	Same as for adults, but see Chapter 6 for special pediatric airway techniques. If performing head-tilt chin-lift, do so without hyperextending the neck.	Same as for children, but see Chapter 6 for special pediatric airway techniques.
Breathing	If respiratory arrest, perform rescue breathing. If depressed mental status and inadequate breathing (slower than 8 per minute), ventilate with BVM and 100% oxygen. If alert and respirations are more than 24 per minute, give 100% oxygen by nonrebreather mask.	Same as for adults, but normal rates for children are faster than for adults. Parent may have to hold oxygen mask to reduce child's fear of mask.	Same as for children, but normal rates for infants are faster.
Circulation	Assess skin, radial pulse, bleeding. If cardiac arrest, perform CPR. See Chapter 21 for how to treat for bleeding and shock.	Assess skin, radial pulse, bleeding, capillary refill. If cardiac arrest, perform CPR. See Chapter 21 for how to treat for bleeding and shock.	Assess skin, brachial pulse, bleeding, capillary refill. If cardiac arrest, perform CPR. See Chapter 21 for how to treat for bleeding and shock.

FIRST take BSI precautions.

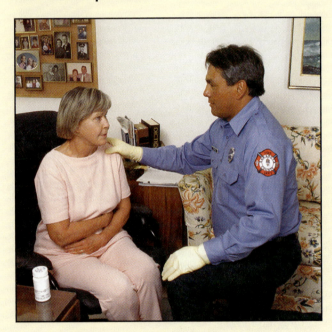

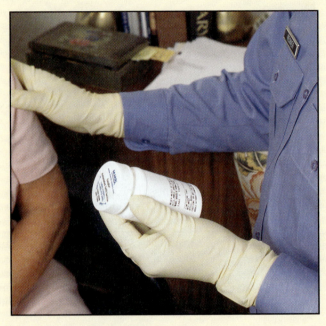

▲ **1. HISTORY OF PRESENT ILLNESS.** Ask the "OPQRST" questions:

Onset
Provokes
Quality
Radiation
Severity
Time

▲ **2. SAMPLE HISTORY.** Ask the SAMPLE questions:

Signs and symptoms
Allergies
Medications
Pertinent past history
Last oral intake
Events leading to the illness

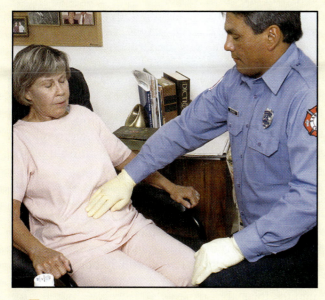

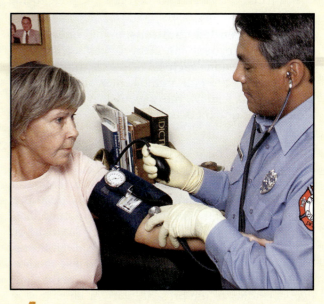

▲ **3.** **Focused Physical Exam.** Perform a quick assessment of affected body part or system:

Head
Neck
Chest
Abdomen
Pelvis
Extremities
Posterior

▲ **4.** **Vital Signs.** Assess the patient's baseline vital signs:

Respiration
Pulse
Skin color, temperature, condition (and capillary refill in infants and children)
Pupils
Blood pressure

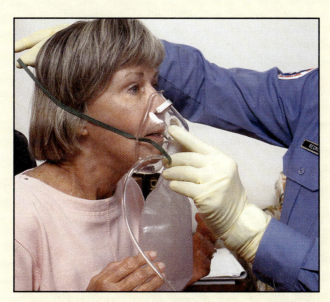

▲ **5.** **Interventions and Transport.** Perform interventions as needed, transport the patient, and contact on-line medical direction as needed.

in a calm, professional manner does wonders in establishing a rapport.

- **Ask how the patient would like to be addressed.** Treat patients with respect by asking them how they would like you to address them. Many of your patients will be older than you, some considerably so. Many elderly patients feel comfortable being on a first-name basis with EMT-Bs, but some prefer being addressed as "Mrs.," "Ms.," or "Mr."
- **Ask open-ended questions.** Avoid questions to which the patient can answer "yes" or "no." By asking questions such as "Where is the pain?" instead of "Is the pain in the center of your chest?" you avoid leading the patient into saying what you want or expect to hear.

SAMPLE History

The SAMPLE history is not exactly the same as the OPQRST history, but they have a lot in common. The "S" for signs and symptoms really acts as a bridge between the history of the present illness (OPQRST) and the past medical history (AMPLE). As you may recall from Chapter 7, the SAMPLE history includes: signs and symptoms, allergies, medications, past medical history, last oral intake, and events leading to the present injury or illness.

Physical Exam

In the responsive medical patient, there is typically little useful information an EMT-B can gain through a physical examination. To a certain extent, this is not unique to EMS but also true in other areas of health care for the medical patient. The history frequently determines what interventions you should provide. There are times, though, when it may be appropriate to examine certain areas based on the patient's chief complaint. For example, if your patient is complaining of abdominal pain, you should gently palpate the four quadrants of the abdomen, looking for tenderness, rigidity, and pulsations.

If your patient has chest pain or shortness of breath, you may wish—or local protocols may direct you—to assess for neck vein distention, ankle edema, and abnormal breath sounds. (If your local protocols direct you to describe abnormal breath sounds, you should have training in this technique and you should review it frequently.) Evaluation of neck veins, ankles, and breath sounds will not change your treatment. However, some systems may wish EMT-Bs to obtain this evaluation for other reasons, such as whether or not to request ALS backup. Follow local protocols.

As appropriate, assess the following areas in responsive medical patients: head, neck, chest, abdomen, pelvis, extremities, and posterior aspect of the patient. (See Chapter 8 for a description of the assessment.)

Baseline Vital Signs

As you do in any assessment, record the patient's pulse, blood pressure, respiration, skin condition, and, as appropriate, pupils. This first set of vital signs will provide a valuable baseline against which to compare later sets. Even if they don't change your management of the patient, they can be valuable to the emergency department staff who will care for the patient after you leave the hospital.

Ongoing Assessment

Your job of assessing the patient does not stop after you have performed appropriate interventions. Keeping a close eye on the patient is an important part of your continuing care, too.

There are five parts to the ongoing assessment: repeating the initial assessment, re-establishing patient priority, reassessing and recording vital signs, repeating a focused assessment regarding the patient's complaint or injuries, and checking interventions you have administered (Skill Summary 9-2).

Perform an ongoing assessment at least every 15 minutes for stable patients and every 5 minutes for unstable patients. You should record the results of your ongoing assessment as soon as possible so that you have an accurate record of changes in the patient's condition that allow you to detect trends.

Repeating the initial assessment means reassessing the patient's mental status, maintaining an open airway, monitoring breathing for rate and quality, reassessing the pulse for rate and quality, and monitoring skin color and temperature. After gathering this information, you can determine whether or not the patient's condition has changed in a way that should alter the priority of the patient.

Repeating vital signs can also tell you if you need to alter your treatment of the patient. In addition, you should reassess the patient's chief complaint. For example, if the patient is having chest pain, ask how the pain is and if it has changed.

Finally, you should check the interventions you have performed. If you have started oxygen, make sure it is still flowing. If the bag on the nonrebreather mask is not filling adequately, make sure the tubing is still attached, the flowmeter is set at the appropriate rate, and there is still oxygen in the tank.

Whenever you check interventions, try to take a fresh look at the patient. Attempt to see the patient as though you had never seen him or her before. This may help you to more objectively evaluate the adequacy of your interventions and adjust them as necessary.

THE UNRESPONSIVE MEDICAL PATIENT

Evaluating an unresponsive patient is more challenging than evaluating a patient who can communicate with you. Since the history of a medical patient can give you more information than a physical exam, it is important that you get one. A responsive patient can give you a history. For the unresponsive patient, you must gather all of the useful information you can find in other ways. This means performing a rapid physical exam and getting as much history as possible from family members or bystanders (Skill Summary 9-3).

Initial Assessment

Your goals in the initial assessment of both unresponsive and responsive medical patients are the same: find and detect immediate threats to life and guide further assessment and treatment. However, in the case of an unresponsive patient, completing an initial assessment will frequently take longer because of the additional steps you must take to secure and maintain an airway.

General Impression

As before, look at the environment and the patient, noting whether the patient is ill or injured and determining the patient's gender and approximate age.

Mental Status

You will not find an unresponsive patient who gets an "A" on the AVPU scale. At best, the patient may respond to verbal stimuli. When describing the mental status of a patient like this, it is important to describe both the stimulus and the patient's response to it. For example, the patient might moan in response to a painful stimulus.

Airway and Breathing

When trauma has been ruled out, open the medical patient's airway with the head-tilt chin-lift maneuver. It should relieve any snoring that is the result of the tongue partially obstructing the airway. Also insert an oral or nasal airway.

Then determine if the patient's breathing is adequate. (You reviewed this in Chapter 6.) This is a skill that is very important in the initial assessment of an unresponsive patient. After seeing a number of patients over the years, an EMT-B can easily be lulled into a false sense of security. Most unresponsive patients you see will be breathing adequately, but you must quickly find the ones who are not and begin ventilating them immediately.

Circulation

Evaluating circulation in responsive and unresponsive patients is the same. Check the radial pulse (brachial pulse in patients under one year of age) for rate and quality. Look for and correct external hemorrhage. Check the patient's skin color, temperature, and condition.

Identification of Priority Patients

Any patient who is unresponsive is a high-priority patient. Remember, the patient's airway is at risk. There are many possible causes of an altered mental status, some of which can be life threatening.

Focused History and Physical Exam— Unresponsive Medical Patient

Since the patient cannot give you a history, get information in other ways. The best sources are a physical exam of the patient and a history from a family member or friend.

Rapid Physical Exam

Examine the patient by inspecting (looking at) and palpating (pressing or touching) these areas: the head, neck, chest, abdomen, pelvis, extremities, and the posterior aspect of the body. Remove any clothing covering the area you are to examine so that you can get a good look at it. Replace clothing after you have finished examining an area.

Baseline Vital Signs

With so little history available, vital signs become even more important than usual. Be sure to assess respirations, pulse, skin, pupils, and blood pressure. Before going any further in your assessment, position the patient to protect the airway. Turn the patient on his or her side so that secretions can drain out of the mouth.

SAMPLE History

Since the patient is unable to give you a history, quickly interview family members or bystanders before you leave the scene. They may have valuable information the emergency department staff would not be able to obtain.

Ongoing Assessment

Check the same things in the ongoing assessment of the unresponsive patient as you would for a responsive patient. However, pay special attention to the unresponsive patient's airway.

FIRST take BSI precautions.

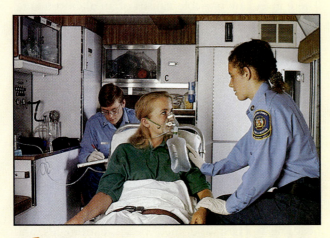

▲ **1.** Repeat the initial assessment. At this time, reevaluate patient priority.

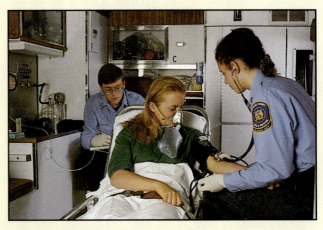

▲ **2.** Reassess and record vital signs.

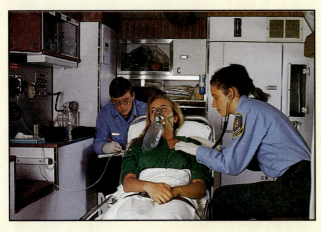

▲ **3.** Repeat focused assessment.

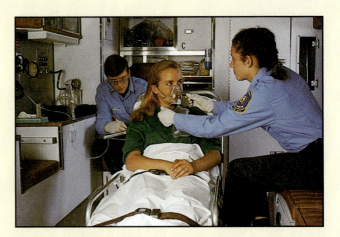

▲ **4.** Check interventions.

FIRST take BSI precautions.

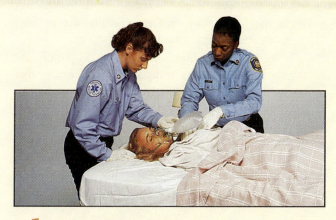

▲ **1.** **RAPID PHYSICAL EXAM.** Perform a rapid assessment of the entire body:

Head
Neck
Chest
Abdomen
Pelvis
Extremities
Posterior

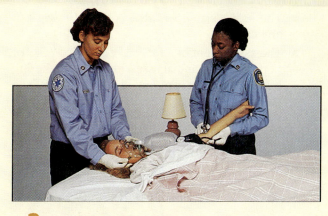

▲ **2.** **VITAL SIGNS.** Assess the patient's baseline vital signs:

Respiration
Skin color, temperature, condition (and capillary refill in infants and children)
Pupils
Blood pressure

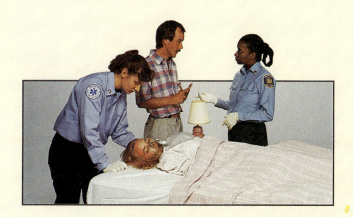

▲ **3.** **SAMPLE HISTORY.** Interview family and bystanders to get as much information as possible about the patient's problem:

Signs and symptoms
Allergies
Medications
Pertinent past history
Last oral intake
Events leading to the illness

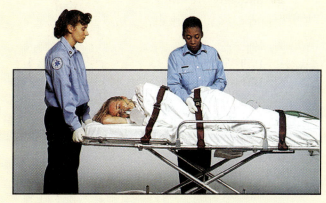

▲ **4.** **INTERVENTIONS AND TRANSPORT.** Contact on-line medical direction as needed, perform interventions as needed, transport the patient.

SUMMARY

- The scene size-up is always the first stage of any call.

- The assessment of a medical patient consists of performing an initial assessment and gathering a history of the present illness (OPQRST), a past medical history (SAMPLE), and a set of vital signs.

- When assessing a responsive medical patient, you can usually get most of your information from the history the patient gives you and from the patient's vital signs.

- Evaluating an unresponsive medical patient includes performing a rapid physical exam and getting as much history as possible from family members or bystanders.

- Performing an ongoing assessment once every 15 minutes for a stable patient and at least once every 5 minutes for an unstable one.

REVIEW QUESTIONS

1. Which of the following does NOT describe a priority responsive medical patient?
   a. chest pain with systolic blood pressure over 110 mm
   b. shock
   c. complicated childbirth
   d. difficulty breathing

2. The "P" in OPQRST stands for:
   a. palliates.
   b. projects.
   c. provokes.
   d. perfuses.

3. Which pulse would you use to check circulation in patients under 1 year old?
   a. radial
   b. tibial
   c. carotid
   d. brachial

REVIEW QUESTIONS *continued*

4. Which of the following steps would you perform first, after initial assessment, with an unresponsive medical patient?
   a. SAMPLE history
   b. rapid physical exam
   c. OPQRST history
   d. baseline vital signs

5. Which of the following steps would you perform first, after initial assessment, with a responsive medical patient?
   a. SAMPLE history
   b. rapid physical exam
   c. OPQRST history
   d. baseline vital signs

WEB MEDIC

Visit Brady's *Essentials of Emergency Care* web site for direct web links. At **www.prenhall.com/limmer,** you will find information related to the following Chapter 9 topics:
- Cardiovascular disease
- Altered mental status
- Syncope
- the Glasgow Coma Score
- the American College of Emergency Physicians

Chapter Ten

ASSESSMENT OF PEDIATRIC AND GERIATRIC PATIENTS

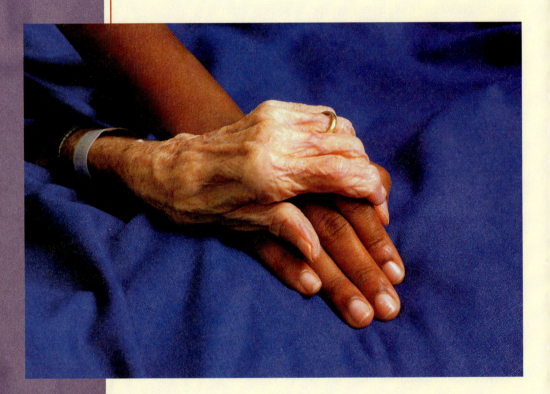

ESSENTIAL ELECTRONIC EXTRAS

CD ESSENTIALS

For preview and review of chapter material, see the student CD-ROM for

- Pretest
- Chapter quizzes
- Posttest

WEB ESSENTIALS

For additional review and enrichment, visit www.prenhall.com/limmer for

- Interactive student quizzes
- Links to online EMS resources
- Online case studies
- Audio glossary

Assessing children and older people is similar to assessing other patients. When your patient is at one of the extremes of age, though, you will need to make some adjustments in how you proceed. Because there are important differences in anatomy, this is especially true about the assessment of infants and small children.

THE PEDIATRIC PATIENT

Differences in Anatomy and Physiology

The Head

Up until about 6 years of age, the heads of children are proportionately larger than those of adults. This disproportionate size increases the potential for head trauma. For example, when children are struck by an automobile, they fly, like a javelin, heavier end (the child's head) first. This larger head size also increases the risk of airway obstruction in the unresponsive supine pediatric patient because the large occiput flexes the neck. As a result, when you must immobilize the spine of a patient in this age group, you should pad behind the shoulders and torso to prevent flexion of the neck.

A baby is born with a skull that has not yet fully fused, which allows for override of the cranial bones so the baby's head can pass through the birth canal. The membranous spaces at the anterior and posterior junctions of these unfused cranial bones are called **fontanels,** or "soft spots." Cranial bones fuse over the posterior fontanel between the ages of 4 and 6 months, but it takes 18 months for bones to fuse and close the anterior fontanel. These "soft spots" are usually flat and soft while the infant is quiet. However, a sunken fontanel may indicate dehydration; a bulging fontanel may indicate that the infant is crying or has increased intracranial pressure.

This importance is highlighted in children because of certain anatomic factors. Remember these key differences (Figure 10-1):

- The mouths and noses of infants and children are smaller and more easily obstructed.
- Their tongues are proportionately larger and take up more space in the mouth.
- Nasal congestion makes it difficult for them to breathe. (Both newborns and infants are obligate nose breathers.)
- The smallest diameter of their airways is located at the cricoid ring in the trachea. (The adult's is smallest at the vocal cords.) A child's cricoid ring forms a physiologic cuff. Due to the diameter of the opening of the cricoid ring, an uncuffed tube is used when an endotracheal tube is inserted in a small child. Since the trachea is relatively narrower than in adults, it is more easily obstructed. This is why "blind" finger sweeps are never used in an infant or child. You could easily push an obstruction further down the narrow trachea.
- Infants and young children have a softer, more flexible trachea than do adults. Hyperextension or flexion of the neck can actually cause airway obstruction. Therefore, as mentioned earlier, place a folded towel under the shoulders and torso of an infant or toddler to keep the airway in a neutral position (Figure 10-2).

PRECEPTOR PEARL

When you are guiding a new EMT-B in the assessment of an infant, be sure to tell the EMT-B to palpate the fontanel gently with the tips of the fingers to avoid inflicting or worsening injury.

The Respiratory System

Just as in adult patients, a patent airway is the highest priority for pediatric patients.

CORE CONCEPTS

In this chapter, you will learn about the following topics:

- Differences in anatomy and physiology between children and adults

- Differences in assessing the injured or ill child

- Special concerns when evaluating the elderly patient

☐ **1.** Perform an initial patient assessment and provide care based on initial assessment findings. (pp. 157–159)

- Summarize the reasons for forming a general impression of the patient. (pp. 157, 159, 162)

- Discuss the methods of assessing altered mental status. (pp. 159, 162)

- Discuss methods of assessing the airway in the adult, child, and infant patient. (pp. 155, 159, 162)

- Describe methods used for assessing if a patient is breathing. (pp. 159, 162)

- Differentiate between a patient with adequate and inadequate breathing. (pp. 159, 162)

- Explain the reason for prioritizing a patient for care and transport. (pp. 159, 162–163)

☐ **2.** Perform a history and physical examination focusing on the specific injury and provide care based on assessment findings. (pp. 159–161, 162–163)

- Discuss the reason for performing a focused history and physical examination. (pp. 159–161, 162–163)

☐ **3.** Perform a detailed physical examination and provide care based on assessment findings. (pp. 160–161, 163)

Airway structures are smaller and more easily obstructed.

Cricoid cartilage is less rigid and less developed.

Tongue takes up more space in pharynx.

Trachea is narrower.

Nose and mouth are smaller.

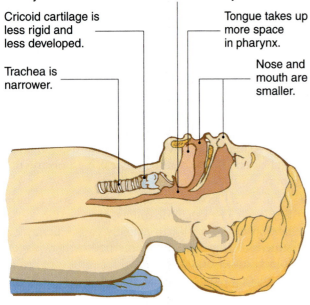

Trachea   Tongue   Nose

Cricoid cartilage

Figure 10-1   Adult and child airways, compared.

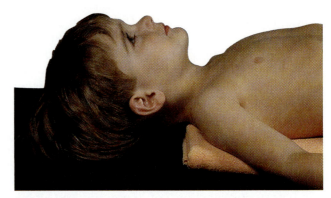

Figure 10-2   To keep the airway aligned, place a folded towel under the shoulders and torso.

■ Since the chest wall is softer, infants and children depend more on the diaphragm for breathing. Therefore, respiratory muscle fatigue occurs more rapidly.

Chest and Abdomen

The muscles and bones in the child's chest and the muscles of the abdomen are not well developed and therefore provide only minimal protection for the underlying organs. Since the chest wall is more elastic, when a child in respiratory distress breathes, the movement of the ribs, sternum, and intercostal muscles makes a dramatic and easily observable general impression. Since young children are abdominal breathers who rely heavily on the movement of the diaphragm, injuries to the chest or abdomen can decrease tidal volume (the amount of inspired air). This is one reason why the abdominal section of the PASG is no longer recommended for use with children.

- State the areas of the body that are evaluated during the detailed physical examination. (pp. 160–161, 163)
- Explain what additional care should be provided while performing the detailed physical examination. (pp. 160–161, 163)

☐ 4. Perform on-going assessments and provide care based on assessment findings. (pp. 161, 163)

- Discuss the reasons for repeating the initial assessment as part of the ongoing assessment. (pp. 161, 163)
- Describe the components of the ongoing assessment. (pp. 161, 163)

✔ **Attitude**

☐ 5. Recognize and respect the feelings that patients might experience during assessment. (pp. 157, 158–159, 161, 162–163)

✔ **Skills**

☐ 6. Demonstrate the steps in performing a focused history and physical on a medical and trauma patient. (pp. 159–161, 162–163)

☐ 7. Demonstrate the skills involved in performing a detailed physical examination. (pp. 160–161, 163)

☐ 8. Demonstrate the skills involved in performing an ongoing assessment. (pp. 161, 163)

PRECEPTOR PEARL

After a child is struck by a vehicle, there may be tire marks on the chest. Since a child's chest is so flexible, there may be no rib fractures. Remind the new EMT-B that the lack of external injury is deceptive and there is a significant risk of contusions and other injuries to the underlying lung and heart that could be devastating.

The Skin

Since a child's body surface is larger in proportion to body mass, children are more prone to heat loss through the skin. Whenever small children are taken out in the cold, they should be wrapped in a blanket. Their heads also should be covered since they lose so much heat from their proportionately larger heads.

The method of calculating the total body surface covered by a burn is different for children, too (see Chapter 22). The head accounts for a larger percentage of body surface area, the legs for a smaller percentage. Some EMT-Bs carry a pocket guide with the pediatric "Rule of Nines" or use the "Rule of Palm" method, which indicates that the size of a child's palm is equal to one percent of the body surface area.

Approaching the Pediatric Patient

Determining a Pediatric Patient's Age

Physicians usually consider children up to the age of 15 to be pediatric patients. Yet it is not unusual for pediatricians to treat young adults throughout their college years and beyond. The American Heart Association defines "infant" as any patient up to one year old, and "child" as any patient from 1 to 8 years old.

This age grouping is based on physical development and the procedures recommended for rescue breathing and CPR.

In emergency care, the following age groups are used to classify children and are based upon anatomical and emotional development:

- **Newborn**—birth to 6 months
- **Infant**—6 months to one year
- **Toddler**—1 to 3 years
- **Preschool**—3 to 6 years
- **School age**—6 to 12 years
- **Adolescent**—12 to 18 years

Tips for Assessing Each Age Group

Since a child's age is not always accessible or evident, you should practice determining children's ages based upon their physical and developmental characteristics. Table 10-1 should be helpful in the assessment and management of pediatric patients in each age group. Keep a card handy with normal pediatric vital signs, weights, and other information you may need in treating pediatric patients (Table 10-2).

Remember, putting the child at ease is an important part of the emergency care you provide. Always kneel or sit at the child's eye level (Figure 10-3). Let the child see your face, and make eye contact without staring at the child.

General Principles of Assessing the Pediatric Patient

Scene Size-Up and Initial Assessment

Scene size-up for pediatric patients is very much like scene size-up for adults.

The initial assessment is very similar, but there are a few things you should keep in mind. When forming a general impression, notice how the child interacts

Table 10-1   Developmental Characteristics of Infants and Children

Age Group	Characteristics	Assessment and Care Strategies
Newborns and infants—birth to 1 year 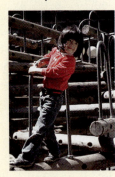	• Infants do not like to be separated from their parents. • There is minimal stranger anxiety. • Infants are used to being undressed but like to feel warm, physically and emotionally. • The younger infant follows movements with his or her eyes. • The older infant is more active, developing a personality. • They do not want to be "suffocated" by an oxygen mask.	• Have the parent hold the infant during assessment. • Be sure to keep the infant warm—warm your hands and stethoscope before touching the infant. • It may be best to observe the infant's breathing from a distance, noting the rise and fall of the chest, the level of activity, and color. • Examine the heart and lungs first and head last. This is perceived as less threatening to infants and therefore less likely to start them crying. • A pediatric nonrebreather mask may be held near the face to provide "blow-by" oxygen.
Toddlers— 1 to 3 years 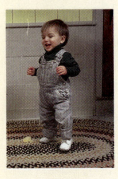	• Toddlers do not like to be touched or separated from their parents. • Toddlers may believe that their illness is a punishment for being bad. • Unlike infants, they do not like having clothing removed. • They frighten easily, overreact, have a fear of needles and pain. • Toddlers may understand more than they communicate. • They begin to assert their independence. • They do not want to be "suffocated" by an oxygen mask.	• Have a parent hold the toddler during assessment. • Assure the child that he or she was not bad. • Remove an article of clothing, examine, and then replace the garment. • Examine in a trunk-to-head approach to help build confidence. (Touching the head first may be frightening.) • Explain what you are going to do in terms the toddler can understand (taking the blood pressure becomes a squeeze or a hug on the arm). • Offer the comfort of a favorite toy. • Consider giving the toddler a choice: "Do you want me to look at your belly or your chest first?" • A pediatric nonrebreather mask may be held near the face to provide "blow-by" oxygen.
Preschool— 3 to 6 years	• Preschoolers do not like to be touched or separated from their parents. • They are modest and do not like their clothing removed. • Preschoolers may believe that their illness is a punishment for being bad. • Preschoolers have a fear of blood, pain, and permanent injury. • They are curious, communicative, and can be cooperative. • They do not want to be "suffocated" by an oxygen mask.	• Have a parent hold the preschooler during assessment. • Respect the child's modesty. Remove an article of clothing, examine it, and then replace it. • Have a calm, confident, reassuring, respectful manner. • Be sure to offer explanations about what you are doing. • Allow the child the responsibility of giving the history. • Explain as you examine. • A pediatric nonrebreather mask may be held near the face to provide "blow-by" oxygen.

(continued)

Table 10-1   Developmental Characteristics of Infants and Children *(continued)*

Age Group	Characteristics	Assessment and Care Strategies
School Age— 6 to 12 years 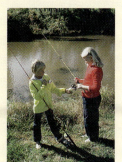	• This age group cooperates but likes their opinions heard. • They fear blood, pain, disfigurement, and permanent injury. • School-age children are modest and do not like their bodies exposed.	• Allow the child the responsibility of giving the history. • Explain as you examine. • Present a confident, calm, respectful manner. • Respect the child's modesty.
Adolescent— 12 to 18 years 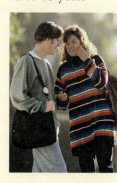	• Adolescents want to be treated as adults. • Adolescents generally feel that they are indestructible but may have fears of permanent injury and disfigurement. • Adolescents vary in their emotional and physical development and may not be comfortable with their changing bodies.	• Although they wish to be treated as adults, they may need as much support as children. • Present a confident, calm, respectful manner. • Be sure to explain what you are doing. • Respect their modesty. You may consider assessing them away from their parents. Have the physical exam done by an EMT-B of the same sex as the patient if possible.

with the environment. A well child is active and interacts with parents. The sick child may be ominously quiet or even unconscious. A well child notices when a stranger (like an EMT-B) enters the room. A sick child frequently is too preoccupied to pay any attention to a stranger. A very sick child may have such poor muscle tone that he or she actually appears limp.

Assessment of mental status is similar, too, but most children are unable to hide their fears and symptoms the way adults can. A healthy child is alert and notices the environment and people nearby, especially strangers. The ill child may have an altered mental status or appear to be oblivious to surroundings. The AVPU method of assessing mental status is still appropriate to use in children as long as you take the child's age and development into account.

Assessing the airway is the same, but remember not to hyperextend the child's neck because of the soft trachea. Assessing breathing is only slightly different. Children are more likely than adults to demonstrate certain signs of breathing difficulty. Nasal flaring and retractions of the sternum and ribs upon inhalation are more common, as is cyanosis.

Keep in mind the normal respiratory rates for children are faster than for adults, but any respiratory rate over 50 is abnormal. Even worse than a rapid respiratory rate is a slow respiratory rate. This frequently occurs just before the child stops breathing.

Assessing circulation is very similar, too, but remember to check capillary refill in children under the age of 6 years.

Priority pediatric patients include those who . . .

- Give a poor general impression.
- Are unresponsive or listless.
- Have a compromised airway.
- Are in respiratory arrest or have inadequate breathing or respiratory distress.
- Have a possibility of shock.
- Have uncontrolled bleeding.

Focused History and Physical Exam

If the child is old enough, let him or her give as much history as possible. Children with medical conditions like asthma and diabetes are sometimes better

Table 10-2 Normal Vital Signs and Weight Ranges, Infants and Children

Normal Respiration Rate (breaths per minute, at rest)

Newborn	30 to 50
Infant, 0-5 months	25 to 40
Infant, 6-12 months	20 to 30
Toddler, 1-3 years	20 to 30
Preschooler, 3-6 years	20 to 30
School age, 6-12 years	15 to 30
Adolescent, 12-18 years	12 to 20

Normal Pulse Rates (beats per minute, at rest)

Newborn	120 to 160
Infant, 0-5 months	90 to 140
Infant, 6-12 months	80 to 140
Toddler, 1-3 years	80 to 130
Preschooler, 3-6 years	80 to 120
School age, 6-12 years	70 to 110
Adolescent, 12-18 years	60 to 105

Blood Pressure Normal Ranges

	Systolic Approx. 80 plus $2 \times$ age	Diastolic Approx. 2/3 systolic
Preschooler, 3-6 years	average 99 (78 to 116)	average 65
School age, 6-12 years	average 105 (80 to 122)	average 69
Adolescent, 12-18 years	average 114 (88 to 140)	average 76

Normal Weight Ranges

Infant, 0-5 months	approx. 3.5 to 7 Kg
Infant, 6-12 months	approx. 8 to 11 Kg
Toddler, 1-3 years	approx. 10 to 15 Kg
Preschooler, 3-6 years	approx. 15 to 20 Kg
School age, 6-12 years	approx. 22 to 37 Kg
Adolescent, 12-18 years	approx. 50 to 65 Kg

Note: A high pulse in an infant or child is not as great a concern as a low pulse. A low pulse may indicate imminent cardiac arrest. Blood pressure is usually not taken on a child under 3 years. In cases of blood loss or shock, a child's blood pressure will remain within normal limits until near the end, then fall swiftly.

informed about their conditions than the adults around them. Keep the questions simple. If the child cannot tell you where it hurts, she can usually still point to the area.

Just as you would for adults, perform a focused history and physical exam for a medical patient and a rapid trauma exam for a trauma patient. Explain to the alert child what you are doing, and do the exam in trunk-to-head order for young children in order to avoid frightening them.

Take and record vital signs, assessing blood pressure only in children older than 3 years, and only using an appropriate-size cuff.

Detailed Physical Exam

Performing the physical examination in head-to-toe order makes sense for older children, but reverse the order on alert infants and small children. By examining the toes or trunk first and working your way toward the head, you will allow the child to become

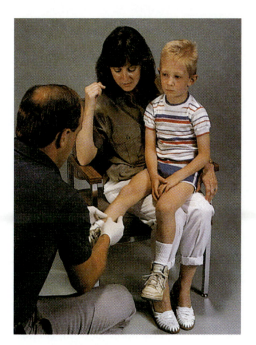

Figure 10-3 Kneel or sit at child's eye level.

accustomed to you and your touch in a less threatening manner.

Unless there are good reasons not to do so, try to examine the child on a parent's lap. A clean toy can help to distract and reassure the child during the physical exam. If it is a stuffed animal or doll, use it as a model to help you explain what you are doing to the patient. Point to an area on the toy to show the child where you must touch during the exam and where you will bandage when you need to provide emergency care. Make sure if you use a toy that it is clean and something the child can keep. A number of civic and public safety organizations provide stuffed animals free of charge to EMS agencies. Do not blow up a latex glove and draw a face on it to soothe a very young child who is anxious. The child may put the glove in his or her mouth, where it may burst and become a potential foreign body obstructing the airway.

Children around 5 to 8 years frequently begin to develop a sense of modesty. Respect this by explaining your actions. Then remove and replace clothing during the physical exam. Since children lose body heat rapidly, if you must expose a significant area, quickly cover the child with a blanket.

Modesty is even more of an issue with the young adolescent. Respect the patient's feelings and do everything you can to minimize embarrassment and discomfort. When possible, have the exam conducted by an EMT-B of the same sex as the patient. If the patient's condition is serious or critical, though, do not delay patient evaluation and care because you or the patient may be embarrassed.

Ongoing Assessment

A pediatric patient's condition can change very quickly. Be sure to keep a close eye on the patient and re-evaluate frequently—at least every 5 minutes for unstable patients and at least every 15 minutes for stable patients.

THE GERIATRIC PATIENT

As the American population ages, EMS responds to more and more calls involving patients over 65 years of age. Despite the impression some EMT-Bs have gained from their experience, the vast majority (almost 95%) of these people do not live in nursing homes. Rather, most elderly people are relatively healthy and live alone or with a spouse. It is true that a sizable portion of this population has medical problems like arthritis, high blood pressure, heart disease, and diabetes, but for the most part they are able to manage these conditions and live fulfilling lives.

The elderly are more likely than other adults to need EMS for medical emergencies like cardiac, respiratory, and neurological problems (such as stroke). Trauma in the elderly is much more likely to be the result of a fall rather than a motor-vehicle collision.

Communicating with the Geriatric Patient

When you assess any patient, it is important for the patient to be able to see and hear you. This can be a challenge with the elderly patient who has a hearing impairment or poor peripheral vision. You may need to speak loudly, but remember that speaking loudly does not mean speaking down to a patient. Treat the patient with respect and dignity (Figure 10-4). Do not assume the patient wishes you to call him by his first name. Ask the patient how he would like you to address him. Whenever possible, position yourself so that the patient does not need to look up or down to see you. Crouch or kneel as necessary.

Patient Assessment

The steps of assessment for geriatric patients are the same as those for other patients. Some particular things to be aware of and to look for are described below.

Scene Size-up

Scene size-up is really the same as for other patients, but take this opportunity to learn more about the geriatric patient's level of activity and mental awareness. When approaching an elderly person's residence, look to see whether or not the house and garden are cared for and evaluate the quality of

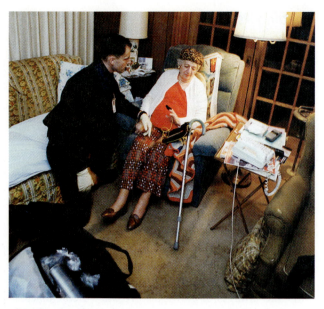

Figure 10-4 Position yourself at the patient's level, make good eye contact, and speak slowly and clearly.

housekeeping. These simple observations can give you important clues to the patient's pre-existing condition. For example, dirty floors or rotting food found on a counter may be the result of decreased strength and ability to get around.

Initial Assessment

When you form a general impression, note the temperature of the environment. The elderly typically need an environment that feels uncomfortably warm to younger people. A temperature that is normal for other adults may cause hypothermia in an elderly person. When you look at the patient, note such things as the level of the patient's distress and the presence or absence of medical appliances such as a hospital bed.

An assessment of mental status can be difficult if the patient's normal mental status is altered. Check with family members or caregivers to find out what is normal for this patient. A useful question to ask is, "How is the patient different from a week ago?"

Airway evaluation is almost the same as for other patients. Some elderly people have arthritis in the neck or spine that can make it difficult to extend the head and flex the neck. If you encounter this, do not try to force the head back, but instead thrust the jaw forward to pull the tongue out of the airway. You may also come across patients with dentures. If they are secure, leave them in. If, however, the dentures are loose or ill-fitting, remove them from the mouth of an unresponsive patient so they do not become an airway obstruction.

Assessing the breathing and circulation of an elderly patient is the same as with other patients, as is the identification of priority patients.

Focused History and Physical Exam

When interviewing the patient, be sure to introduce yourself, speak slowly and clearly, and position yourself where the patient can easily see you. If the patient is answering your questions slowly and your initial assessment did not reveal any immediate threats to life, give the patient additional time. Be sure to ask just one question at a time. Similarly, if the patient's speech is slurred but still understandable, don't rush him. Doing so could easily fluster the patient, delaying responses even more, and destroying any rapport you have established. If the patient's speech is difficult to understand because dentures are not in place, ask him to put them in if appropriate.

Occasionally you may find that the family tells you the patient was wrong in some of his or her responses. This is sometimes a result of a neurological condition, but it can also be caused by medications the patient is taking, especially if there are many of them or the dose is too high for some of them (Figure 10-5).

This points out the importance of gathering information from family members and others who are familiar with the patient's condition. If the patient lives with a spouse or other family members, they can frequently be an excellent source of information about the patient's medications, SAMPLE history, and even history of the present illness. Similarly, visiting nurses can provide a great deal of this information.

When performing a physical exam on an older person, keep in mind the patient's dignity. Explain what you are going to do before you do it and replace any clothing you remove as soon as possible. Many older people have a high threshold for pain. An extremity that is obviously fractured may cause very little discomfort to some patients. However, others have a very low threshold for pain. You will need to judge this for yourself when doing a physical exam.

Taking baseline vital signs is similar to taking those of other adults, with only a few exceptions. As we age, the systolic blood pressure has a tendency to increase. It usually does not require treatment. Many older patients you meet will be on medication for hypertension, usually defined as a diastolic pressure over about 90 mm of mercury. These medications can have significant side effects, including weakness and dizziness, especially when the patient stands up quickly from a sitting or supine position.

The skin loses much of its elasticity as we age, leading to dry skin that is thin and fragile. Applying too much pressure, even with just your fingertips, can be enough to cause the skin to tear. So be as gentle as possible and very careful when pulling or lifting a patient.

The pupils are not round and reactive to light in some older patients. Eye surgery or pre-existing con-

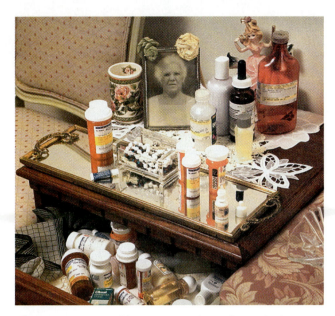

Figure 10-5 Older patients often take multiple medications.

ditions may have given the pupil an abnormal shape or the inability to react to light normally. Certain eye drops can also prevent normal reactions to light. When you find this condition, inquire as to whether it is normal for your patient before assuming he or she has a serious condition based on this sign.

Detailed Physical Exam

The detailed physical exam for older patients is the same as for other adults. You may come across some unusual findings because of the patient's age or condition, though. The neck may be stiff and the head may be far forward of where it normally is because of changes in the spine. This can be a challenge to deal with when you suspect a neck injury and must immobilize the patient. Use folded towels or other materials to keep the head in its normal position, prevent hyperextension, and make the patient more comfortable.

The chest and abdomen are not commonly injured, but keep in mind the decreased sensitivity to pain that many older people have. Serious abdominal problems that would cause a younger person agony may produce only slight discomfort for older patients.

The hip or proximal femur is commonly fractured in a fall, especially in women. This is partly because women live longer than men, but even more so because women are very prone to loss of calcium from bone. This leads to so much weakening of the bone itself that it is sometimes the cause of a fall rather than a result. Other areas on the extremities are also injured sometimes because of this weakening of the bone.

The back may be injured in a fall, but it is very commonly injured in motor-vehicle collisions. Again, because of abnormal curvature that sometimes accompanies aging, immobilizing these patients can be very challenging. Do your best to keep the vertebrae in alignment and to reduce the patient's discomfort as much as possible.

Ongoing Assessment

Elderly patients can deteriorate suddenly, but often they experience a slow, steady decline in condition. Do not let yourself be lulled into a false sense of security by the lack of sudden changes. Perform an ongoing assessment at regular intervals and evaluate your findings for trends.

Additional Concerns During Assessment

Do not underestimate the significance of a fall in an elderly person. Of older patients seen in an emergency department for a fall, one-quarter will die within a year. Death may not be a direct result of the fall, but instead may be a result of complications from the fall. For example, while recuperating from bruised ribs sustained in a fall, a 74-year-old man may not breathe as deeply as normal because of the pain associated with inhalation. As a result of not coughing and other changes in the lungs associated with aging, if this patient comes down with pneumonia, he is more likely to die from complications of the disease.

Often, a fall is just an indication of a more serious problem. A number of older people fall because of abnormal heart rhythms. Others fall because of a stroke or internal bleeding from an ulcer. Whenever possible and when time allows, assess the patient not only for injuries, but also for a cause of the fall.

It is difficult for younger adults to understand how disruptive a serious injury or illness can be to an older person. Years of independence can vanish in an instant, leaving the patient in the care of strangers. Even worse, he or she goes to a hospital where many friends and perhaps a spouse may have died. The EMT-B can ease this transition by treating the patient in a respectful, dignified manner. Do not minimize the patient's fears and concerns. Instead, acknowledge them and try to put them in perspective.

Ask the patient if he or she would like you to lock up before you leave the house. Inquire about the care of any pets and if there is a trusted neighbor who can take care of them for a while. A friendly hand on the patient's hand or forearm, if you feel the patient will accept it, can be very reassuring. Asking the patient during transport about what he or she has done over the course of a lifetime can be not only therapeutic for the patient, but enlightening for you as well. Above all, treat the patient in a respectful, empathetic manner.

SUMMARY

- Estimate a child's age before you establish contact with the patient and use this information to guide your assessment of and communication with the patient.

- Consider the normal range of vital signs for the age of a child since the signs are very different from those of an adult.

- Family members can be valuable sources of information about the patient, but let the patient answer your questions if he or she is able.

- Handle older patients gently when possible to avoid inflicting injury.

- Consider carefully the possible causes of an elderly patient's fall and report your findings to emergency department staff.

REVIEW QUESTIONS

1. Based on anatomical and emotional development, a 1- to 3-year old is classified as a(n):
   a. infant.
   b. toddler.
   c. newborn.
   d. preschooler.

2. Normal respiratory rate for a 5-year-old patient at rest is _____ breaths per minute.
   a. 30 to 50
   b. 25 to 40
   c. 20 to 30
   d. 12 to 20

3. The normal systolic blood-pressure range for school-age children is:
   a. 78 to 116.
   b. 90 to 150.
   c. 80 to 122.
   d. 120 to 160.

REVIEW QUESTIONS continued

4. When the friend of an elderly patient tells you that the patient is giving you incorrect information, you should:

a. ask the friend to leave.

b. ask about current medications.

c. suspect alcoholism in your patient.

d. suspect Alzheimer's disease in your patient.

5. Which of the following statements about elderly patients is NOT true?

a. Their skin tends to be dry, thin, and fragile.

b. Their systolic blood pressure tends to decrease.

c. Their pupils are not round and as reactive to light.

d. Their abdominal problems may cause only slight discomfort.

WEB MEDIC

Visit Brady's *Essentials of Emergency Care* web site for direct web links. At **www.prenhall.com/limmer,** you will find information related to the following Chapter 10 topics:

- American Academy of Pediatrics
- Hearing-impaired children
- EMSC Resource Center
- Falls and hip fractures among geriatric patients
- American Association of Retired People

Correlates with the U.S. DOT "EMT-Basic National Standard Curriculum" Lessons 3-7 and 3-8

Chapter Eleven

COMMUNICATION AND DOCUMENTATION

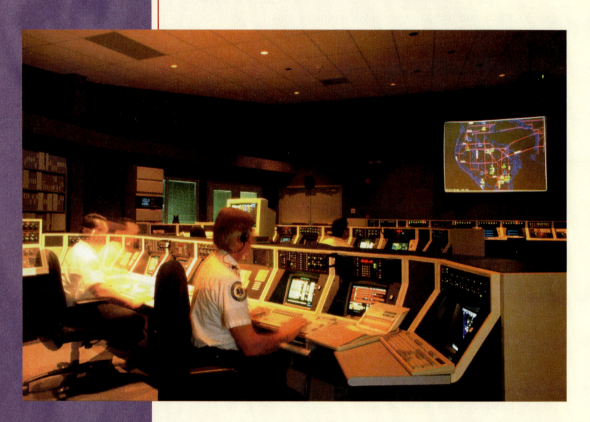

ESSENTIAL ELECTRONIC EXTRAS

CD ESSENTIALS

For preview and review of chapter material, see the student CD-ROM for

- Pretest
- Chapter quizzes
- Posttest

WEB ESSENTIALS

For additional review and enrichment, visit www.prenhall.com/limmer for

- Interactive student quizzes
- Links to online EMS resources
- Online case studies
- Audio glossary

There are many different ways in which an EMT-B communicates on the job. Understanding and speaking to patients, family members, and bystanders require excellent interpersonal communication skills. Communicating with other health-care providers also requires special skill.

Radio transmissions help to inform other members of the health care team about a patient in your care. As you know, assessing a patient thoroughly and delivering quality care are two major tasks of the EMT-B. However, excellent prehospital care cannot be continued in the hospital if the emergency department is unprepared for the patient's arrival. Therefore, by providing information in an orderly, efficient manner, the EMT-B can help ensure that the patient will continue to receive quality care.

The prehospital care report you complete also is an important link in the chain of communication for your patient. To continue quality care, the hospital staff needs critical information about what happened to the patient before arrival. They can learn this information only if you document your assessment findings and treatment in an organized, comprehensive way.

When members of the health-care team are able to give and receive information about a patient in a clear, concise manner, communication leads to improved patient care. Such vital communication starts in the dispatch phase of a call, ending only after completion of transport. As an EMT-B and member of the patient's health-care team, you must have excellent verbal and written communication skills to assure that the appropriate individuals receive the information they need to treat the patient. In fact, the continuum of patient care is dependent upon effective and efficient communication skills.

COMMUNICATIONS

General Principles of Communication

There are many ways human beings communicate. Verbal and written forms of communication are especially important to EMT-Bs. However, there are nonverbal methods of communication that you must also use when dealing with a patient, family member, friend, bystander, public safety officer, or fellow EMS provider. Particularly when dealing with patients, keep in mind the following simple principles:

- **Make eye contact with the patient.** Remember that some cultures discourage eye contact. If there are ethnic enclaves in your community, find out more about these cultures to ensure that you can appropriately communicate with patients from those areas.
- **When practical, position yourself at a level lower than the patient.** Do this only when the scene is safe (Figure 11-1).
- **Be honest with the patient.** If a patient asks you a direct question, give the best answer you can.

- **Use language the patient can understand.** Asking a patient if he has ever had an "MI" is not likely to be as effective as asking if he has ever had a heart attack or heart problem.
- **Be aware of your own body language.** Taking a defensive stance can sometimes make you appear to be unapproachable.

CORE CONCEPTS

In this chapter, you will learn about the following topics:

- Delivery and format of a patient care radio report
- Principles of radio use
- Purposes and principles of documentation of patient assessment and care
- Documentation of special incidents

☐ 1. Complete a prehospital care report. (pp. 170–176)

- Apply the components of the essential patient information in a written report. (pp. 170–179)

☐ 2. Communicate with the patient, bystanders, other health care providers, and patient family members while providing health care. (pp. 167–170)

- Discuss the communication skills that should be used to interact with the patient. (pp. 167–168)

- Discuss the communication skills that should be used to interact with the family, bystanders, individuals from other agencies, and hospital personnel while providing patient care, and the difference between skills used to interact with the patient and those used to interact with others. (pp. 167–170)

☐ 3. Provide a report to medical direction of assessment findings and emergency care given. (pp. 168–170)

- Explain the importance of effective communication of patient information. (pp. 170–175)

✔ **Attitude**

☐ 4. Recognize and respect the feelings that patients might experience during assessment. (pp. 167–168)

☐ 5. Explain the rationale for providing efficient and effective radio and written patient care reports. (pp. 168–169, 170–171)

✔ **Skills**

☐ 6. Complete a prehospital care report. (pp. 170–174)

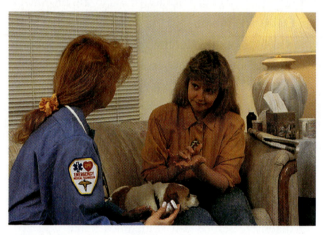

Figure 11-1 If possible, position yourself at or below the patient's eye level to be less intimidating and to aid communication.

- **Speak clearly, slowly, and distinctly.**
- **Use the patient's proper name, either first or last, depending on the circumstances.** Ask the patient what he or she wishes to be called.
- **If a patient has difficulty hearing, speak clearly with your lips visible.**
- **Allow the patient enough time to answer a question before asking the next one.** When you are trying to move quickly and spend as little time on scene as possible, it is easy to appear rushed. This can fluster patients, making it even harder for them to describe their chief complaints. It also can antagonize an already anxious patient.
- **Act and speak in a calm, confident manner.** Even if you don't feel confident, look and act that way. A patient wants to feel that you know what

you are doing. If you appear unsure, the patient may avoid talking to you, waiting instead to talk to the doctor at the hospital.

LIFESPAN DEVELOPMENT

Children can be a communication challenge. It is especially important that you speak to a child at the child's level. Kneel, if necessary, to make eye contact and use words the child will understand. You should be extremely careful to be honest with children. They sense falsehoods more quickly than do many adults.

Radio Use

Although the information that follows is intended to describe the use of radios, much of it also applies to the use of cellular telephones. Your system should have guidelines on what equipment to use under different circumstances (Table 11-1).

The dispatcher plays a pivotal role in EMS. He or she gets essential information from the caller about the nature and location of the call, as well as keeps track of certain events. To accomplish this, the dispatcher must be kept informed. In particular, you need to notify the dispatcher when:

- You have received the call.
- You are en route.
- You arrive at the scene.

TABLE 11-1 Principles of Radio Communication

Follow these principles when using the EMS radio system.

- Make sure your radio is on and volume is adjusted properly.
- Reduce background noise by closing the vehicle window when possible.
- Listen to the frequency and ensure that it is clear before beginning a transmission.
- Press the "press to talk" (PTT) button, then wait one second before speaking. This prevents cutting off the first few words of your transmission.
- Speak with your lips about two to three inches from microphone.
- When calling another unit or base station, use their unit number or name followed by yours. "Dispatcher, this is Ambulance 2."
- The unit being called will signal when transmission should start by saying "go ahead" or another accepted term: "Ambulance 2, this is the dispatcher. Go ahead." If you are told to "stand by," wait until they tell you they are ready to take your transmission.
- Speak slowly and clearly.
- Keep transmissions brief. If a transmission takes longer than 30 seconds, at that point pause for a few seconds so emergency traffic can use the frequency if necessary.
- Use plain English. Avoid codes and slang.
- Do not use phrases like "be advised," which serve no purpose.

- Courtesy is assumed, so there is no need to say "please," "thank you," and "you're welcome."
- When transmitting a number that might be unclear (15 may sound like 16 or 50), give the number, then repeat the individual digits. Say "15, one five."
- Anything said over the radio can be heard by the public on a scanner. Do not use the patient's name over the radio. Also do not use profanities or statements that may slander any person. Use objective, impartial statements.
- Use "we" instead of "I." As an EMT-B, you will rarely be acting alone.
- "Affirmative" and "negative" are preferred over "yes" and "no" because the latter are difficult to hear.
- Give assessment information about your patient, but avoid offering a diagnosis of the patient's problem. For example, say "Patient complains of chest pain," but do not say "Probably having a heart attack."
- After transmitting, say "Over." Wait for acknowledgment that your message was heard.
- Use only authorized codes and abbreviations.
- Use EMS frequencies only for authorized EMS communication.

- You leave the scene.
- You arrive at the hospital.
- You leave the hospital.
- You are back at quarters.

In many rural areas, EMS notifies the local hospital when responding to a call. This allows the limited staff to make contingency plans so that they are not overwhelmed.

In some systems, EMT-Bs receive medical direction through the receiving hospital. In others, medical direction is at a separate site. In either case, EMT-Bs need to contact medical direction to get orders for administering certain medications and occasionally to obtain additional advice about patient care. When communicating with medical direction, the EMT-B needs to make the radio transmissions organized, concise, and pertinent. Since the physician will base the decision on whether to order medications and additional procedures on the information you provide, you must make sure this information is accurate.

When you receive an order for a medication or procedure (or denial of such a request), repeat the order back to the physician word for word. This ensures that the order you are about to implement is the one the physician intended. If you receive an order that is unclear or that appears to be inappropriate, ask the physician to repeat the order again. If it is still unclear, discuss it with the physician until it is clear and you feel comfortable. At times like this, the telephone may be the preferred method of communication. It allows you to speak more comfortably and to say certain things that are not appropriate over the radio airwaves or are confidential (e.g., the patient's name). Moreover, an ordinary telephone is superior to a cellular phone if you are going to discuss confidential information since cellular phone transmissions are not confidential.

Many new EMT-Bs are understandably very nervous about speaking for the first time on the radio. They probably know that thousands of people are listening to scanning radios at any given time. This can make the first radio transmission a very stressful experience. There are several things you can do to help the new person get through this. First, select a call where the patient's condition is not critical. Make sure you have plenty of time before arrival at the hospital so the new EMT-B has time to prepare. If the EMT-B is extremely nervous, give reassurance by saying you will not let him make a fool of himself. Then put your finger on the power button and let him know that if he says something inappropriate you will turn the radio off before the problem is compounded. Alternatively, arrange a hand signal to indicate that he needs to stop transmitting. Since the natural reaction to this situation is for the new person to hold his breath, encourage him after he is finished to take a deep breath or two.

The information you provide about a patient allows the receiving hospital to prepare for the patient's arrival, which includes selecting the right room, equipment, and personnel. Your report should include the following information, in the order shown (unless local protocol dictates otherwise):

- ID and level of certification of provider
- Estimated time of arrival (ETA)
- Patient's sex and age
- Chief complaint
- Brief, pertinent history of the present illness
- Major past illnesses
- Mental status
- Baseline vital signs
- General impression
- Pertinent findings of the physical exam
- Emergency medical care given
- Response to emergency medical care

This same information (with the exception of the ETA) is what the EMT-B should relay to an ALS provider who will be taking over care of the patient.

As part of your ongoing assessment, you will reevaluate the patient frequently. In accordance with local protocol, advise the hospital of updated vital signs. If the patient's condition takes a turn for the worse, you must notify the hospital so that the patient will get the appropriate care upon arrival.

Remember to always be objective and impartial when describing a patient over the airwaves. Making disparaging remarks about a patient may result in the EMT-B being charged with slander.

Reporting to the Hospital Staff

After you arrive at the hospital, you should give a verbal report to the staff. Oftentimes, the nurse who receives the patient has not obtained all of the information you gave in your radio report. When done properly, your verbal report shows the emergency department staff that you did a good assessment and gave quality care. Start by introducing the patient by name. Summarize the information you gave over the radio next. Then describe information that was not appropriate or necessary for a radio transmission: additional history, additional vital signs, and any other treatments you have given the patient.

DOCUMENTATION

Prehospital Care Report (PCR)

As an experienced EMT-B, you have had considerable experience in preparing prehospital care reports. You are also aware that these reports vary from system to system. As you learned in Chapter 1 of this textbook, the U.S. Department of Transportation has developed a minimum data set—the elements recommended for inclusion on a prehospital care report. (See Chapter 1, Table 1-1.) Each EMS system is encouraged to collect at least this much information so that system evaluation and quality improvement can occur.

Functions

The prehospital care report (PCR) has many functions. They include:

- **Continuity of care.** It is easy for EMT-Bs to feel that no one in the hospital reads the prehospital care report because in the emergency department it is often not read immediately. However, at a later time a nurse or physician may read it more carefully. If the patient is admitted, staff on the floor or in a critical care unit may depend on your PCR to gain information about the scene and the patient's initial condition. This is information that was available only to you and, if not documented, may be lost to the hospital staff forever.

- **Legal document.** Many EMT-Bs consider this function of the PCR to be the most important one because the form may be used in court proceedings. The form does not go to court alone; the person who completed it ordinarily also must appear in court. The best way to avoid legal problems with a PCR is to do a good job completing it.

A clear, comprehensive, and well-written report documents the condition of the patient upon EMS arrival, the emergency medical care the patient received, any changes in the patient's condition, and the status of the patient upon arrival at the hospital. The report should include both objective and subjective information. An example of objective information is a description of the patient's appearance. Subjective information could include the patient's SAMPLE history. The PCR should avoid the EMT-B's opinions on any non-medical findings.

- **Educational.** Selected PCRs (with information that might identify a patient deleted) can demonstrate not only proper documentation techniques, but also how to handle unusual and uncommon cases.
- **Administrative.** Agencies that bill for their services need accurate information in order to get reimbursement. Many services also compile statistics that help them to determine the best locations for their vehicles and to maintain adequate staff and equipment.
- **Research.** Advancing the quality of EMS is virtually impossible without adequate information. If a service or region enters data into a computerized database, it becomes much easier to determine where promising areas of research lie.
- **Evaluation and continuous quality improvement.** These areas are closely related to research and just as dependent on data. Without a system to identify problems, an EMS system is not fulfilling all of its responsibilities. Progressive systems go further and try to prevent problems from occurring by carefully evaluating all of the information at their disposal.

Principles of Completion

Most EMS agencies use the traditional paper form for recording information about a call (Figures 11-2 and 11-3). Some services use a computerized version, which can take the form of an "electronic clipboard" (Figure 11-4). Other services enter data on personal computers at a hospital or in quarters. Some areas, like North Carolina, enter data through a web-based system. The user logs on to a particular site through a secure connection, types in the information, and prints out a report. With computer technology advancing rapidly, it is difficult to determine what the PCR of the future will look like.

Regardless of the way information is collected, there are certain characteristics all of these approaches have in common. There are two sections of the form, one for run data and one for patient data. The run data section includes the date, times, service, unit, and names of crew members. It is important

that clocks used to record times be accurate and synchronous. If your dispatcher's clock is five minutes different from your wristwatch, then administrative times (call received, arrival at scene, etc.) and patient times (e.g., vital signs) may conflict.

The patient data section includes:

- Patient name, address, date of birth, and sex
- Insurance information
- Nature of call
- Mechanism of injury
- Location of patient
- Treatment administered prior to arrival of EMT-B
- Signs and symptoms
- Baseline vital signs
- SAMPLE history
- Care administered
- Changes in patient condition

There may be three ways to record this information: check boxes, fill-in boxes, and open-ended narrative. Check boxes or fill-in boxes are not only quick to complete, they also make gathering statistics easier. But patients don't always fit into all the categories on any one form. So the narrative section allows you to explain things and to go into more detail. Be sure to fill in check boxes completely, and avoid stray marks if your form will be scanned into a computer.

If your form has a narrative section, there are a number of important principles to keep in mind:

- Describe, don't conclude.
- Include pertinent negatives (for example, a patient with chest pain denies difficulty breathing).
- Record important observations about the scene (suicide note, weapon, etc.).
- Avoid radio codes.
- Use abbreviations only if they are standard.
- When information of a sensitive nature is documented, note the source of that information (for example, certain communicable diseases).
- Be sure to spell words correctly, especially medical words. If you do not know how to spell a word, find out or use a different one.
- Every time you reassess the patient, record the time and your findings.
- Be sure to fulfill all other state and local requirements.
- Confidentiality is a vital issue in documentation. This is particularly true in light of the Health Information Portability and Accountability Act (HIPAA). This federal law puts certain obligations on health care agencies and providers to protect the confidentiality

MAINE ✦EMS **PRESS DOWN, YOU ARE MAKING THREE COPIES.**

RUN REPORT #	Mo.	Day	Year	M T W Th	F S Sun	SERVICE NAME		SERVICE NO.	VEHICLE NO.	ALS ☐ Performed ☐ Back-up called	SERVICE RUN NO.
746118											

NAME	BILLING INFORMATION

STREET OR R.F.D.

CITY/TOWN	STATE	ZIP

AGE/DATE OF BIRTH	☐ Male ☐ Female	PHONE

INCIDENT LOCATION:	ADDRESS	CITY/TOWN

TRANSPORTED TO:	TREATING/FAMILY PHYSICIAN	CREW LICENSE NUMBERS

TRANSPORTATION/COMMUNICATIONS PROBLEMS

☐ Medical   ☐ Trauma   ☐ Code 99

☐ Cardiac
☐ Poisoning/OD
☐ Respiratory
☐ Behavioral
☐ Diabetic
☐ Seizure
☐ CVA
☐ OB/Gyn
☐ Other _____

☐ Multi-Systems Trauma
☐ Head
☐ Spinal
☐ Burn
☐ Soft Tissue Injury
☐ Fractures
☐ Other _____

☐ MEDICATIONS   ☐ ALLERGIES

CHIEF COMPLAINT:

R	L	LUNG SOUNDS
☐	☐	CLEAR
☐	☐	ABSENT
☐	☐	DECREASED
☐	☐	RALES
☐	☐	WHEEZE
☐	☐	STRIDOR

TYPE OF RUN
☐ Emergency Transport
☐ Routine Transfer
☐ Emergency Transfer
☐ No Transport
☐ Refused Transport

TIME	CODE		ODOMETER
		Call Received	
		Enroute	
		At Scene	
		From Scene	
		At Destination	
		In Service	

TIME	PULSE	RESP	BP	PUPILLARY RESPONSE	SKIN	VERBAL RESPONSE	MOTOR RESPONSE	EYE-OPENING RESPONSE	CAPILLARY REFILL
						5 4 3 2 1	6 5 4 3 2 1	4 3 2 1	☐ Normal ☐ None ☐ Delayed
						5 4 3 2 1	6 5 4 3 2 1	4 3 2 1	☐ Normal ☐ None ☐ Delayed
						5 4 3 2 1	6 5 4 3 2 1	4 3 2 1	☐ Normal ☐ None ☐ Delayed

☐ MVA   ☐ Concern AOB/ETOH   SEAT BELTS: ☐ Used   ☐ Not Used   ☐ N/A   ☐ Helmet Used

MUTUAL AID: Assisted/Assisted by Service # _____   Time Called: _____

	☐ Medication Administered	☐ Defib Lic.# _____	**MEDICAL CONTROL**	☐ Written Order/Protocol ☐ Verbal Order/Protocol
PATIENT'S SUSPECTED PROBLEM: **746118**	☐ Monitor	☐ Chest Decomp	**IV** ☐ SUC LIC.# _____	Total Attempts
	☐ Pacing	☐ Cricothyrotomy	☐ UNSUC LIC.# _____	

Cleared Airway	Extrication	
Artificial Respiration/BVM	Cervical Immobilization	**EOA** ☐ SUC LIC.# _____ Total Attempts
Oropharyngeal Airway	KED/Short Board	
Nasopharyngeal Airway	Long Board	☐ UNSUC LIC.# _____
CPR–Time:	Restraints	
Bystander CPR	Traction Splinting	
AED	General Splinting	
Suction	Cold Application	
Oxygen–LPMin ___ ☐ Nasal ☐ Mask	MAST Inflated	
Pulse Oximetry		
Autovent		

ET ☐ SUC LIC.# _____ Total Attempts
☐ UNSUC LIC.# _____

LIC #	EKG RHYTHM	TIME	MEDS/DEFIB/C-VERT	DOSE W/S	ROUTE

NAME OF E.D. TREATING PHYSICIAN _____   SIGNATURE OF CREW MEMBER IN CHARGE _____   **COPY 1 HOSPITAL**

Figure 11-2   An example of a prehospital care report with check boxes, fill-in boxes, and a narrative space.

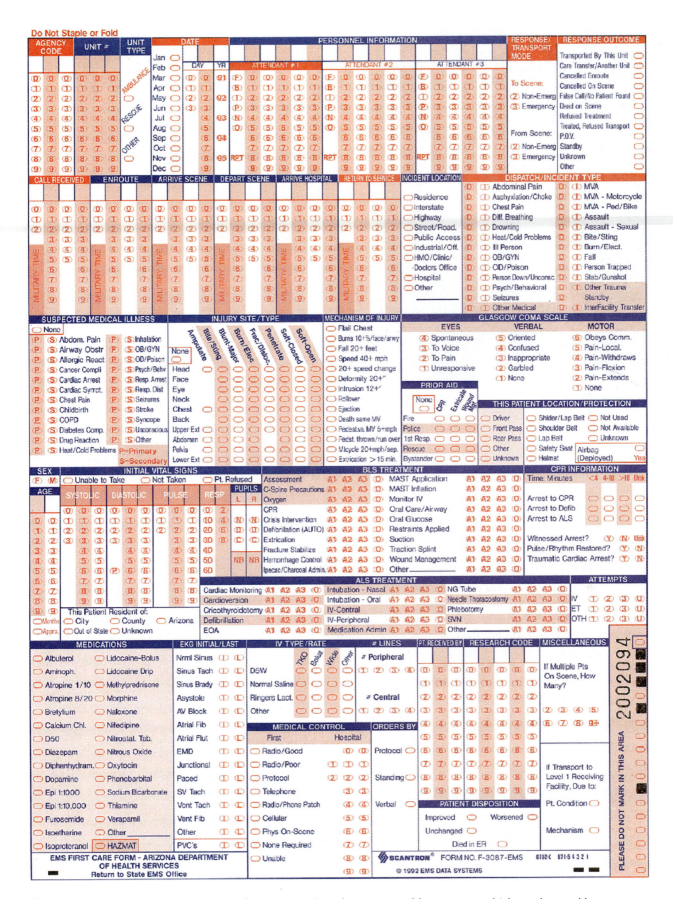

Figure 11-3 The Arizona prehospital care report form has a scannable segment, which can be read by computer.

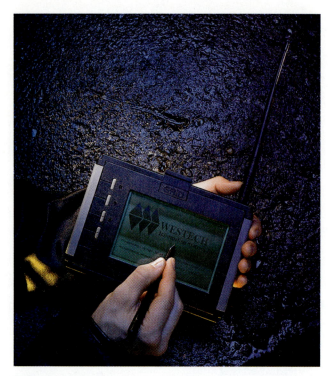

Figure 11-4 A pen-based computer can read handwriting and convert it to computer text.

of patient information. Although the PCR itself is considered confidential, it is important to remember that the information on the form is also considered confidential.

After you complete the PCR, you will need to distribute different copies of the form to different individuals or agencies. Generally, the service retains the original copy and one copy is inserted in the patient's hospital medical record. In some areas, another copy is used for data collection and still another goes to the medical director or quality improvement coordinator.

Be familiar with local protocol and procedures that describe where the different copies of the form should be distributed.

Falsification

An **error of omission** is the failure to do something for the patient, in either assessment or treatment. An **error of commission** is doing something for or to the patient, but doing it poorly or in a manner that is harmful to the patient. When either of these errors occurs, never try to cover it up. Instead, document what did or did not happen and what steps you took (if any) to correct the situation. You are not expected to be perfect; attempting to cover up a mistake usually makes the situation a lot worse than admitting an error occurred.

Falsification of information on the PCR may lead not only to suspension or revocation of the EMT-B's certification or license, but also to poor patient care. Other health-care providers who depend on the form get a false impression of what findings were discovered in patient assessment or what treatment was given.

One of the areas in which it may be tempting to "make up" information is in the recording of the patient's vital signs. It is essential to quality patient care to document only the vital signs that were actually taken. In the area of treatment, it can also be tempting to document, for example, that you administered oxygen when you actually forgot to do it. Do not chart that you gave the patient a treatment unless you actually did.

Correction of Errors

There are two times you can discover an error on a PCR: while you are completing the form and after you have distributed the copies of the form. For example, you thought you were writing "albuterol," but someone was talking about nitroglycerin as you began writing. When you check the form, you discover you wrote the wrong medication name. To correct this, draw a single horizontal line through the error, initial it, and write the correct information beside it. Do not try to obliterate the error, because it may be interpreted as an attempt to cover up a mistake.

If you discover an error after you submit the report form, the procedure is a little different. Draw a single line through the error (preferably in a different color ink), initial and date it, and add a note with the correct information. If you neglected to include some important information, add a note with the correct information, the date, and your initials.

Special Situations

There are several instances where the usual principles of documentation do not meet the needs of the situation. These can include charting patient care at multiple-casualty incidents and documenting unusual incidents.

Multiple-Casualty Incidents (MCIs)

There are days when your service is very busy and you do not have time to complete a form immediately after each call. Although everyone would like to avoid these situations, they are sometimes inevitable in EMS. When you don't have enough time to complete the form before the next call, keep your notes and fill out the report later.

Multiple-casualty incidents (MCIs) are special cases. The very nature of an MCI prevents you from completing the form immediately after you have transported a patient. Fortunately, good local MCI plans include some means of recording important medical information temporarily (like a triage tag) that can be used later to complete the form (Figure 11-5). The standard for documentation in an MCI is not the same as for a typical call. Your local plan should have guidelines.

Special Situation Reports

Unusual events occur from time to time that do not fit into the system of documenting patient care. When an EMS provider is stuck by a contaminated needle, for example, special care must be taken to document the incident, preferably on a form made for this purpose. Other types of injuries to crew members need to be documented, too. There are other events that you may need to report to local authorities, and occasionally you may need to explain an unusual event on a call.

Whatever the nature of the unusual incident, you should submit any required report in a timely manner to the authority described by local protocol. The report should be accurate and objective, with careful attention to the facts of the case. Be very careful about speculation. Note that it is prudent for you to keep a copy of the report for your own records.

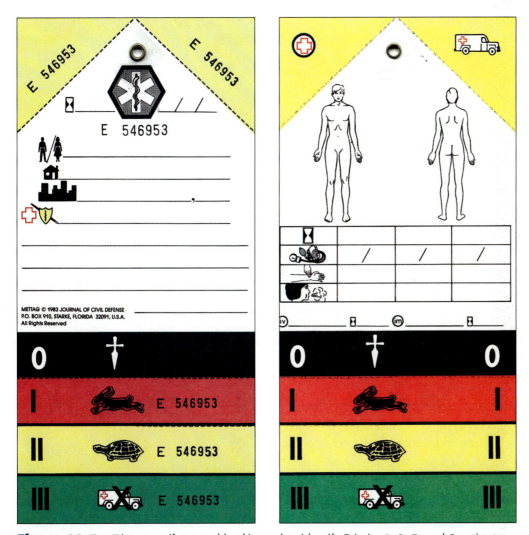

Figure 11-5 Triage tag (front and back) used to identify Priority 1, 2, 3, and 0 patients.

CHAPTER REVIEW

Summary

- Use both verbal and nonverbal means of communication with your patients.
- Organize your radio reports so that they are clear, concise, and organized.
- Take care when writing your PCR to improve its usefulness in the continuity of care, evaluation, and quality improvement.

Review Questions

1. Which of the following is NOT one of the basic principles you should follow when communicating with a patient?
   a. Position yourself at a lower level than the patient when it is practical.
   b. Avoid eye contact.
   c. Speak clearly, slowly, and distinctly.
   d. Use language the patient can understand.

2. If you receive an order over the radio from the medical direction physician that is unclear, you should:
   a. ask the physician to repeat the order.
   b. confer with your partners at the scene.
   c. consult written protocols
   d. use your own judgment as to what was meant.

3. Which of the following is NOT part of the patient information that should be included in the EMT-B's radio report?
   a. patient's age and sex
   b. general impression of the patient
   c. patient's chief complaint
   d. patient's Social Security number

4. Your verbal report to the medical or nursing staff at the hospital should include:
   a. additional vital signs and suspected diagnosis.
   b. summary of radio transmission and insurance information.
   c. general impression, chief complaint, and major illnesses.
   d. introduction of the patient and summary of the radio transmission.

REVIEW QUESTIONS *continued*

5. If you discover an error on a PCR after you have submitted the form, you should:

a. tell your medical director.

b. tell your superior.

c. write a new report and replace the old one with it.

d. draw a line through the error, initial it and date it, and add the correct information.

WEB MEDIC

Visit Brady's *Essentials of Emergency Care* web site for direct web links. At **www.prenhall.com/limmer,** you will find information related to the following Chapter 11 topics:

- the Federal Communications Commission
- the Association of Public Safety Communications Officials International
- Body language
- Medical abbreviations

Correlates with the U.S. DOT "EMT-Basic National Standard Curriculum" Lesson 4-1

Chapter Twelve

GENERAL PHARMACOLOGY

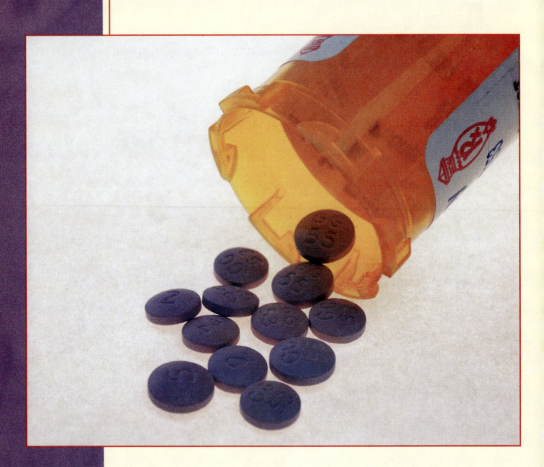

As an EMT-B, you carry several medications on your EMS unit that you can give a patient under specific conditions. You also are permitted to assist the patient in taking certain prescribed medications with medical direction's approval.

Being able to give the proper medication to a patient in an emergency can prove to be life-saving. This section provides basic information on what you need to know in order to assist a patient with prescribed medications, provided your medical director agrees that is the most appropriate course of action.

Generally, the medications that an EMT-B may administer are: activated charcoal, oral glucose, oxygen, prescribed inhalers, nitroglycerin, and epinephrine. The information below is a brief review of each of them.

MEDICATIONS

Medications Carried on the Ambulance

As an EMT-B, you carry three types of medication in your ambulance: activated charcoal, oral glucose, and oxygen.

Activated Charcoal

Activated charcoal is a powder prepared from charred wood, usually pre-mixed with water (Figure 12-1). It is used to treat a poisoning or overdose where a substance was ingested and is in the patient's digestive tract. Activated charcoal absorbs poisons and prevents them from being absorbed by the body. (The procedure for administering activated charcoal is included in Chapter 17.)

Oral Glucose

Glucose is a kind of sugar. Oral glucose is a form of glucose that is taken by mouth to treat a patient with an altered mental status and a history of diabetes. The brain is very sensitive to low blood sugar, often caused by poorly managed diabetes, and this can cause an altered mental status. Oral glucose usually comes in a tube of gel (Figure 12-2). You can apply the gel to a tongue depressor and then place it between the patient's cheek and gum. This area is very vascular, and the glucose is easily absorbed into the bloodstream and carried to the brain. This may begin to reverse a patient's life-threatening condition. (The procedure for administering oral glucose is included in Chapter 15.)

Oxygen

Oxygen is a gas commonly found in the atmosphere. Pure oxygen is used as a drug to treat any patient whose medical or traumatic condition causes him or her to be, or potentially to be, hypoxic (Figure 12-3). Throughout your EMS training you have learned many situations in which oxygen should be administered. (The procedure for administering oxygen therapy is included in Chapter 6.)

Prescribed Medications

Three medications—prescribed inhalers, nitroglycerin, and epinephrine—are drugs that an EMT-B may assist the patient in taking. You need permission from medical direction by phone or radio or there may be standing medical orders that permit you to assist a patient with their prescribed medications. Always comply with the protocols of your EMS system.

CORE CONCEPTS

In this chapter, you will learn about the following topics:

- Medications that are carried on the ambulance

- Medications the EMT-Basic can assist a patient in taking

- What EMT-Basics must know when giving medications

✔ Knowledge

☐ 1. Provide treatment for a patient in respiratory distress. (pp. 180–181)

  • Recognize the need for medical direction to assist in the emergency medical care of the patient with breathing difficulty. (pp. 180-181)

☐ 2. Provide care to a patient experiencing chest pain/discomfort. (p. 181)

  • List the indications for the use of nitroglycerin. (p. 181)

☐ 3. Provide care of the patient experiencing an allergic reaction. (p. 181)

  • State the generic and trade names, medication forms, dose, administration, action, and contraindications for the epinephrine auto-injector. (p. 181)

✔ Attitude

☐ 4. 1. Defend the rationale for the EMT-Basic to carry and assist with medications. (pp. 179-183)

✔ Skills

☐ 5. Given medical scenarios, demonstrate the ability to properly assess the patient and demonstrate the ability to properly utilize the intervention to include inhaler, nitroglycerin, oral glucose, and activated charcoal. (pp. 179-183)

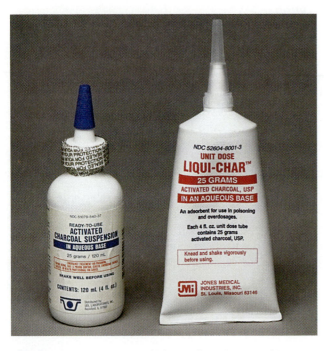

Figure 12-1 Activated charcoal is often used in poisoning cases.

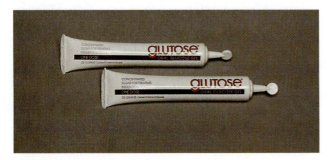

Figure 12-2 Oral glucose may help a patient with diabetes.

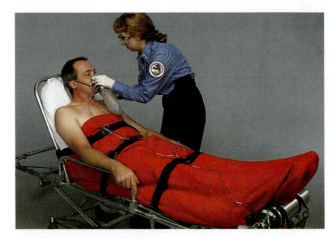

Figure 12-3 Oxygen is the drug most frequently administered by EMT-Bs.

Prescribed Inhalers

There are various medications that patients may carry to help them through a period of breathing difficulty. According to the CDC, the number of Americans with asthma will double in the next 20 years. Most often patients with a history of emphysema or chronic bronchitis (COPD) or asthma carry a "bronchodilator," which is a drug designed to dilate the constricted bronchial tubes in order to make breathing easier. Many of these medications can be carried in an inhaler, which contains an aerosol form of a drug in a spray device with a mouthpiece so the patient can spray the medication directly into the airway (Figure 12-4).

Since many bronchodilators also have some effect on the heart, an increased heart rate or patient jitteriness are common side effects of treatment.

You need permission from medical direction to help a patient self-administer a prescribed inhaler. Be

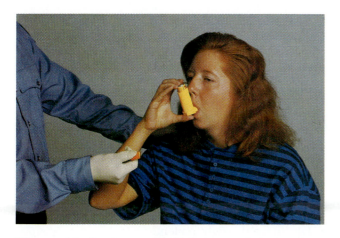

Figure 12-4 A prescribed inhaler may help a patient with certain respiratory problems.

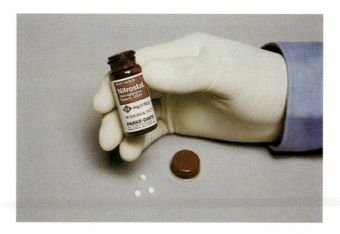

Figure 12-5 Nitroglycerin is often prescribed for chest pain.

sure to determine that the inhaler is actually the patient's and not that of a family member or bystander. (The procedures for assisting a patient with an inhaler are included in Chapter 13.)

Nitroglycerin

Many patients with cardiac problems, such as recurrent chest pain or a history of heart attack, carry nitroglycerin pills or spray (Figure 12-5). Nitroglycerin is a drug that reduces the work of the heart and helps to dilate the coronary vessels that supply the heart muscle with blood. It is often called "nitro." This drug is taken by the patient when he begins to have chest pain he believes to be cardiac in origin. It is not uncommon for EMT-Bs to treat patients who have already taken a nitro pill or who are carrying a bottle of nitroglycerin pills and have not thought to try one.

You need permission from medical direction to help the patient self-administer nitroglycerin. Be sure to determine that the nitroglycerin is actually the patient's and not that of a family member or bystander.

Since nitro causes a dilation of blood vessels, a drop in blood pressure is a potential side effect of administration. If this occurs, lay the patient flat and recontact medical direction. (The procedures for assisting a patient with nitro are covered in Chapter 14.)

Epinephrine Auto-Injectors

When a patient is highly allergic to substances such as shellfish, peanuts, penicillin, or bee stings, he or she may have a very severe reaction, which could cause airway obstruction and cardiovascular collapse. This anaphylactic reaction can be reversed by epinephrine.

Epinephrine is a medication that will help to constrict the blood vessels, correct heart rhythm problems, and relax airway passages. Because severe allergic reactions are almost immediately life-threatening,

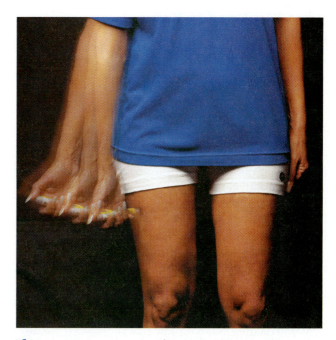

Figure 12-6 An epinephrine auto-injector can reverse a severe allergic reaction.

epinephrine must be administered quickly. Many patients who are prone to severe allergic reactions carry an epinephrine auto-injector (Figure 12-6). This is a syringe with a spring-loaded needle that will release and inject epinephrine into the muscle when the auto-injector is pushed against the thigh. If you need to assist a patient with the use of an epinephrine auto-injector, be sure to determine that it is actually the patient's and not that of someone else.

Since epinephrine has a potent effect on the heart and vascular system, increased heart rate and blood pressure commonly occur after epinephrine administration. (The procedures for assisting a patient with epinephrine are covered in Chapter 16.)

GENERAL INFORMATION ABOUT MEDICATIONS

Drug Names

Each drug is found in the *U.S. Pharmacopoeia (USP),* a comprehensive government publication, listed by its generic name ("generic" means a general name that is not the brand name of any manufacturer). Actually, each drug has at least three names: the chemical name, the generic name, and one or more trade (brand) names. For example, "epinephrine" is a generic drug name. Its chemical name is B-(e,4 dihydroxyphenyl)-a-methylaminoethanol. (Chemical names are technical formulas used only by scientists or manufacturers.) "EpiPen®" is the trade name of an epinephrine auto-injector.

What You Need to Know to Give a Medication

Every drug has **indications,** or specific circumstances, when it is appropriate to administer the drug to a patient. For example, nitroglycerin is indicated when a patient has squeezing, dull pressure chest pain.

Each drug also has **contraindications,** or specific circumstances when it is not appropriate, and may be harmful, to administer to a patient. For example, nitroglycerin is contraindicated if the patient has low blood pressure, because nitroglycerin, in dilating the coronary arteries, causes a slight drop in the systolic blood pressure.

Some drugs have side effects. A **side effect** is any action of a drug other than the desired actions. Some side effects are predictable, like the drop in blood pressure from nitroglycerin. If you were not aware of this side effect and gave the drug to a patient who started out with low blood pressure, the results could be devastating. The patient's blood pressure might "bottom out," which is definitely not a desirable effect for a cardiac patient.

Forms of Medications

Medications come in different forms. A few examples are:

- Compressed powders or tablets, such as nitroglycerin pills
- Liquids for injection, such as the epinephrine in an auto-injector
- Gels, such as the paste in a tube of oral glucose
- Suspensions, such as the thick slurry of activated charcoal in water
- Fine powder for inhalation, such as that in a prescribed inhaler

- Gases for inhalation, such as oxygen
- Sublingual (under-the-tongue) sprays, such as a nitro spray
- Liquid that is vaporized, such as a fixed-dose nebulizer

Medication Administration Rights

Before administering a drug to any patient, you must confirm the order, write it down, and then check the "rights." Do this by asking yourself the following questions as you select the drug and confirm that it is not expired:

- Do I have the right patient?
- Is this the right medication?
- Is this the right dose? (Generally, a dose is given in milligrams.)
- Am I giving this drug by the right route of administration?

Some sources also suggest that you consider as "rights" the right time of administration and the right documentation of the medication you administer.

The route of drug administration affects the rate at which the drug enters the bloodstream and arrives at its target organ to achieve its desired effect. Methods of administration include:

- Oral, or swallowed
- Intravenous, or injected into a vein
- Intramuscular, or injected into a muscle
- Sublingual, or dissolved under the tongue
- Subcutaneous, or injected into the tissues beneath the skin
- Endotracheal, sprayed into the ET tube and absorbed by the lungs
- Inhaled, or breathed into the lungs in tiny aerosol particles from an inhaler or mask
- Rectal, or placed into the rectum.

After any drug is given to a patient, it is important that you reassess the patient to see how the drug has affected him or her. Obtain another set of vitals and compare them to the baseline vitals you took before administering the drug. The ongoing assessment should include an evaluation of the changes in the patient's condition and vital signs after administration of a medication. Be sure to always document the patient's responses to each drug intervention (for example, "The respiratory distress decreased after 5 minutes of oxygen by nonrebreather mask").

Medications Patients Often Take

It would be impossible to memorize all the types of medications your patients may be taking. For example, a person might be taking insulin for diabetes, or Dilantin® to control seizures, or morphine for pain, or Inderal® for a heart rhythm disorder. The drugs a patient is taking are often a clue to a pre-existing medical condition or, if improperly used, may be a cause of his or her current problem.

It is a good idea to have a resource from which you can find out additional information about a patient's medications en route to the hospital. Many ambulances carry a *Physicians' Desk Reference,* or *PDR,* for this purpose. EMT-Bs should carry a pocket guide, such as the *Pocket Reference for the EMT-B and First Responder* available from Brady, that contains information such as generally used abbreviations. These guides list commonly prescribed medications along with the general category of that drug to help you understand what it is used for.

LIFESPAN DEVELOPMENT

Some patients, particularly the elderly, are being treated for multiple medical conditions. In these cases, it would not be surprising to find the patient is taking a number of prescriptions as well as over-the-counter drugs. In some instances, the patient may have gone to numerous physicians and the patient's care may not have been well coordinated.

If the patient produces a bagful of drug bottles, be sure to bring them along and try to determine what he or she takes on a regular basis. In these situations, patients sometimes take the following: expired medications, too many medications that have additive effects or that enhance another drug's effects, or medications whose effects counteract another drug's desired actions.

The list in Table 12-1 gives the seven common categories of drugs you find in the field that are relevant to patient care, with a few examples of drugs in each category. (The trade names are capitalized; the generic names are not.) There are many other categories in addition to those listed in the table.

Table 12-1 Medications Patients Often Take

Analgesics
Drugs prescribed for pain relief

- propoxyphene (Darvon)
- nalbuphine (Nubain)
- morphine (Astramorph PF, Duramorph, MS Contin, Roxanol)
- acetaminophen (Anacin-3, Panadol, Tempra, Tylenol)
- ibuprofen (Actiprofen, Advil, Excedrin IS, Motrin, Novoprofen, Nuprin)
- aspirin (Ecotrin, Emprin)
- codeine

Antiarrhythmics
Drugs prescribed for heart rhythm disorders

- digoxin (Lanoxin)
- propranolol (Inderal)
- verapamil (Calan, Calan SR, Isoptin, Isoptin SR, Verelan)
- procainamide (Procan SR, Promine, Pronestyl)

(continued)

Table 12-1   Medications Patients Often Take *(continued)*

Anticonvulsants
Drugs prescribed for prevention and control of seizures

- atenolol (Tenorim)
- carbamazepine (Epitol, Tegretol)
- phenytoin (Dilantin)
- primidone (Mysoline)
- phenobarbital (Phenobarbital, Phenobarbital Sodium, Solfoton)
- valoproic acid (Depakene)

Antihypertensives
Drugs prescribed to reduce high blood pressure

- captopril (Capoten)
- clonidine (Catapres)
- guanabenz (Wytensin)
- hydralazine (Apresoline, Hydralazine HCL)
- hydrochlorothiazide (Esidrix, HydroDiuril, Oretic)
- methyldopa (Aldomet)
- nifedipine (Adalat, Adalat CC, Procardia)

Bronchodilators
Drugs that relax the smooth muscles of the bronchial tubes.
These medications provide relief of bronchial asthma and allergies affecting the
respiratory system.

- albuterol (Proventil, Ventolin, Volmax)
- ipratropium bromide (Atrovent)
- isoetharine (Bronkometer, Bronkosol)
- metaproterenol (Alupent, Metaproterenol Sulfate, Metaprel)
- terbutaline (Brethaire, Brethine, Bricanyl)
- theophylline (Theo-Dur, T-Phyl, Uniphyl)

Antidiabetic agents
Drugs prescribed to diabetic patients to control hyperglycemia (high blood sugar)

- chlorpropamide (Diabinese)
- glipizide (Glucotrol)
- glyburide (DiaBeta, Glynase Prestab, Micronase)
- insulin (Humulin, Novolin, NPH, Humalog)
- metformin (Glucophage)

Table 12-1 *(continued)*

Antidepressant agents
Drugs prescribed to help regulate the emotional activity of the patient to minimize the peaks and valleys in their psychological and emotional state

- amitriptyline (Elavil)
- amoxapine (Asendin)
- bupropion (Wellbutrin)
- clomipramine (Anafranil)
- desipramine (Desipramine HCl, Norpramin)
- doxepin (Adapin, Sinequan, Sinequan Concentrate)
- fluoxetine (Prozac)
- imipramine (Tofranil, Tripamine)
- nefazodone (Serzone)
- nortriptyline (Aventyl, Pamelor)
- paroxetine (Paxil)
- protriptyline (Vivactil)
- sertraline (Zoloft)
- trimipramine (Surmontil)

Note: Generic names are lowercase. Trade names are capitalized.

SUMMARY

- Medications carried on the ambulance that the EMT-B may administer are activated charcoal, oral glucose, and oxygen.
- Medications that patients may have in their possession that the EMT-B may assist them in taking are prescribed inhalers, nitroglycerin, and epinephrine auto-injectors.
- Medical direction, defined by your local protocols, is required to assist patients with these medications.

- There are many medications that patients may be taking which offer clues to their medical history or presenting problem. The EMT-B should carry a pocket guide such as the *Pocket Reference for the EMT-B and First Responder* (Brady), which lists many commonly prescribed medications.

REVIEW QUESTIONS

1. Which of the following may the EMT-B assist the patient in taking?
   a. codeine
   b. insulin
   c. acetaminophen
   d. nitroglycerin

2. Which of the following medications does the EMT-B carry in the ambulance?
   a. activated charcoal
   b. albuterol
   c. nitroglycerin
   d. epinephrine

3. What effect does a prescribed inhaler have on a patient with a breathing emergency?
   a. It constricts blood vessels.
   b. It dilates the bronchial tubes.
   c. It dilates the coronary arteries.
   d. It constricts the bronchial tree.

4. EMT-Bs, in most EMS systems, can administer _____ with permission from medical direction for a patient with chest pain.
    a. nitroglycerin
    b. taxol
    c. epinephrine
    d. albuterol

5. Epinephrine is a _____ drug name.
    a. brand
    b. generic
    c. trade
    f. registered

WEB MEDIC

Visit Brady's *Essentials of Emergency Care* web site for direct web links. At **www.prenhall.com/limmer,** you will find information related to the following Chapter 12 topics:
*   How medications are classified
*   Reactions between the medications nitro and Viagra
*   Where to get information on drugs

RESPIRATORY EMERGENCIES

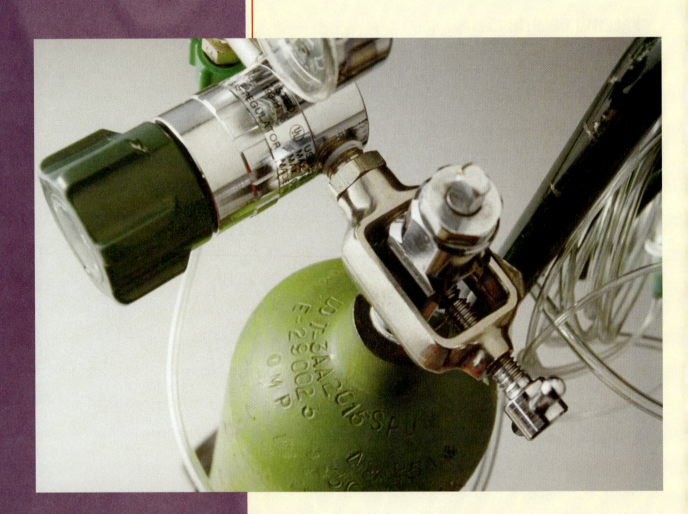

ESSENTIAL ELECTRONIC EXTRAS

CD ESSENTIALS

For preview and review of chapter material, see the student CD-ROM for

- Pretest
- Chapter quizzes
- Posttest

WEB ESSENTIALS

For additional review and enrichment, visit www.prenhall.com/limmer for

- Interactive student quizzes
- Links to online EMS resources
- Online case studies
- Audio glossary

The EMT-B curriculum discusses only one respiratory condition: respiratory distress. As an experienced EMT-B, you know that there are many diseases and conditions that can cause respiratory distress including emphysema, asthma, and chronic bronchitis. What is important to remember is that the treatment for each of these conditions is essentially the same.

RESPIRATORY SYSTEM

Respiratory anatomy and physiology consists of external and internal structures. The nose and mouth are external portions of the respiratory system. The oropharynx and nasopharynx lie posteriorly to the mouth and nose respectively. The trachea, also known as the windpipe, has cartilage rings to support its structure. The structure at the superior portion of the trachea is the larynx, or voice box. It is protected by the epiglottis, which folds over the laryngeal opening to prevent items from being aspirated into the lungs. The cricoid cartilage is a ring-shaped structure that forms the lower portion of the larynx.

The trachea splits, or bifurcates, into two bronchi. These bronchi continue to divide until they reach the alveoli, the tiny sacs where actual gas exchange with the cells takes place.

The actual process of breathing uses the diaphragm as well as muscles in the chest (Figure 13-1). During inhalation, the diaphragm and intercostal muscles contract. The diaphragm moves downward while the ribs move upward and outward, increasing the size of the thoracic cavity. This increase in the size of the chest cavity draws air into the lungs.

On exhalation, the opposite happens. The diaphragm and intercostal muscles relax, decreasing the size of the chest cavity. The end result is air flowing out of the lungs.

Gases are exchanged at the alveolar level of the lungs. Oxygen is turned over to the red blood cells while carbon dioxide is taken from the cells to be removed from the body. The oxygen-rich blood travels to the capillaries, where oxygen is turned over to the cells of the body and carbon dioxide is picked up for transport to the lungs. (You can review the anatomy and physiology of respiration in greater detail in Chapters 4 and 6.)

Adequate vs. Inadequate Breathing

Breathing is not an all-or-nothing proposition. In the past, EMS students were taught that the patient would either be breathing

---

LIFESPAN DEVELOPMENT

Remember that there are differences between the airway anatomy of the adult and infant or child patients (refer to Chapter 10, Figure 10-1). In the infant or child:

- **All structures are smaller and therefore more easily obstructed.**
- **The tongue takes up proportionally more space in the mouth.**
- **The trachea is more narrow and flexible.**
- **The cricoid cartilage is less developed and therefore less rigid.**
- **The chest wall of children is softer, and they tend to rely more heavily on the diaphragm for breathing.**

---

or not breathing. Over the years, we have come to realize that this is not always the case. Therefore, the terms "adequate breathing" and "inadequate breathing" describe the patient's respiratory status more accurately. For example, there are patients who are breathing but not at a rate or depth adequate to support life. These patients must be treated aggressively with artificial ventilation. The signs of adequate and inadequate ventilations are described in Table 13-1.

CORE CONCEPTS

In this chapter, you will learn about the following topics:

- How to recognize adequate and inadequate breathing

- How to assist a patient with breathing difficulty with a prescribed inhaler

DOT OBJECTIVES

✔ **Knowledge**

☐ 1. Provide treatment for a patient in
   respiratory distress. (pp. 191–192)

   • List the signs and symptoms of
     breathing difficulty. (p. 191)

• Describe the emergency medical care of the patient with
  breathing difficulty. (p. 192)

• Recognize the need for medical
  direction to assist in the emergency medical care of the patient with breathing difficulty.
  (pp. 190–192)

• State the generic name, medication forms, dose, administration, action, indications, and
  contraindications for the prescribed inhaler. (p. 194)

INSPIRATIONS AND EXPIRATIONS

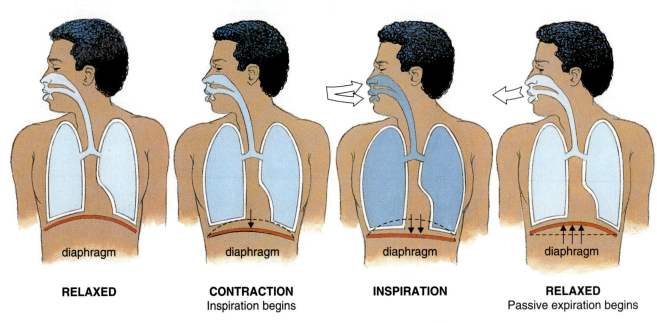

| RELAXED | CONTRACTION
Inspiration begins | INSPIRATION | RELAXED
Passive expiration begins |

Figure 13-1 The process of respiration. During inspiration, the diaphragm and rib muscles contract, causing air to flow into the lungs. During expiration, the muscles relax, causing air to flow out of the lungs.

PRECEPTOR PEARL

The concept of adequate vs. inadequate breathing is one that must be stressed to new EMT-Bs. The mere thought of providing artificial ventilation to a person who has some respiratory effort is confusing. In fact, ventilating a nonbreathing patient is difficult, let alone one that is breathing. Explain to new EMTs that they should work with the patient's respiratory effort and coach the patient when appropriate.

Recognizing and effectively treating inadequate breathing could be the most important skill you possess as an EMT-B. It is also important to determine if artificial ventilations (pocket face mask or BVM) are being performed adequately.

If these ventilations are being performed adequately:

■ The chest rises and falls with each ventilation.
■ The rate is sufficient (12 per minute for adults, 20 per minute for children and infants).
■ The heart rate may return to normal.
■ The patient's skin color improves toward normal.

Artificial ventilation is inadequate when:

■ The chest does not rise and fall with each ventilation.
■ The rate is too slow or too fast.
■ The heart rate does not return to normal.
■ The patient's skin color becomes gray or blue.

Table 13-1 Adequate and Inadequate Breathing

	Adequate Breathing	Inadequate Breathing
Rate	Adult: 12–20/min Child: 15–30/min Infant: 25–50/min	Above or below normal rates for patient's age group
Rhythm	Regular	May be irregular
Quality—breath sounds	Present and equal	Diminished, unequal, or absent
Quality—chest expansion	Adequate and equal	Inadequate or unequal
Quality—effort of breathing	Unlabored, normal respiratory effort	Labored; increases respiratory effort; use of accessory muscles (may be pronounced in infants and children and involves nasal flaring, seesaw breathing, grunting, and retractions between the ribs and above the clavicles)

Breathing Difficulty

All respiratory complaints are placed in a single category called "breathing difficulty." While we may learn about the patient's history, or even a specific cause for the complaint, emergency medical care will be essentially the same.

Patient Assessment

Breathing Difficulty

The following are signs and symptoms of breathing difficulty (Figure 13-2):

- Shortness of breath
- Restlessness
- Increased pulse rate
- Abnormal breathing rate (too fast or too slow)
- Skin color changes (cyanotic, pale, flushed)
- Noisy breathing, including crowing, wheezing (whistling sounds), gurgling, snoring, and stridor
- Inability to speak or inability to speak full sentences
- Retractions (the visible sinking in of the soft tissues of the chest between the ribs and above and below the sternum)
- Altered mental status
- Coughing
- Irregular breathing rhythm
- Abdominal breathing (diaphragm only)
- Patient in tripod position, feet dangling, leaning forward
- Unusual anatomy (barrel chest)
- Agonal respirations (slow, gasping breaths)

Use the pertinent elements of the OPQRST mnemonic to determine the respiratory history. Since it may be possible to assist the patient with his or her own prescribed medications, be sure to ask which interventions, if any, have been used.

There are acute respiratory diseases in children which may cause partial or total obstruction of the airway. Asthma attacks in the pediatric patient also may be severe. Many of these medical conditions can resemble a foreign body airway obstruction (FBAO). A key to differentiation is the patient's history: Patients who have a sudden onset of distress or obstruction without prior fever or history of disease may have an FBAO, especially if small objects are found where the child is playing. If a patient has been ill, feverish, drooling, or has a history of respiratory disease, consider this possibility. Remember that nothing is set in stone. Children with respiratory diseases may still have FBAOs. Always consider all possibilities.

Patient Care

Breathing Difficulty

Emergency care for breathing difficulty includes the following:

1 **Assess breathing.** Determine if the patient is breathing adequately.

2 **Position the patient.** If the patient is breathing adequately, place him or her in a position of comfort.

3 **Apply high-concentration oxygen,** and be prepared for changes in respiratory status throughout the call. Assist ventilations as necessary.

4 **Consult medical direction or follow standing orders,** if the patient has a prescribed inhaler. Find out if you may facilitate its use.

5 **Perform an ongoing assessment** every 5 minutes for the unstable patient. ✳

There are many respiratory diseases and conditions. While it is not necessary to diagnose these conditions in the field, it is sometimes helpful to know what each disease entails so that you can intelligently communicate with your patient and other health professionals. Table 13-2 describes common respiratory diseases and conditions.

PRECEPTOR PEARL

Patients with chronic obstructive pulmonary disease (COPD) may over time lose the normal ability to use the body's blood carbon dioxide levels as a stimulus to breathe. When this occurs, the COPD patient's body may use low blood oxygen as the factor that stimulates him or her to breathe. Because of this so-called hypoxic drive, we have for years been trained to administer only low concentrations of oxygen to COPD patients for fear of increasing the patient's blood oxygen levels and wiping out their "drive to breathe." This is an area a new EMT-B may find very confusing. Assure the EMT that it is now widely agreed that more harm is done if high-concentration oxygen is withheld.

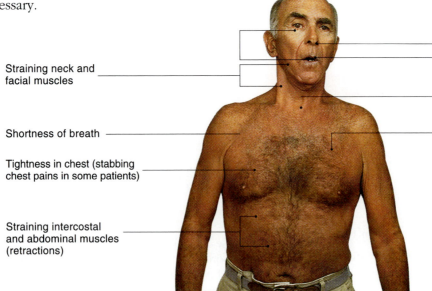

Straining neck and facial muscles

Shortness of breath

Tightness in chest (stabbing chest pains in some patients)

Straining intercostal and abdominal muscles (retractions)

Flaring nostrils
Pursed lips

Coughing

Noisy breathing
• Wheezing
• Crowing
• Gurgling
• Snoring
• Stridor

Numbness or tingling in hands and feet

Altered levels of awareness, unconsciousness, dizziness, fainting, restlessness, anxiety, confusion, combativeness

Figure 13-2 Some signs and symptoms of breathing dificulty.

Table 13-2   Common Respiratory Diseases and Conditions

Disease or Condition	Description
Emphysema	A chronic obstructive pulmonary disease (COPD) that causes the walls of the alveoli to break down and lose elasticity. Excess secretions and damaged alveoli trap stale air in the lungs.
Chronic Bronchitis	A chronic obstructive pulmonary disease (COPD), in which the lining of the bronchiole is inflamed. Mucus production prevents the cilia (small hairs that provide a sweeping motion) from clearing the mucus from the bronchioles.
Asthma	Asthma is *not* a chronic pulmonary disease. Triggered by an allergen, exercise, or emotional stress, asthma affects young and old patients. Asthma is episodic. Attacks occur at irregular intervals. The patient is free of symptoms between attacks. During an attack, bronchioles in the lungs constrict and mucus is produced. This causes wheezing and severe difficulty breathing.
Congestive Heart Failure	This is usually a condition that is caused by the heart but affects the lungs. The heart fails to pump properly and blood actually backs up into the pulmonary circulation and into the lungs (pulmonary edema). Patients will have difficulty breathing, rapid pulse, moist skin that is pale or cyanotic, and swollen ankles. In extreme cases the patient may cough up pink frothy sputum.

NOTE: The diseases and conditions presented in this table are for your information only. Patients with respiratory distress receive similar treatment in the field. It is not necessary for you to diagnose specific conditions to provide proper treatment.

Prescribed Inhaler

You may be called to a patient with respiratory distress who has a prescribed inhaler. Being unable to breathe can be frightening. If your EMS system allows you to assist the patient with the inhaler, it may ease the patient's distress and be a tremendous benefit.

As much of a benefit as medications can be, they also may be a hazard. Administering or facilitating the administration of medications is a major responsibility. It must always be taken seriously and handled responsibly.

Before administering any medication, be sure that it is indicated. The patient must meet certain criteria—in this case, signs of respiratory distress must be present (Skill Summary 13-1). The patient must have an inhaler that is actually prescribed to him or her. If your system requires, contact medical direction before you assist with administration of the inhaler.

There are also contraindications to medications—situations in which the medication must not be used. For the prescribed inhaler, contraindications include: the patient is not able to use the device, the inhaler is not prescribed to the patient, medical direction has not given approval, and the patient already used the maximum prescribed dose(s). The type of drug contained in prescribed inhalers may cause tremors, nervousness, and increased pulse rate, especially if the maximum dose is exceeded.

Always check the "rights" as they apply to your situation: right patient, right medication, right dose, right route, right time, and right documentation.

Use of the prescribed inhaler requires the cooperation of the patient (Skill Summary 13-2). This may not be an easy task if the patient is anxious—a condition frequently seen in respiratory distress. It is important to have the patient exhale deeply before activating the inhaler. Then, when the inhaler is activated, the patient should inhale deeply. Instruct the patient to hold his or her breath for a reasonable time so the medication may be absorbed. The dose may be repeated if allowed or ordered by medical direction.

You may observe a spacer device attached to the patient's inhaler. It helps the patient inhale more of the medication.

Monitor the patient carefully after administration of any medication. The ongoing assessment should be performed, including vital signs, chief complaint, and effects of the medication.

Note that home medication nebulizer devices have become more common in the treatment of patients with respiratory disease. (Nebulizers cause a gas such as oxygen to flow through a liquid medication, turning it into a vapor that can be continuously inhaled.) These devices deliver the same types of medications as inhalers, but over a long period of time. Your local medical direction may authorize you to assist patients in the use of nebulizers.

FIRST take BSI precautions.

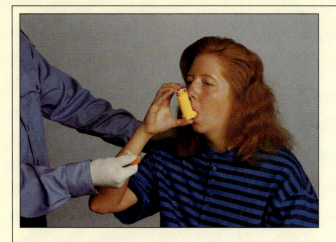

MEDICATION NAME

- Generic: albuterol, isoetharine, metaproterenol, ipratropium.
- Trade: Proventil®, Ventolin®, Bronkosol®, Bronkometer®, Alupent®, Metaprel®, Atrovent®.

INDICATIONS

All of the following criteria must be met:
- Patient exhibits signs and symptoms of respiratory emergency.
- Patient has physician-prescribed hand-held inhaler.
- Medical direction gives specific authorization to assist in administration of the medication.

CONTRAINDICATIONS

- Patient is unable to use device (e.g., not alert).
- Inhaler is not prescribed for patient.
- No permission has been given by medical direction.
- Patient has already taken maximum prescribed dose prior to EMT-B's arrival.

MEDICATION FORM

Hand-held metered dose inhaler.

DOSAGE

Number of inhalations based on medical direction's order or physician's order.

ADMINISTRATION

1. Obtain order from medical direction, either on-line or off-line.
2. Assure right patient, right medication, right dose, right route, right time, right documentation. Patient also should be alert enough to use inhaler.
3. Check expiration date of inhaler.
4. Check to see if patient has already taken any doses.
5. Assure inhaler is at room temperature or warmer.
6. Shake inhaler vigorously several times.
7. Have patient exhale deeply.
8. Have patient put lips around the opening of inhaler.
9. Have patient depress the inhaler as she inhales deeply.
10. Instruct patient to hold her breath for as long as she comfortably can so that medication can be absorbed.
11. Put oxygen back on patient.
12. Allow patient to breathe a few times and then repeat dose, if so ordered by medical direction.
13. If patient has a spacer device for use with inhaler, it should be used. (A spacer is attached between inhaler and patient to allow for more effective use of medication.)

ACTIONS

Beta agonist bronchodilator dilates bronchioles, reducing airway resistance.

SIDE EFFECTS

- Increased pulse rate
- Tremors
- Nervousness

REASSESSMENT STRATEGIES

1. Gather vital signs.
2. Perform focused reassessment of chest and respiratory function.
3. Observe for deterioration of patient. If breathing becomes inadequate, provide artificial ventilations.
4. Record assessments.

FIRST take BSI precautions.

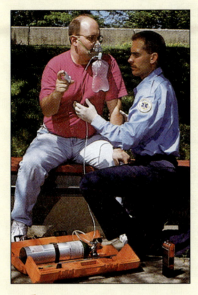

▲ **1.** The patient has the indications for use of an inhaler.

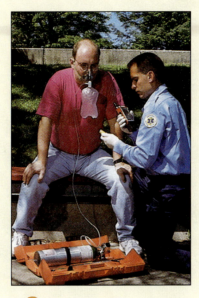

▲ **2.** The EMT-B contacts medical direction to obtain an order to assist the patient with the prescribed inhaler.

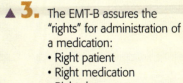

▲ **3.** The EMT-B assures the "rights" for administration of a medication:
- Right patient
- Right medication
- Right dose
- Right route
- Right time
- Right documentation.

EMT-B also checks expiration date, shakes inhaler, makes sure inhaler is room temperature or warmer, and makes sure patient is alert.

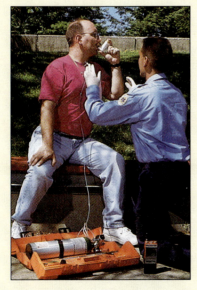

▲ **4.** The EMT-B coaches the patient in use of inhaler: exhale deeply, press the inhaler to activate spray as you begin to inhale, hold in your breath so the medication can be absorbed.

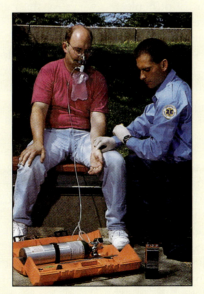

▲ **5.** After use of inhaler, EMT-B reassesses the patient: takes vital signs, does a focused exam, determines if breathing is adequate.

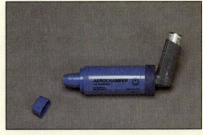

▲ **6.** A "spacer" device between inhaler and patient allows more effective use of medication. If the patient has a spacer, it should be attached to the inhaler before use. The patient should then follow the manufacter's instructions. It is important to note two things about using a spacer: (1) timing is not as critical as long as the patient presses the inhaler *before* inhaling, and (2) the patient should inhale deeply but *slowly*.

Respiratory Emergencies

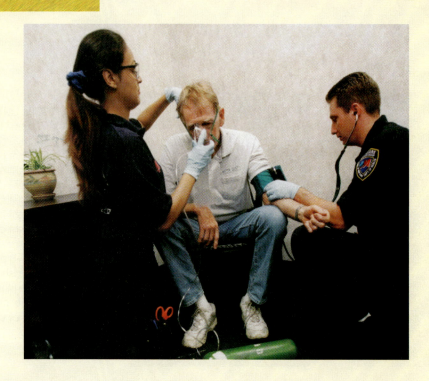

Dispatch Information: 1425 McGregor Circle   **Difficulty Breathing   2237 hrs**

Your ambulance is dispatched to a senior citizen housing complex for a report of difficulty breathing. You approach the scene scanning for dangers and find none. As you walk into the building, you see an open door at the end of the hallway.

The patient's labored breathing can be heard even before you round the corner into the room. He is sitting in a chair and appears to be using his whole upper body to breathe. Your general impression is that of a male in his 60s in considerable respiratory distress with poor skin color. This is enough for you to assign him a high priority for transport.

You find he is by himself in the apartment. He gives his name as Glen McDougal and says that he would like your help and transportation to the hospital. He tells you he has been there before on two occasions, both for heart attacks. Your partner indicates that he will begin to give the patient oxygen by nonrebreather mask while you perform a history and obtain vital signs. You notice that Mr. McDougal is anxious.

The patient states that he had been feeling weak for the past day or so and that he had a bit of difficulty breathing last night, but nothing serious. He tried to retire early tonight but couldn't lie down without having trouble breathing. It is now difficult to breathe in any position. He takes furosemide, Lanoxin, K-Dur, and naproxen. He denies pain or discomfort in his chest, neck, back, or arms. He has not been diagnosed with emphysema, chronic bronchitis, or asthma.

His vital signs are: pulse 96 and slightly irregular; respirations 24 and labored; blood pressure 142/92; skin pale, cool, and moist; and pupils equal and reactive to light. The patient has equal lung sounds bilaterally, and you can't help but notice moist crackling sounds as you evaluate his breathing. The patient's ankles appear somewhat swollen. He denies having had a fever, cough, or other respiratory infection recently.

After putting an oxygen mask on the patient, your partner prepares him for transport by bringing the stretcher inside and moving it alongside the chair. You move Mr. McDougal to the stretcher and then to the ambulance in a sitting position and begin transport. En route, you perform an ongoing assessment and repeat vitals. The oxygen has helped the difficulty breathing; and vitals remain essentially the same.

CASE DISCUSSION

The patient appeared to be in respiratory distress. His poor skin color and anxiousness add to the picture and suggest a potentially serious condition. This patient is indeed a high priority. His history of previous heart attacks and medications indicate a possible cardiac cause of the problem, although diagnosis isn't critical since your treatment would be the same regardless of the cause.

The patient was provided with immediate high-concentration oxygen, and transport was initiated promptly. An adequate history was obtained, but the effort to gather it was not prolonged because prompt transport was crucial.

Name: Glen McDougal
Age: 66
Chief Complaint: *"I am really having a hard time breathing."*

ASSESSMENT INFORMATION	RELEVANCE TO THIS PATIENT
History of heart attacks	• This history points to the possibility of this call being cardiac related, even without chest pain (silent heart attack). • Care givers should be alert for possible cardiac or respiratory arrest throughout this call.
Physical examination	• Swollen ankles may indicate fluid accumulation. • Pale skin and anxiety indicate hypoxia.
Medications	• Furosemide (also called Lasix) is a diuretic (water pill). • K-Dur is a potassium supplement used in conjunction with the water pill. • Lanoxin is a cardiac medication. • Naproxen is an anti-inflammatory. Its use should prompt questions about arthritis or previous skeletal injury.
Other considerations	• The patient's increase in breathing difficulty when lying down is significant and also may indicate fluid build up in the lungs. • He appears to be a patient with a serious condition (cardiac/respiratory). He looks bad and should be treated as a high priority.

CHAPTER REVIEW

SUMMARY

- It is a main responsibility of an EMT-B to identify inadequate or absent breathing and provide immediate respiratory support or artificial ventilation.

- Patients with breathing difficulty are often anxious, with labored respirations, abnormal respiratory rates, poor skin color, and other symptoms.

- The EMT-B may assist a patient with breathing difficulty who has a prescribed inhaler as long as local protocols are followed.

- Be especially alert for signs and symptoms of breathing difficulty in children because they can become unstable very quickly.

REVIEW QUESTIONS

1. Which of the following is true regarding the child's airway as opposed to the adult's?

  a. The trachea is wider and less flexible.

  b. The tongue takes up proportionally more space in the mouth.

  c. The cricoid cartilage is more rigid.

  d. The chest wall is firmer.

2. The proper rate of artificial ventilation for adult/child patients is:

  a. 8/18.

  b. 12/20.

  c. 20/12.

  d. 20/30.

3. Which of the following is NOT a sign of breathing difficulty?

  a. coughing

  b. restlessness

  c. decreased pulse rate

  d. abdominal breathing

4. Which of the following is NOT a side effect associated with use of a prescribed inhaler?

  a. cyanosis

  b. increased pulse rate

  c. tremors

  d. nervousness

REVIEW QUESTIONS continued

5. Which of the following is NOT an indication to assist a patient in using a hand-held inhaler?

a. The patient shows signs and symptoms of respiratory emergency.

b. The patient has a physician prescribed hand-held inhaler.

c. Medical direction gives authorization to assist in use of the inhaler.

d. The patient is not alert.

WEB MEDIC

Visit Brady's *Essentials of Emergency Care* web site for direct web links. At **www.prenhall.com/limmer,** you will find information related to the following Chapter 13 topics:

- American Lung Association
- Asthma
- Bronchitis
- American Cancer Society

Chapter Fourteen

CARDIAC EMERGENCIES

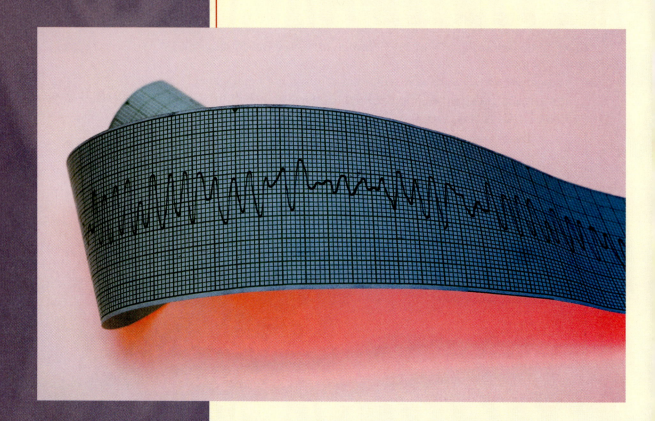

ESSENTIAL ELECTRONIC EXTRAS

CD ESSENTIALS

For preview and review of chapter material, see the student CD-ROM for

- Pretest
- Chapter quizzes
- Posttest

WEB ESSENTIALS

For additional review and enrichment, visit www.prenhall.com/limmer for

- Interactive student quizzes
- Links to online EMS resources
- Online case studies
- Audio glossary

More than a half million people die from cardiovascular disease in the United States every year. Many of these deaths occur before the patient reaches a hospital. However, defibrillation, if performed early enough, can prevent some of them. Rapid defibrillation is the single most important factor in increasing survival from cardiac arrest caused by ventricular fibrillation.

For patients who are not in cardiac arrest but who are experiencing cardiac-related chest pain, EMT-Bs can now, in addition to oxygen administration, assist them in taking their own nitroglycerin. This can sometimes relieve pain and the anxiety that accompanies it. When patients meet certain conditions, it should be safe for the EMT-B to assist them in taking this medication. NOTE: Your ability to assist a patient with the administration of nitroglycerin will be determined by local medical direction.

CARDIAC COMPROMISE

Like "breathing difficulty," "cardiac compromise" is also a general term. There are many diseases and conditions that can cause chest pain. You have undoubtedly heard other health professionals talking about terms like "angina pectoris," "myocardial infarction," and "pulmonary edema." These are only some of the many conditions that affect the heart. There are also other conditions that can mimic heart problems. Problems with the lungs or the muscles around the chest have led patients to believe they were having heart attacks. Diagnosing these conditions can be perplexing even to an emergency physician with a battery of laboratory tests available. Since EMT-B treatment for all the potential causes of cardiac compromise is the same, a specific diagnosis is not important.

Patient Assessment

Cardiac Compromise

Cardiac compromise is characterized by any of a number of signs and symptoms, such as:

- Pain or a squeezing, dull pressure in the chest, commonly radiating down the arms or up to the jaw
- Difficulty breathing
- Feeling of impending doom
- Epigastric (upper abdominal) pain or discomfort
- Nausea and vomiting
- Sudden onset of sweating

These signs and symptoms can arise for a number of reasons. When the heart is functioning normally, both the mechanical and electrical aspects function in a coordinated manner. When one of these

systems malfunctions, the patient can experience any one of a number of conditions that fall into the category of cardiac compromise. ✱

However, before you consider these conditions, briefly review the anatomy and physiology of the heart. The normal heart has four chambers, an atrium and a ventricle on both the left and right sides. Blood comes into the atrium, flows into the ventricle, and is then pumped out of the heart. The left side of the heart pumps blood out through the aorta where it then is channeled through arteries, arterioles, and capillaries throughout the body. When the blood gets to the capillaries, it gives oxygen and nutrients to the cells, and picks up carbon dioxide in exchange. The blood then travels through venules and veins to the right side of the heart. Here it is pumped out through the pulmonary arteries to the capillaries surrounding the alveoli in the lungs. Again, oxygen and carbon dioxide are exchanged and the blood returns via the

CORE CONCEPTS

In this chapter, you will learn about the following topics:

- How to assess, recognize, and manage cardiac emergencies
- How to assist a patient in taking his or her nitroglycerin
- How to attempt resuscitation of a patient in cardiac arrest by administering CPR and applying an automated external defibrillator (AED)

✔ **Knowledge**

☐ 1. Provide care to a patient experiencing chest pain/discomfort. (p. 203)

- Describe emergency medical care of the patient experiencing chest pain/discomfort. (p. 203)

- Discuss the position of comfort for patients with various cardiac emergencies. (p. 203)

- Recognize the need for medical direction or protocols to assist in the emergency medical care of the patient with chest pain. (p. 203)

- List the indications for the use of nitroglycerin. (pp. 203, 204)

☐ 2. Attempt to resuscitate a patient in cardiac arrest. (pp. 209–210)

- Discuss the circumstance which may result in inappropriate shocks. (p. 208)

- Explain the considerations for interruption of CPR when using the automated external defibrillator. (p. 217)

- List the steps in the operation of the automated external defibrillator. (pp. 209–210, 211–214)

- Discuss the need to complete the Automated Defibrillator: Operator's Shift Checklist. (p. 218)

- Explain the role medical direction plays in the use of automated external defibrillation. (p. 218)

✔ **Skills**

☐ 3. Given medical scenarios, demonstrate the ability to properly assess the patient and demonstrate the ability to properly utilize the intervention to include nitroglycerin. (pp. 220–221)

☐ 4. Given a cardiac arrest scenario, demonstrate the use of the AED. (pp. 209–210, 220–221)

pulmonary veins to the left side of the heart where it begins the cycle again.

Like any muscle, the heart needs oxygen and nutrients and a way to get rid of carbon dioxide and wastes. This is done through the coronary arteries, a system of blood vessels that come off the aorta immediately after it leaves the heart. If one or more of these arteries become blocked, the patient may (or may not) experience symptoms. If the blockage is sufficient to cut off enough of the blood supply to cause death of heart tissue, the patient has had a **myocardial infarction (MI),** or heart attack (Figure 14-1). Depending on the location and extent of the damage, the patient may sustain a cardiac arrest, or experience chest pain, epigastric distress, sudden onset of weakness and sweating, shortness of breath, or nothing at all.

If some of the heart tissue has its blood supply temporarily restricted (but not to the point of causing cell death), the patient has **angina pectoris.** Typically during one of these episodes, the patient experiences chest pain that is relieved by stopping strenuous activity, taking nitroglycerin, or increasing the percentage of oxygen intake. However, not all cases of angina are typical or respond to these measures. Differentiating MI from angina can be difficult at times—even for experienced physicians.

Congestive heart failure (CHF) is another common cardiac problem seen in EMS systems. This condition is characterized by buildup of fluid in the lungs or other areas of the body. It results from an inability of one or both sides of the heart to pump out all the blood that is coming in. If the trouble is on the left side (as often happens), the blood coming into the

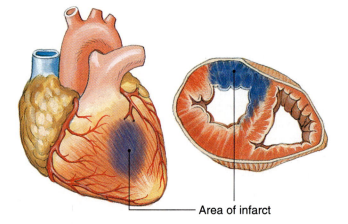

Area of infarct

Figure 14-1 Cross-section of heart showing myocardial infarction.

left side of the heart from the lungs begins to back up. The pressure in the pulmonary veins increases, causing the pressure in the capillaries surrounding the alveoli to increase also. The distance between a capillary and an alveolus is extremely small in order to allow oxygen and carbon dioxide to pass through. When fluid pressure in the capillaries increases significantly, this short distance allows fluid to pass into the alveoli, obstructing the airway. This is why you sometimes see patients with severe CHF or pulmonary edema coughing up pink, frothy sputum.

If the right side of the heart is experiencing difficulty, blood backs up into the systemic circulation. In this case, you may see distended neck veins and edema in the ankles, among other things.

The electrical system of the heart is an integral part of this activity. The heart has specialized fibers that conduct electrical impulses that stimulate the cells in the heart to contract. Ordinarily, the heart's own natural pacemaker in the right atrium, called the **sinoatrial node,** is the starting point for these impulses, which simultaneously travel to both the atria and the ventricles. The atria immediately contract and squeeze blood into the ventricles, providing them with about 10% to 20% more blood than if the atria did not do this. The impulses to the ventricles do not arrive until about one- to two-tenths of one second later, allowing time for this "priming" of the pump to occur. An abnormality with the conduction system can cause a number of different problems. For example, the patient's heart rate may become extremely fast or extremely slow.

Sometimes, the heart's electrical system loses all ability to regulate these impulses, and the cells all fire randomly (**ventricular fibrillation, or VF**). The patient's heart then no longer beats in a coordinated fashion and the patient experiences cardiac arrest.

As you can see, there are many different presentations that patients with cardiac problems can have. However the patient presents, you will still need to perform an initial assessment, a focused history and physical exam including baseline vital signs, and an OPQRST and SAMPLE history.

Patient Care

Cardiac Compromise

The mainstay of management of cardiac compromise is oxygen. A commonly administered medication, oxygen can correct the hypoxia that sometimes accompanies cardiac emergencies. There is virtually no risk to the patient and the potential benefit is very high.

The other medication that may be appropriate is **nitroglycerin (NTG)** (Skill Summary 14-1). Nitroglycerin is a very powerful drug that dilates blood vessels and reduces the workload of the heart. This reduces the heart's demand for oxygen and can prevent further hypoxic damage to the heart. Because nitroglycerin is so powerful and has significant side effects (like hypotension), it is not for every patient. It should be safe to administer nitroglycerin to a patient who has been evaluated by a physician and received a prescription for it. Even then, it is taken only for specific reasons (e.g., chest pain or discomfort) and can still occasionally produce serious side effects.

Emergency care steps include the following shown in Skill Summary 14-2.

1 Place the patient in a position of comfort. Typically this is sitting up. Patients who are hypotensive (systolic blood pressure less than 90) will usually feel better lying down. This position allows more blood to flow to the brain. Occasionally, you will see a patient who has both difficulty breathing and hypotension, in which case it may not be easy to find a good position. The best way to determine this is to ask the patient what position will relieve his or her difficulty breathing without causing weakness or lightheadedness.

2 Apply high-concentration oxygen through a nonrebreather mask. If the patient has or develops an altered mental status, you will need to open and maintain the airway. If the patient is not breathing adequately, you will also need to ventilate. Always be prepared for the patient to go into cardiac arrest.

3 Call ALS, if it is available in your EMS system.

4 If the patient has any one of the following, transport promptly:
- No history of cardiac problems.
- History of cardiac problems, but does not have nitroglycerin.
- Systolic blood pressure of less than 100.

5 If all of the following conditions are met, give the patient (or help the patient take) nitroglycerin:
- Patient complains of chest pain.
- Patient has a history of cardiac problems.
- Patient's physician has prescribed nitroglycerin (NTG).
- Patient has the nitroglycerin with him or her.
- Systolic blood pressure is greater than 100.
- Medical direction authorizes administration of the medication.

6 If all of the following conditions are met after giving one dose of the nitroglycerin, repeat another dose in 3 to 5 minutes:
- Patient experiences no relief.
- Systolic blood pressure remains greater than 100.
- Medical direction authorizes another dose of the medication.

Administer up to a maximum of three doses of nitroglycerin, reassessing vital signs and chest pain after each dose. If the blood pressure falls below 100 systolic, treat the patient for shock (hypoperfusion), and transport promptly. ✳

FIRST take BSI precautions.

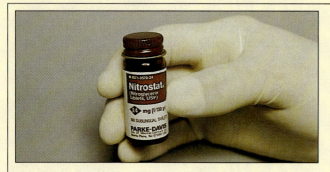

MEDICATION NAME
- Generic: nitroglycerin.
- Trade: Nitrostat®, Nitrolingual® Spray.

INDICATIONS
All of the following conditions must be met:
- Patient complains of chest pain.
- Patient has history of cardiac problems.
- Patient's physician has prescribed nitroglycerin (NTG).
- Systolic blood pressure is greater than 100 systolic.
- Medical direction authorizes administration of the medication.

CONTRAINDICATIONS
- Patient has hypotension or a systolic blood pressure below 100.
- Patient has a head injury.
- Patient is an infant or child.
- Patient has already taken the maximum prescribed dose.
- No permission has been given by medical direction.

MEDICATION FORM
Tablet, or sublingual (under the tongue) spray.

DOSAGE
One dose, repeat in 3 to 5 minutes. If there is no relief, systolic blood pressure remains above 100, and if authorized by medical direction, assist in administering up to maximum of three doses.

ADMINISTRATION
1. Perform focused assessment for cardiac patient.
2. Take blood pressure. (Systolic must be above 100.)
3. Contact medical direction, if there are no standing orders.
4. Assure right medication, right patient, right dose, right route. Be sure patient is alert enough to take medication.

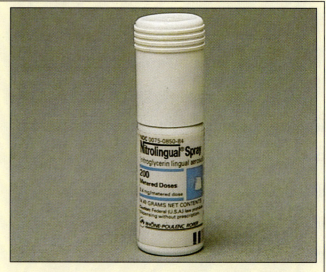

5. Check expiration date of medication.
6. Question patient on last dose taken and effects. Assure understanding of route of administration.
7. Ask patient to lift tongue and place tablet or spray dose under tongue.
8. Have patient keep mouth closed with tablet under tongue (without swallowing) until it dissolves and is absorbed.
9. Recheck blood pressure within 2 minutes.
10. Record name, dose, route, and time of administration of the medication.
11. Perform reassessment.

ACTIONS
- Relaxes blood vessels
- Decreases workload of heart

SIDE EFFECTS
- Hypotension (lowers blood pressure)
- Headache
- Pulse rate changes

REASSESSMENT STRATEGIES
1. Monitor patient's blood pressure.
2. Ask patient about effect on pain relief.
3. Seek medical direction before assisting in administration of another dose.
4. Record assessments.

Chest Pain Management

FIRST take BSI precautions.

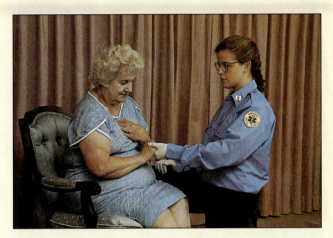

▲ **1.** Perform an initial assessment.

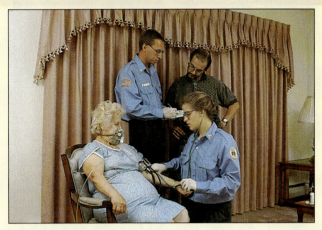

▲ **2.** Provide high-concentration oxygen by nonrebreather mask. Perform a focused history and physical exam for a medical patient. Document findings.

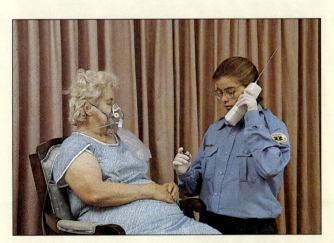

▲ **3.** If patient meets nitroglycerin criteria and has pre-scribed nitroglycerin, ask the patient about the last dose taken. Consult medical direction with regard to assisting the patient in taking medication.

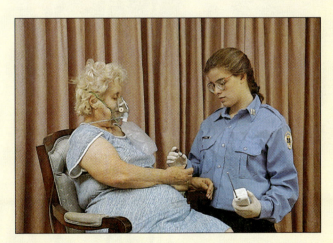

▲ **4.** Check the four rights: right patient, right drug, right dose, right route. Also check the expiration date.

(continued)

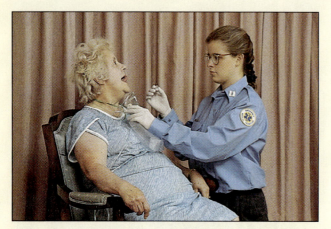

▲ **5.** Remove the oxygen mask. Ask the patient to open her mouth and lift her tongue.

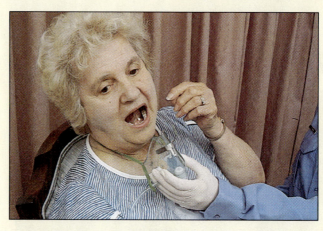

▲ **6.** Place the nitroglycerin tablet under the patient's tongue.

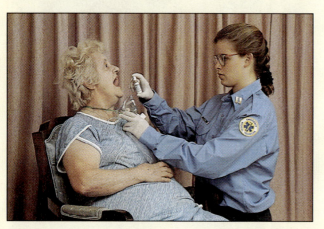

▲ **7.** . . . Or if the nitroglycerin is in spray form, spray the medication under the tongue according to label directions.

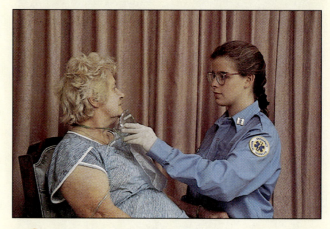

▲ **8.** Have the patient close her mouth and hold the nitroglycerin under the tongue, where the medication will be quickly absorbed.

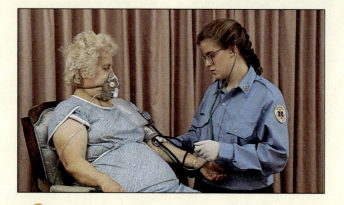

▲ **9.** Replace the oxygen mask, reassess the patient, and document findings.

CARDIAC ARREST

Only 1 to 2 percent of the emergency calls in a typical EMS system are cardiac arrests, but many systems dedicate a significant amount of their resources to handling those cases. This is probably related to both the ancient desire to bring someone back from the dead and the recent advances in technology that sometimes allow us to actually accomplish this.

Chain of Survival

For the patient in cardiac arrest to have the greatest possible chance of survival, the EMS system must be configured properly and EMS responders must act quickly and efficiently. The American Heart Association has summarized the four major factors that affect the likelihood of recovery from cardiac arrest: early access, early CPR, early defibrillation, and early advanced care. Together, these elements make up the "chain of survival" (Figure 14-2).

Early access means that someone who sees a patient collapse, or finds the patient already collapsed, notifies EMS quickly. This depends on having a well-educated public, an easy-to-remember phone number (like 911), and an efficient dispatch system.

Early CPR depends on having either a CPR-trained bystander nearby or being able to send an EMS-trained First Responder. This is where the value of training lay people in CPR becomes apparent.

Early defibrillation means delivering the first defibrillatory shock while it can still do some good. Every minute a heart remains in VF (ventricular fibrillation) without being defibrillated reduces the patient's chance of survival by 8% to 12%. This is why virtually no one is resuscitated if the response time of the person with the defibrillator is more than 8 minutes. Automated defibrillation keeps to a minimum the time from arrival of the defibrillator to delivery of the first shock.

A few patients arrest after the arrival of EMS. This is why you must always be prepared for the patient to go into cardiac arrest. Most patients you see in cardiac arrest, though, are already pulseless when EMS receives the call.

Early advanced care refers to interventions such as endotracheal intubation and administration of medications. Strengthening the first three elements in the chain of survival can produce significant improvements. Strengthening the fourth element—early advanced care—may improve the survival rate even further.

As an EMT-B, your responsibilities at a cardiac arrest include not only performing one- and two-rescuer CPR, but also:

- Using an automated external defibrillator.
- Requesting ALS backup when appropriate (or prompt transport to an emergency department).
- Ventilating with a bag-valve-mask or flow-restricted, oxygen-powered ventilation device.
- Lifting and moving the patient.
- Suctioning and using airway adjuncts.
- Interviewing family members and bystanders to obtain information related to the arrest.

Types of Defibrillators

Defibrillators are either manual or automated. A manual defibrillator is the kind typically found in an emergency department. The operator interprets the electrocardiographic (ECG) rhythm and makes the decision whether to shock.

An automated external defibrillator (AED), on the other hand, has a microprocessor that interprets the rhythm and determines whether or not it is appropriate to deliver a shock. A fully automated defibrillator operates without the need for any action by the operator except to turn on the power and attach the monitoring/defibrillation pads to the patient. A semi-automatic defibrillator, after analyzing the rhythm, advises the EMT-B to deliver a shock, if appropriate. Semi-automatic defibrillators are sometimes called shock advisory defibrillators. (See Figure 14-3 for examples of AEDs.)

Chain of Survival

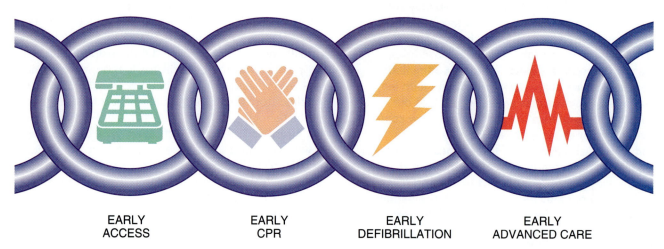

EARLY
ACCESS

EARLY
CPR

EARLY
DEFIBRILLATION

EARLY
ADVANCED CARE

Figure 14-2 The American heart Association has identified the elments of the "chain of survival.".

Another way in which defibrillators differ is in the kinds of shocks they deliver. The traditional direct current shock goes from one electrode to the other. This is called monophasic. A newer type of AED provides biphasic defibrillation, in which the energy goes in one direction, then reverses itself and moves in the opposite direction between the two electrodes.

Research suggests that biphasic shocks are at least equal to monophasic shocks, and they hold the promise of causing less damage to the heart. A biphasic AED typically determines the impedance or resistance of the tissue between the two electrodes and adjusts the size of the shock accordingly. This allows a biphasic AED to deliver a first shock to patients smaller than the traditional 200 joules with lower impedance. The need for less energy has also resulted in smaller, lighter batteries in these devices.

Using a biphasic AED is just like using a monophasic AED. The only difference you might notice is that the machine is lighter than the monophasic AED you may have carried in the past.

Using an AED

Automated defibrillators have been extremely accurate in discriminating between patients who do and do not need shocks. The most common reason for an incorrect decision by an AED is improper use by the person operating the machine (e.g., attaching an AED to a patient who has a pulse or not charging the batteries). Occasionally, an AED will make an error that is not the result of operator error. In this case, the machine will almost always fail to deliver a shock rather than deliver an inappropriate shock.

LIFESPAN DEVELOPMENT

Infants and children rarely go into cardiac arrest because of ventricular fibrillation. In adults, cardiac arrest is often the result of a problem with the heart, the most common cause being myocardial infarction. In infants and children, cardiac arrest is typically the end result of a respiratory problem, which causes the heart to slow, gradually leading to asystole (straight line). Rarely do they go into VF.

Since defibrillation is the appropriate treatment for VF, this means a defibrillator has very limited value in the treatment of a pediatric arrest patient. The best treatment for an infant or child in arrest is CPR, with special attention to the airway and ventilation, along with prompt transport to an appropriate facility. Using an AED on a child will delay transport without any reason to believe that it will help the patient.

An EMT-B should *not* attach an AED to a patient who has a pulse because many defibrillators advise shocks for ventricular tachycardia when the rate exceeds a certain value (for example, above 180 beats per minute). You should attach an AED *only* to an unresponsive, pulseless, nonbreathing patient to avoid delivering inappropriate shocks.

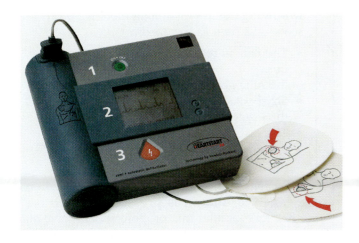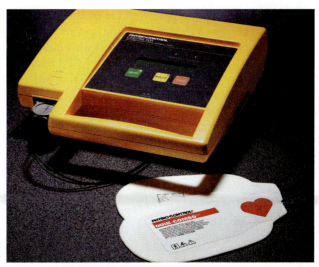

Figure 14-3 Automated external defibrillators (AEDs). Units capable of administering proper shocks to children are now available.

Patient Assessment

Cardiac Arrest

As with all calls, you should protect yourself from infectious diseases by taking BSI precautions. This is especially important in the case of a cardiac arrest, where blood and other body fluids are commonly found.

- Perform the initial assessment. If a bystander is doing CPR when you arrive, have the bystander stop. Verify pulselessness and apnea. Look for external blood loss.

- After you have started or resumed CPR, you should perform a focused history and physical exam. Inquire about onset, trauma, and signs and symptoms that were present before the patient collapsed. Get a SAMPLE history if you can. Do not let history gathering interfere with or slow down defibrillation. ✳

Patient Care

Cardiac Arrest

Refer to Skill Summary 14-3 as you read the steps that follow.

1. **Begin or resume CPR.**

2. **Determine whether or not the patient is a candidate for the AED:** If the patient is an adult (defined as at least 8 years old or 55 pounds for the purpose of defibrillation) who has not sustained trauma, proceed with the AED. If the patient is less than 8 years old and less than 55 pounds OR the patient has sustained trauma, do not attach the AED unless

you are ordered to do so by medical direction. Continue CPR and transport.

3. **Turn on the defibrillator power.**

4. **Begin the narrative,** if the AED has a voice recorder. You should describe who you are, what the situation is, and what you are doing as you do it. However, do not delay your actions in order to describe them.

5. **Attach the monitoring/defibrillation pads to the cables.**

6. **Bare the patient's chest** (if not already done), and place the pads so that the one attached to the white cable is in the angle between the sternum and the right clavicle and the one attached to the red cable is over the lower left ribs ("white to right, red to ribs"). Press the pads firmly on the chest to ensure good contact. Once in a while, you may have a male patient whose chest is so hairy that the pads do not make good contact. Use a hospital razor to quickly shave some of the hair away, and use a new pair of pads.

7. **Stop CPR and clear the patient** (make sure no one is touching the patient).

NOTE: About half of all patients in cardiac arrest have nonshockable heart rhythms. If this is the case, when you press the "analyze" button, the AED will give a "No shock" message. In other cases, the AED may give you a "Deliver shock" message and then, after one or more shocks are delivered, will give a "No shock" message on a subsequent try. (When the AED gives a "No shock" message, it may be very bad news: the patient has a nonshockable heart rhythm and cannot be helped by the defibrillator. Or it may be very good news: the electrical rhythm of the patient's heart has responded successfully to earlier shocks. In the latter case, even though the heart's electrical activity has recovered, another stint of CPR may be required to get enough oxygen into the muscle cells of the heart to start it beating again.) If your AED shows a heart rhythm, remember: just because the patient's heart shows electrical activity on the screen, that does not mean there is a pulse!

If a "Deliver shock" message is received each time you press the "analyze" button:

8 **When you get a "Deliver shock" message:**

- Deliver the first shock.
- Press the "analyze" button to re-analyze the rhythm. If you get a "Deliver shock" message, deliver a second shock.
- Press the "analyze" button to re-analyze the rhythm. If you get a "Deliver shock" message, deliver a third shock.

The set of shocks you have just delivered is called a "set of three stacked shocks"— "stacked" because they are delivered with no pause for a pulse check or CPR between shocks. Pulse checks should not occur during rhythm analysis. They would slow down defibrillation and are not necessary.

9 **Check the carotid pulse** after the first set of three stacked shocks. If the patient has a pulse, check breathing. If the patient is breathing adequately, give high-concentration oxygen by nonrebreather mask and transport. Or, if the patient is not breathing adequately, provide artificial ventilations with high-concentration oxygen and transport.

10 **If the patient does not have a pulse, resume CPR for 1 minute. Then:**

- Press the "analyze" button to analyze the rhythm. If you get a "Deliver shock" message, deliver the fourth shock.
- Press the "analyze" button to re-analyze the rhythm. If you get a "Deliver shock" message, deliver a fifth shock.
- Press the "analyze" button to re-analyze the rhythm. If you get a "Deliver shock" message, deliver a sixth shock.

You have now completed the second set of three stacked shocks.

11 **Transport the patient when any one of the following occurs** (assuming there is no on-scene ALS such as paramedics):

- The patient regains a pulse (determined during the pulse check before CPR or after the AED gives a "No shock" message), or . . .
- Six shocks have been delivered (two sets of three stacked shocks), or . . .
- The machine gives three consecutive messages (separated by one minute of CPR) that no shock is advised.

If a "No shock" message is received when the "analyze" button is pressed (whether it is the first time or after one or more shocks have already been delivered), check the patient's pulse. If the patient has a pulse, check breathing. If the patient is breathing adequately, give high-concentration oxygen by nonrebreather mask and transport. Or if the patient is not breathing adequately, artificially ventilate with high-concentration oxygen and transport.

If the patient has no pulse, resume CPR for one minute, then analyze the rhythm a second time. If the AED gives a "Deliver shock" message, deliver up to two sets of three stacked shocks (a total of six shocks), with 1 minute of CPR separating the two sets. (Do not deliver more than a total of six shocks, including those you gave before receiving the "No shock" message. Consider that your first sequence was interrupted by the "No shock" message and now, having received a "Deliver shock" message, you are going to continue the sequence. This will be your second try at completing the sequence of six shocks.)

If you get a "No shock" message at any point during the sequence and there is no pulse, resume CPR for one minute. Analyze the rhythm a third time. If the AED gives a "Deliver shock" message, deliver up to two sets of three stacked shocks separated by 1 minute of CPR. (Do not deliver more than a total of six shocks, including all those already delivered to this point. This will be your third try at completing the sequence of six shocks.) If you get a "No shock" message again and if there is no pulse, resume CPR and transport. Do not request any further analyses or deliver any further shocks with the AED.

NOTE: Whenever you perform CPR, ventilate with 100% oxygen (or as close as you can get). If you are authorized to intubate the trachea, also do so at this time. ✳

Assessing and Managing a Cardiac Arrest Patient

FIRST take BSI precautions.

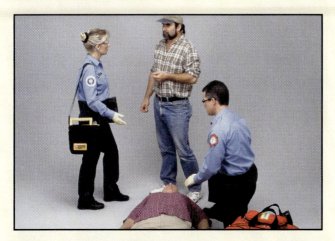

▲ **1.** On arrival, briefly question those present about arrest events. (If a rescuer on scene is performing CPR, direct him to stop.).

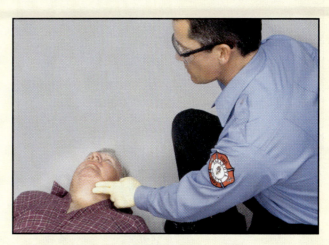

▲ **2.** Verify absence of spontaneous pulse.

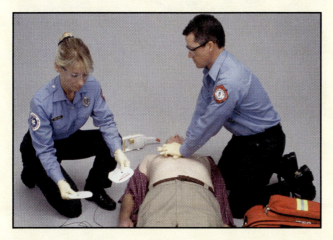

▲ **3.** One EMT-B provides CPR; the other sets up AED.

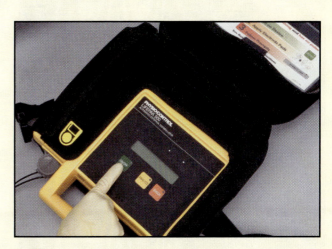

▲ **4.** Turn on the AED power.

NOTE: At earliest opportunity, call for ALS intercept.

(continued)

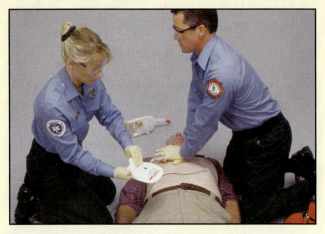

▲ **5.** Connect the two defibrillator pads to cables, following color code. Remove backing. Place one pad on upper right chest, one on lower left ribs.

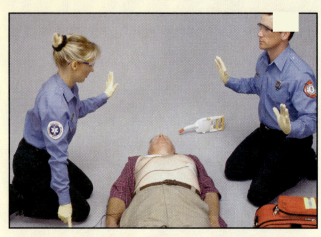

▲ **6.** Say "Clear!" Ensure that all individuals are clear of patient.

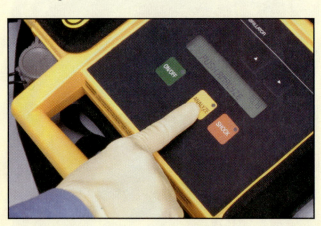

▲ **7.** After everyone is clear, press the "analyze" button and wait for the AED to analyze the rhythm.

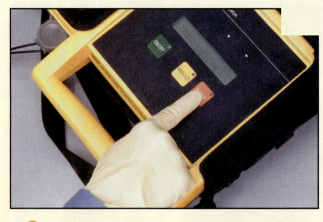

▲ **8.** If advised by the AED, press button to deliver a shock. Repeat analysis and shock delivery until three shocks have been delivered.

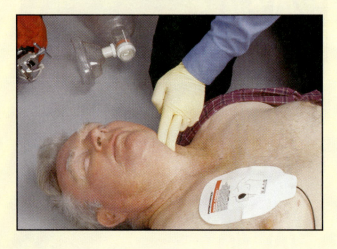

▲ **9.** Verify presence or absence of a spontaneous carotid pulse.

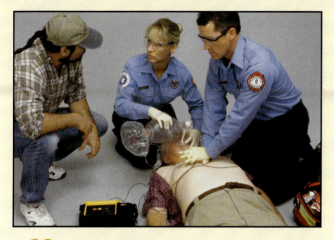

▲ **10.** If pulse is absent, direct resumption of CPR. Gather additional information on arrest events.

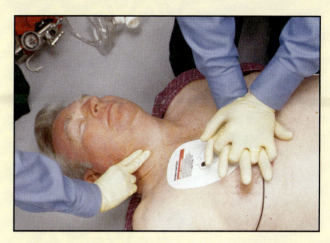

▲ **11.** Check patient's pulse during CPR to confirm effectiveness of compressions.

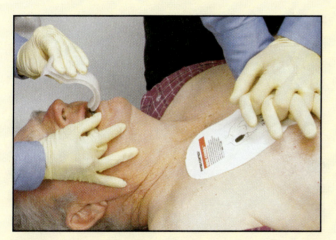

▲ **12.** Direct insertion of airway adjunct.

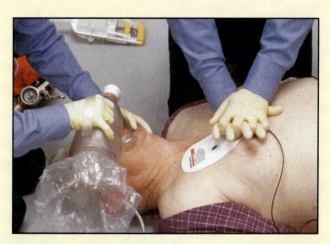

▲ **13.** Direct ventilation of patient with high-concentration oxygen.

(continued)

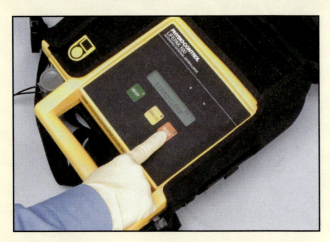

▲ **14.** After 1 minute of CPR, have all individuals stand clear and repeat sequence of three analyses and shocks by AED.

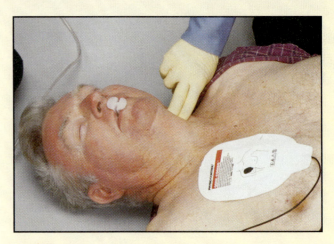

▲ **15.** Check patient's carotid pulse.

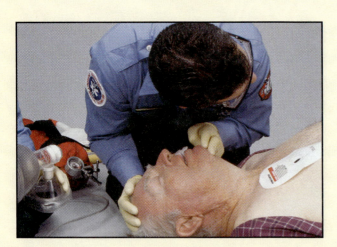

▲ **16.** If there is a spontaneous pulse, check patient's breathing. Note that in many cases, even when a pulse has returned, the patient will require ventilatory assistance.

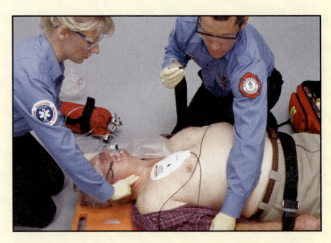

▲ **17.** If breathing is adequate, provide high-concentration oxygen by nonrebreather mask. If breathing is inadequate, ventilate patient with high-concentration oxygen. Transport without delay.

If you wish to review CPR skills, please refer to Table 14-1. For a visual summary of the AED cardiac arrest treatment sequence, see Figure 14-4.

Advantages of AEDs

Use of an AED is an easy skill to learn (in fact, probably easier than CPR), but it still requires an investment of time and energy both initially and later in continuing education. You must know the protocol used in your EMS system so that you can deliver care quickly and efficiently. The American Heart Association has recommended that anyone who operates an AED should receive continuing education and demonstrate competency in the skill at least once every 6 months.

An AED is very fast. An EMT-B can frequently deliver the first shock within 1 minute of arrival at the patient's side. This has been shown to be almost 1 minute faster than EMTs operating manual defibrillators.

Defibrillation with an AED includes the use of adhesive monitoring-defibrillation pads. By making automated defibrillation a "hands-off" skill, the pads improve safety, allow for more consistent electrode placement, and provoke less anxiety among EMT-Bs.

Persistent Ventricular Fibrillation

If you function in a system that does not have ALS or you respond to an arrest patient when ALS is not available, you should prepare the patient for transport after you have:

- Delivered six shocks, or . . .
- Received three "No shock" messages separated by one minute of CPR, or . . .
- The patient regains a pulse.

Although you can use an AED without ALS and see an increase in survival, having ALS may increase the patient's chance of survival even more. If you work in a system where ALS is available, it is important that you know how and when to call. If you can call for ALS, you should do so as soon as possible. Local protocol will guide you in the decision as to whether it is best to wait for ALS at the scene, arrange an intercept, or transport directly to a hospital. Local protocols also will describe who has the responsibility for coordination of the scene at different stages of the call. Ordinarily, this is the person who is able to give the highest level of care.

Safety

When you operate an AED, it is your responsibility to make sure that the patient is cleared during all rhythm analyses and shocks. This means that no one

TABLE 14-1 CPR for Adults, children, and Infants

	Adult	Child	Infant
Age	8 years and older	1 to 8 years	Birth to 1 year
Compression depth	1½ to 2 inches	1 to 1½ inches (approx. ⅓ to ½ the depth of the chest)	½ to 1 inch (newborn ⅓ the depth of the chest)
Compression rate	100/min	100/min	at least 100/min (newborn 120/min)
Each ventilation	1½ to 2 seconds	1 to 1½ seconds	1 to 1½ seconds
Pulse check location	carotid artery (throat)	carotid artery (throat)	brachial artery (upper arm)
One-rescuer or two-rescuer CPR compressions-to-ventilations ratio	15:2	5:1	5:1 (newborn 3:1)

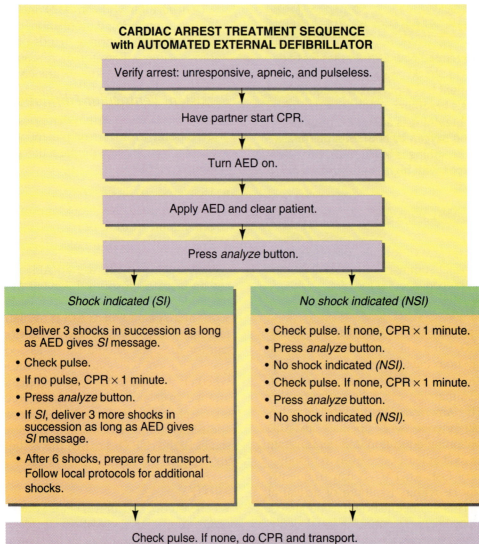

**CARDIAC ARREST TREATMENT SEQUENCE
with AUTOMATED EXTERNAL DEFIBRILLATOR**

Verify arrest: unresponsive, apneic, and pulseless.

↓

Have partner start CPR.

↓

Turn AED on.

↓

Apply AED and clear patient.

↓

Press *analyze* button.

Shock indicated (SI)

- Deliver 3 shocks in succession as long as AED gives *SI* message.
- Check pulse.
- If no pulse, CPR × 1 minute.
- Press *analyze* button.
- If *SI*, deliver 3 more shocks in succession as long as AED gives *SI* message.
- After 6 shocks, prepare for transport. Follow local protocols for additional shocks.

No shock indicated (NSI)

- Check pulse. If none, CPR × 1 minute.
- Press *analyze* button.
- No shock indicated *(NSI)*.
- Check pulse. If none, CPR × 1 minute.
- Press *analyze* button.
- No shock indicated *(NSI)*.

Check pulse. If none, do CPR and transport.

Notes:

Whenever a *no shock indicated (NSI)* message appears, check for a pulse.

If the patient regains a pulse, check breathing. Ventilate with high-concentration oxygen, or give oxygen by nonrebreather mask as needed.

If you initially shock the patient and then receive an *NSI* message before giving six shocks, follow the steps in the above right-hand column.

If you initially receive an *NSI* message and then on a subsequent analysis receive a *shock indicated (SI)* message, follow the steps in the above left-hand column.

Occasionally you may need to shift back and forth between the two columns. If this happens, follow the steps until one of the indications for transport (described below) occurs.

Transport as soon as one of the following occurs:

• You have administered six shocks.

• You have received three consecutive *NSI* messages (separated by one minute of CPR).

• The patient regains a pulse.

If you shock the patient out of cardiac arrest and he arrests again, start the sequence of shocks from the beginning.

Figure 14-4 AED cardiac arrest treatment sequence.

should be touching the patient or anything conductive that the patient is touching. This ensures that during a rhythm analysis the AED is evaluating the patient's rhythm and not someone else's. When a shock is delivered, being clear prevents other rescuers from being injured by a shock.

Clearing a patient means more than just saying "Clear!" It means saying "Clear!" loudly enough for all involved to hear it and looking from the patient's head to toes to make sure no one is touching him or her. This is especially important when the patient is in contact with water or something metallic (like the frame of an ambulance stretcher).

Since no one can touch the patient during these times, you must interrupt CPR to allow rhythm analysis and shocks. This can mean no CPR for up to 90 seconds in order to deliver three shocks. But since defibrillation is more effective than just CPR in resuscitating a patient, this interruption of CPR is actually for the patient's benefit.

An AED cannot accurately analyze a patient's ECG rhythm when in a moving vehicle. Road bumps cause movement in some of the patient's muscles. This leads to extra electrical signals that can obscure the patient's ECG and even imitate some ECG rhythms.

If a patient goes into cardiac arrest in the ambulance (or arrests again after regaining a pulse previously), you must bring the vehicle to a complete stop in order to analyze the rhythm. It also is unsafe to defibrillate in a moving ambulance, because the driver may have to swerve or stop suddenly in order to avoid a collision. If this happens when you are pressing the shock button, someone can fall on the patient as the shock is being delivered.

Another potential hazard with defibrillation is medication patches. These devices allow for the slow administration of some medications through the skin. The hazard apparently lies in the plastic in the patch, which can melt and even explode when a shock is delivered. The patch may also interfere with the delivery of the shock, which would lead to a short circuit of the current and skin burns to the patient.

The most common medication delivered by a patch is nitroglycerin, but any medication patch has the potential to become a hazard. The only patches that have caused problems to date have been on patients' chests. For this reason, if you see a patch on a patient's chest, remove it (with gloved hands so you do not absorb the medication through your skin). After it is removed, wipe away any residue from the skin.

An additional hazard involves implanted pacemakers or implanted defibrillators, which can malfunction unless the AED electrodes are placed 4 to 5 inches away from them.

Single Rescuer with an AED

Since defibrillation is much more likely than CPR to bring a patient back, if you are alone with a patient in cardiac arrest and an AED, you should:

- Perform an initial assessment and assure unresponsiveness, apnea, and pulselessness but do not start chest compressions.
- Turn on the AED.
- Attach the device.
- Press the "analyze" button.
- Deliver up to three stacked shocks.

After you have delivered three shocks or you have received a "No shock" message:

- Check for a carotid pulse.
- Activate the EMS system.
- Start CPR if there is no pulse.

The shocks are stacked, just as when you are working with a partner, so do not check for a pulse between the stacked shocks.

Post-Resuscitation Care

Once you have completed the defibrillation protocol, the patient will be in one of three conditions. The most common situation is he or she will have no pulse and the AED will give a "No shock" message. Sometimes the patient will have no pulse and the AED will signify that further shocks may be indicated. The third possibility is that he or she will have a pulse. If this is the case, you must be aggressive in maintaining the airway. If breathing is adequate, administer high-concentration oxygen by nonrebreather mask and transport the patient on his or her side. If breathing is inadequate, ventilate with 100% oxygen and transport. You should leave the AED on the patient until you arrive at the hospital. As time allows, perform a focused assessment and ongoing assessment en route.

Recurrent Ventricular Fibrillation

A patient who has just recovered a spontaneous pulse is not stable. Despite your attempts to oxygenate and ventilate the patient and transport promptly, he or she may go back into cardiac arrest. If the patient is unconscious and you are providing ventilations, it may not be immediately obvious that the patient no longer has a pulse. To avoid this, check the patient's pulse frequently (at least every 30 seconds). If a pulse is absent, tell your driver to stop the vehicle, press the analyze button, and deliver shocks as described by your local protocol. Only if the defibrillator is not immediately ready should you start CPR before using it. This rarely should be the case.

Defibrillator Maintenance

A defibrillator can save a life only if it is working properly. You must check the machine frequently and maintain it in accordance with the manufacturer's recommendations. A special task force of the Food and Drug Administration (FDA) has compiled a list of steps to be taken every shift to ensure that a defibrillator is ready when needed (Figure 14-5). The checklist must be completed at least daily if it is to accomplish its purpose.

When the FDA's task force looked at defibrillator failures, they found that the most common cause of problems was improper device maintenance, usually battery failure. As part of completing the checklist, you must make sure that the battery in the AED is charged.

If your AED has a built-in clock that records the time of each shock, it should be synchronized with dispatch clocks. This allows for accurate documentation of the time from dispatch to defibrillation.

Quality Improvement

Quality improvement (QI) is essential to the success of any EMS system, but especially to a defibrillation program. Simply undergoing AED training and buying an AED by no means guarantees success. A good QI program involves both the individuals who use AEDs and the EMS system in which the machines are used.

As someone using an AED, you have the responsibility to use it quickly and efficiently. You must take care to maintain the skills of CPR, airway maintenance, automated defibrillation, and lifting and moving patients. Because skills that are used infrequently deteriorate over time, most systems permit a maximum of 90 to 180 days between AED practice sessions.

Medical direction is an essential component of any defibrillation program. Successfully completing AED training in an EMT-Basic course does not necessarily mean you are automatically allowed to use the device. You are subject to the requirements of state laws and rules as well as local medical direction.

One of the roles of the medical director is to review every event in which an AED is used. Depending on the size of your EMS system, the medical director may delegate some or all of this task, but he or she bears responsibility for your actions and should have the authority to match that responsibility.

The medical director may use a number of different sources of information in reviewing AED cases, including your written report, solid-state memory modules, magnetic-tape recordings, and voice-ECG-tape recordings. The brand of machine you use will determine what information is available. The review will look to determine that protocols were followed, that good basic life support care was given, that shocks were appropriate, and that transport occurred in a timely way.

Public Access Defibrillation

A recent initiative by the American Heart Association has promoted public access defibrillation (PAD), the concept of expanding the numbers and types of people trained and equipped to use an AED. This has resulted in AED training for people like firefighters, police officers, flight attendants, athletic trainers, and members of the general public. If your EMS agency coverage area includes sites with AEDs where nonmedically trained responders may use them, you should know where the devices are, who is qualified to use them, what brands and models are being used, and whether they are compatible with the AED you use. Ideally, your service has a good relationship with these PAD organizations and you have procedures approved by your medical director for the transition of care from a PAD provider to an EMS provider. This will vary from place to place, depending upon the compatibility of the AEDs and the pads they use, the qualifications of the PAD providers, and the level of comfort they have in dealing with emergencies. Follow your local protocols.

OPERATOR'S CHECKLIST

HEARTSTREAM FR2 Model No.: _____ Serial No.: _____

HEARTSTREAM FR2 Location or Vehicle ID: _____

DATE							
SCHEDULED FREQUENCY							
Heartstream FR2							
Clean, no dirt or contamination; no signs of damage							
Supplies Available							
* Two sets defibrillation pads, sealed, undamaged, within expiration date * Acilllary supplies (hand towel, scissors, razor) * Spare battery, within "Install Before" date * Data cards, undamaged, and spare data card tray							
Status Indicator							
Shows alternating hourglass/square; selftest passed.							
Inspected by							
Signature or initials of operator completing the maintenance inspection							
Remarks, Problems, Corrective Actions							

Figure 14-5 An AED checklist from Laerdal.

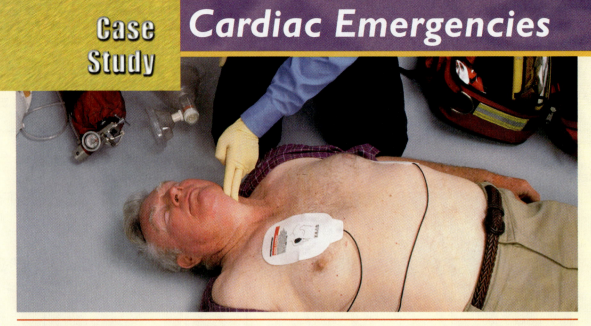

Dispatch Information 1452 Lowell Street, Apartment 2C   **Chest pain   1934 hrs**

Your ambulance is dispatched to a 58-year-old man complaining of chest pain. When you are 2 minutes away from the scene, dispatch advises that the patient's wife has called again. The patient is now unresponsive, and the dispatcher is giving her instructions in CPR. This is a BLS system, so ALS is not available.

Shortly after the update, you arrive on the scene of a small apartment building. Police have just arrived and are securing the scene. You proceed upstairs to apartment 2C where you find a middle-aged woman doing CPR on a moderately obese middle-aged male on the living room floor. You quickly check for and find a carotid pulse with each compression before your partner takes over ventilations and compressions. There is no spontaneous breathing or palpable pulse when compressions are stopped. This is obviously a case with a high priority.

You apply the AED, instruct everyone to clear, check that no one is touching the patient, and press the "analyze" button. After delivering the first shock in the second set of stacked shocks, the AED advises "check pulse." A quick check reveals a weak carotid pulse. The patient's repirations do not resume, however, so you continue ventilations while a police officer assists in packaging him to a long backboard. Meanwhile, you learn from the wife that the patient, Chester Tate, started having some mild pain in the center of his chest about an hour ago while he was at rest. He has no history of cardiac problems (before now) and takes Glucophage for diabetes.

Mr. Tate is now secured to the backboard so he will not slide off when you carry him down the stairs. A quick carotid pulse check before you leave the apartment verifies that Mr. Tate still has a carotid pulse. The patient is not breathing spontaneously, however, so your partner continues to ventilate him with high-concentration oxygen.

After a workout carrying Mr. Tate down the stairs, you put the patient on the stretcher and wheel him into the ambulance. Your EMS agency has a close working relationship with the police department, so the officer drives the ambulance as you and your partner tend to the patient.

As your partner continues to ventilate Mr. Tate, you check the carotid pulse again. It is stronger than before, so after you advise the hospital of your patient's condition, you check the patient's vital signs. He has a pulse of 104 and irregular, a blood pressure of 94/64, assisted respirations at 12 per minute, and pupils that are equal and reactive, though a bit sluggish. He does not yet respond to verbal or painful stimuli.

When Mr. Tate vomits a minute later, you assist your partner in positioning and suctioning. With his airway clear, you arrive at the emergency department. As you bring him to the resuscitation room, you give a report to the doctor and nurse. You and your partner, with a few helping hands from emergency department staff, move the patient from your stretcher to theirs.

On a call later that shift, you learn that Mr. Tate started breathing on his own a little while after you left. By the time he was going to the intensive care unit, he was starting to wake up.

CASE DISCUSSION

This case presents many of the challenges an EMT-B faces in the field. You are expected to do CPR, use an AED, strap a patient onto a board, carry him down a staircase, and continue resuscitation efforts en route, all without ALS or other additional EMS personnel. But you and your partner have trained for this kind of situation, so you know who is going to do what and how it is going to get done. This includes taking advantage of the police officer's training and offer to assist.

Most prehospital patients don't recover from cardiac arrest, frequently because too much time has elapsed before help arrives. In this case, Mr. Tate had a lot of things going for him. He arrested in front of a witness just before you arrived, who kept her wits about her and called early for the appropriate type of help. Mrs. Tate also was able to follow the CPR instructions of the dispatcher. Upon arrival, you were able to shock his heart into beating spontaneously. You then got the patient down a staircase and into the ambulance safely. The police officer on scene was able and willing to drive the ambulance, and you and your partner were able to maintain the patient's airway despite vomiting.

Three of the four links in the chain of survival (early access, early CPR, and early defibrillation) were enough to bring this man back from the dead. This was the result, not of coincidence, but of dedicated efforts over many years by many people to build a strong EMS system.

Name: Chester Tate **Age:** 58 **Chief Complaint:** cardiac arrest	
ASSESSMENT INFORMATION	**RELEVANCE TO THIS PATIENT**
Timing and progression of symptoms	• Because the patient arrested just before you arrived, you know he has been down a short time, that someone was doing CPR early, and that the chance of successful resuscitation is good. • Even though the patient had only mild pain before he arrested, the severity of chest pain in myocardial infarction is not a good indicator of the severity of the episode or amount of damage to the heart.
SAMPLE History	• The patient has several risk factors for heart disease: male sex, middle age, obesity, and diabetes.
Physical examination	• The patient is large and on the second floor, so you will have to strap him securely to something flat and rigid that will allow you to carry him downstairs without injuring him or you.
Other considerations	• Because your agency had worked with the police department providing CPR and driver training to the officers, you and your partner were able to both tend the patient. • Most EMS patients who regain a pulse in the field do not go back into cardiac arrest, but it does happen, so you frequently check the carotid pulse while your partner ventilates. • The emphasis in ventilating these patients is not on hyperventilating them (at a faster than normal rate), but on providing good ventilations at a normal rate (about 12 per minute).

SUMMARY

- Treat patients with signs and symptoms of cardiac compromise as though they actually do have cardiac problems, even though they may not.

- You may be able to assist a patient in taking his or her own nitroglycerin to relieve some or all of the pain; however, you must know how to give the medication, as well as when (and when not) to do so.

- If you understand the use of the AED and practice it until you are confident and competent, you may be able to save a life.

REVIEW QUESTIONS

1. The mainstay for management of cardiac compromise is:
   a. nitroglycerin.
   b. glucose.
   c. oxygen.
   d. epinephrine.

2. The maximum number of doses of nitroglycerin an EMT-B can assist a patient with administration of is:
   a. 2.   c. 4.
   b. 3.   d. 5.

3. The first link in the American Heart Association's cardiac "chain of survival" is:
   a. early CPR.
   b. early access.
   c. early ALS.
   d. early defibrillation.

4. Which of the following is NOT a characteristic of a patient to whom an EMT-B should attach an AED?
   a. nonbreathing
   b. diaphoretic
   c. pulseless
   d. unresponsive

5. On which of the following patients should an AED be used?
  a. a trauma patient
  b. a patient weighing less than 55 pounds
  c. a patient over 6 feet 6 inches tall
  d. a patient younger than 8 years old

WEB MEDIC

Visit Brady's *Essentials of Emergency Care* web site for direct web links. At **www.prenhall.com/limmer,** you will find information related to the following Chapter 14 topics:

• Cardiovascular disease in women
• Sudden cardiac arrest and AED use
• Public access defibrillation
• Cardiac catherization
• Prehospital fibrinolytics

Chapter Fifteen

DIABETIC EMERGENCIES AND ALTERED MENTAL STATUS

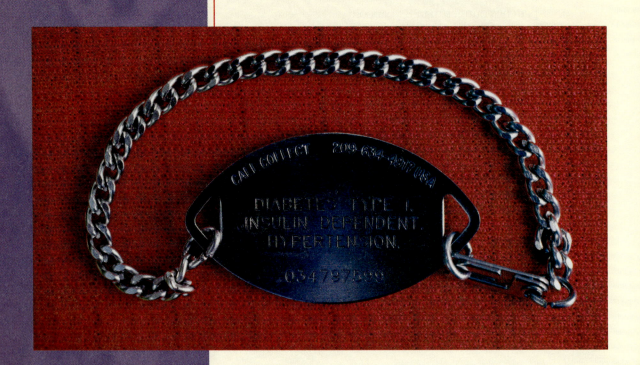

ESSENTIAL ELECTRONIC EXTRAS

CD ESSENTIALS

For preview and review of chapter material, see the student CD-ROM for

- Pretest
- Chapter quizzes
- Posttest

WEB ESSENTIALS

For additional review and enrichment, visit www.prenhall.com/limmer for

- Interactive student quizzes
- Links to online EMS resources
- Online case studies
- Audio glossary

Common causes of altered mental status include traumatic conditions such as head injury, as well as medical conditions such as brain tumor, infection, and hypoxia. Three frequent causes of altered mental status—diabetic conditions, seizures, and stroke—are reviewed in this chapter.

ALTERED MENTAL STATUS

Simply stated, an **altered mental status** is any mental status that is not normal or expected for that patient. Note that some patients may not be fully responsive normally. For example, a patient who has experienced a prior stroke may have some diminished mental status to begin with. It is important to determine what is normal for a person on a daily basis and then determine if there has been any change from that baseline.

Altered mental status may be caused by a wide variety of conditions. Although it is not necessary to determine the cause, there are some interventions that may help the patient (such as glucose or activated charcoal). Some of the main causes of altered mental status may be remembered by using the "4H" mnemonic:

H — Hypoglycemia or hyperglycemia

H — Hypoxia

H — Hypovolemia (shock)

H — Head injury

Other causes include infection, seizures, poisoning, and alcohol or drug use. A thorough scene size-up and history may reveal clues to the causes of altered mental status.

General principles of care include a thorough initial assessment with suctioning and ventilations if necessary, oxygen administration, spinal precautions if trauma is suspected, reassurance, and transport. Be sure to document your findings, including vital signs and mental status, before and after assisting with any medications.

DIABETIC EMERGENCIES

Glucose is a primary fuel for the body. If the body has too much or too little glucose in the bloodstream, a diabetic emergency is taking place. If a patient meets specific criteria, glucose—a medication carried by the EMT-B—may be administered. The rapid improvement of the patient with **hypoglycemia** (low blood sugar) after administration of glucose is an amazing sight and a truly rewarding experience.

Hypoglycemia is the most common medical emergency for someone with diabetes. It occurs when he or she does any of the following:

- Takes too much insulin or oral medication used to treat diabetes.
- Decreases sugar levels by not eating.
- Overexercises and uses sugar faster than normal.
- Vomits and empties the stomach of food and sugar.

Administering Oral Glucose

Available as gel in toothpaste-type tubes, oral glucose increases the patient's blood sugar. With the approval of medical direction, oral glucose is given when all of the following criteria are met:

- The patient presents with an altered mental status.
- The patient has a history of diabetes.
- The patient is alert enough to swallow.

CORE CONCEPTS

In this chapter, you will learn about the following topics:

- Recognition and management of diabetic emergencies, including the use of oral glucose

- Recognition and management of seizures

- Recognition and management of stroke

✔ **Knowledge**

☐ **1.** Provide care to a patient with an altered mental status. (pp. 225–228)

- State the steps in the emergency medical care of the patient taking diabetic medicine with an altered mental status and a history of diabetes. (p. 226)

- Evaluate the need for medical direction in the emergency medical care of the diabetic patient. (pp. 225–226)

✔ **Attitude**

☐ **2.** Recognize and respond to the feelings of the patient who may require interventions to be performed. (pp. 226–228)

✔ **Skills**

☐ **3.** Given medical scenarios, demonstrate the ability to properly assess the patient and demonstrate the ability to properly utilize the intervention of oral glucose. (pp. 225–226)

Patient Assessment

Diabetic Emergencies

Remember that it is not important for you to distinguish between hypoglycemia (low blood sugar) and hyperglycemia (high blood sugar). The prehospital treatment is the same. (Hypoglycemic emergencies are much more common than hyperglycemic emergencies.) Signs and symptoms of a diabetic emergency include:

- Altered mental status; if the patient is conscious, he or she may appear to be intoxicated, anxious, combative.
- Slurred speech
- Staggering walk
- Rapid heart rate
- Cold, clammy skin
- Hunger
- Seizures

To obtain accurate findings for a diabetic emergency, first perform the initial assessment. Assess mental status using the AVPU scale. If a life-threatening condition exists, treat it immediately. Then, if your patient is responsive, perform a focused history and physical exam. Be sure to gather a history of the present illness as well as a SAMPLE history. (When you ask about current medications, note that insulin might be found in the patient's refrigerator.) Assess vital signs. Provide emergency care as per local protocols. In some jurisdictions, oral glucose may be given before vital signs are taken.

If your patient is unresponsive, perform a focused history and physical exam, including a rapid trauma assessment. Gather a SAMPLE history from bystanders or family. Assess vital signs. Provide emergency care. ✳

Patient Care

Diabetic Emergencies

EMT-B care for a patient having a diabetic emergency includes the following (Skill Summary 15-1):

1 After completing the appropriate assessment steps, obtain an order from medical direction either by radio or by protocols to administer oral glucose. Consider a request for advanced life support.

2 Assure that the patient has an altered mental status, a history of diabetes, and is conscious and can swallow. (Do not administer glucose if the patient lacks a gag reflex.)

3 Administer glucose.

4 Perform an ongoing assessment.

If your patient loses consciousness or seizes, remove the tongue depressor, secure the airway, and provide artificial ventilations as necessary. ✳

Administer glucose by squeezing it from the tube onto a tongue depressor. Most patients will be confused or frightened. Explain the procedure you are about to perform. A calm, reassuring approach both relaxes the patient and helps to instill confidence in your treatment efforts. Next, place the tongue depressor between the patient's cheek and gum. The patient typically responds with an improved mental status in several minutes. When oral glucose is given properly, there are no side effects. Note that aspiration of the glucose into the trachea may occur in patients without a gag reflex. Therefore, make sure that the patient can swallow before administration.

If there is no response to the oral glucose or if the patient loses consciousness or seizes, remove the tongue depressor. Suction the airway as needed. Contact medical direction about whether or not to administer additional glucose.

Always take BSI precautions first.

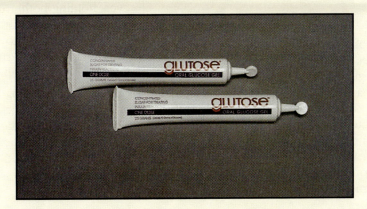

MEDICATION NAME

- Generic: glucose, oral.
- Trade: Glutose®, Insta-glucose.

INDICATIONS

All of the following conditions must be met:
- Patient has an altered mental status.
- Patient has history of diabetes mellitus.
- Medical direction authorizes administration of the medication.

CONTRAINDICATIONS

- Patient is unconscious.
- Patient is a known diabetic who has not taken insulin for days.
- Patient is unable to swallow.
- No permission has been given by medical direction.

MEDICATION FORM

Gel, in toothpaste-type tubes.

DOSAGE

One tube

ACTIONS

1. Obtain order from medical direction, either on-line or off-line.
2. Assure signs and symptoms of an altered mental status with a known history of diabetes.
3. Assure patient is conscious and able to swallow.
4. Administer glucose:
   a. Place on tongue depressor between cheek and gum.
   b. Self-administered between cheek and gum.
5. Record the name, dose, route, and time of administration of the medication.
6. Perform reassessment.

ACTIONS

Increases blood sugar

SIDE EFFECTS

None when given properly. May be aspirated by the patient who has no gag reflex.

REASSESSMENT STRATEGIES

If patient loses consciousness or seizes, remove tongue depressor from the patient's mouth.

NOTE: Since many diabetic patients monitor their blood sugar levels with a glucose monitor, the patient's family may have the device and the training to use it. This can be very helpful in distinguishing a hypoglycemic emergency from other conditions with similar signs and symptoms, but it has limited applicability when the only intervention a provider can administer is oral glucose. A few EMS systems train EMT-Bs in the use of this device and carry it on the ambulance. Follow your local protocol.

SEIZURES

If the normal functions of the brain are upset by injury, infection, or disease, the electrical activity of the brain can become irregular. This irregularity can bring about a sudden change in sensation, behavior, or movement called a **seizure.** Some seizures involve uncontrolled muscular movements, or convulsions. The most common reason for EMS calls involving seizures in adults is failure to take anti-seizure medication. The most common cause of seizures in infants and children six months to three years of age is high fever.

The emergency medical care for seizures includes assuring patency of the airway, positioning the patient on his or her side if there is no possibility of cervical-spine injury, having suction ready, and transporting. If the patient exhibits signs of inadequate breathing, assure an open airway and artificially ventilate.

STROKE

Stroke, or cerebrovascular accident, is a condition where blood flow to a portion of the brain is interrupted. The most common mechanisms of stroke are ruptured blood vessels and clots. The extent of a stroke depends on several factors including the type of stroke, the extent of the area left without oxygen, and the age and physical condition of the patient.

Patient Assessment

Stroke

Signs and symptoms of stroke include confusion, impaired or slurred speech, weak or drooping facial muscles, dizziness, numbness, or paralysis (usually on one side of the body), seizures, and more. Although stroke is a frequent cause of altered mental status, it rarely causes true coma. Some patients may complain of a headache but not all.

The Cincinnati Prehospital Stroke Scale (Table 15-1) is a means of helping to determine if a patient has had a stroke. The scale consists of three tests:

- **Facial droop.** Have the patient show his or her teeth or smile. A normal response occurs when both sides of the patient's face move equally. An indicator of stroke is the inability to move one side or the inability to move one side as well as the other.

- **Arm drift.** Have the patient close his or her eyes, holding both arms out in front. A normal response is when both arms move the same or both arms do not move at all. Indicators of stroke include one arm drifting down or one arm not moving at all.

- **Speech.** Have the patient say "You can't teach an old dog new tricks." A normal response occurs when the patient uses correct words and no slurring. Indicators of stroke include the inability to speak, use of inappropriate words, and slurring. ✳

The American Heart Association has begun a major initiative to educate lay people about the signs and symptoms of stroke. Patients usually call an ambulance or go to the emergency department 12 hours or longer after the onset of stroke symptoms. This greatly reduces and may even prohibit the use of new and beneficial stroke treatments. Be prepared to do your part in educating people on the signs and symptoms of stroke.

Patient Care

Stroke

To provide emergency care to a patient with suspected stroke, calm and reassure him or her. Remember that the loss of function of body parts or the inability to communicate can be terrifying to the patient. Administer high-concentration oxygen by nonrebreather mask, and transport promptly. Conscious patients may be transported in a semi-sitting position. Be alert for the development of inadequate breathing, and assist ventilations as needed. Report your suspicions of stroke to the emergency department staff so they can be prepared to receive the patient. ✳

The term **brain attack** is now being promoted to instill in people's minds a sense of urgency regarding the treatment of stroke. For a heart attack, we know that time is of the essence. Special clot-busting drugs

Table 15-1 Cincinnati Prehospital Stroke Scale

Test	Normal Response	Abnormal Response
Facial Droop (Patient smiles or shows teeth.)	Both sides of face move equally well.	One side of face does not move as well as other side.
Arm Drift (Patient closes eyes and holds both arms out.)	Both arms move the same or both arms do not move at all (other findings, such as pronator grip, may be helpful).	One arm does not move or one arm drifts down compared to the other.
Speech (Patient says "You can't teach an old dog new tricks.")	Patient uses correct words with no slurring.	Patient slurs words, uses inappropriate words, or is unable to speak.

NOTE: Definitive diagnosis of stroke occurs in the hospital emergency department. Always transport patients to the emergency department promptly when there is any possibility that a stroke has occurred.

Adapted from American Heart Association's "1997-99 Handbook of Emergency Cardiovascular Care for Healthcare Providers."

(thrombolytics) may be administered if a heart attack is recognized quickly and the patient is promptly transported to a hospital emergency department.

Great strides have been made in the management of strokes in recent years. A decade ago, only minimal acute interventions were available to stroke patients, leaving many interventions until weeks or months into post-stroke rehabilitation. Newer acute stroke interventions, such as the administration of thrombolytics like those used in acute myocardial infarctions, are becoming more widespread. Research is showing that the time from the onset of symptoms to arrival at the hospital is even more critical to stroke patients than to heart-attack patients who need clot busters. Where heart-attack patients often receive clot busters up to 6 hours after the onset of symptoms, stroke patients must receive such medications within 3 hours of the onset of symptoms. Most centers will not give these medications to stroke patients after more than 3 hours because of the risk of complications after that time. For this reason, if there is uncertainty about when the symptoms began, stroke victims will usually be excluded from these medications.

Thus it is vital that you get the patient to definitive care and the beginning of therapy and that you learn when the stroke symptoms began. Perhaps your most important role as an EMT-B in stroke care, beyond ensuring the ABCs, is determining from family members or bystanders the exact time the stroke symptoms began. Ask, "When did you last see him in his normal condition?" or "When did you first notice her slurred speech?" Obtaining such a history and conveying it to the emergency department staff will save valuable time and may allow the patient the chance at a rapid reversal of the stroke through the use of thrombolytics.

Since the stroke patient must receive a thorough evaluation including a computer assisted tomographic scan of the brain within a very short time, EMT-Bs may have specific local protocols regarding management and transport of patients with symptoms suggestive of a stroke. Unfortunately, many conditions can mimic stroke, including brain tumor, seizure disorder, and hypoglycemia. This makes the emergency physician's job of diagnosing stoke quite difficult at times.

Because a patient who receives a thrombolytic is at risk of intracerebral hemorrhage, it is critical that only patients meeting certain strict criteria undergo this treatment. A number of people in the health care community question whether the benefit is real and whether it is achievable in the "real world" outside of academic medical centers participating in a research study. They feel the risk of thrombolytics outweighs their benefits and thus feel that thrombolytics are too risky for stroke patients given our present knowledge. Early aggressive rehabilitation, on the other hand, has been shown to improve the condition of stroke patients about as much as thrombolytics do, but at much less risk.

A number of hospitals are now providing advanced CVA care, and they are participating in clinical trials of other experimental drugs for stroke. Your medical director should let you know if this might affect your management of potential stroke patients. Follow your local protocol.

Altered Mental Status Emergencies

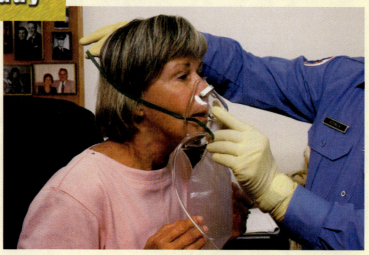

Your ambulance is dispatched to a residence for an elderly woman who is weak and having difficulty speaking. As you walk up to the house, you see a small, well-kept residence with well-tended flower beds and lawn. There are no dangers apparent to you. Upon entering the house, you find the patient in the living room.

You see an elderly woman sitting in a chair, leaning toward her left side. Her eyes appear open, but she is not speaking. An elderly man with a walker is near her and appears very concerned. You don't have enough information to make a definitive determination of priority, but you see enough to make you think this may be a high-priority patient.

The elderly man, who is the patient's husband, tells you he noticed about 10 minutes ago that his wife was not behaving normally. She became sluggish when answering questions and seemed unable to get out of the chair. The patient's husband was out of the room for about an hour before he noticed this, so he doesn't know how long she has been in this condition. She complains of a headache that started last night, but denies any other pain or difficulty breathing.

The patient takes insulin for diabetes, propranolol for high blood pressure, Synthroid for a thyroid condition, and aspirin for arthritis. As the patient's husband gives you his wife's medical history, he informs you that he suspected she might be having a diabetic problem, so he checked her blood sugar just before he called for EMS. It was 142.

Vital signs include the following: pulse 104 and regular; blood pressure 160/92; respirations 20, regular and unlabored; skin pale and slightly sweaty; left pupil briskly reactive to light and right pupil slightly sluggish in response to light. You notice on examination of the patient that she is leaning onto her left side, so much so that if the chair didn't have a high back, she might fall off of the chair. When you ask the patient to smile, the right side of her face moves appropriately while the left side barely moves at all. She is not drooling and appears able to maintain her airway on her own. When you ask her to hold her arms out in front of her, she is unable to lift the left one more than a few inches. Her answers to your questions are slow and a little difficult to understand because her speech is slurred. She is oriented to person and place, but not time. Her left-hand grip is very weak, while the right is strong.

Your partner applies oxygen by nonrebreather mask at 10 liters per minute. You transport her in a semi-sitting position, taking special care to support her left side. Transport to the emergency department is expeditious yet gentle.

CASE DISCUSSION

Like many elderly patients, this patient was on multiple medications, had several medical conditions, and was at risk for a number of different problems. Since there are so many causes of altered mental status (whole books have been written about the subject), the EMT-B must focus on searching for and correcting immediate threats to life, then looking for conditions for which the EMT-B has some kind of treatment. This generally means oxygenation, ventilation, and oral glucose.

Although this patient had classic signs of a stroke, there are many diseases that can mimic stroke. For example, a seizure with a prolonged postictal period could very easily present a picture of a patient with slurred speech, confusion, and even weakness that is greater on one side of the body than the other.

The key to the management of this patient was monitoring of the ABCs, thorough assessment, consideration of oral glucose, and transport. This patient's history of insulin-dependent diabetes, together with her altered mental status, warranted at least a brief reflection on whether oral glucose might be appropriate. A recent blood sugar reading in the normal or high range makes hypoglycemia very unlikely. This assumes, of course, that the monitor has been properly maintained and the person using it is employing good technique. These are reasonable questions to ask when a patient or family member gives you a blood glucose reading.

In this case, since the patient's blood glucose level was above normal, it was not necessary to administer oral glucose. Transport with high-concentration oxygen to a facility capable of caring for this patient's problem is the best option for her.

Name: Henrietta Bourgault
Age: 72
Chief Complaint: Headache and left-sided weakness

ASSESSMENT INFORMATION	RELEVANCE TO THIS PATIENT
Timing and progression of symptoms	• A headache that started last night rules out any possibility of thrombolytic administration in the hospital because onset cannot definitively be determined to be less than 3 to 6 hours. • The change the husband noticed about 10 minutes ago reflects how much a patient's condition can change and shows the importance of ongoing assessment.
SAMPLE History	• Diabetes and high blood pressure are risk factors for stroke. • Aspirin is good at relieving pain, but also at preventing clotting, so this patient is at risk of intracerebral hemorrhage.
Physical Examination	• Lack of drooling suggests the patient is able to maintain her airway on her own, but you will need to watch her airway en route in case that changes and she needs suctioning. • One-sided weakness, a sluggish pupil, facial asymmetry (inability to move muscles on both sides of the face), and slurred speech are all classic signs of a stroke.
Other considerations	• Blood sugar of 142 indicates the patient is not hypoglycemic. • One-sided deficits strongly suggest a neurological problem like stroke, but occasionally a hypoglycemic patient presents with signs and symptoms like the ones this patient is experiencing. • Since the patient's husband uses a walker, he may have limited ability to drive; if possible, make sure a neighbor or relative can assist him if he does not go to the hospital in the ambulance.

SUMMARY

- Altered mental status means that the patient does not have the same level of orientation or awareness that he or she normally has.

- Diabetes is one of the more frequent causes of altered mental status. You may administer oral glucose to the conscious patient with signs and symptoms of a diabetic emergency, if you are allowed to do so by medical direction.

- Emergency care for stroke and seizures includes assuring patency of the airway and adequate breathing and transportation to the emergency department.

REVIEW QUESTIONS

1. The "4H" mnemonic for the main causes of altered mental status includes all of the following EXCEPT:
   a. hypovolemia.
   b. hyphema.
   c. head injury.
   d. hypoxia.

2. What is the chief action of oral glucose?
   a. It raises blood oxygen levels.
   b. It encourages water retention.
   c. It increases blood sugar.
   d. It serves as a neurotransmitter.

3. Which of the following is NOT an indication for use of oral glucose?
   a. a patient with a history of diabetes
   b. a patient with the ability to swallow
   c. a patient with a history of diabetes who has not taken insulin for several days
   d. a patient with an altered mental status

4. The most common reason for EMS calls involving seizures in adults is:
   a. hypoglycemia or hyperglycemia.
   b. allergies to environmental toxins.
   c. stroke or cerebrovascular accident.
   d. failure to take anti-seizure medication.

5. The term _____ is defined as a condition in which blood flow to a portion of the brain is interrupted.

a. stroke

b. seizure

c. hunger

d. hypoxia

WEB MEDIC

Visit Brady's *Essentials of Emergency Care* web site for direct web links. At **www.prenhall.com/limmer,** you will find information related to the following Chapter 15 topics:

- National Diabetes Foundation
- National Stroke Association
- Cincinnati Prehospital Stroke Scale
- Insulin
- Epilepsy

ALLERGIES

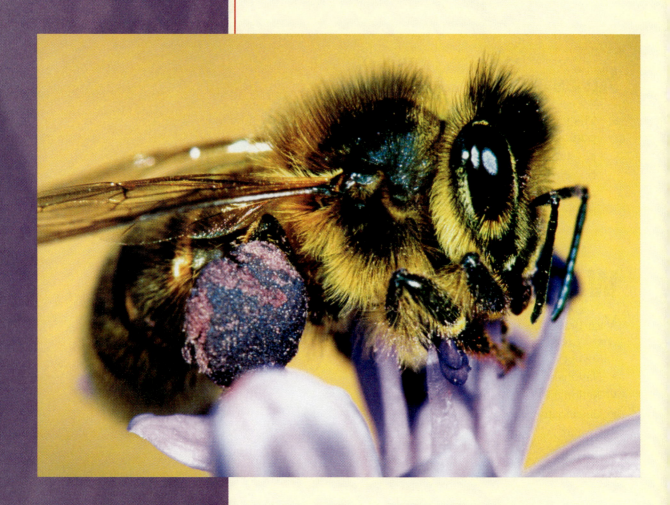

Allergic reactions are often serious, occasionally fatal. The EMT-B is allowed to assist with another prescribed medication for an allergic reaction—the epinephrine auto-injector.

ALLERGIC REACTIONS

An allergic reaction is an exaggerated response of the body's immune system to any substance. Common causes of these reactions include insect bites and stings, foods, plants, and medications, among others (Figure 16-1).

All EMT-Bs should be aware that latex is a potential allergen. One group of people likely to develop a sensitivity to latex are patients who have a history of diseases or conditions that require multiple surgeries, such as spina bifida patients. These patients face repeated exposure to the latex in surgical gloves, which can contribute to the development of the problem. This is important to understand because EMS providers often wear latex gloves and use many latex supplies in the care of patients. The manufacturers of medical equipment and supplies can provide guidance and substitutes for latex products. Be sure to discuss the policy and procedures on dealing with a patient who may have a latex allergy with your service's medical director.

The other group of people who may be susceptible to latex sensitivity can be health care providers themselves. If you find that you develop a rash from the gloves being used for BSI, speak with your medical director about alternate products that can be used.

Allergic reactions range from mild to severe, life-threatening anaphylactic reactions. In anaphylaxis, exposure to an allergen will cause blood vessels to dilate rapidly, resulting in a drop in blood pressure. The more serious attacks usually begin rapidly after exposure to the allergen, although the reaction can be delayed for up to 30 minutes. There is no way to predict the course of an allergic reaction, so each event must be treated seriously. The greatest danger to the patient is compromise of the airway due to swelling in the airway from edema (fluid accumulation).

Patient Assessment

Allergic Reaction

After performing an initial assessment, perform a focused history and physical exam to determine:

- The patient's history of allergies
- What the patient was exposed to
- How the patient was exposed
- What effects the exposure has caused
- The progression of the signs and symptoms
- What interventions have been used by the patient so far
- Baseline vital signs
- SAMPLE history ✳

The signs and symptoms of an allergic reaction vary from person to person and range from mild to severe. In mild allergic reactions, the patient may only complain of itchy, watery eyes. Severe allergic reactions include signs and symptoms throughout the body, such as:

CORE CONCEPTS

In this chapter, you will learn about the following topics:

- How to identify a patient experiencing an allergic reaction

- Differences between a mild allergic reaction and anaphylaxis

- How to treat the patient experiencing an allergic reaction

- Who should be assisted with an epinephrine auto-injector

✔ **Knowledge**

☐ 1. Provide care of the patient experiencing an allergic reaction. (pp. 235–240)

• Recognize the patient experiencing an allergic reaction. (pp. 235–236)

• Describe the emergency medical care of the patient with an allergic reaction. (p. 236)

• State the generic and trade names, medication forms, dose, administration, action, and contraindications for the epinephrine auto-injector. (pp. 237–238)

• Evaluate the need for medical direction in the emergency medical care of the patient with an allergic reaction. (p. 237)

• Differentiate between the general category of those patients having an allergic reaction and those patients having an allergic reaction and requiring immediate medical care, including immediate use of the epinephrine auto-injector. (pp. 235–236)

✔ **Skills**

☐ 1. Demonstrate the use of an epinephrine auto-injector. (pp. 239–240)

INSECT STINGS

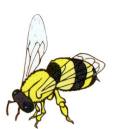

FOOD

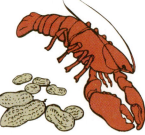

MEDICATIONS

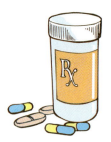

PLANTS

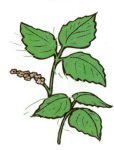

Figure 16-1   Substances that may cause allergic reactions

Skin
■ Itching, hives, flushing, red skin
■ Swelling of the face, hands, neck, or tongue
■ Cool and clammy to touch if shock (hypoperfusion) is present

Tongue
■ Warm or tingling feeling

Respiratory system
■ Tightness in the throat, chest
■ Rapid, labored, or noisy breathing
■ Stridor, hoarseness
■ Wheezing, cough

Cardiovascular system
■ Increased heart rate
■ Decreased blood pressure

Generalized
■ Itchy, watery eyes
■ Headache
■ Runny nose

Level of consciousness
■ Altered mental status
■ Signs and symptoms of shock

Patient Care

Allergic Reaction

Emergency care of a patient having an allergic reaction includes the following:

1. **Administer high-concentration oxygen** through a nonrebreather mask in the initial assessment, if the patient complains of breathing difficulty. Airway assessment and care are very important since respiratory compromise may develop initially or at any time throughout the call.

2. **Determine if the patient has an epinephrine auto-injector available.** If so, contact medical direction if necessary to facilitate its use. Be sure to record the administration of the epinephrine auto-injector.

3. **Perform an ongoing assessment** every 5 minutes.

4. **Transport the patient immediately.** Consider ALS backup, especially if the patient does not have or does not respond to the epinephrine injection. ✳

Some patients exposed to a substance that may cause an allergic reaction will not exhibit signs and symptoms of shock or respiratory distress. These patients should not receive epinephrine. Monitor them carefully in case more serious signs develop.

On your prehospital care report (PCR), be sure to document the patient's history of allergies, all signs and symptoms observed, and the progression of the allergic reaction. Note if any medications were given and the patient's response to them.

EPINEPHRINE AUTO-INJECTOR

For years, the epinephrine auto-injector has been prescribed to patients who experience severe allergic reactions. The epinephrine works by dilating the bronchioles, which decreases respiratory distress, and constricting blood vessels, thus lessening shock. The auto-injectors come in two sizes: adult and infant/child. The adult syringe contains 0.3 mg of epinephrine while the infant/child injector contains 0.15 mg. The entire syringe is administered. Information about epinephrine auto-injectors is given in Skill Summary 16-1.

The indications for use of an epinephrine auto-injector are:

■ Signs and symptoms of a severe/serious allergic reaction (including shock or respiratory distress).

■ Medication is prescribed by a physician.

■ On- or off-line medical direction approves use of the device.

Since the drug is already prescribed to the patient and is used only in an extreme emergency, there are no contraindications for its use. There is the possibility of the injector causing side effects such as an increased heart rate, pallor, dizziness, headache, or chest pain. Nausea, vomiting, and excitability have also been reported.

Follow this procedure for administering the auto-injector (Skill Summary 16-2):

1. Determine that the patient shows signs of an allergic reaction (including shock or respiratory distress).

2. Obtain permission from medical direction (on- or off-line).

3. Obtain the patient's auto-injector. Verify that it is prescribed to the patient and the solution is not cloudy.

4. Remove the cap from the auto-injector.

5. Place the auto-injector firmly against the patient's thigh. (The skin should be bared prior to the injection.) Hold it in place for 10 seconds to allow the medication to inject.

6. Dispose of the injector in a biohazard (sharps) container.

7. Record activity and time.

8. Monitor the patient. Reassess to determine what effect the epinephrine has had.

LIFESPAN DEVELOPMENT

Allergic reactions are common in older children. Fortunately, many children grow out of their allergies as they mature. The epinephrine pen comes in two sizes. The adult size contains 0.3 mg and the child size contains 0.15 mg. It is suggested that the child size be used for children who are less that 66 pounds. It would be rare that the child size would be used on an infant, since an anaphylactic reaction would be rare because the immature immune system usually does not have the types of antibodies that produce such reactions.

As with any unstable patient, frequent reassessment is important. The main focus of the reassessment is airway, breathing, and circulation. If the signs and symptoms worsen or do not improve, you may be called upon by medical direction to repeat the use of an auto-injector. The injectors are single-use, so be sure to take any extras the patient has available with you to the hospital in case they are needed. If the patient fails to respond or if the condition continues to worsen, as may happen in serious reactions, call for ALS backup if possible, and be prepared to assist ventilations, perform CPR, and use the AED if necessary.

PRECEPTOR PEARL

Epinephrine auto-injectors are devices that use needles to administer epinephrine. Injectable drugs are not commonly used at the EMT-B level. However, this truly life-saving drug is an exception. There are two important points to stress to a new EMT-B: 1. After the auto-injector is prepared and placed against the patient's thigh, it must be held in place to allow the medication to be injected. Simply pressing and immediately removing the device will be ineffective. 2. After the device is used, it must be properly disposed of in a sharps container. The injector must be considered a contaminated sharp and treated accordingly!

Epinephrine Auto-Injector

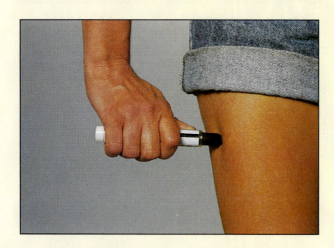

MEDICATION NAME

- Generic: epinephrine.
- Trade: Adrenalin®, EpiPen®.

INDICATIONS

All of the following conditions must be met:
- Patient exhibits signs of a severe allergic reaction, including either respiratory distress or shock (hypoperfusion).
- Medication is prescribed for this patient by a physician.
- Medical direction authorizes administration of the medication.

CONTRAINDICATIONS

No contraindications when used in a life-threatening situation.

MEDICATION FORM

Liquid administered by an auto-injector, which is an automatically injectable needle-and-syringe system.

DOSAGE

- Adult: one adult auto-injector (0.3 mg)
- Infant or child: one infant/child auto-injector (0.15 mg)

ADMINISTRATION

1. Obtain patient's prescribed auto-injector and ensure that the prescription is written for the patient who is experiencing the severe allergic reaction and that medication is not discolored (if visible).
2. Obtain order from medical direction, either on-line or off-line.
3. Remove cap from auto-injector.
4. Place tip of auto-injector against patient's thigh (the lateral portion, midway between waist and knee).
5. Hold the injector in place until the medication is injected (at least 10 seconds).
6. Record the name, dose, route, and time of administration of the medication.
7. Dispose of the injector in a biohazard container.

ACTIONS

- Dilates the bronchioles
- Constricts blood vessels

SIDE EFFECTS

- Increased heart rate
- Pallor
- Dizziness
- Chest pain
- Headache
- Nausea
- Vomiting
- Excitability, anxiety

REASSESSMENT STRATEGIES

1. Continue focused assessment of airway, breathing, and circulation.
2. If patient's condition continues to worsen (decreasing mental status, increasing breathing difficulty, decreasing blood pressure):
   a. Obtain medical direction for an additional dose of epinephrine.
   b. Treat for shock (hypoperfusion); place in Trendelenburg position.
   c. Prepare to initiate basic life support procedures (CPR, AED).
3. If patient's condition improves, provide supportive care:
   a. Continue oxygen.
   b. Treat for shock (hypoperfusion); place in Trendelenburg position.

Always take BSI precautions first.

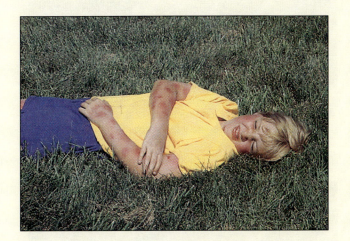

Patient suffers a severe allergic reaction.

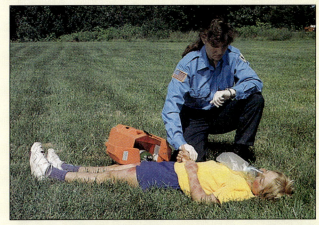

▲ **1.** Perform an initial assessment. Provide high-concentration oxygen by nonrebreather mask.

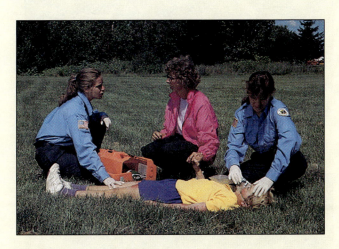

▲ **2.** Perform a focused history and physical exam, including a SAMPLE history.

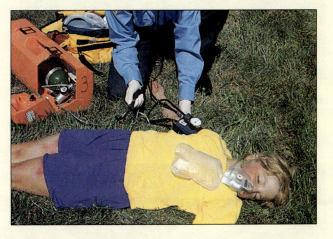

▲ **3.** Take the patient's vital signs.

(continued)

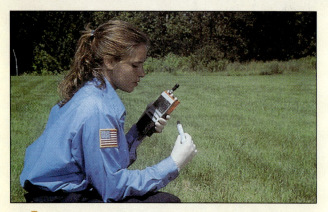

▲ **4.** Find out if the patient has a prescribed epinephrine auto-injector. Check to be sure it is prescribed for this patient. Check expiration date, and check for cloudiness or discoloration, if liquid is visible. Contact medical direction.

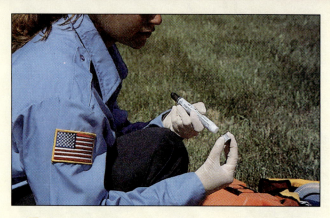

▲ **5.** If medical direction orders use of the epinephrine auto-injector, prepare it by removing the safety cap.

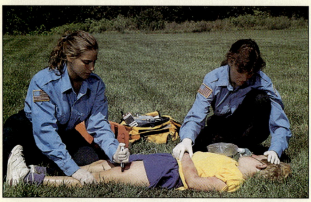

▲ **6.** Then press injector against the patient's thigh to trigger release of the spring-loaded needle, and inject the dose of epinephrine into patient.

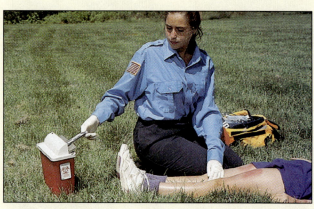

▲ **7.** After holding the injector against the thigh for at least 10 seconds, dispose of it in a biohazard container.

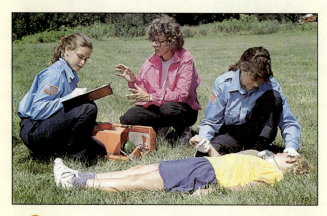

▲ **8.** Document the patient's response to the medication.

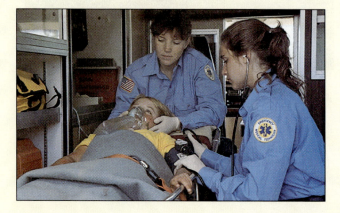

▲ **9.** Perform an ongoing assessment, paying special attention to the patient's ABCs and vital signs en route to the hospital.

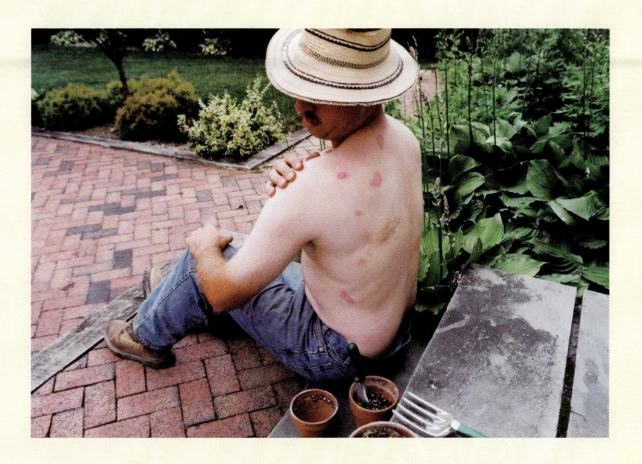

Dispatch: 1280 Freeland Road   Difficulty Breathing   1530 hrs

Your ambulance is dispatched to a private residence on the outskirts of town for the report of a patient having difficulty breathing. You pull up in front of a big, old farmhouse and are meet by the patient's wife, who is waving for you to come to a shed in the rear of the house. You approach the scene scanning for dangers and observe none.

The patient's wheezing can be heard as you approach the shed. He is sitting on the steps in the garden. He has his shirt off, which is not unusual on a warm day, and his chest and neck are all hives. Your general impression is that of a male in his middle 30s who is having difficulty breathing. This is enough for you to assign him a high priority for transport.

The patient is able to speak in short, choppy sentences and manages to tell you that he was moving some rose bushes when he came across a bee hive. His wife interrupts and says that he is very allergic to bees and has an EpiPen® in the house. Your partner indicates that he will start the patient on oxygen by nonrebreather mask while you send the wife to get the EpiPen®. You perform a history and obtain vital signs, noticing that the patient is cold and clammy and has a weak, rapid radial pulse. He also seems very anxious.

The man states that he lost count of the number of times he was stung. He says that his throat seems like it is swelling, that his chest is becoming tight, and that he feels very dizzy. You lay him down with his feet elevated as the wife returns with his EpiPen®. She tells you that he takes Benadryl occasionally and Allegra daily and is also allergic to certain foods as well. He has no other relevant medical disorders or recent hospitalizations.

His vital signs reveal a pulse of 120 and regular, respirations of 24 and labored, BP of 108/74, a moist and pale skin, except for the area where there are hives, and pupils equal and reactive to light. The patient has equal lung sounds bilaterally with both inspiratory and expiratory wheezing. You observe at least five areas where he was stung that are already swollen and inflamed.

After putting the oxygen on the patient, your partner prepares for transport by getting the stretcher from the back of the ambulance. You look closely at the EpiPen® and observe that it is prescribed for this patient, not yet expired, and that the a situation meets the criteria of your local EMS system's standing orders for assisting a patient with his EpiPen®. You then quickly help the patient in injecting the medication into his right thigh. Next, you and your partner move the patient onto the stretcher and then to the ambulance. Just prior to leaving the scene, your partner is able to obtain a second EpiPen® from the wife as you notice the patient's wheezing is getting quieter and his color is looking better. En route, you perform an ongoing assessment and repeat the vital signs. The oxygen and epinephrine have helped, and the patient states that he feels some improvement in his breathing.

You get on the radio and inform medical direction of the patient and his condition, what you found on assessment, your treatment, and your estimated time of arrival at the hospital.

CASE DISCUSSION

The patient is experiencing a severe allergic reaction to the bee stings. An allergic reaction that involves a systemic response involving breathing difficulty, wheezing, and hypotension is referred to as anaphylaxis. The rapid onset of hives and swelling in the airway as well as bronchoconstriction are early clues that this condition can be life threatening. This patient is definitely a high priority and, if this was a system where ALS is available, it should be called to the scene or to meet your ambulance en route to the emergency department. The fact that the patient's physician had prescribed an EpiPen® is an indication that this is not the first time the patient has had a brush with death from a bee sting. Most people have a mild local reaction to bee stings. Patients who are allergic can have both the local reaction as well as a severe systemic reaction as was the case in this patient.

The patient was provided with immediate high-concentration oxygen, placed in the Trendelenburg position, and assisted with his EpiPen® following your local treatment protocols. An adequate history was obtained but you did not delay transport to obtain it. Asking the wife to get a second EpiPen® was a smart move because in some cases it is necessary to administer another dose en route to the hospital if your protocol or medical direction allows.

Name: Bill Rafferty
Age: 35
Chief Complaint: *"My throat is swelling up, and it's hard to breathe."*

ASSESSMENT INFORMATION	RELEVANCE TO THIS PATIENT
History of allergic reaction	• This increases the likelihood of this being caused by a reaction to the bee stings. • It also increases the likelihood that this patient could have another severe reaction. • The speed of the onset of the symptoms is sometimes an indicator of severity also.
Physical examination	• The rash and multiple stings may indicate how fast the patient is reacting to the allergen. • The wheezing lung sounds indicate broncho-constriction. • The pale and clammy skin indicates hypoperfusion.
Medication	• The fact that the patient's physician has pre-scribed an EpiPen® for him indicates that the patient has previously had a serious reaction and the physician was concerned about another reaction occurring. • Benadryl is a medication that is often taken for less serious allergies. • Allegra is a medication taken daily to help patients with allergies breathe easier.
Other considerations	• The fact that the patient is dizzy is an indicator that the brain is not perfusing well from the hypoperfusion or shock. The Trendelenburg position may be helpful as well as the oxygen. Monitor this patient's vital signs very closely and do not stand him up!

SUMMARY

- Allergic reactions can run from a small rash to a life-threatening condition.

- Patients may experience allergic reactions to food, medications, insects, and plants.

- Signs and symptoms of allergic reactions include itching, hives, swelling of the hands, face, and tongue, respiratory distress, wheezing, a cough, an increased heart rate, and decreased BP.

- Treatment for the allergic reaction depends on the severity of the reaction.

- A mild allergic reaction requires little emergency care, but patients should be monitored carefully to be sure that a severe reaction does not develop.

- A severe reaction, also called anaphylaxis, should be treated with oxygen and by assisting the patient with a prescribed epinephrine auto-injector.

- Auto-injectors contain epinephrine, which is a potent medication that can reverse the effects of anaphylaxis.

- Epinephrine should only be given if authorized by medical direction.

REVIEW QUESTIONS

1. The greatest danger to patients with severe allergic reactions is:
   a. liver damage.
   b. internal hemorrhage.
   c. stroke.
   d. compromise of the airway due to edema.

2. The standard dose delivered by an epinephrine auto-injector is:
   a. .3 mg.
   b. .5 mg.
   c. .7 mg.
   d. 1 mg.

3. Which of the following is a contraindication to the use of an epinephrine auto-injector with an allergic reaction patient in a life-threatening situation?
   a. head injury
   b. inability to swallow
   c. systolic blood pressure below 100
   d. no contraindications in life-threatening situations

4. Which of the following is an action caused by the epinephrine auto-injector?
   a. dilation of bronchioles
   b. dilation of blood vessels
   c. decreased heart rate
   d. increased gastric motility

5. For administration of its dose, the auto-injector should be placed against the patient's:
   a. lower arm.
   b. upper arm.
   c. thigh.
   d. calf.

WEB MEDIC

Visit Brady's *Essentials of Emergency Care* web site for direct web links. At **www.prenhall.com/limmer,** you will find information related to the following Chapter 16 topics:

- Stinging insects
- Food allergies
- Anaphylaxis
- Latex allergies

Chapter Seventeen

POISONING AND OVERDOSE EMERGENCIES

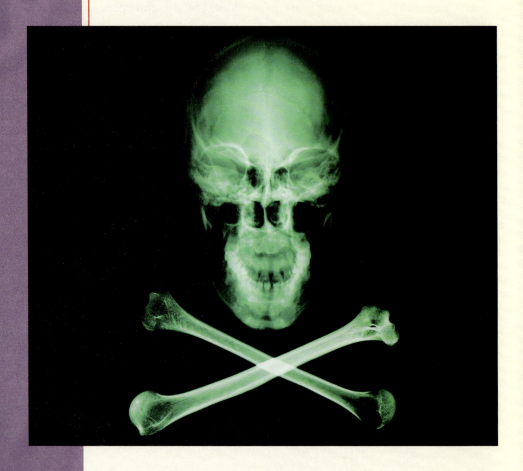

ESSENTIAL ELECTRONIC EXTRAS

CD ESSENTIALS

For preview and review of chapter material, see the student CD-ROM for

- Pretest
- Chapter quizzes
- Posttest

WEB ESSENTIALS

For additional review and enrichment, visit www.prenhall.com/limmer for

- Interactive student quizzes
- Links to online EMS resources
- Online case studies
- Audio glossary

Poisons may enter the body in many ways. Some of these ways are accidental, some through occupational exposure, and others intentionally. Unlike other medical emergencies which are frequent in older adults, accidental poisoning is common in children. Poisoning calls will require competent patient care and your ability to size up the scene in order to quickly and accurately identify the poisons involved. The following chapter will help you to review these skills.

POISONING AND OVERDOSE EMERGENCIES

How Poisons Enter the Body

A poison is any substance that can harm the body by altering cell structure or functioning. Poisons may enter the body in four ways:

- Ingestion (swallowing)
- Inhalation (breathing in)
- Absorption (through unbroken skin)
- Injection (through the skin, by a needle, snake fangs, or insect stinger)

Administering Activated Charcoal

Research now suggests that the most effective means of managing many ingested poisons includes the administration of activated charcoal. In some cases, dilution of ingested poisons is also recommended. Poison-control experts no longer consider syrup of ipecac the medication of first choice. Ipecac's disadvantages are slowness and relative ineffectiveness; syrup of ipecac may take longer than 15 or 20 minutes to work. During this delay, a patient can become drowsy or lose consciousness. This increases the chances of aspiration of vomitus in a nonalert patient. Regarding ipecac's effectiveness, studies indicate that, on the average, less than a third of the patient's stomach contents are removed following vomiting. Due to these disadvantages, activated charcoal replaces ipecac as the first drug of choice for certain ingested poisons.

How does activated charcoal work? Activated charcoal binds with many ingested poisons and drugs and prevents absorption into the body. It is pre-mixed in water, and it typically is available in a plastic bottle. Veteran EMTs may remember the messiness of the powder form of activated charcoal. Powdered charcoal should not be used in the field.

Generally, contact medical direction early in the poisoning call because different poisons are treated differently. Some are absorbed by activated charcoal, while others are not.

To provide proper administration of activated charcoal, follow the instructions given to you by medical direction. Occasionally, medical direction may request dilution of an ingested poison. Dilution with water may delay the absorption rates of some poisons; dilution with milk may soothe an upset stomach. Be sure to consult medical direction before you dilute any ingested poison.

Note that activated charcoal will permanently stain clothes and is otherwise very difficult to clean if spilled. Dispose of unused portions in an impenetrable container.

PRECEPTOR PEARL

Sometimes it can be very difficult to convince a patient to drink a pre-mixed solution of activated charcoal. It looks like mud. Providing a covered container and straw to the patient may make it easier to drink. As mentioned previously, it is important to acknowledge any fear or apprehension your patient is experiencing. Your calm, professional demeanor helps gain a patient's trust and respect in your ability to administer medication in the appropriate manner. Remember, too, that activated charcoal may be given to the patient while en route to the receiving facility.

CORE CONCEPTS

In this chapter, you will learn about the following topic:

- Recognition and management of poisoning and overdose emergencies, including administration of activated charcoal

✔ **Knowledge**

☐ **1.** Provide care to a suspected poison/overdose patient. (pp. 247–248, 252)

- Describe the steps in the emergency medical care for the patient with suspected poisoning. (pp. 247–248, 252)

- Discuss the emergency medical care for the patient with possible overdose. (p. 248)

✔ **Attitude**

☐ **2.** Recognize and respond to the feelings of the patient who may require interventions to be performed. (pp. 247, 252)

✔ **Skills**

☐ **3.** Given medical scenarios, demonstrate the ability to properly assess the patient and demonstrate the ability to properly utilize the intervention of activated charcoal. (pp. 248, 253–254)

Patient Assessment

Poisoning and Overdose Emergencies

A rapid, organized approach to patient assessment is essential in cases of possible ingested poisoning. Before you contact medical direction, you should perform an initial assessment. Look for an altered mental status. Assess ABCs. If a life-threatening condition exists, treat immediately. Then, if your patient is responsive:

- Perform a focused history and physical exam. When you gather the history, be sure to ask: What substance was ingested? When was the substance ingested? How much was ingested? Over what time period did the ingestion occur? What interventions have the patient, family, or bystanders taken? How much does the patient weigh? Has the patient vomited?

- Assess vital signs.

- Provide emergency care. Be sure to check with medical direction.

Or if your patient is unresponsive, perform a focused history and physical exam, including a rapid trauma assessment. Gather a SAMPLE history from bystanders or family. Assess vital signs, and provide emergency care.

The following signs and symptoms are frequently associated with a poisoning or overdose emergency:

- Nausea
- Vomiting
- Diarrhea
- Altered mental status
- Abdominal pain
- Chemical burns around or inside the mouth
- Rapid pulse
- Abnormal breath odors ✳

Patient Care

Poisoning and Overdose Emergencies

Emergency care of a patient with a poisoning emergency includes the following:

1 **Perform an initial assessment.** Immediately treat life-threatening problems. Request advanced life support when appropriate.

2 **Perform a focused history and physical exam.** Be sure to remove any pills, tablets, or fragments from patient's mouth.

3 **Assess baseline vital signs.**

4 **Consult medical direction about the administration of activated charcoal** (Skill Summary 17-1). If directed by medical direction, dilute the poison with water or milk.

5 **Bring all poison containers, bottles, and labels to receiving facility.**

6 **Conduct an ongoing assessment en route to the emergency department.** ✳

Be sure to include in your prehospital care report (PCR) a thorough documentation of observations at the scene, changes in the patient's mental status, and treatment given.

For the other types of poison exposures (inhaled, absorbed, or injected poisons), apply the assessment techniques learned in this chapter. Treatment for these poison exposures remains the same (Skill Summaries 17-2 and 17-3 on the following pages).

ADMINISTERING ACTIVATED CHARCOAL

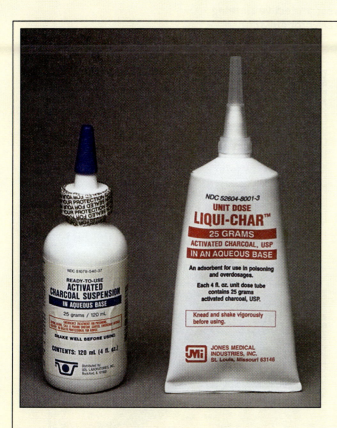

MEDICATION NAME
- Generic: activated charcoal.
- Trade: Actidose™, LiquiChar™.

INDICATIONS
Poisoning by mouth.

CONTRAINDICATIONS
- Altered mental status
- Ingestion of acids or alkalis
- Inability to swallow

MEDICATION FORM
- Premixed in water, frequently available in plastic bottle containing 12.5 grams of activated charcoal.
- Powder, which should be avoided in the field.

DOSAGE
- Adults and children: 1 gram activated charcoal/kg of body weight.
- Usual adult dose: 25 to 50 grams
- Usual pediatric dose: 12.5 to 25 grams

ADMINISTRATION
1. Consult medical direction.
2. Shake container thoroughly.
3. Since medication looks like mud, patient may need to be persuaded to drink it. Providing a covered container and a straw will prevent patient from seeing the medication and so may improve patient compliance.
4. If patient does not drink the medication right away, the charcoal will settle. Shake or stir it again before administration.
5. Record the name, dose, route, and time of administration of the medication.

ACTIONS
- Adsorbs (binds) certain poisons and prevents them from being absorbed into the body.
- Not all brands of activated charcoal are the same. Some absorb much more than others. Consult medical direction about the brand to use.

SIDE EFFECTS
- Black stools
- Some patients, particularly those who have ingested poisons that cause nausea, may vomit. If patient vomits, repeat the dose once.

REASSESSMENT STRATEGIES
Be prepared for the patient to vomit or further deteriorate.

SAFETY NOTE: In the presence of hazardous fumes or gases, wear protective clothing and self-contained breathing apparatus or wait for those who are properly trained and equipped to enter the scene and bring the patient out.

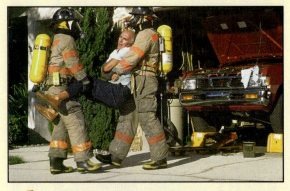

▲ **1.** Remove the patient from the source of poison.

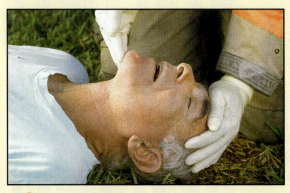

▲ **2.** Establish an open airway.

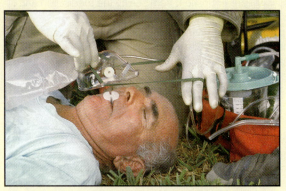

▲ **3.** Insert an oral airway and administer high-concentration oxygen by nonrebreather mask.

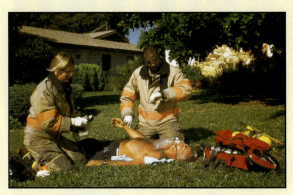

▲ **4.** Perform a focused history and physical exam, and take vital signs.

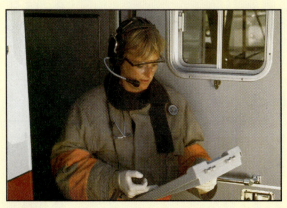

▲ **5.** Contact medical direction.

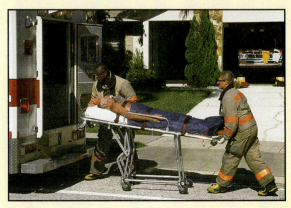

▲ **6.** Transport.

Absorbed Poisons

SAFETY NOTE: Take care to protect your skin from contact with poisonous substances. Wear protective clothing. If necessary, have firefighters or others who are properly protected hose off the patient before you touch him or her. The procedure shown below is for a patient with a small exposure to a substance that is not dangerous to the EMT-Bs.

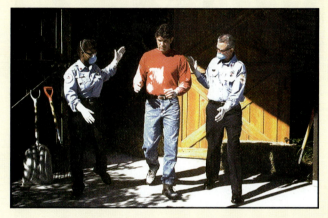

▲ **1.** Remove patient from source or remove source from patient. Avoid contaminating yourself with the poison.

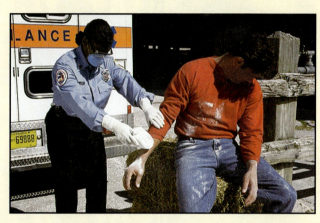

▲ **2.** Brush powders from the patient. Be careful not to abrade the patient's skin.

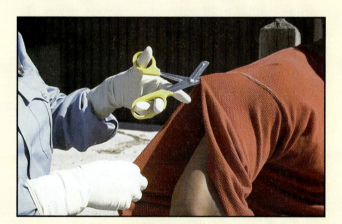

▲ **3.** Remove contaminated clothing and other articles.

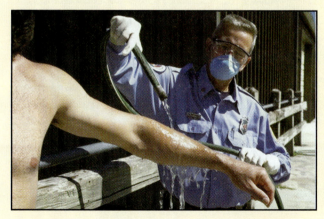

▲ **4.** After any powders have been brushed away, wash with clear water. (Catch contaminated run-off and dispose of safely.)

(continued)

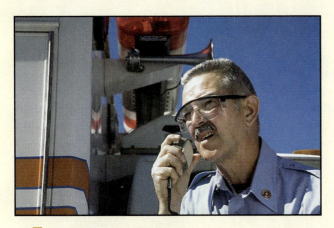

▲ **5.** Contact medical direction.

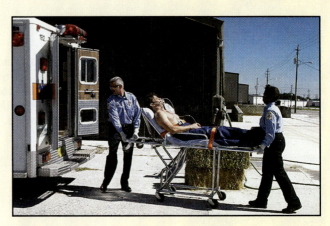

▲ **6.** Transport the patient.

LIFESPAN DEVELOPMENT

Accidental ingestion of poison occurs most frequently with children. No matter how horrible something tastes, children will sometimes drink the same poison on more than one occasion. Also, with children it is very difficult to determine how much of a poison has been ingested. Always treat for the worst possible ingestion. Remember, before appropriate care is provided, you will need to give medical direction the child's approximate weight.

INJECTED POISONS

Injected poisons come primarily from injected drugs of abuse and through the venom of snakes and in-sects. Information on bites and stings may be obtained in Chapter 18, "Environmental Emergencies."

Injected drugs and medications range from therapeutic insulin to illegal and dangerous heroin. The signs and symptoms the patient will exhibit depend on the medication taken. Accidental overdose of insulin will result in signs and symptoms of severe hypoglycemia. Injected illegal drugs may cause a variety of signs and symptoms.

Patient care begins with a thorough scene size-up. If illegal drugs are involved, the scene has many inherent hazards such as dangerous individuals. Persons who inject drugs may keep their hypodermic needle on their persons or close by. This poses a grave risk of accidental needle stick and subsequent infection.

Care for the patient is largely supportive. Make the patient comfortable and provide reassurance. Treat any respiratory difficulty with oxygen and assisted ventilations if necessary. Gather what information you can from the scene about the injected substance for hospital personnel.

Poisoning and Overdose Emergencies

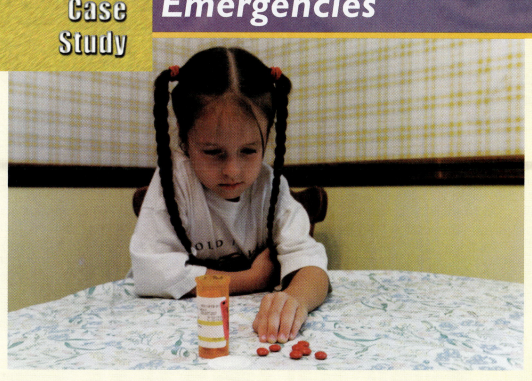

Dispatch: 121 Wilkinson Dr.   Possible Poisoning   1645 hrs

Your ambulance is dispatched to a 5-year-old girl who ingested some medication. As you pull up to the scene, you observe a house in a new development. There are no dangers visible, so you enter the house and find an anxious mother with her crying 5-year-old daughter. Your general impression is that the patient is alert and not in any acute distress. For the moment, you decide this is not necessarily a high-priority call, keeping in mind that you don't yet know the effects of the medication involved.

Five-year-old Michelle is visiting with her mother, brother, and two sisters, along with two of her siblings' friends. One of the friends has Tourette's syndrome and had put his bottle of 1 mg Tenex tablets on the kitchen table before getting a drink of water. Michelle loves candy and will do almost anything to get it. Not being one to miss an opportunity like this, she grabbed the attractive red pill and popped it into her mouth. The friend came back, discovered what had happened, and immediately told Michelle's mother. She called the poison control center, where they told her to bring the girl to the local emergency department. The mother has no idea where the hospital is and her brother, who she is visiting, is not home at the moment.

Michelle is not in any acute distress. She is alert and crying, with no apparent immediate threats to airway, breathing, or circulation. The ingestion occurred about 10 minutes ago. She is not complaining of any signs or symptoms. She is a healthy little girl who takes no medications (of her own, that is), gets an occasional ear infection, and has no known allergies to medications. The patient has a pulse rate of 108; BP 84/56; respirations 26; skin warm, pink and dry; pupils equal and reactive. She weighs about 30 pounds, her mother tells you, and you see no hives or other external signs of a problem.

When you call the emergency department to find out more about the ingestion and recommended treatment, you discover the poison control center has already called with preliminary information about the case. Tenex is usually prescribed for high blood pressure, but like many medications is sometimes prescribed for other problems, in this case, Tourette's syndrome. Because of the drug's effects, there is a risk of significant hypotension, particularly in a small 5-year-old. They advise administration of activated charcoal, approximately 1 gm/kg of body weight. Thirty pounds, they tell you, is about 14 kg, so your bottle of 25 gm of activated charcoal should do just fine.

You begin transport, and, en route, you and Michelle's mother attempt to coax her into sucking some of the activated charcoal through a straw. She is quite resistant for someone who just took some medicine she wasn't supposed to take, so you are limited in your success. You also check her vital signs again, verifying that her blood pressure has not fallen. On arrival at the emergency department, she is perfusing well, her blood pressure is unchanged, and she has swallowed an amount of activated charcoal you estimate as one fifth of the bottle, or 5 gm.

Case Discussion

Poisoning cases typically involve small children, usually in the 2- to 3-year old age group. A 5-year-old generally knows better than to take a pill that isn't hers, but this patient looked at it as candy, not medicine. This is one of the risks of candy manufacturers making candy that looks like medicine and pharmaceutical companies making medicine that tastes like candy.

A 30-pound child may have severe blood-pressure-lowering effects from an adult dose of an anti-hypertensive medication, so careful and repeated evaluation of blood pressure is warranted for this patient. But blood pressure doesn't tell the whole story, so it is appropriate to keep an eye on other signs of perfusion like skin, capillary refill, and mental status.

Activated charcoal doesn't look or taste pretty. Disguising it, e.g., with a covered cup and a straw, is likely to make this difficult task a little easier.

Name: Michelle Anderson	
Age: 5	
Chief Complaint: Ingested Tenex	
ASSESSMENT INFORMATION	**RELEVANCE TO THIS PATIENT**
History of the present illness	• Few medications have life-threatening effects in 10 minutes, particularly when only one tablet is involved. • You are able to determine no more than one tablet could have been taken, so the risk of problems is less than it might have been. • A child in this situation is likely to deny the ingestion after the surrounding adults become anxious and begin questioning her. • The poison center has already been informed of this case and has suggested a course of treatment
SAMPLE history	• The patient is healthy.
Physical examination	• The patient is asymptomatic right now, but that could change, so you monitor her blood pressure and signs of perfusion very carefully and diligently. • A blood pressure of 84/56 is in the normal range for a 5-year-old.
Other considerations	• You receive medical direction from the emergency department, so the appropriate place to call for treatment advice is there, not the poison center. • Check calculations like weight conversions with the emergency department staff, especially if you are not familiar with them.

SUMMARY

- Poisons can enter the body through inhalation, injection, ingestion, or absorption.
- Emergency care is aimed at minimizing the effects of the poison.

- Substances on the skin are brushed and/or washed away, patients are removed from toxic environments, and activated charcoal may be used to prevent absorption of ingested poisons.

REVIEW QUESTIONS

1. How does activated charcoal work?
   a. by diluting certain poisons
   b. by eliminating certain poisons
   c. by negating certain poisons
   d. by binding to and preventing the absorption of certain poisons

2. Which of the following is NOT one of the ways poisons enter the body?
   a. inhalation
   b. absorption
   c. injection
   d. emulsion

3. Which of the following is a contraindication for the use of activated charcoal in a poisoning by mouth?
   a. diarrhea
   b. altered mental status
   c. abdominal pain
   d. rapid pulse

4. The standard dose of activated charcoal to administer to adults and children in cases of accidental poisoning is _____ grams of charcoal per kilogram of body weight.
   a. 0.5
   b. 1
   c. 3
   d. 10

5. The age-group among which accidental ingestion of poisons occurs most frequently is:
   a. children
   b. teenagers
   c. middle-aged adults
   d. geriatrics

WEB MEDIC

Visit Brady's *Essentials of Emergency Care* web site for direct web links. At **www.prenhall.com/limmer,** you will find information related to the following Chapter 17 topics:

- the American Association of Poison Control Centers
- Use of ipecac
- Activated charcoal
- Poisonings
- Home carbon monoxide detectors

Correlates with the U.S. DOT "EMT-Basic National Standard Curriculum" Lesson 4-7

Chapter Eighteen

ENVIRONMENTAL EMERGENCIES

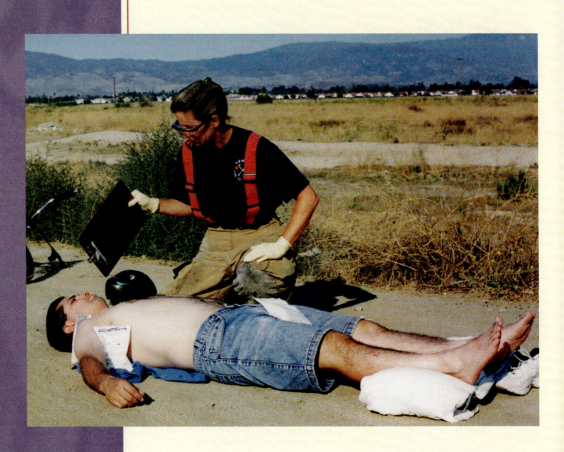

ESSENTIAL ELECTRONIC EXTRAS

CD ESSENTIALS

For preview and review of chapter material, see the student CD-ROM for

- Pretest
- Chapter quizzes
- Posttest

WEB ESSENTIALS

For additional review and enrichment, visit www.prenhall.com/limmer for

- Interactive student quizzes
- Links to online EMS resources
- Online case studies
- Audio glossary

Environmental emergencies cover a wide range of conditions, including heat exposure, cold exposure, water emergencies, and bites and stings. Some of these problems, like heat exposure, occur more often in some areas of the country than others, but there are certain conditions—like hypothermia—that you may encounter no matter where you are located.

TEMPERATURE REGULATION

The human body does an amazing job of keeping internal temperature constant despite a bewildering array of environmental conditions. Whether a person lives in the sub-zero Arctic or a tropical jungle, body temperature is kept close to 98.6°F (37°C). The body accomplishes this by balancing the amount of heat generated internally and the amount of heat lost externally.

When someone is exposed to cool or cold temperatures, the body conserves heat by constricting blood vessels, especially the ones in and near the skin surface, thereby limiting the amount of heat given off. At the same time, the person feels cold and puts on clothing to prevent further heat loss. If the temperature dips lower, the person generally puts on more layers of clothing or seeks shelter. If the body temperature drops below normal despite these measures, the person experiences hypothermia.

On the other hand, when someone is exposed to warm or hot temperatures, the body attempts to lose heat through dilation of the blood vessels in and near the skin surface. The person removes clothing to accelerate heat loss. There comes a point, though, when there is no more clothing to remove. Fortunately, there are other means of promoting cooling: conduction, convection, radiation, evaporation, and breathing. If body temperature rises above normal despite these efforts, the person experiences hyperthermia.

Conduction occurs when two objects of different temperatures touch. The warmer object will transfer heat to the cooler object. An example of this is the summertime hiker who stops and sits on a large rock in the shade. The hiker can become much cooler in a surprisingly short time. For *convection* to work, there must be air currents to carry heat away. This is part of the reason why fans make people feel cooler. *Radiation* of heat occurs when the sun warms the earth or a person stands in the sunshine. There is no need for any medium to carry the heat from the source to the object being warmed. *Evaporative* heat loss occurs through the cooling power of evaporating water or sweat. This is the other reason why fans make people feel cooler in the summer. Finally, breathing, or *respiration,* is the last means of losing heat. This is usually apparent only in colder weather (for example, the condensation of breath on a cold day).

An understanding of these mechanisms of heat loss can help you not only to protect yourself from extremes of temperature, but also to give your patients better care.

EXPOSURE TO COLD

Cold exposure can cause either generalized or localized problems. If the patient's body temperature is lower than normal, he or she has a generalized condition called **hypothermia.** If only a part of the body is cooled to the point where tissues freeze, this is a localized cold injury commonly called **frostbite.**

There are many factors that can predispose a patient to cold injury, including the environment, the patient's age and medical condition, and drugs or poisons.

CORE CONCEPTS

In this chapter, you will learn about the following topics:

- The effects of heat and cold on the body

- The treatments for conditions caused by heat and cold

- The personal safety concerns in water emergencies

- The signs, symptoms, and treatment of a near-drowning patient

- The signs, symptoms, and treatment of patients who have experienced bites and stings

Hypothermia

It is easy to see how a cold environment can induce hypothermia, but what is less obvious is just how easily this can occur. The body temperature of someone who is suddenly immersed in cold water can drop quickly despite all of the body's attempts to prevent it. Less apparent, but more common, is the case of someone old or ill who is exposed to room-temperature air with little clothing for protection. This kind of hypothermia occurs fairly often but can be difficult to recognize because of the subtlety of its presentation.

Many medical conditions affect the body's ability to regulate temperature. Shock (hypoperfusion) typically causes sweating, which increases heat loss. So does significant hypoglycemia. A serious head injury sometimes causes a high temperature with significant vasodilation. If the patient is not protected against excessive heat loss, this can eventually cause hypothermia. Burns, because they interfere with the normal function of the skin, prevent the normal mechanisms of heat preservation from working. A generalized infection can cause a fever that leads to so much heat loss that hypothermia develops. An injury to the spinal cord can cause enough vasodilation to produce the same result.

Certain drugs and poisons interfere with the body's ability to respond to changes in temperature. This may be the result of either an overdose or, sometimes, just the proper dose of medication.

The signs and symptoms of hypothermia are progressive. As the patient's core temperature drops, this will usually be reflected in the way he or she presents. Subtle signs at the beginning of hypothermia become more and more obvious as body temperature continues to go down (Table 18-1).

LIFESPAN DEVELOPMENT

The extremes of age present another risk factor for hypothermia. Very old and very young patients have a reduced ability to compensate for variations in temperature. Infants and young children, like many elderly people, have thinner skin and less body fat. Shivering may not be as effective because of relatively small muscle mass, especially in infants, who do not shiver at all. Like elderly people who have limited mobility, infants need help putting on additional clothing. Children and infants also have proportionally more body surface area that puts them at additional risk of losing heat.

TABLE 18-1   Stages of Hypothermia

Core Body Temperature		Symptoms
99°F—96°F	37.2°C—35.5°C	Shivering.
95°F—91°F	35.5°C—32.8°C	Intense shivering. If conscious, patient has difficulty speaking.
90°F—86°F	32.2°C—30.0°C	Shivering decreases and is replaced by strong muscular rigidity. Muscle coordination is affected, and erratic or jerky movements are produced. Thinking is less clear, general comprehension is dulled, possible total amnesia. Patient generally is able to maintain the appearance of psychological contact with surroundings.
85°F—81°F	29.4°C—27.2°C	Patient becomes irrational, loses contact with environment, and drifts into stuporous state. Muscular rigidity continues. Pulse and respirations are slow and cardiac arrhythmias may develop.
80°F—78°F	26.6°C—25.5°C	Patient loses consciousness and does not respond to spoken words. Most reflexes cease to function. Heartbeat becomes erratic.

Hypothermia

For a generalized cold emergency, consider the impact of the following factors:

- Air temperature, wind chill and/or water chill

- The patient's age

- Whether or not the patient's clothing is adequate

- Health of the patient including underlying illness and existing injuries

- How active the patient was during exposure

- Whether or not the patient may have used alcohol or drugs.

Be sure to document this and all assessment findings on your prehospital care report (PCR).

- Perform an initial assessment.

- Perform a focused history and physical exam of pertinent areas. Include a history of the present illness and a SAMPLE history. For all environmental emergencies, in addition to the usual OPQRST information, obtain the following: What is the source of the problem (for potentially toxic environmental exposures)? If there is alcohol or other drug involvement, what is the exact name of the substance? What route was involved? What is the environment like? What are the temperature and humidity? Was the patient immersed at any time? Was there a loss of consciousness? If so, how long? What effects is the patient experiencing?

- Obtain a complete set of vital signs.

The signs and symptoms of hypothermia include the following. Note that decreasing mental status and decreasing motor function both correlate with the degree of hypothermia.

- Shivering in early stages when core body temperature is above 90°F. In severe cases, shivering decreases or is absent.

- Numbness, or reduced-to-lost sensation to touch.

- Stiff or rigid posture in prolonged cases.

- Drowsiness and/or unwillingness or inability to do even the simplest activities. In prolonged cases, the patient may become irrational, drift into a stuporous state, or actually remove clothing.

- Rapid breathing and rapid pulse in early stages. Slow-to-absent breathing and pulse in prolonged cases. Blood pressure may be low to absent.

- Loss of motor coordination, such as staggering or inability to hold things.

- Joint/muscle stiffness, or muscular rigidity.

- Decreased mental status, from confusion to unresponsiveness. In extreme cases the patient has a "glassy stare."

- Cool abdominal skin temperature. (To assess, place the back of your hand inside the clothing and against the patient's abdomen.)

- Skin may appear red in early stages. In prolonged cases, skin is pale to cyanotic. In most extreme cases, some body parts are stiff and hard (frozen). ✳

During initial assessment, be sure to check an awake patient's orientation to person, place, and day. (Can the patient tell you his name? Where he or she is? What day it is?) Perform a focused history and physical exam to help you estimate the extent of hypothermia. Assume a case of severe hypothermia if shivering is absent.

For your prehospital care report (PCR), be sure to document the patient's condition when found; skin temperature, color, and condition; whether or not the patient was shivering; time exposed to the cold, and so on.

Passive and Active Rewarming

Passive rewarming involves simply covering the patient and taking other steps to prevent further heat loss, allowing the body to rewarm itself. Active rewarming includes application of an external heat source to the body. All EMS systems permit passive rewarming. Some EMS systems allow the active rewarming of a hypothermic patient who is alert and responding appropriately. However, many do not.

Active rewarming can prove to be dangerous due to a too-rapid rise in the patient's body temperature. If you are allowed to rewarm a patient with hypothermia who is alert and responding appropriately, do not delay transport. Rewarm the patient while en route. *The emergency care steps that follow assume a protocol that permits active rewarming of a patient who is alert and responding appropriately. Follow your local protocols.*

Patient Care

Hypothermic Patient, Alert and Responding Appropriately

For the hypothermic patient who is alert and responding appropriately, proceed with active rewarming:

1 Remove all of the patient's wet clothing. Keep him dry, dress him in dry clothing, or wrap him in dry warm blankets. Keep the patient still and handle him very gently. Do not allow the patient to walk or exert himself. Do not massage extremities.

2 During transport, actively rewarm the patient. Gradually and gently apply heat to the patient's body in the form of heat packs, hot-water bottles, electric heating pads, warm air, radiated heat, and even your own body heat. Do not warm the patient too quickly. Rapid warming will circulate peripherally stagnated cold blood and rapidly cool the vital organs, possibly causing cardiac arrest. If transport is delayed, move the patient to a warm environment if at all possible.

3 Provide emergency care for shock. Provide oxygen, which should be warmed and humidified, if possible.

4 Give the alert patient warm liquids slowly. When warm fluids are given too quickly, circulation patterns change, sending blood away from the core to the skin and extremities. Do not allow the patient to eat or drink stimulants, such as coffee or tea.

5 Transport the patient, except in the mildest of cases (shivering). Continue to provide high-concentration oxygen and monitor vital signs. Never allow a patient to remain in, or return to, a cold environment.

Take the following precautions when actively rewarming a patient.

- **Rewarm the patient slowly.** Handle the patient with great care, the same as you would if there were unstabilized cervical-spine injuries.

- **Use central rewarming.** Heat should be applied to the lateral chest, neck, armpits, and groin. You must avoid rewarming the limbs. If they are warmed first, blood will collect in the extremities due to vasodilation and may cause a fatal form of shock.

- **If transport must be delayed, a warm bath is very helpful.** However, you must keep the patient alert enough so that he or she does not drown. Again, do not warm the patient too quickly.

- **Keep the patient at rest.** Do not allow the patient to walk, and avoid rough handling of the patient. Such activity may set off severe heart problems, including ventricular fibrillation. Since the patient's blood is coldest in the extremities, exercise or unnecessary movement could also quickly circulate the cold blood and lower the core body temperature. ✳

Patient Care

Hypothermic Patient, Unresponsive or Not Responding Appropriately

A patient with a cold emergency who is unresponsive or not responding appropriately has severe hypothermia. For this patient, provide passive rewarming. Do not try to actively rewarm the patient with severe hypothermia. Remove the patient from the environment and protect him or her from further heat loss. Active rewarming may cause the patient to develop ventricular fibrillation.

For the patient with severe hypothermia, you should provide emergency care by following these steps:

1 Assure an open airway.

2 Provide high-concentration oxygen. The oxygen should be passed through a warm-water humidifier if possible. If necessary, the oxygen that has been kept warm in the ambulance passenger compartment can be used. If there is no other choice, oxygen from a cold cylinder may be used.

3 Wrap the patient in blankets. If available, use insulating blankets. Handle the patient as gently as possible. Rough handling may cause ventricular fibrillation. Do not allow the patient to eat or drink stimulants. Do not massage extremities.

4 Transport immediately. ✳

Extreme Hypothermia

In extreme cases of hypothermia, you will find the patient unresponsive, with no discernible vital signs. In extreme hypothermia, the heart rate can slow to less than 10 beats per minute, and the patient will feel very cold to your touch (core body temperature may be below 80°F). Even so, be aware that it is possible that the patient is still alive or can be resuscitated.

To provide emergency care, assess the carotid pulse for 30–45 seconds. If there is no pulse, start CPR immediately. (If you do detect a pulse, do not start CPR.) Apply the AED and transport immediately. ✳

Because the hypothermic patient may not reach biological death for over 30 minutes, the staff at the hospital emergency department will not pronounce a patient dead until after he or she is both rewarmed and resuscitative measures have failed. This means you cannot assume that a severe hypothermia patient is dead on the basis of body temperature and lack of vital signs. As medical personnel point out, "You're not dead until you're warm and dead!"

Local Cold Injury

When the temperature drops low enough, ice crystals form and tissue freezes. This is most likely to occur in cold, windy environments, affecting the nose, ears, cheeks, and tips of the fingers and toes. Smoking, like anything that causes constriction of the blood vessels near the skin surface, can increase the risk of local cold injury.

Early or Superficial Local Cold Injury

Early or superficial local cold injuries (sometimes called "frostnip") are brought about by direct contact with a cold object or exposure of a body part to cold air. Wind chill and water chill also can be major factors. Tissue damage is minor and the response to care is good. The tip of the nose, the tips of the ears, the upper cheeks, and the fingers (all areas that are usually exposed) are most susceptible to early or superficial local cold injuries. The injury, as its name suggests, is localized, with clear demarcation of its limits.

Early or Superficial Local Cold Injury

Patients are often unaware of the onset of an early local cold injury until someone indicates that there is something unusual about their skin color. The affected area of patients with light skin at first reddens; dark skin lightens. Both then blanch (whiten). Once blanching begins, the color change can take place very quickly. The affected area also feels numb to the patient. ✳

Early or Superficial Local Cold Injury

Emergency care for early local cold injury is simple. Get the patient out of the cold environment. Warm the affected area. If the injury is to an extremity, splint and cover it. Do not rub or massage it, and do not re-expose it to the cold. ✳

Usually, the patient can apply warmth from his or her own bare hands, blow warm air on the site, or, if the fingers are involved, hold them in the armpits. During recovery from an early local cold injury, the patient may complain about tingling or burning sensations, which is normal. If the condition does not respond to this simple care, begin to treat for a late or deep local cold injury.

Late or Deep Local Cold Injury

Late or deep local cold injury (also known as "frostbite") develops if an early or superficial local cold injury goes untreated (Figure 18-1). In late or deep local

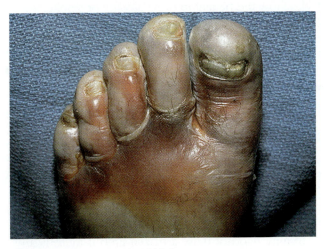

Figure 18-1 Local cold injury.

cold injury, the skin and subcutaneous layers of the body part are affected. Muscles, bones, deep blood vessels, and organ membranes can become frozen.

Patient Assessment

Late or Deep Local Cold Injury

In frostbite, the affected area of the skin appears white and waxy. When the condition progresses to actual freezing, the skin turns mottled or blotchy, the color turns from the blanched color of early cold injury to grayish yellow and finally to grayish blue. Swelling and blistering may occur.

With frostbite, the affected area feels frozen, but only on the surface. The tissue below the surface is still soft and has its normal resilience, or "bounce." With freezing, the tissues are not resilient and feel frozen to the touch. (Note: Do not squeeze or poke the tissue. The condition of the deeper tissues can be determined by gently feeling the affected area. Do the assessment as if the affected area had a fractured bone.) ✳

Patient Care

Late or Deep Local Cold Injury

Initial emergency care for late or deep local cold injury—frostbite and freezing—is the same:

1. **Administer high-concentration oxygen.**

2. **Transport to a medical facility without delay,** protecting the frostbitten or frozen area by covering it and handling it as gently as possible.

3. **If transport must be delayed, get the patient indoors and keep him or her warm.** Do not allow the patient to drink alcohol or smoke, because constriction of blood vessels and decreased circulation to the injured tissues may result. Rewarm the frozen part per local protocol, or request instructions from medical direction.

Important: Never listen to myths or folktales about the care of frostbite. Never rub a frostbitten or frozen area. Never rub snow on a frostbitten or frozen area. There are ice crystals at the capillary level; rubbing the injury site may cause them to seriously damage the already injured tissues. Do not break blisters or massage the injured area. Do not allow the patient to walk on an affected extremity. Do not thaw a frozen limb if there is any chance it will be refrozen. ✳

Active Rapid Rewarming of Frozen Parts

Active rewarming of frozen parts is seldom recommended. The chance of permanently injuring frozen tissues with active rewarming is too great. Consider it only if local protocols recommend it, if you are instructed to do so by medical direction, or if transport will be severely delayed and you cannot reach medical direction for instructions. If you are in a situation where you must attempt rewarming without instructions from a physician, follow the procedure described here.

You will need warm water and a container in which you can immerse the entire site of injury without the limb touching the sides or bottom of the container. If you cannot find a suitable container, fashion one from a plastic bag supported by a cardboard box or wooden crate (Figure 18-2). Proceed as follows:

1. **Heat the water.** It should be heated to a temperature between 100°F and 105°F. You should be able to put your finger into the water without experiencing discomfort.

2. **Fill the container with the heated water.** Then bare the injured part by removing clothing, jewelry, bands, or straps.

3. **Fully immerse the injured part.** Do not allow the injured area to touch the sides or bottom of the container. Do not place any pressure on the affected part. Continuously stir the water. When the water cools below 100°F, remove the affected part and add more warm water. The patient may complain of moderate pain as the affected area rewarms, or the patient may experience some period of intense pain. The presence of pain is usually a good indicator of successful rewarming.

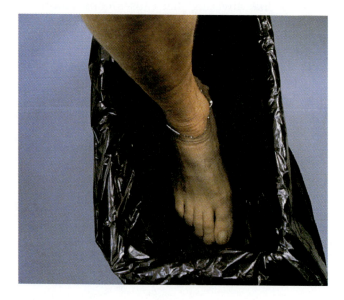

Figure 18-2   Rewarming the frozen part.

4. **When rewarming is complete, remove the affected part.** When the affected part is completely rewarmed (it no longer feels frozen and is turning red or blue), gently dry the affected area and apply a dry sterile dressing. Place dry sterile dressings between fingers and toes before dressing hands and feet. Next, cover the site with blankets or whatever is available to keep the affected area warm. Do not allow these coverings to come in direct contact with the injured area or to put pressure on the site. It is best if you first build some sort of framework on which the coverings can be placed.

5. **Keep the patient at rest.** Do not allow the patient to walk if a lower extremity has been frost-bitten or frozen.

6. **Keep the entire patient warm, without overheating.** Cover the patient's head with a towel or small blanket to reduce heat loss. Leave the patient's face exposed.

7. **Continue to monitor the patient.** Assist circulation according to local protocol. Do not allow the limb to refreeze.

8. **Transport as soon as possible,** with the affected limb slightly elevated.

EXPOSURE TO HEAT

A patient who is exposed to high temperatures is no longer able to lose heat through radiation. This leads to excessive sweating (up to one liter per hour or more) and dehydration. When high temperature is combined with high humidity, the body has even less ability to get rid of excessive heat. In this situation, sweating does not work because the air is already saturated with water. This can lead to life-threatening increases in body temperature.

Just as certain conditions increase the risk of cold injury, there are conditions that predispose patients to heat injury. Again, the extremes of age are considerable risk factors—for the reasons mentioned under hypothermia. Pre-existing illnesses such as heart disease, obesity, fatigue, or diabetes also put the patient at increased risk, as do certain medications.

Patient with Moist, Pale, Normal-to-Cool Skin

Prolonged exposure to excessive heat can create an emergency in which the patient presents with moist pale skin that may feel normal or cool to the touch. The individual perspires heavily, often drinking large quantities of water. As the sweating continues, salts are lost by the body, bringing on painful muscle cramps (sometimes called "heat cramps"). A person who is actively exercising can lose more than a liter of sweat per hour.

Healthy individuals who have been exposed to excessive heat while working or exercising may experience a form of shock brought on by loss of fluid and salt. This is seen among firefighters, construction workers, dock workers, and those employed in poorly ventilated warehouses. It is more of a problem during the summer and reaches a peak during prolonged heat waves. This condition is sometimes known as "heat exhaustion."

Patient Assessment

Heat-Emergency Patient with Moist, Pale, Normal-to-Cool Skin

Signs and symptoms include the following:

- Muscular cramps, usually in the legs and abdomen
- Weakness or exhaustion, sometimes dizziness or periods of faintness
- Rapid, shallow breathing
- Weak pulse
- Moist pale skin that may feel normal to cool
- Heavy perspiration
- Loss of consciousness is possible

Patient Care

Heat-Emergency Patient with Moist, Pale, Normal-to-Cool Skin

Emergency care includes the following:

1. **Remove the patient from the hot environment.** Place him or her in a cool environment, such as the back of an air-conditioned ambulance.

2. **Administer oxygen** by nonrebreather mask at 15 liters per minute.

3. **Help cool the patient.** Loosen or remove clothing, and fan the patient without chilling him. Watch for shivering.

4. **Position the patient.** Put him at rest and in a supine position with legs elevated.

5. **Transport.**

If the patient is unresponsive or vomiting, transport to the hospital with patient on his left side. If the patient is responsive and not nauseated, have him drink water (Figure 18-3). If the patient experiences muscular cramps, apply moist towels over cramped muscles. ✳

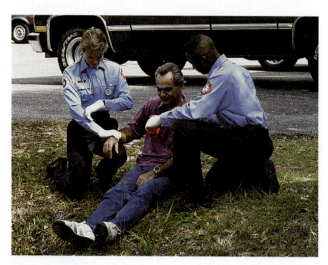

Figure 18-3 Move the heat-emergency patient into the shade. If he is responsive and not nauseated, have him drink water.

Patient with Hot Skin (Dry or Moist)

When a person's temperature-regulating mechanisms fail and the body cannot rid itself of excessive heat, you will see a patient with hot, dry or possibly moist skin. When the skin is hot—whether dry or moist—a true emergency exists. It is a condition that is sometimes called "heat stroke." The problem is compounded when, in response to loss of fluid and salt, the patient stops sweating, which prevents heat loss through evaporation. Athletes, laborers, and others who exercise or work in hot environments commonly develop this condition. So do the elderly who live in poorly ventilated apartments without air conditioning, and children left in cars with the windows rolled up.

Most cases of patients with hot, dry skin are reported on hot, humid days. However, many cases occur from exposure to dry heat.

<table>
<tr><td style="background:#E8541E; color:white">**Patient Assessment**</td></tr>
</table>

Heat-Emergency Patient with Hot Skin (Dry or Moist)

Signs and symptoms include:

- Rapid, shallow breathing
- Full, rapid pulse
- Generalized weakness
- Hot, dry or possibly moist skin
- Little or no perspiration
- Altered mental status, from confusion to unresponsiveness
- Dilated pupils
- Possible seizures; no muscle cramps

<table>
<tr><td style="background:#2E3A87; color:white">**Patient Care**</td></tr>
</table>

Heat-Emergency Patient with Hot Skin (Dry or Moist)

Emergency care includes the following:

1. **Remove the patient from the hot environment.** Place him in a cool environment, such as in the air-conditioned ambulance with air conditioner running on high.

2. **Help cool the patient.** Remove clothing, and apply cool packs to neck, groin, and armpits. Keep the skin wet by applying water by sponge or wet towels. Fan aggressively.

3. **Administer oxygen** by nonrebreather mask at 15 liters per minute.

4. **Transport immediately.** Should transport be delayed, find a tub or container, immerse the patient up to the neck in cooled water. Monitor vital signs throughout process.

WATER EMERGENCIES

Drowning occurs when someone dies after being immersed in water. A patient has experienced a "near-drowning" if he or she has been immersed but is still alive. In this case, the patient may have no pulse (for the moment), may have a pulse but no breathing, may be unconscious and breathing, or may be alert and in no distress.

Drowning is asphyxiation which results from submersion in water and the death of the patient in the first 24 hours. The term near-drowning is used to define an incident that is potentially fatal from a submersion in water but that does not result in a death within the first 24 hours. In the United States each year there are approximately 4,500 deaths due to drowning. Almost 40 percent of these deaths that occur to children under 5 years of age could be prevented by closer supervision and the wearing of personal floatation devices whenever people are near pools or bodies of water.

The process of drowning begins as a person struggles to keep afloat in the water. The person gulps in large breaths of air while thrashing about. When he can no longer keep afloat and starts to submerge, he tries to take and hold one more deep breath. As he does, the water enters the airway. The patient then inhales and swallows additional water. When the water flows past the epiglottis, it triggers a reflex known as a laryngospasm. This spasm caps the glottic opening to minimize the amount of water that enters the lungs. Unconsciousness quickly develops from hypoxia or asphyxiation. When a significant amount of water fails to enter the lungs, it is called a "dry drowning." If the laryngospasm does not occur and a large amount of water enters the lungs, it is a "wet drowning." Studies have shown that approximately 10 percent of drownings are dry drownings.

All EMT-Bs should be aware of the order of procedures for a water rescue. In fact, they should receive practical skills training in the shore-based techniques, the use of a personal flotation device (PFD), and community resources that should be called to respond to and carry out in-water techniques. The order of water rescue procedures follow the sequence of reach, throw and tow, and row as shown in Figure 18-4. Then, only if properly trained, should a responder "go" to the patient.

■ **Reach.** When the patient is responsive and near the shore or poolside, try to reach him or her by holding out an object for the patient to grab. This should always be done while you are wearing a PFD and from a secure position so you are not pulled or fall into the water. Objects such as a vacuum pole, pike pole, an oar, a long board splint, or a tree branch can be useful.

■ **Throw and tow.** If the patient is conscious and alert, yet too far to reach with an object, attempt to throw him or her an object that will float such as a ring buoy, boogie board, large beach ball, plastic milk jugs, or a PFD (not yours). Once the conscious patient has a flotation device, use a rope to tow him or her to the shore. This is done from a safe position on shore. It is a good idea for all emergency vehicles that respond to bodies of water to carry a rope throw bag with 50 to 100 feet of polypropylene line. If such equipment is carried, EMT-Bs should practice rapidly deploying the rope with accuracy. Do not enter the water unless you are a good swimmer and experienced and trained in water rescue.

■ **Row.** When the patient is too far from the shore for you to throw a rope or is unresponsive, the next approach would be for the trained team to row a boat over to the patient. Do not attempt to lift the patient into a small boat if he or she is alert. Instead have the patient hang on to the side of the boat. All personnel in the rescue boat should wear a PFD at all times.

■ **Go.** The last resort, when all other means have failed, is to enter the water and swim to the patient. This should only be done by persons who have been trained in water rescue and lifesaving.

During the winter, you may respond to a call for a patient who has fallen into a hole in the ice. Call for the ice-rescue team immediately. You should not attempt to go out on the ice unless you are properly trained and wearing a cold-water submersion suit and a PFD. Attempts at shore-based rescue by throwing a rope to the patient will have little value once hypothermia sets in and the patient is no longer able to grasp the rope. The priority should be to limit additional rescuers and bystanders from going out on the ice and to get the ice-rescue team to the scene as soon as possible.

Once you have reached the patient, you must be aggressive in your treatment. This is obviously true for the unconscious patient, but is just as important in the patient who is alert and denying any difficulty. A number of patients who look fine shortly after near-drowning episodes deteriorate hours later. Urge all of these patients to accept your offer of treatment and transportation.

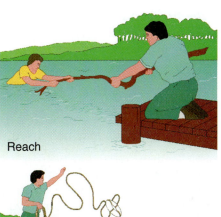

Reach

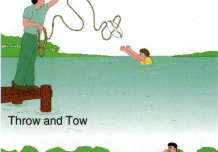

Throw and Tow

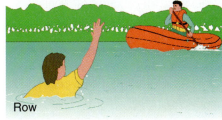

Row

Figure 18-4 First try to *reach* and pull the patient from the water. If that fails, *throw* anything that will float and *tow* the patient from the water. If that fails, *row* to the patient. If all the above fail, the rescuer may swim to the patient, but only if he or she is an experienced swimmer with rescue training.

Water Emergencies

Learn to look for the following problems in water-related accident patients:

- **Airway obstruction.** This may be from water in the lungs, foreign matter in the airway, or swollen airway tissues. Spasms of the larynx may be present in cases of near-drowning.

- **Cardiac arrest.** This is often related to respiratory arrest or occurs before the near-drowning.

- **Signs of heart attack.** Through overexertion, the patient may have greater problems than the obvious near-drowning. Some untrained rescuers too quickly conclude that chest pains are due to muscle cramps as a result of swimming.

- **Injuries to the head and neck.** These are expected to be found in boating, water-skiing, and diving accidents, but they also occur in swimming accidents.

- **Internal injuries.** While doing the focused physical exam, stay on the alert for musculoskeletal injuries, soft-tissue injuries, and internal bleeding (which may be missed during the first stages of emergency care).

- **Generalized cooling, or hypothermia.** The water does not have to be very cold and the length of stay in the water does not have to be very long for hypothermia to occur. In some cases of near-drowning, the patient may have a better chance for survival in cold water.

- **Substance abuse.** Alcohol and drug use are closely associated with adolescent and adult drownings. Elevated blood alcohol levels have been found in over 30 percent of drowning victims. The screening for drug use has not been as extensive as that done for alcohol, but research indicates that drugs are a contributory factor in many water-related accidents.

- **Drowning or near-drowning.** The patient may be discovered under or face down in the water. He or she may be unconscious and without discernible vital signs or may be conscious, breathing, and coughing up water. ✳

Water Emergencies

Emergency care of a patient with a water emergency includes the following:

1. **Ensure the safety of all rescue personnel.**

2. **Suspect spine injury,** if the patient was diving or if diving cannot be ruled out.

3. **Resuscitate the patient if necessary.** If the patient has been submerged in cold water, be aggressive in your resuscitation efforts. Any pulseless, nonbreathing patient who has been submerged in cold water should receive resuscitation efforts unless medical direction orders otherwise.

4. **Take spinal precautions if necessary.** If the patient is in the water and you suspect spine injury, apply neutral in-line manual stabilization of the head and cervical spine (Skill Summary 18-1). Remove the patient from the water with a backboard.

5. **Position the patient properly.** If there is no reason to suspect a spine injury, place the patient on his left side to allow water, vomitus, and secretions to drain from the upper airway.

6. **Maintain an open airway.** Suction as needed.

7. **Administer oxygen** if you have not already done so during the initial assessment.

NOTE: If you are unable to ventilate the patient because of gastric distention, place the patient on his left side. With suction immediately available, place your hand over the epigastric area of the abdomen and apply firm pressure to relieve the distention. Do this only if the gastric distention interferes with ventilation. ✳

BITES AND STINGS

Animals that bite and sting far outnumber human beings on this planet, and it is only natural to expect some of them to be toxic. Fortunately, most of them cause no more than transient discomfort or mild pain. There are a few, however, that can cause more serious problems, sometimes from an allergic or anaphylactic reaction. (You reviewed the recognition and treatment of this condition earlier in Chapter 16.) At other times, the problem results from a poisonous or venomous sting or bite.

The specific signs and symptoms you will see depend not only on the particular animal, but also on

SAFETY NOTE: Unless you are a very good swimmer and trained in water rescue, do not go into the water to save someone.

Head-Chin Support

Two Rescuers in Shallow Water

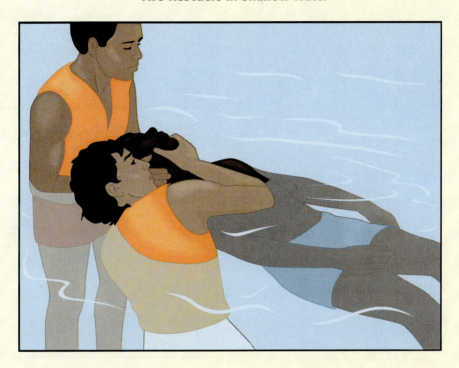

▲ When there are two rescuers present, perform the head-chin support technique to provide in-line stabilization of a patient in shallow water.

(continued)

Head-Splint Support

One Rescuer in Shallow Water

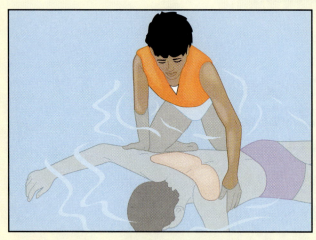

▲ **1.** When you find a patient face down in shallow water, position yourself alongside the patient.

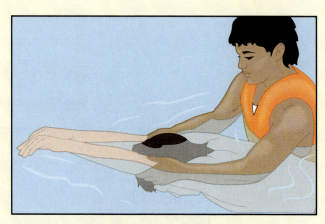

▲ **2.** Extend the patient's arms straight up alongside his or her head to create a splint.

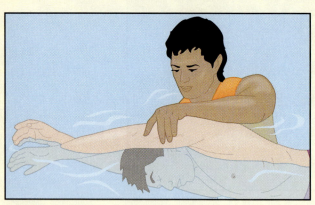

▲ **3.** Begin to rotate the torso toward you.

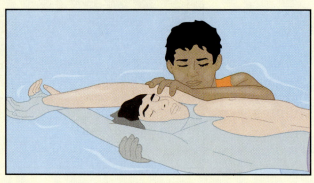

▲ **4.** As you rotate the patient, lower yourself into the water.

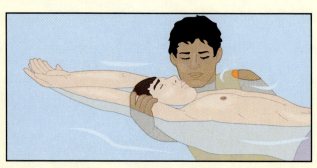

▲ **5.** Maintain manual stabilization by holding the patient's head between his arms.

Head-Chin Support Technique

One Rescuer in Deep Water

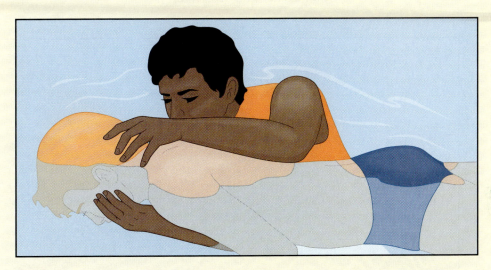

▲ **1.** When you find a patient face down in deep water, position yourself beside him. Support his head with one hand and his mandible with the other.

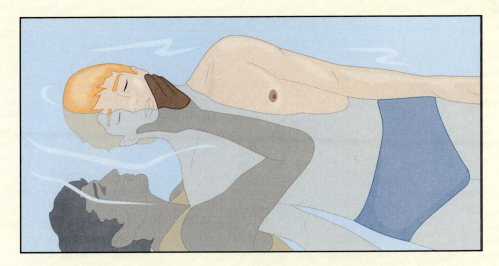

▲ **2.** Then rotate the patient by ducking under him.

(continued)

Head-Chin Support Technique

One Rescuer in Deep Water

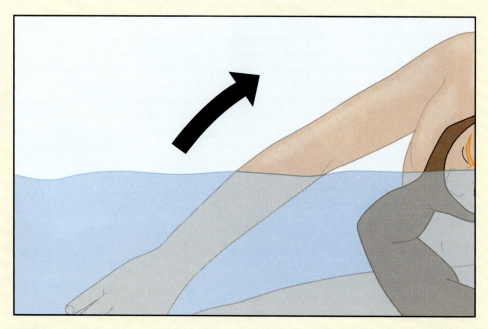

▲ **3.** Continue to rotate until the patient is face up.

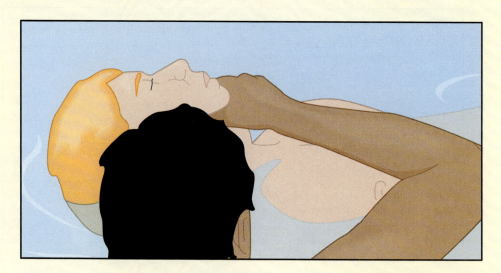

▲ **4.** Maintain in-line stabilization until a backboard is used to immobilize the patient's spine.

the patient and the circumstances surrounding the exposure. A very young or very old patient may react more strongly to a sting, for example, as may someone who has a pre-existing illness.

All spiders are poisonous, but most species cannot get their fangs through human skin. The black widow spider and the brown recluse, or fiddleback, spider (Figure 18-5) are two that can, and their bites produce medical emergencies. Almost all brown recluse bites are painless, with the patients not remembering being bitten. The lesion shown in Figure 18-6 only appears in about 10 percent of the cases and takes about 12 or more hours to develop. EMS is seldom called to respond to a brown recluse bite. Black widow bites cause a more immediate reaction.

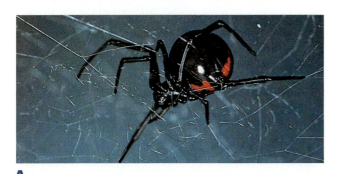

A

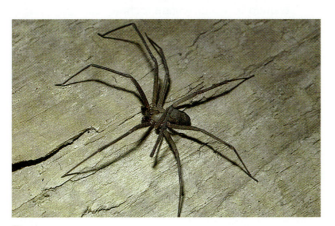

B

Figure 18-5 (A) Black widow spider, and (B) a brown recluse spider.

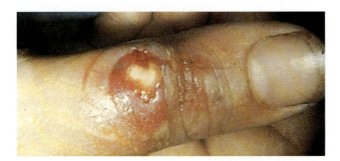

Figure 18-6 Brown recluse spider bite.

Patient Assessment

Bites and Stings

- Perform an initial assessment.
- Perform a focused history and physical exam, including a SAMPLE history.
- Obtain a complete set of vital signs.
- Evaluate the patient for the following signs and symptoms:
  - History of bite (spider, snake) or sting (insect, scorpion, marine animal)
  - Redness and swelling at the site
  - Weakness and dizziness
  - Chills and fever
  - Localized pain or itching
  - Altered mental state
  - Blotchy skin (mottled skin)
  - Numbness in a limb or body part
  - Nausea and vomiting
  - Bite marks
  - Stinger ✳

Patient Care

Bites and Stings

Emergency care consists of the following:

1. **Remove the stinger,** if one is present. Scraping is a traditional method of removing a stinger. Use the edge of a credit card to scrape the stinger out. Follow your local protocols when removing a stinger .
2. **Wash the area gently.**
3. **Remove jewelry** from the injured area before swelling begins, if possible.
4. **Position the injection site** slightly below the level of the patient's heart.

If the wound is a snakebite, consult medical direction about whether to apply a constricting band. Do not apply cold to snakebites. Be sure to observe the patient for development of signs and symptoms of an allergic reaction, and treat appropriately. ✳

SUMMARY

- The human body loses heat through the mechanisms of conduction, convection, radiation, evaporation, and breathing.

- A person whose body temperature is lower than normal is said to be suffering from hypothermia.

- Signs and symptoms of hypothermia include: shivering; numbness or reduced sensation; stiff or rigid posture; drowsiness; irrationality; breathing changes; loss of motor coordination; joint/muscle stiffness; decreased mental status; cool abdominal skin temperature; skin color changes from red to pale to cyanotic.

- Treatment for hypothermia, in addition to ensuring the ABCs, includes removing the patient from the cold environment and rewarming him or her actively or passively.

- Ice crystals forming in tissues produce local cold injuries, which can be early or superficial (frostnip) or late and deep (frostbite).

- Treatment for local cold injuries includes removing the patient from the cold environment and covering the injured area, allowing it to warm. With late or deep injuries, transport to a medical facility.

- When the body is no longer able to lose excess heat, the patient may suffer a heat emergency—heat cramps in milder cases or heat stroke in more severe ones.

- Signs and symptoms of heat emergencies may in less severe cases include muscular cramps; weakness or exhaustion; rapid, shallow breathing; weak pulse; moist pale skin; heavy perspiration; loss of consciousness. In more severe cases, symptoms might include full, rapid pulse; hot and either dry or moist skin; little or no perspiration; altered mental status; dilated pupils; possible seizures.

- In water emergencies, use the rescue technique steps of reach, throw and tow, row, and go. Always use a personal floatation device when attempting a water rescue and only go into the water to a patient if you have been trained in water rescue techniques.

- Suspect spine injury in water emergencies in which diving cannot be ruled out; take spinal precautions.

- Bites and stings from animals and insects are common reasons for emergency calls. Obtain the history of the bite. Common symptoms of bites and stings include a history of a bite; redness and swelling at the site; weakness and dizziness; chills and fever; localized pain or itching; altered mental state; blotchy skin; numbness; nausea and vomiting; bite marks; stinger.

- Remove insect stingers; consult with medical direction on snakebite.

REVIEW QUESTIONS

1. When a patient suffers damage from the cold to muscles, bone, deep blood vessels, or organ membranes, the condition is termed:
   a. late or deep local cold injury.
   b. generalized cold injury.
   c. traumatic cold injury.
   d. internal cold injury.

2. A patient with a hot and dry or moist skin suffering from a heat emergency may have a condition called heat:
   a. cramps.
   b. aphasia.
   c. stroke.
   d. debility.

REVIEW QUESTIONS *continued*

3. For a heat emergency, you should apply cool packs to the neck, groin, and armpits if the patient's skin is:

a. hot and dry or moist.

b. cool, pale, and moist.

c. normal temperature but moist.

d. pale and dry.

4. A victim of a water emergency has gastric distention. When relieving this condition, you should place the patient:

a. on his left side.

b. in a sitting position.

c. face down on his stomach.

d. face up on his stomach.

5. With an insect bite or sting, you should position the injection site:

a. slightly below the level of the patient's heart.

b. on a level with the patient's heart.

c. as far above the patient's heart as possible.

d. in a position of comfort for the patient.

WEB MEDIC

Visit Brady's *Essentials of Emergency Care* web site for direct web links. At **www.prenhall.com/limmer,** you will find information related to the following Chapter 18 topics:

- Heat and cold emergencies
- Aquatic safety and water rescue

Chapter Nineteen

BEHAVIORAL
EMERGENCIES

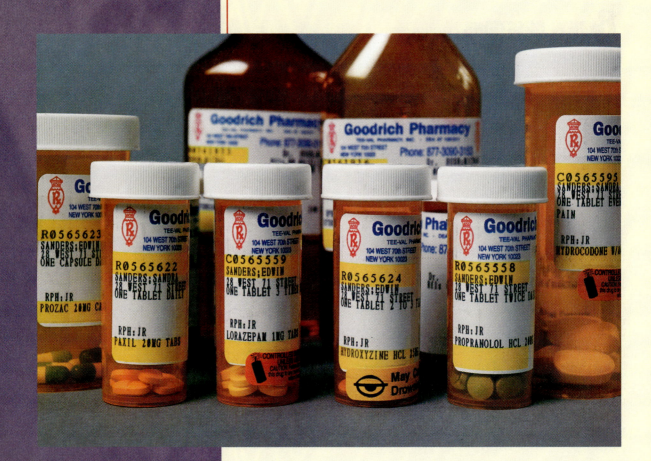

ESSENTIAL ELECTRONIC EXTRAS

CD ESSENTIALS

*For preview and review of
chapter material, see the
student CD-ROM for*

- Pretest
- Chapter quizzes
- Posttest

WEB ESSENTIALS

*For additional review
and enrichment, visit
www.prenhall.com/limmer for*

- Interactive student quizzes
- Links to online EMS
  resources
- Online case studies
- Audio glossary

Behavioral emergencies can involve a wide range of patient problems, including attempted suicide, depression, or unusual behavior. As an EMT, you will be called upon to evaluate and care for these patients as you would any other—but with behavioral emergencies you will rely on your "people" skills more than your medical skills to communicate with the patient to assess and treat his or her condition effectively.

BEHAVIORAL EMERGENCIES

A behavioral emergency is a situation in which a patient exhibits behavior that is alarming, unacceptable, or intolerable to the patient, family, or community. This behavior may be due to a number of potential causes, including psychiatric conditions, medical problems, and acute reactions to stress.

It is best to consider all patients who appear to be psychiatric patients as having an altered mental status until proven otherwise. It is not uncommon for a patient who is a diabetic to display bizarre behavior as a result of low blood sugar. If this patient were treated as a psychiatric patient and restrained, he or she could die. You should also consider the fact that psychiatric patients are often prescribed potent medications that when used therapeutically are beneficial. Overdose of these drugs can also cause altered mental status. Finally, never discount the fact that a patient with a long psychiatric history may actually be having a medical problem.

With all the cautions noted in the paragraph above, it is also quite safe to assume you have treated psychiatric patients in the past and will treat more in the future. While it is relatively simple to identify and treat a laceration or chest pain, psychiatric emergencies are often a cause for concern for the EMT-B for many reasons. These patients pose a challenge because the EMT-B's assessment and communication skills are put to the test. Many EMTs do not feel confident in the assessment and care skills needed for psychiatric patients. Often, too, they are concerned with the potential for violence they feel these patients present.

Scene safety should be the primary concern on every call. Psychiatric patients add an element of danger on some calls. It is important to keep the danger in perspective. Not all psychiatric patients will be out to harm you. However, some patients, due to their altered perceptions or suicidal intentions, may actually be a danger. A patient who is hallucinating or experiencing delusions is not responding to reality and could be dangerous. For example, a patient who has attempted suicide with carbon monoxide has created an unsafe atmosphere that should not be entered.

Another area of concern in dealing with psychiatric patients is the terminology of conditions and diseases. While you may have been taught about cardiac and respiratory conditions in your initial EMT training, you may not have received detailed information on psychiatric emergencies. Table 19-1 provides some of the more common psychiatric signs, symptoms, and diseases you will encounter. Remember that it is not necessary to diagnose a patient's condition (just as it is not necessary to attempt to differentiate angina pectoris from a myocardial infarction), but learning some of this information will help you when communicating with patients and mental health professionals and to understand the patient's condition.

CORE CONCEPTS

In this chapter, you will learn about the following topics:

- How to assess the patient with a psychiatric presentation

- How to differentiate between an altered mental status caused by a psychiatric condition from one caused by medical or traumatic conditions

- How to provide care for the patient with a psychiatric presentation

- How to provide restraint safely and effectively

✔ **Knowledge**

☐ **1.** Provide care to a patient experiencing a behavioral problem. (p. 278)

- Discuss the characteristics of an individual's behavior which suggest that the patient is at risk for suicide. (p. 280)

- Discuss the special considerations for assessing a patient with behavioral problems. (pp. 275–278)

- Discuss the general principles of an individual's behavior which suggest that he is at risk for violence. (pp. 277–278)

- Discuss methods to calm behavioral emergency patients. (p. 278)

✔ **Attitude**

☐ **2.** Recognize and respond to the feelings of the patient who may require interventions to be performed. (pp. 277, 278, 281–283)

The Mental Status Examination

Mental health personnel use a mental status examination (MSE) when examining psychiatric patients. This would be the equivalent of a focused physical examination for a medical or trauma patient, but in this case it focuses on the patient's psychiatric or mental status. Components of the exam include observations of the patient, evaluation of thought processes, and social factors.

As background to the MSE, you will be aware of the chief complaint or why EMS was called. You should also learn of the patients' history, including psychiatric history and living conditions. The living conditions may be an important cause of behavioral problems (e.g., a care giver may no longer be living with the patient, which causes worsening of living conditions. Or residents of a house next door erecting a satellite dish, which causes a paranoid patient to believe that the device is being used by the government to eavesdrop on him.) Remember that there are certain conditions, such as living arrangements, that will not be seen by mental health personnel at

---

TABLE 19-1   Common Psychiatric Terms and Conditions

Term	Definition
Anxiety	State of apprehension, uneasiness, discomfort or restlessness
Bipolar disorder	Involves swings between mania (excitement or excessive activity) and depression (previously called manic-depressive disorder)
Delusion	False belief. Examples include: • Delusions of grandeur—patient believes he or she is a famous person, religious figure, or other prominent person he or she is not. • Paranoid or persecution—patient believes people or things (e.g., aliens) are following, out to get him or her, etc.
Hallucinations	False perceptions having no relation to reality. May be visual (often seen with drug use), auditory (classic in schizophrenics), tactile, gustatory, or olfactory
Phobia	Excessive or unreasonable fear that interferes with functioning
Psychosis	Impaired dealing with reality resulting in unusual behavior
Schizophrenia	Serious and chronic condition with significant changes in behavior often involving psychosis, delusions, and hallucinations

the hospital. It is critical to report and document your observations of the scene; doing so may help the patient later in his or her care.

The elements of the MSE are:

- **Mental status** (AVPU)
- **General description**—How does the patient appear? What is his or her affect (outward behavior—e.g., flat, depressed, outrageous?) How is the patient dressed? How is his or her hygiene?
- **Perceptions**—How is the patient perceiving reality? Does he or she feel persecuted or paranoid?
- **Thought content**—Are the patient's thoughts organized? Do they flow logically? How is his or her speech? Does it match the conversation? Is it pressured? (Is the patient speaking so rapidly that it seems almost as if he or she is under pressure?)
- **Behavior**—What is the patient's behavior like? Aggressive? Meek?
- **Emotions**—Is the patient experiencing any emotions (or lack of emotions) such as sadness, excitement?
- **Insight and judgement**—Are the patient's actions reasonable? Examples of poor judgement would be a lack of concern for the weather or traffic. Failing to care for children is another example.

The mental status examination is a part of overall patient assessment and should be performed only after the scene size-up and initial assessments have been completed as part of a focused assessment of a psychiatric patient. Suggestions for communicating with a patient during the mental status exam, or at any time during a behavioral emergency, are given in Table 19-2.

TABLE 19-2 Communicating with Patients Experiencing a Behavioral Emergency

- Identify yourself and your crew.
- Tell the patient you are there to help him or her.
- Speak slowly and clearly.
- Listen to the patient.
- Avoid fast movements or unexplained movements toward the patient.
- When safe to do so, position yourself on the same level as the patient.
- Be empathetic but do not patronize the patient.
- Use positive body language.

PRECEPTOR PEARL

Assessment and care of the behavioral emergency patient require a high level of caution. Experienced EMT-Bs know that anything can happen at any time. Newly certified EMT-Bs should be reminded to maintain a safe distance when managing all behavioral emergency patients. Tell them that management of the behavioral emergency takes a while, and as EMT-Bs, they must be prepared to spend time with the patient. Encourage them to remember that these types of calls require that the care giver become "patient with the patient."

Patient Assessment

Behavioral Emergencies

- Ask for police assistance if, prior to your emergency response to the scene, you know the patient is displaying destructive, violent, or unpredictable behavior or if weapons are involved.

- Conduct a scene size-up, and ensure personal safety. Ask yourself: Is the patient in an unsafe environment? Are there unsafe objects in the possession of or in reach of the patient? Scenes in which patients have barricaded themselves (those locked in a room or house) are very dangerous. Other indicators for the risk of violence include:
  —Loud voices, shouting
  —Physically aggressive behavior
  —Threatening words
  —History of violence
  —Unusual or intense glancing or staring
  —Inappropriate silence or "brooding"
  —Alcohol or drug use

- Perform the initial assessment only after it is safe to approach the patient. Remember that there are other causes of altered mental status.

- Perform a focused history and physical exam. For the SAMPLE history, consider the following common causes of behavioral changes:
  —Lack of oxygen
  —Low blood sugar
  —Head trauma
  —Mind-altering drugs
  —Inadequate blood flow to the brain

—Excessive cold or heat
—Depression

- Assess vital signs.
- Use the mental status examination to gain further information on the patient's psychological condition.

For the unresponsive patient:

- Perform a focused history and physical exam, including a rapid trauma assessment. Gather a SAMPLE history from bystanders or family.
- Assess vital signs.

Experienced EMTs know that the signs and symptoms of a behavioral emergency are highly variable. Look for the following signs and symptoms:

- Panic
- Agitation
- Anxious, combative attitude
- Sadness, crying, depression
- Bizarre thinking and behavior
- Threatening behavior
- Self-destructive behavior ✳

Patient Care

Behavioral Emergencies

Emergency care of a patient with a behavioral emergency includes the following:

1. **Perform a scene size-up.** Make certain that the scene is safe before entering.

2. **Perform a patient assessment.** Be sure to identify yourself, and let the patient know you are there to help. Question him or her in a calm, reassuring, nonjudgmental manner. Acknowledge the patient's feelings. Listen to what the patient says, and repeat back what you have heard.

3. **Calm the patient.** Tell the patient you wish to help, and encourage him or her to express problems. Be sure to tell the truth. While doing so, use good eye contact. Do not make quick moves, and maintain a comfortable distance.

    Remember that your body language, tone of voice, and actions will have a tremendous influence on the way the patient responds to you. Do not make rapid movements that might startle the patient. Speak in a soothing voice. Listen to the patient, and show empathy and

concern. Avoid statements such as "I know how you feel" and "I understand" because you probably don't. Do not play along with a patient's hallucinations.

4. **Restrain the patient if necessary.** Skill Summary 19-1 demonstrates the restraint process. Follow local protocol for restraint procedures.

5. **Transport.** If you suspect overdose, bring any drugs or medications you find to the receiving facility. ✳

Restraint

There are certain medical/legal issues that must be considered when treating patients with behavioral emergencies. The principle of consent requires that the patient be mentally competent to refuse care. This may apply to some behavioral emergency patients. Not all patients who experience behavioral emergencies will be irrational or incompetent, but some will.

Other patients will have the desire to hurt or kill themselves or others. In cases such as this, law enforcement and certain mental health authorities may have the legal power to order a person to be taken into custody. Be sure you know who has that authority in your region. Also know your agency's policy in assisting involuntary transport to a hospital or appropriate mental health facility.

When restraint may legally be used, it must be done safely. The following guidelines apply to restraining patients:

- Develop a plan before approaching the patient. Often personnel are assigned to control the limbs closest to them. Use a proper number of people to accomplish the restraint (usually four). Too few will likely cause injury to the patient or to the EMTs. Too many will cause confusion and inefficiency.

- Use humane restraints such as wide roller gauze or restraints designed for the purpose. Do not use handcuffs because they are likely to cause injury. If the handcuffs are only partially applied and the patient wiggles away, they may be used as weapons.

- Restrain the patient in a face-up position if possible and monitor the patient's airway while he or she is restrained. If a patient who was agitated suddenly becomes quiet, be sure that the patient is still conscious and alert. Positional asphyxia is a situation in which a restrained patient suddenly dies. Monitor the patient constantly during transport (Skill Summary 19-1).

Always take BSI precautions first.

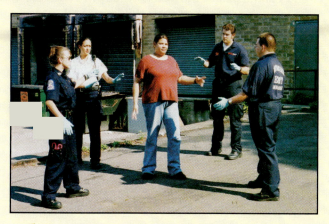

▲ **1.** Plan your approach to the patient in advance and remain outside the range of his arms and legs until you are ready to act.

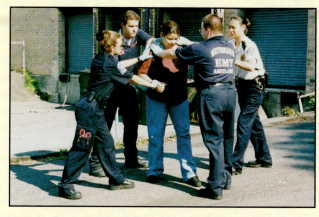

▲ **2.** Assign one EMT-B to each limb, and approach the patient at the same time.

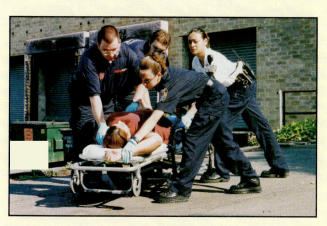

▲ **3.** Place the patient on the stretcher as his condition and local protocols indicate. Do not let go until he is properly secured.

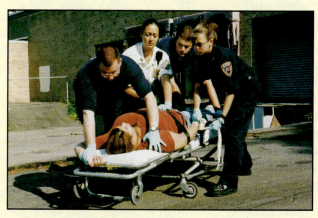

▲ **4.** Use multiple straps or other soft restraints to secure the patient to the stretcher.

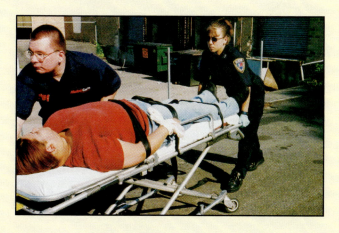

◄ **5.** When the patient is secure, assess his distal circulation and monitor his airway and breathing continually.

- Never "hog tie" the patient. This practice is also linked to positional asphyxia and death in restrained patients. If the patient is hog-tied or hobbled, respirations may be restricted to the point of death.

- Restraint must never be punitive. Use only the amount of force necessary to accomplish the restraint (even if the patient spat on you and insulted your mother). Then monitor the patient carefully en route to the hospital.

- Remember that it may not be your responsibility to restrain violent patients. Follow local protocols and request police assistance immediately.

Suicide

Suicide is the ninth leading cause of death in the United States. It is the third leading cause of death in the 15 to 24 age group, falling behind only intentional and non-intentional trauma. Suicide in the elderly population has also increased dramatically. Risk factors for suicide include:

- Being single, widowed, or divorced
- Alcohol or drug abuse
- History of depression
- Prior suicide attempts
- Family member who has committed suicide

Additionally, patients who have a detailed suicide plan (a definite course of action set up to cause death) have a higher rate of successfully killing themselves.

Care for the suicidal patient involves providing medical care for self-inflicted injuries as well as providing emotional care and support. Injuries from attempted suicides can be severe (gunshot wounds) to minor (superficial lacerations).

LIFESPAN DEVELOPMENT

In the geriatric population suicide rates have risen dramatically. Science has lengthened the average life expectancy but with this comes potential problems. Quality of life often fades dramatically in later years. Elderly patients may attempt or commit suicide rather than face the long and painful stages of cancer; or may not wish to become dependent on their children or others to care for them when they are unable to care for themselves. Depression is also common in the geriatric population as they observe their friends die off. Patients themselves become isolated and often are unable to drive. Many older people live below the poverty level.

PRECEPTOR PEARL

Patients who have made what appear to be half-hearted attempts at suicide are often labeled as "looking for attention" rather than actually being suicidal. This labeling is dangerous and is poor medical care. Any person who has taken steps toward ending his or her life or has made threats to do that should be taken seriously and evaluated by a mental health professional. As an experienced EMT-B, you should give the message to others you work with that compassion and professionalism are mandatory toward any patient who has expressed thoughts or made actions toward suicide.

Behavioral Emergencies

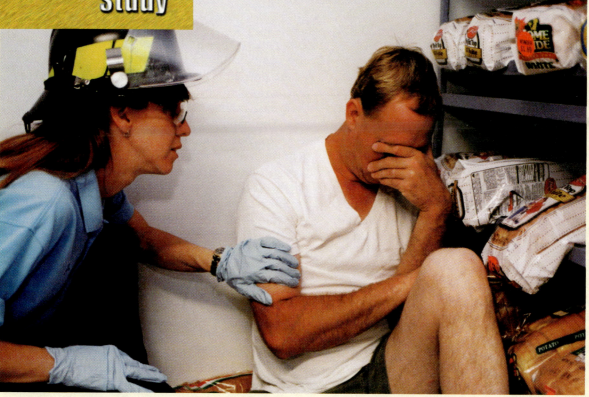

Dispatch: 4101 Short Street   **Psychiatric patient   1435 hrs**

On a hot July day, your ambulance is called to Eddie's Supermarket at 4101 Short Street for a psychiatric patient. You approach the scene carefully and observe two police cars in front. The dispatcher tells you that the police have asked you to bring your stretcher to the bakery aisle. The scene is safe.

You arrive at the bakery aisle and find loaves of bread and dozens of packages of rolls scattered about the aisle. The patient is sitting on the floor by the police officers. One officer is crouched down and talking with the patient. The patient's eyes are darting around at the people and the surroundings. The second police officer comes to you and gives this report: "This guy was in the aisle here and thought that someone was following him. Then he thought that there could be listening devices behind the bread and stuff. He decides to look for them—and here we are.

We couldn't get any information initially. Once we got his ID, we called his house and spoke to his parents. He is schizophrenic. Has been for many years. He leaves the house for weeks at a time and lives on the street. His mother doesn't think he has taken his meds in at least a week. He's 27 years old. Jimmy Thornton is his name."

You note the history given by the police officer and ask a few questions of your own. "Do you know if he has a history of other medical problems? Do you know what medication he was on?"

The officer has his dispatcher call the mother back to get the information while you are introduced to the patient. Jimmy has agreed to be transported to the local medical center, which has a psychiatric facility where the patient has been admitted previously. The officers do not believe the patient will be

(continued)

a problem, but one officer will follow you to the hospital just in case. Jimmy has not been violent toward any individuals.

You introduce yourself to Jimmy and kneel down to his level. You tell him that you understand that he was talking to the police and that he will be going to Mercy Medical Center. Jimmy agrees. You carefully and slowly describe what you are going to do, and then complete your focused assessment and taking of vital signs. The patient has an open airway and is breathing. There are no bleeding wounds and the patient's skin color is good. His clothes are filthy, and he smells quite bad. You suspect he hasn't bathed in some time.

Jimmy denies injury or illness. He appears oriented to person, place, and day. He admits to the psychological condition but claims to have no other medical problems or allergies. He hasn't eaten in about 24 hours. He relates the same events as told to you by police but is "tired of talking about it now." You respect his wishes and obtain a set of vital signs. His pulse is 88 strong and regular; respirations 16 and adequate; blood pressure 118/82; pupils equal and reactive to light, and his skin is warm and dry. You begin to note these findings, and the patient becomes suspicious of your writing. Observing this, you explain to the patient what you are doing and why. He relaxes somewhat, but you note that you must carefully explain things for the rest of the trip.

The police officers get a message from the dispatcher that the patient is on Tegretol. Otherwise, he is healthy. You place the patient on the stretcher and bring him to the ambulance. The police follow you to the hospital. A reassessment in the ambulance does not reveal any changes. Jimmy is transported without incident to the hospital.

CASE DISCUSSION

This patient appeared to have paranoid delusions and has a history of schizophrenia. In many cases where you are called to patients with schizophrenia, it is common to have the patients not taking their medications as a potential cause of the problem. The nature of psychiatric medications is that it takes some time (often several weeks) to achieve a therapeutic effect. When the medications do take effect, patients often feel that they do not need to take them any longer. Patients who are hospitalized are given medications and have a structured environment while in the hospital. Upon discharge, patients often do not continue their medications. Significant side effects of these medications also play a role in the resistance of some patients to taking their medications.

The police were on the scene at this call. In such cases, their role is to assure safety as well as to provide patient restraint if necessary. In most areas, the police are the only ones who can transport or order transport of a patient against his or her will. A physician may also have this authority.

In this case, it was critical to explain things to the patient. He became nervous when he observed you writing. While you know you were simply writing down his vital signs, he could look at the situation differently (e.g., as part of a conspiracy against him). Explaining what you were doing was helpful. This may also become an issue when you write more or when you call the hospital with your radio report.

Be alert in behavioral emergency cases for signs of agitation or impending outbursts that could become violent. If the patient begins to act in a bizarre manner, has increased anxiety, begins to raise his voice, or shows other signs of potential violence, notify the police immediately.

Name: Jimmy Thornton

Age: 27

Chief Complaint: Altered mental status/psychiatric condition (reported by police)

ASSESSMENT INFORMATION	RELEVANCE TO THIS PATIENT
Scene safety	You observed for safety as well as checking with the police as you arrived. It is also important to realize that things may change throughout the call. There is no guarantee that the patient will remain calm simply because he is calm now.
Altered mental status	It is important to remember that all patients who present with an apparent psychiatric problem may actually have an underlying medical problem causing their symptoms (e.g., diabetes, hypoxia). In this case, you not only asked for a history from the patient but you also verified it with his mother via police dispatcher.
Mental status examination	You received many bits of information which are part of the mental status examination and which helped to paint a picture of the patient and some of the reasons he was found as he was. These include: • He is experiencing paranoid delusional thoughts. • He believes people are listening or monitoring him. • His behavior was wild. He began emptying shelves in a supermarket because of his belief that he was being listened to and followed.
Patient assessment	The patient received an assessment like any other patient. The basics of your assessment should not change simply because this is a patient with a psychiatric complaint. This patient received an initial assessment, focused history, SAMPLE history (from various sources), and vital signs.

SUMMARY

- Behavioral emergencies are situations where a patient's behavior becomes alarming or unreasonable to the patient, his family, or others.

- All patients with an apparent psychiatric illness should be considered altered mental status patients until proven otherwise. Other causes of altered mental status which may mimic a psychiatric emergency include low blood sugar (hypoglycemia), low oxygen content in the blood (hypoxia), head trauma, alcohol, and drugs

- Safety is a primary concern due to the unpredictable nature of psychiatric emergencies.

- Signs of danger include loud voices or shouting, aggressive behavior, threats, history of violence, intense staring or glaring, and alcohol or drug use

- The mental status examination is a method of identifying and documenting signs and symptoms of psychiatric illness.

- Patient care is largely supportive. Good communication techniques, listening, taking your time, avoiding fast movements, using positive body language, and being empathetic are all part of proper patient care.

- Restraint may be necessary. If it is, use soft, flexible restraints and position the patient face up. Use enough rescuers to restrain safely and efficiently. Never use hog-tie or hobble restraints.

- Monitor all restrained patients constantly.

REVIEW QUESTIONS

1. A situation in which a patient exhibits behavior that is alarming, unacceptable, or intolerable to the patient, the family, or the community is a:

  a. burnout.

  b. stressout.

  c. behavioral emergency.

  d. breakdown.

2. A serious and chronic condition with significant changes in behavior often involving psychosis, delusions, and hallucinations is:

  a. depression.   c. phobia.

  b. schizophrenia. d. delusion.

3. If you must restrain a behavioral emergency patient, it is a good idea to use:

  a. handcuffs.

  b. leather straps.

  c. wide roller gauze.

  d. thick nylon cord.

REVIEW QUESTIONS *continued*

4. When restraining a behavioral emergency patient, you should NEVER:
  a. hog tie the patient.
  b. use more than two rescuers to subdue the patient.
  c. place the patient in a face-up position.
  d. speak to the patient.

5. In the United States, the third leading cause of death in the 15 to 24 age group is:
  a. drug overdose.
  b. automobile accidents.
  c. suicide.
  d. anorexia.

WEB MEDIC

Visit Brady's *Essentials of Emergency Care* web site for direct web links. At **www.prenhall.com/limmer,** you will find information related to the following Chapter 19 topics:

- Suicide
- Depression
- American Association of Geriatric Psychiatry
- Schizophrenia
- American Academy of Child and Adult Psychiatry

Correlates with the U.S. DOT "EMT-Basic National Standard Curriculum" Lesson 4-9

OBSTETRICS AND GYNECOLOGY

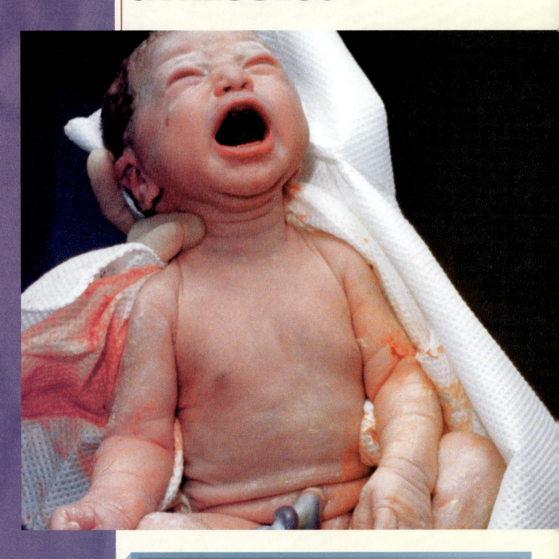

ESSENTIAL ELECTRONIC EXTRAS

CD ESSENTIALS

For preview and review of chapter material, see the student CD-ROM for

- Pretest
- Chapter quizzes
- Posttest

WEB ESSENTIALS

For additional review and enrichment, visit www.prenhall.com/limmer for

- Interactive student quizzes
- Links to online EMS resources
- Online case studies
- Audio glossary

Time has changed many of the things we have practiced as EMTs. The theories behind the use of a PASG and capillary refill have changed, as have our patient assessment practices. One thing that has not changed significantly (over thousands of years) is the process of childbirth. This section will review the anatomy relating to childbirth, childbirth procedures, complications, and other special considerations.

ANATOMY OF CHILDBIRTH

The **uterus** is the organ which contains the **fetus,** or developing child. Contractions of the uterus expel the infant during labor. Within the uterus is the **amniotic sac,** which contains the amniotic fluid in which the fetus "floats" for protection during development.

The **placenta** is attached to the wall of the uterus. It is responsible for distribution of oxygen, nutrients, and other substances between the mother and fetus. It also serves to remove waste products from the fetus. The fetus and placenta are connected by the **umbilical cord.**

The **cervix** is the inferior opening of the uterus. The birth canal includes the cervix and the vagina, from which the baby is born. The **perineum** is the area of skin between the vagina and anus which may be torn during delivery. The anatomy of pregnancy is shown in Figure 20-1.

At some time around the beginning of labor, a **bloody show** may be seen. This mixture of blood and mucus comes from the cervix and is considered normal. **Crowning** occurs when the presenting part presses against the vaginal opening. This causes the vagina to appear as if it were bulging and is the first appearance of the infant.

The part of the infant that appears at the vaginal opening first is called the **presenting part.** In most cases this is the head. In an abnormal delivery, an arm, leg, the buttocks, or the umbilical cord may present first.

Labor is a process in which uterine muscles go through a series of contractions resulting in the delivery of the infant and eventually the placenta. The stages of labor are shown in Figure 20-2.

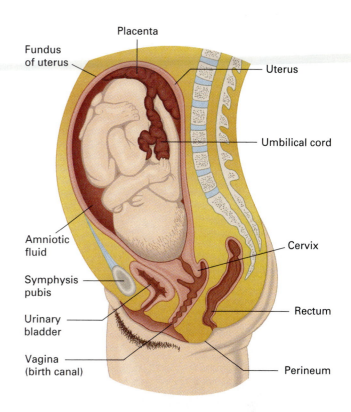

FIGURE 20-1 Anatomy of pregnancy.

CORE CONCEPTS

In this chapter, you will learn about the following topics:

- How to deal with predelivery emergencies

- Normal and abnormal deliveries

- How to treat gynecological emergencies

DOT OBJECTIVES

✔ **Knowledge**

☐ **1.** Assess and provide care to the obstetric patient. (pp. 288–294)

☐ **2.** Assist with the delivery of an infant. (pp. 290–294)

☐ **3.** Assess and provide care to the newborn. (pp. 291–294)

☐ **4.** Assess and provide care to the mother immediately following delivery of a newborn. (p. 291)

- Identify predelivery emergencies. (pp. 288–290)
- State the steps to assist in the delivery. (pp. 290–294)

- Discuss the steps in the delivery of the placenta. (p. 291)
- List the steps in the emergency medical care of the mother post-delivery. (p. 291)
- Summarize neonatal resuscitation procedures. (p. 294)

First stage:
beginning of contractions to full cervical dilation

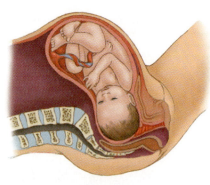

Second stage:
baby enters birth canal and is born

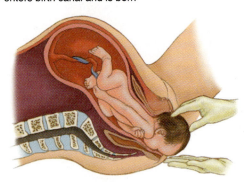

Third stage:
delivery of the placenta

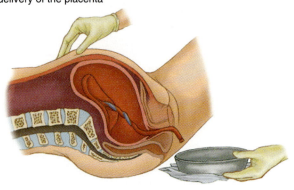

Figure 20-2   Three stages of labor.

PREDELIVERY EMERGENCIES

There are several emergencies that may occur during the nine months of pregnancy and before the actual delivery. These include miscarriage, seizures during pregnancy, and trauma.

Miscarriage (Spontaneous Abortion)

A **miscarriage** is a delivery of the fetus (or products of conception) before the baby can live outside the mother's body. If this happens on its own, it is called a **spontaneous abortion.** Induced abortions are those in which intentional actions are taken to terminate the pregnancy.

Signs and symptoms of a miscarriage may include the following:

- Abdominal pain which may resemble labor or menstrual pains
- Vaginal bleeding
- Discharge of tissue and blood from the vagina

Patient Care

Miscarriage

Emergency care steps include:

1 Complete a patient assessment including vital signs.

2 Apply high-concentration oxygen, and be alert for shock.

3 Use vaginal pads to absorb blood. Do not pack the vagina.

4 Save all tissue that has been expelled from the vagina and bring it to the hospital.

5 Transport as soon as possible.

6 Provide emotional support.

- Describe the procedures for the following abnormal deliveries:
  —Prolapsed umbilical cord (p. 295)
  —Breech presentation (p. 295)
  —Limb presentation (p. 295)

✔ **Skills**

☐ **5.** Demonstrate steps to assist in the normal cephalic delivery. (pp. 290–291)

☐ **6.** Demonstrate post delivery care of the mother. (p. 291)

Seizures During Pregnancy

Seizures may occur because of a pregnancy-related condition called **eclampsia.** They usually occur late in the course of the pregnancy and are associated with elevated blood pressure and **edema** (fluid accumulation), which may be seen in the extremities. Seizures also may occur because of non-pregnancy-related conditions such as epilepsy and hypoglycemia.

Signs and symptoms include:

- Elevated blood pressure.
- Excess weight gain
- Extreme swelling of the face, hands, ankles, and feet
- Headache

Patient Care

Seizures During Pregnancy

Emergency care steps include:

1. Maintain an open airway, and administer oxygen.
2. Complete a full patient assessment.
3. Transport the patient positioned on her left side.
4. Handle her gently. Rough handling may increase the chance of seizure.
5. Have suction and a delivery kit ready. ✳

Trauma During Pregnancy

Trauma may occur to anyone, including those who are pregnant. There are just a few differences in patient assessment or emergency care because the patient is pregnant.

Patient Assessment

Trauma During Pregnancy

- Perform the full patient assessment sequence.
- You may be able to observe a patient and determine if she is pregnant. The fact that a woman is pregnant will usually be volunteered because of concern for the baby.
- Shock (hypoperfusion) may be more difficult to assess in the pregnant patient. The pulse may be naturally 10–15 beats per minute faster than in the non-pregnant female. Additionally, due to an increase in blood volume of up to 48%, signs of shock may not appear until a considerable blood volume has been lost. ✳

Patient Care

Trauma During Pregnancy

Emergency care steps include the following:

1. Perform emergency care based on the signs and symptoms exhibited by the patient. A general rule is "What's good for the mother is good for the baby."
2. Since the patient's oxygen demand is higher (due to pregnancy), administer high-concentration oxygen by nonrebreather mask.
3. Transport as soon as possible.

The patient should be transported on her left side. This is because a near-term fetus will press against the mother's inferior vena cava which runs along the right side of the spine. Compression of this major vein will reduce blood flow to the heart with a resulting decrease in blood pressure. Placing the mother on the left eliminates this potential complication. If the mother must be immobilized, as is often the case, secure the mother firmly to the spine board and place padding under the right side of the board, which causes a shift to the left but still maintains immobilization.

Remember to provide emotional support. The mother will naturally worry about her unborn child. ✳

CHILDBIRTH

Normal Delivery

Childbirth is a natural process. Unlike many other situations encountered by an EMT-B, childbirth is not a result of a disease state or injury. At the scene of a call for impending childbirth, your main functions will be to determine whether or not there is time for transport to the hospital before delivery and/or to support and assist the mother during delivery.

Predelivery Considerations

In general, it is best to transport the mother and have the delivery occur at a hospital. This will be done in many cases. In other cases, delivery will be performed at the scene for two reasons: the delivery is imminent, or factors such as severe storms prevent you from transporting the patient to the hospital in a reasonable amount of time. Asking the questions below and performing a brief physical examination will help you make a transportation decision:

- Are you pregnant? How long have you been pregnant? Is this your first pregnancy?
- Have there been any complications with this pregnancy?
- Are there any contractions or pain?
- Have you observed any bleeding or discharge?
- Do you feel the need to push?
- Do you feel as if you are having a bowel movement?
- When is the baby due?
- Are you expecting one baby or more?

During first pregnancies, women may be in labor for 16 hours or longer. However, not all first pregnancies will take that long. Subsequent pregnancies generally have shorter periods of labor. When labor pains are 2 or 3 minutes apart and last 30 seconds to 1 minute, delivery of the baby may be imminent.

It will not be unusual to find clear or slightly bloody fluid coming from the vagina during the process of labor. The fluids may be the "bloody show," which is the mucus plug separating from the cervix, or the rupturing of the "bag of waters" (amniotic sac). These are both normal events.

You also will need to examine the patient for:

- Frequency and duration of contractions.
- Crowning, or bulging of the presenting part from the vagina during contractions. *This is a sign of imminent delivery.*
- Contraction of the uterus that may be felt through the skin. This area will feel more rigid as the delivery of the baby nears.

Remember that your actions may cause alarm or be embarrassing for the mother, father, and anyone else present. Do your best to explain everything you do and to protect the patient's modesty.

With few exceptions, it will not be necessary to place your hand or fingers in the patient's vagina. It is never necessary to check for cervical dilation.

> ## PRECEPTOR PEARL
>
> Tell new EMT-Bs that it is not uncommon to find patients and family members who are very nervous. This is to be expected. This emotion will make examination of the patient and subsequent decision making very difficult. The patient or her family may want to rush to the hospital, or they may have the opposite feeling that there just isn't enough time. Encourage new EMT-Bs to carefully and objectively examine the patient and obtain a history. This is the proper basis for a transportation decision. Assure the patient and family that you are equipped and trained both to evaluate the situation and to handle the delivery at home or in the ambulance.

When preparing for delivery, take BSI precautions. Gloves, eye protection, face mask, and a gown are appropriate. Also have a childbirth delivery kit at your side (Table 20-1).

There are a few "don'ts" involved in the delivery of a child:

- Don't let the mother go to the bathroom.
- Don't hold the mother's legs together.
- Don't touch the patient's vaginal area except during delivery and with a partner present.

Remember to follow local protocols for signs of impending delivery. Medical direction should be consulted if required by protocol or if advice is needed.

Delivery

The following steps outline the procedure for assisting with childbirth (Figure 20-3).

1. Take BSI precautions (gloves, mask, eye protection, and gown).

2. Have the mother lie with knees drawn up and spread apart. Elevate the buttocks with a blanket or pillow.

3. Create a sterile field around the vaginal opening. This may be done with drapes or towels found in the OB kit (Figure 20-4).

4. When the infant's head appears (crowning), very gently place your fingers on the bony part of the infant's skull. This will prevent an explosive delivery. Do not place your fingers on the soft fontanelles or face.

5. As the infant's head appears, make sure the amniotic sac is broken. If it is intact, break the membrane and pull it away from the infant's face. As the head continues to emerge, make sure the umbilical cord is not wrapped around the infant's neck. If this is the case, slip the cord over the infant's shoulder. If this is not possible, clamp the cord in two places, cut between the clamps, and unwrap the cord immediately.

6. After the infant's head delivers, support the head and use the bulb syringe found in the OB kit to suction the mouth two or three times, then the nostrils. (It is important to suction the mouth before the nose, because suctioning the nose first may cause the infant to gasp and suck fluid from the mouth into the lungs.) Expel air from the bulb syringe before introducing it into the infant's nose or mouth. Be sure to avoid contact with the back of the infant's mouth.

7. Support the torso, body, and legs of the infant as each appears. Use both hands. Securely hold the baby and with sterile gauze wipe the blood and mucus from the mouth and nose. Use the bulb syringe again on the mouth and nose (Figure 20-5).

8. Warmth is very important. Wrap the infant in a warm blanket. Position on his or her side at the level of the vagina until the cord is cut. The infant's head should be slightly lower than the trunk.

9. When the pulsations cease in the umbilical cord, place two clamps (or thick ties) on the cord, the first being approximately four finger widths from the infant. Cut between the clamps. Your partner should continue to monitor and care for the infant.

10. While preparing for transportation, watch for delivery of the placenta. If it delivers, wrap it in a towel, then place it in a plastic bag. Bring the placenta to the hospital with the mother and infant.

11. There may be vaginal bleeding after delivery. Up to 500 cc is not considered unusual. Do not let normal amounts of bleeding put undue stress on you and the new family. Place a sterile pad over the vagina and have the mother lower and hold her legs together.

12. Record time of delivery and begin transport.

13. If bleeding is profuse, massaging the uterus may help to control it (Figure 20-6). Place your open hand on the mother's abdomen above the pubis. Massage in a kneading motion over the area. The uterus should feel like a grapefruit-size ball within the abdomen. Treat for shock (hypoperfusion) and transport, performing the massage en route.

Care of the Newborn

Care of the newborn after delivery is very important. Although seemingly small tasks, drying and keeping the infant warm are crucial. Wrap the infant in blankets and cover the top of the head. Place the infant in a position on his or her side with the head slightly lower than the trunk. Repeat suctioning as necessary.

Assessment of the Newborn

There are five areas in which the newborn should be assessed. Ideally, this should be done 1 minute after birth and again 5 minutes after birth. This assessment should not take the place of resuscitation or care of the newborn. It may be performed by yourself or by a partner while care is ongoing:

■ **Appearance.** The infant may be pink, blue, or some combination of the two colors. A baby that is all blue should be evaluated carefully for the

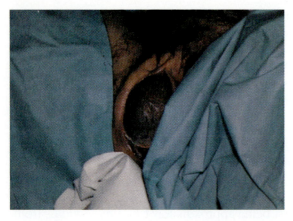

A. Crowning.

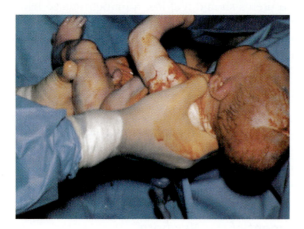

B. Head delivers and turns.

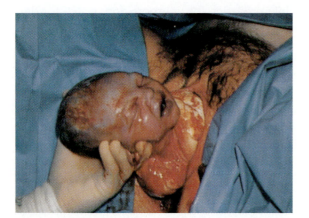

C. Shoulders deliver.

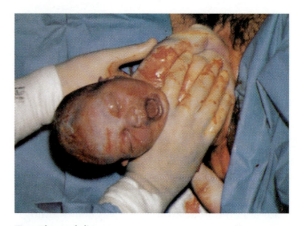

D. Chest delivers.

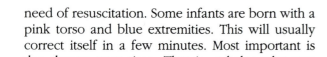

E. Infant delivered.

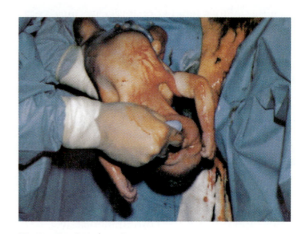

F. Suctioning the airway.

Figure 20-3 Delivery of an Infant *(continued on next page)*

need of resuscitation. Some infants are born with a pink torso and blue extremities. This will usually correct itself in a few minutes. Most important is the change over time. That is, a baby who was bluish and becomes pink is doing better, while a baby who shows no change or becomes bluer requires urgent care.

■ **Pulse.** The pulse may be determined with a stethoscope over the heart. An infant should have a pulse of at least 100/minute, but it may be as high as 180/minute. It is considered a problem when the pulse gets below 100/minute. (The discussion on resuscitation of the newborn that follows explains this in more detail.)

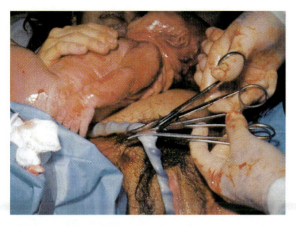

G. Cutting the cord.

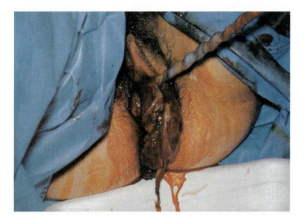

H. Placenta begins delivery.

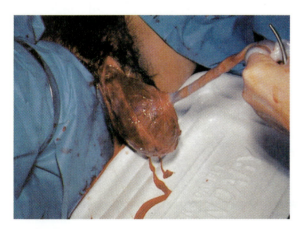

I. Placenta delivers.

Figure 20-3 Delivery of an Infant *(concluded)*

- **Grimace.** When the infant is flicked on the foot, there should be some response. The ideal response is vigorous motion and crying. You may see some motion or crying or no response at all.
- **Activity.** There should be some movement of the extremities. This may range from no movement to some slight flexion to active motion.

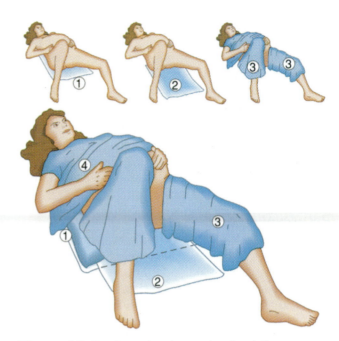

Figure 20-4 Preparing the mother for delivery.

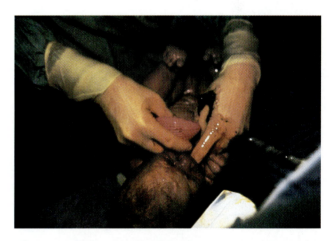

Figure 20-5 Suction the mouth first and then the nose of the newborn.

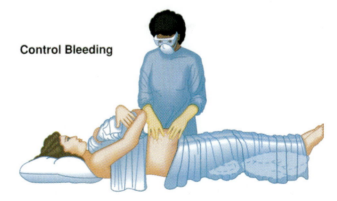

Control Bleeding

Figure 20-6 After delivery of the placenta, massaging the area over the uterus helps control vaginal bleeding.

■ **Respiratory effort.** This is an observation of the ease of breathing. The infant's crying helps make this determination. Strong crying requires air movement and indicates adequate breathing. Notice chest expansion and the effort required by the baby to breathe.

These five elements make up the APGAR score. It has little practical value in the field as long as you assess the newborn appropriately. If your EMS system uses this scoring method associated with the APGAR score, become familiar with it.

Resuscitation of the Newborn

True resuscitation of the newborn is rarely required. In most cases, some very simple measures will cause the newborn to respond and thrive.

An inverted pyramid is used to describe the actions taken in order during resuscitation (Figure 20-7). The pyramid shape is broader on the top indicating that the most commonly successful interventions are the least invasive. As you work down through the levels of the pyramid, the procedures become more invasive. The following steps outline the procedure for resuscitation of the newborn:

1. **Assess breathing.** The infant should begin breathing within about 30 seconds. If breathing does not begin spontaneously, stimulate the infant to breathe by gently, but vigorously, rubbing the infant's back. If this fails, flick the soles of the infant's feet with your finger.

2. **If the infant's breathing is absent, shallow, or slow, begin artificial ventilation.** Use gentle puffs if using a mouth-to-mask technique, or a gentle squeeze on an infant BVM. Ventilate at a rate of 40 to 60 ventilations per minute. Reassess the infant's respiratory effort frequently.

3. **Assess the infant's heart rate.** If the infant's heart rate is below 100/minute, assist ventilations. If the heart rate is below 80/minute and has not increased after ventilations, begin chest compressions. Begin compressions immediately at a rate of 120/minute on any infant with a pulse below 60 (Figure 20-8).

It may seem unusual to provide compressions in the presence of a pulse. However, low pulse rates are dangerous for an infant, and compressions will help maintain circulation. The infant may regain adequate pulse and respirations after ventilations and compressions.

In cases where there are adequate pulse and respirations but the infant has cyanosis (especially of the torso), use oxygen tubing to deliver 10 to 15 lpm by way of the "blow-by" method. That is, place the tubing near, but not directly into, the infant's face to provide supplemental oxygen to the infant.

Abnormal Deliveries

While most deliveries are considered normal, there are many situations that are termed abnormal. These include prolapsed umbilical cord, breech birth, and limb presentation.

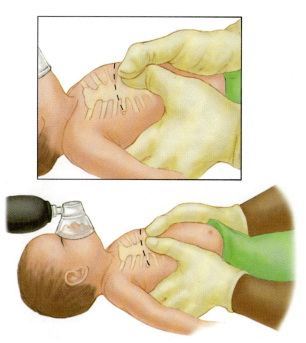

Figure 20-8 Deliver chest compressions at 120 per minute, midsternum with two thumbs, at a depth of 1/2 to 3/4 inches. For a very small infant (inset), the thumbs may be overlapped.

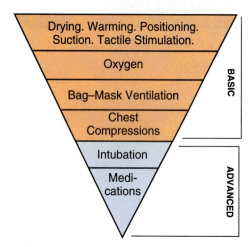

Figure 20-7 The inverted pyramid of neonatal resuscitation shows approximate relative frequencies of neonatal care and resuscitative efforts. Note that a majority of infants respond to the simple measures described at the top wide part of the pyramid.

Prolapsed Umbilical Cord

When the umbilical cord presents through the birth canal before delivery of the head, this is known as a **prolapsed umbilical cord.** This is a serious emergency which endangers the life of the infant. Emergency care is as follows:

1. **Position the mother in a head-down position.**
2. **Administer high-concentration oxygen.**
3. **Insert a sterile, gloved hand into the vagina.** This is one of the few situations where it is appropriate to do this. The purpose is to push the presenting part of the fetus off the cord. When this is successful, you should be able to feel pulsations in the cord. This action is critical to the survival of the baby.
4. **Immediately transport the patient.** Do not release pressure until relieved at a medical facility.

Breech Presentation

A **breech birth** occurs when the buttocks or lower extremities are the presenting part (Figure 20-9). While it is not impossible for a breech baby to deliver, the complication rate is high. The risk of a breech delivery is higher when the cord is prolapsed.

For emergency care, place the mother in a head-down position. If a prolapsed cord exists, begin care for that emergency. Administer high-concentration oxygen, and begin immediate transportation.

Limb Presentation

A **limb presentation** is identified by a single limb (arm or leg) protruding from the vagina. It requires immediate intervention by an obstetrician. Delivery should not be attempted in the field.

For emergency care, place the mother in a head-down position with pelvis elevated. Administer high-concentration oxygen, and initiate immediate transportation.

Complications of Childbirth

Meconium

Normal amniotic fluid is clear in color. A thick green, brownish-yellow, or dark tarry substance in the amniotic fluid is **meconium.** Meconium is the result of fetal defecation and is usually a sign of fetal distress.

Meconium must be suctioned immediately. If this substance is observed, thoroughly suction the baby's mouth, then nose, before any more of the infant delivers. Never stimulate breathing until the infant has been suctioned thoroughly. Infants born with meconium in the amniotic fluid are at greater risk for respiratory complications after birth. So document it and verbally report it to the emergency department staff.

Multiple Births

Multiple births are not a complication of pregnancy, provided the deliveries are normal. When a woman has been under a doctor's care, she will very likely

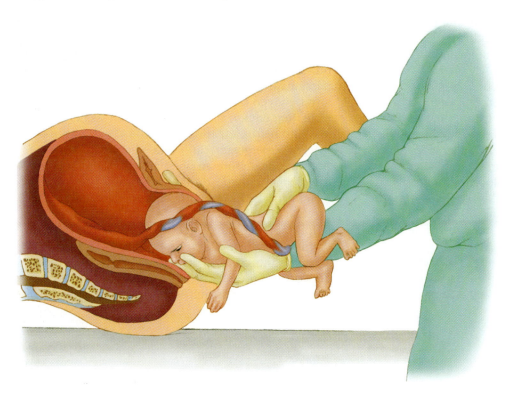

Figure 20-9   Breech delivery.

be aware that she is carrying more than one baby. Other indicators of impending multiple births are an abnormally large abdomen or an abdomen that remains abnormally large after the delivery of the first infant.

Twins are the most frequent multiple birth. The procedure for delivery of each infant is identical to that of a single birth. The mother may remain in labor to deliver the second child. After each delivery, clamp and cut the umbilical cord. Note that there may be either one or two placentas.

An infant who is one of multiple births typically has a smaller birth weight than a single birth baby. Make sure that the infants are kept warm. In the event that they require resuscitation, remember that you may have to resuscitate two (or more) infants as well as care for the mother. Additional help may be required. Call for assistance early if necessary.

Premature Births

Premature births are those that occur before the 37th week of gestation or when infants are born weighing less than 2500 grams (about 5-1/2 pounds). You may determine the birth is premature from information the mother tells you and your observation of the infant. Premature infants have heads that are larger in proportion to the rest of their bodies than are those of full-term infants. Their bodies are also smaller, thinner, and redder.

Premature infants are at increased risk for hypothermia, even more so than a full-term infant. Many EMS systems use foil or insulating plastic wrap in addition to blankets for warmth. However, never let sharp surfaces of the foil come in contact with the infant's skin.

Provide resuscitation as needed, based on the inverted pyramid described earlier. There may be some cases where an infant is so premature that resuscitation cannot be performed. In these situations, follow local protocols and contact medical direction.

Occasionally after a delivery there is some blood loss from the umbilical cord. Since the premature infant has limited blood supply, this blood loss must be stopped. If blood is leaking from the end of the cord, tie the cord again, this time closer to the infant to stop the bleeding.

Administer blow-by oxygen. Take steps to reduce contamination of the infant since it will be susceptible to infection. Transport immediately.

Follow your local protocols for childbirth and delivery. Remember to contact medical direction for information on delivery of normal births, abnormal births, and complications you may encounter.

GYNECOLOGICAL EMERGENCIES

Vaginal Bleeding

Bleeding from the vagina may range from very minor to severe. Vaginal bleeding may occur in nonpregnant women or at any time during pregnancy. It is important to remember that the cause of the bleeding may not be determined in the field. Field priorities are the prevention, recognition, and treatment for shock (hypoperfusion).

For emergency care, take BSI precautions. Assure an adequate airway. Administer high-concentration oxygen. Treat for shock, and transport immediately.

Trauma to the External Genitalia

Traumatic injuries to the female external genitalia may result in profuse bleeding and severe pain. Consider the patient's modesty when examining and caring for a wound to this area.

For emergency care, assure an open airway and administer oxygen. Be alert for signs of shock. Control any bleeding with direct pressure, but do not pack or insert anything into the vagina.

Sexual Assault

A patient who has experienced sexual assault requires care for all physical injuries as well as compassionate psychological care. Consideration must also be given to preservation of evidence when possible. Remember, since this is a crime scene, be sure it is safe before entering.

For emergency care, take the appropriate BSI precautions. Assure an open airway. Maintain a nonjudgmental attitude during the history and physical examinations. Examine the external genitalia only if profuse bleeding is present. A female EMT-B may be helpful. Discourage the patient from voiding, bathing, or cleaning wounds. However, actions to preserve the crime scene should never take precedence over life-saving care. Follow local reporting requirements for assault/sexual assault cases.

Obstetrical and Gynecological Emergencies

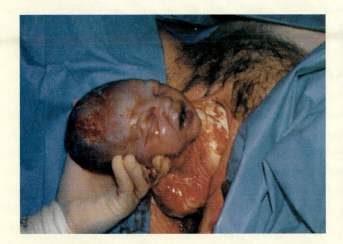
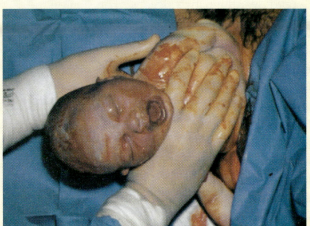

Dispatch: 263 Arbor Way   **Woman in labor   0132 hrs**

Your ambulance is dispatched to a woman in labor. The scene appears safe as you arrive at a small house on the edge of town. Upon entering, you are directed to the bedroom by an excited man who identifies himself as Paul Lasker, the patient's husband. An approximately 30-year-old woman is lying on the bed with another woman standing next to her. The sweaty, flushed patient, whose name is Karen, is huffing and puffing as she shouts, "It's coming!" One quick glance confirms her medical judgment: you see what appears to be a head just starting to crown. Your general impression is that Karen is going to have her baby very soon.

As you open the OB kit, your partner completes the initial assessment and informs you that Karen's ABCs are as expected for a woman in labor. In determining her priority, you consider that Karen is experiencing a common, normal event. Most childbirths occur without incident, but complications do occur on occasion, and both mother and child can be at risk. You decide this patient is not critical, but you would like to get her to a hospital as soon as possible in case something unexpected happens. It does not appear, though, that you will be able to transport before birth occurs.

As you position yourself and your childbirth supplies, you find out from Karen, Paul, and their neighbor that this is the patient's third child. Karen is healthy, has been getting regular prenatal care, and has had no complications. A few days ago, her midwife told her that she is not carrying twins and she was due in two weeks. Labor began about a half-hour ago. Contractions are about a minute long with only a few minutes apart. Karen has an urge to move her bowels, and you see that her membranes have ruptured by the wet area of the bed under her.

The baby's head is now emerging, so you support it as you check for the umbilical cord around the neck. To your surprise, you find it there. A little bit of rearranging allows you to slip the cord over the baby's neck, so you suction the baby's mouth and nose. You see no meconium in the fluid around the mother or in what you are removing from the baby's airway. With the next contraction, a slippery baby emerges completely and you support her on your forearm.

Your partner helps to suction the airway again, dry the baby, and put her on a blanket as you inform the happy parents that they have a daughter. As you clamp and cut the umbilical cord, the newborn is crying and breathing well with a respiratory rate of about 40. She is pink, except for a little bit of cyanosis in the hands and feet. Her apical pulse rate is 140. Your general impression is of a healthy, normal newborn. She is not a high priority, although you would still like to transport her soon.

As Karen cradles her baby, you deliver the placenta with a gush of blood that you estimate at about 200 cc. You pick it up with a towel and place it in a plastic bag. Now that you have the time, your partner is able to get a complete set of vital signs, which are within the range you would expect for a woman who has just given birth.

You package mother and child for transport and monitor both of them on a happy, uneventful trip to the hospital.

CASE DISCUSSION

In EMS, we are much more likely to see someone leave this world than come into it. Childbirth is a wonderful exception to this. To assist a mother in giving birth to her baby is one of the most uplifting experiences an EMT-B can have. Fortunately, the vast majority of births occur without incident. Occasionally, however, a complication arises that the EMT-B must be prepared to deal with. This includes low birth weight, multiple births (which are likely to be associated with low birth weight), meconium aspiration, breech or limb presentation, an umbilical cord wrapped around the neck, a prolapsed cord, excessive bleeding, and a newborn in need of resuscitation. The EMT-B must be prepared to deal with any of these situations, even though they are usually not needed.

Name: Karen Lasker
Age: 29
Chief Complaint: Labor

ASSESSMENT INFORMATION	RELEVANCE TO THIS PATIENT
Timing and progression of symptoms:	• Labor began only a half-hour ago, but the patient has an urge to move her bowels and says, "It's coming!" Contractions are about a minute long and only a few minutes apart.
SAMPLE history:	• This is a singleton (not multiple births) delivery. The mother has been getting regular prenatal care and has had no complications in this pregnancy. The mother has had two previous deliveries
Physical examination:	• Crowning indicates imminent delivery; if the head is crowning, you should not have to deal with a breech or limb presentation • The wet bed under the patient suggests the patient's membranes have already broken. • The lack of meconium is a good sign that the baby has not been stressed unduly. • It is important to check for the umbilical cord around the baby's neck as soon as the head emerges. • Cyanosis of the hands and feet is common in newborns; if it does not resolve on its own within a few minutes, administer oxygen.
Other considerations:	• Up to 500 cc blood loss is considered normal during childbirth. • You would like to transport as soon as possible, but that is unlikely under the circumstances present in this case. • If you can loosen the cord around the baby's neck, you will not have to clamp and cut it in place.

SUMMARY

- Treat seizures in pregnant patients as you would in nonpregnant patients.

- Transport a woman with an advanced pregnancy on her left side; if she is on her back, shift her to the left side.

- Assess the newborn's airway, breathing, and circulation and treat accordingly.

- Abnormal deliveries are uncommon and typically require definitive care in a hospital.

- Treat both the physical and psychological needs of a patient who has been sexually assaulted.

REVIEW QUESTIONS

1. A pregnant trauma patient should be transported in which position?
- a. on her left side.
- b. on her right side.
- c. with her legs elevated.
- d. supine.

2. The first thing you should do after the infant's head has delivered is:
- a. suction the infant's mouth and nose.
- b. place him or her on the mother's belly.
- c. check for the cord around the neck.
- d. wipe the head dry with sterile gauze.

3. If you deliver and suction the airway of an infant and breathing does not begin simultaneously, the next step is to:
- a. begin CPR immediately.
- b. do nothing at this time.
- c. provide mouth-to-mouth resuscitation.
- d. rub the baby's back or flick the soles of his or her feet.

4. If an infant's breathing is absent, shallow, or slow, begin artificial ventilation at _____ ventilations per minute.
- a. 10 to 15
- b. 40 to 60
- c. 65 to 80
- d. 80 to 100

5. For emergency care of trauma to the external genitalia of a woman, do NOT:
   a. administer oxygen.
   b. apply direct pressure.
   c. give her anything by mouth.
   d. insert anything into the vagina.

WEB MEDIC

Visit Brady's *Essentials of Emergency Care* web site for direct web links. At **www.prenhall.com/limmer,** you will find information related to the following Chapter 20 topics:

- Low birth weight
- APGAR
- Pregnancy and childbirth
- Complications of pregnancy
- National Women's Health Information Center

Chapter Twenty-One

BLEEDING AND SHOCK

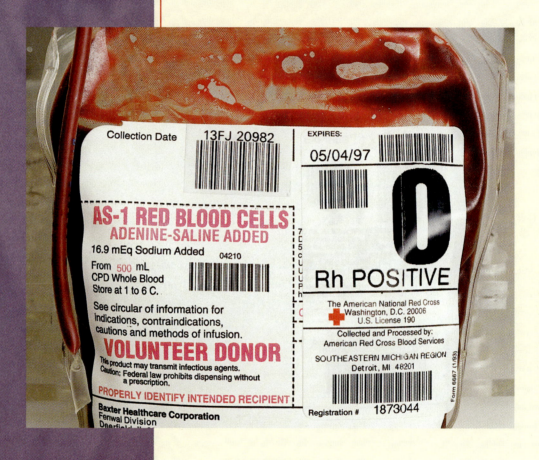

Collection Date 13FJ 20982

EXPIRES:
05/04/97

O
Rh POSITIVE

AS-1 RED BLOOD CELLS
ADENINE-SALINE ADDED

16.9 mEq Sodium Added   04210

From 500 mL
CPD Whole Blood
Store at 1 to 6 C.

See circular of information for
indications, contraindications,
cautions and methods of infusion.

VOLUNTEER DONOR
This product may transmit infectious agents.
Caution: Federal law prohibits dispensing without
a prescription.

PROPERLY IDENTIFY INTENDED RECIPIENT

Baxter Healthcare Corporation
Fenwal Division
Deerfield, Illinois

The American National Red Cross
Washington, D.C. 20006
U.S. License 190

Collected and Processed by:
American Red Cross Blood Services

SOUTHEASTERN MICHIGAN REGION
Detroit, MI 48201

Registration #   1873044

ESSENTIAL ELECTRONIC EXTRAS

CD ESSENTIALS

*For preview and review of
chapter material, see the
student CD-ROM for*

- Pretest
- Chapter quizzes
- Posttest

WEB ESSENTIALS

*For additional review
and enrichment, visit
www.prenhall.com/limmer for*

- Interactive student quizzes
- Links to online EMS
  resources
- Online case studies
- Audio glossary

Whether internal or external, bleeding can be serious and lead to hypoperfusion, also known as shock. It will be a key part of your responsibilities as an EMT to identify potentially serious conditions involving bleeding and internal injuries and to treat and transport these patients promptly. Identifying these conditions may involve examination of the patient; at other times, clues at the scene will give clues about a serious mechanism of injury. One thing is certain. It will be your assessment, care, and prompt transportation to a trauma center that will mean the difference between life and death for the patient.

BLEEDING

Circulatory System Review

The circulatory system is responsible for circulating blood throughout the body in order to supply it with nutrients and rid it of wastes. It has three major components: the heart (pump), the blood vessels (pipes), and the blood (fluid).

The Heart

The heart is a four-chambered, muscular pump about the size of a fist, lying beneath and slightly to the left of the sternum. The right side of the heart receives oxygen-depleted blood from the body and pumps it to the lungs. The left side receives oxygen-rich blood from the lungs and pumps it throughout the body. The two upper chambers of the heart are called the atria. The lower chambers are called the ventricles.

The Blood Vessels

There are three major types of blood vessels—arteries, veins, and capillaries (Figure 21-1). **Arteries** are blood vessels that carry oxygen-rich blood away from the heart and supply it to the body. The exception is the pulmonary artery, which carries oxygen-depleted blood to the lungs. Arteries are composed of three different layers containing muscle and elasticized tissue that allow for dilation or constriction depending on the system's needs.

Veins are the blood vessels that carry oxygen-depleted blood back to the heart. The exception is the pulmonary vein, which carries oxygen-rich blood from the lungs to the left atrium. Since blood in the veins is under less pressure than the blood in the arteries, the veins contain valves at various points to prevent back flow of blood.

The larger arteries gradually branch to smaller and smaller vessels called **arterioles,** which lead to the **capillaries**—a

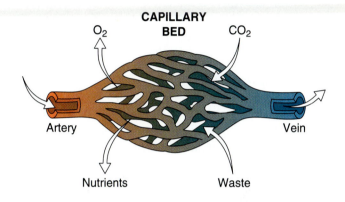

Figure 21-1 The blood vessels.

functional network of tiny, one-cell-thick blood vessels that are found in all parts of the body. The **venules,** the smaller branches of larger veins, lead away from the capillaries. This thin-walled capillary network that connects arterioles and venules allows for the exchange of oxygen and nutrients for carbon dioxide and other wastes, thus ensuring that all body cells are nourished and wastes are removed.

CORE CONCEPTS

In this chapter, you will learn about the following topics:

- Body substance isolation when handling patients who are bleeding

- Identifying and controlling external bleeding

- Identifying and treating internal bleeding

- Hypoperfusion and its progressive stages

DOT OBJECTIVES

✔ **Knowledge**

☐ 1. Provide care to a patient with shock (hypoperfusion). (pp. 307–311)

- State methods of emergency medical care of external bleeding. (pp. 304–307, 308, 311)

- List signs and symptoms of shock (hypoperfusion). (pp. 309–310)

- State the steps in the emergency medical care of the patient with signs and symptoms of shock (hypoperfusion). (pp. 309–311)

✔ **Attitude**

☐ 2. Explain the sense of urgency to transport patients that are bleeding and show signs of hypoperfusion. (p. 309)

✔ **Skills**

☐ 3. Demonstrate care of the patient experiencing external bleeding. (p. 308)

☐ 4. Demonstrate care of the patient exhibiting signs and symptoms of shock (hypoperfusion) (pp. 310, 311)

Blood Composition

Approximately 8 percent of the body's total weight is blood. Thus, a 50-pound preschooler has about 4 pints of blood, a 150-pound adult about 12 pints, and a 200-pound adult about 16 pints.

Blood is composed of red blood cells, white blood cells, plasma, and platelets. **Red blood cells** give the blood its color, carry oxygen to the body's cells, and pick up carbon dioxide and carry it away from the body's cells and back to the lungs. **White blood cells** are part of the body's immune system, which defends against infections. **Plasma** is the serum, or fluid, that carries the blood cells and nutrients to the body's cells. Plasma also carries away the waste products that are the result of cell metabolism. **Platelets** are essential to the clotting of blood and aid in the prevention of blood loss. Normal clotting of the blood takes 6 to 7 minutes.

The Pulse

As the heart's left ventricle contracts, it sends a wave, or pulsation, of blood through the arteries. A **pulse** can be felt, or palpated, at any location where an artery passes over a bone near the skin surface. The most common **pulse points** are found in the wrist over the **radial artery** and in the neck over the **carotid artery.** Other pulse points include the **brachial artery** in the upper arm, the **femoral artery** in the groin, the **popliteal artery** behind the knee, the **dorsalis pedis** on the top of the foot, and the **posterior tibial** found behind the medial ankle.

Blood Pressure

Blood pressure may be defined as the pressure exerted against the arterial walls during circulation. The **systolic** pressure is the pressure exerted against the arterial walls during contraction of the left ventricle. The **diastolic** pressure is the pressure exerted against the arterial walls during relaxation of the left ventricle.

Perfusion

Perfusion is the supply of oxygen to—and removal of wastes from—the cells and tissues of the body as a result of the flow of blood through the capillaries. **Hypoperfusion,** or shock, is the inadequate perfusion of the cells and tissues of the body caused by insufficient flow of blood through the capillaries. Two major causes of hypoperfusion are low blood volume (hypovolemia) or insufficient pumping action by the heart (pump damage).

Since all parts of the body require some level of perfusion, a loss of blood volume as a result of bleeding has a devastating effect on perfusion. No body part can exist for indefinite periods without receiving its normal level of nutrients and ridding its wastes. The heart requires a constant flow of blood, or it will not function properly. The brain and spinal cord cannot withstand a lack of perfusion for more than 4 to 6 minutes before irreversible damage begins. Lack of perfusion in the kidney for more than 45 minutes leads to kidney damage. Skeletal muscle can withstand lack of perfusion for about 2 hours before permanent damage begins to occur.

External Bleeding

There are three types of external bleeding: arterial, venous, and capillary (Figure 21-2). **Arterial bleeding** is characterized by bright red, spurting blood, which indicates that an artery has been damaged or severed. In some cases, arterial bleeding is difficult to control because of the higher pressure in the arteries. **Venous bleeding** is characterized by a dark red, steady flow of blood, which indicates a vein is severed or damaged. Venous bleeding can be profuse and life threatening. However, it is usually easier to control due to the lower pressure in the veins. Dark red blood oozing slowly from a wound is a sign of **capillary bleeding.** Damage to the capillaries usually is not life

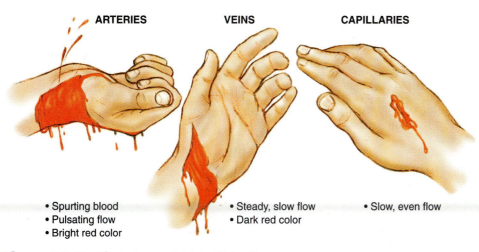

ARTERIES   VEINS   CAPILLARIES

- Spurting blood
- Pulsating flow
- Bright red color

- Steady, slow flow
- Dark red color

- Slow, even flow

Figure 21-2   Three types of external bleeding.

threatening. However, if there is an extensive amount of capillary damage due to injury to a large area of body surface, blood loss may be severe.

Importance of BSI

Before caring for bleeding patients, you must take BSI precautions to avoid contact with the patient's blood and body fluids. By using gloves, eye protection, mask, gown, and proper handwashing techniques, you can dramatically reduce your chances for contracting an infectious disease. The amount of personal protective equipment (PPE) needed correlates directly to the degree of exposure to blood and other body fluids. If there is a slight risk of exposure, then only gloves are needed. If there is any greater potential for exposure, such as occurs in emergency childbirth, endotracheal intubation, or major trauma, all PPE must be worn. Always wash your hands thoroughly after every call.

Severity of Bleeding

To get a general impression of the severity of a patient's bleeding, assess:

- *Severity of blood loss.* The loss of one liter or 1000 cc of blood is considered serious (Table 21-1).
- *Signs or symptoms.* If the patient is presenting with signs or symptoms of shock (hypoperfusion), the bleeding is considered serious.
- *Rate of blood flow.* The larger the blood vessel, the more bleeding there will be.
- *Type of bleeding.* Arterial bleeding is more rapid and profuse; venous is slower.

Patient Assessment

External Bleeding

Begin patient assessment with scene size-up, considering the need for BSI precautions, making sure the scene is safe, determining the mechanism of injury and number of patients, and calling for additional resources if needed. Upon arrival at the scene, quickly consider the mechanism of injury and if there are multiple patients. Consider questions such as: What caused the patient's injury? Did the patient fall and is there a possibility for spine injury? Is there a weapon or other item that caused the patient's injury?

The next step, the initial assessment, includes rapidly identifying and "treating as you go" any life-threatening problems by assessing the patient's ABCs, mental status, and the need for manual stabilization of the spine. Form a general impression of the patient to assist you in setting priorities and making early transport decisions for critical patients. Severe or profuse arterial or

TABLE 21-1   The Body's Response to Significant Blood Loss

Organ	Response to Blood Loss	Resulting Signs and Symptoms
Brain	Decrease of perfusion in higher centers of thinking in order to maintain cardiac and respiratory control centers	Altered mental status —Confusion —Restlessness —Anxiety
Cardiovascular system	Heart pumps faster; blood vessels constrict	Increased pulse rate Increased breathing rate Rapid, weak pulse Low or falling blood pressure Delayed capillary refill time (pediatric patients)
Gastrointestinal organs	Decrease of perfusion in the digestive tract	Nausea and vomiting
Kidneys	Reduction in function to conserve the body's salt and water	Decreased urine production Increased thirst
Skin	Marked loss of perfusion as blood vessels to the skin constrict	Cool, clammy, pale skin Pallor Cyanosis
Extremities	Marked loss of perfusion	Weak or absent peripheral pulses Decreased blood pressure

venous bleeding is usually detected and controlled immediately in the initial assessment.

Treatment of shock (hypoperfusion) and bleeding is performed after the initial assessment and a rapid transport decision is made. Generally, any non-life-threatening bleeding will be detected and treated during the rapid trauma exam, which is part of the focused history and physical exam for the trauma patient. ✳

Patient Care

External Bleeding

Always take the appropriate BSI precautions whenever you must control a patient's bleeding. Also, remember to always expose the wound area to completely assess the injury.

The major steps for bleeding control are: direct pressure, elevation of an extremity, and use of pressure points (Skill Summary 21-1). Other methods include the use of splints or pneumatic pressure devices and, as a last resort, tourniquets.

- **Direct pressure.** Apply pressure directly over a wound with a sterile gauze pad, or dressing. If a dressing is not readily available, use your gloved hand. Use a bandage to snugly hold the dressing in place and to provide pressure over the wound. Bandage distal to proximal, and leave fingertips (or toes) exposed so circulation may be monitored. A large gaping wound may require extra dressing material to pack it in order to control bleeding.

  If bleeding continues, remove all layers of dressings, except the layer that is actually touching the wound (it is part of the clot), and apply additional layers of dressing material.

- **Elevation.** Combine elevation of an injured extremity with direct pressure to control bleeding. Raise the injured extremity above the level of the heart to slow the flow of blood. However, if the extremity is painful, swollen, or deformed, avoid this technique.

- **Pressure points.** Use pressure points if direct pressure and elevation fail to control bleeding. A pressure point is a site where a main artery lies near the surface of the body and directly over a bone (Figure 21-3). Compressing the

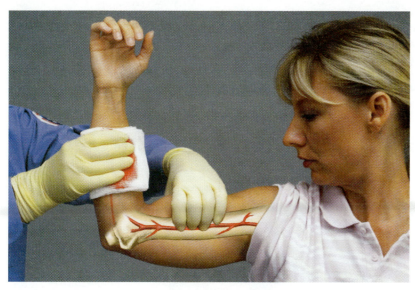

Figure 21-3 The use of pressure points can stop profuse bleeding from an arm or leg if direct pressure and elevation fail. The artery is constricted by pressing it firmly against the bone.

artery over the bone slows or reduces the blood flow to the injured area. The two most commonly used pressure points are on the brachial and femoral arteries.

- **Supplemental oxygen.** Remember that since blood loss reduces perfusion and the supply of oxygen to the tissues, the use of supplemental oxygen is vital. Oxygen should be administered after the bleeding has been controlled. Never delay the manual methods of bleeding control to set up or deliver oxygen to the patient.

Use splints and pneumatic pressure devices to control bleeding from painful, swollen, or deformed extremities (suspected fractures). Bleeding occurs when the jagged bone ends or fragments damage the tissue and blood vessels that surround the bone. Splinting the body part stabilizes the bone ends or fragments and thus aids in controlling bleeding. Pneumatic pressure devices, such as an air splint or pneumatic antishock garment (PASG), apply pressure over a wound area. Use a PASG in the presence of massive soft-tissue injury to the lower extremities and associated shock, by inflating the leg compartments. Remember that an air splint will not have enough pressure to control arterial bleeding.

Use tourniquets to control bleeding only when all other bleeding control methods fail. Tourniquets have the potential to cause nerve damage and injure soft tissues and may result in the loss of the injured limb. Remember, once a tourniquet is applied, it should never be loosened or removed without approval from medical direction. ✳

Special Considerations

When a trauma patient is bleeding from the ears or nose, suspect a possible skull fracture. Do not try to stop the flow of blood. Attempting to control bleeding would increase pressure inside the skull. Instead, place a loose dressing over the area to collect any drainage and to reduce the risk of further contamination.

Internal Bleeding

Internal bleeding, while not always evident, results from blunt and penetrating trauma, abnormal clotting mechanisms within the body, rupture of a blood vessel, or long bone and pelvic fractures. It may progress into life-threatening shock. The severity of internal bleeding depends on its source, as well as the patient's overall medical condition and age. Blood loss from internal bleeding can ultimately lead to death. During the scene size-up, you should have a high index of suspicion for internal bleeding based upon the patient's mechanism of injury (MOI).

Patient Assessment

Internal Bleeding

- During the scene size-up, evaluate the scene, looking for mechanisms of injury such as impact marks or fallen ladders.

- Your general impression and evaluation of the patient's ABCs during the initial assessment will also lend support to a suspicion for internal bleeding.

Always take BSI precautions first.

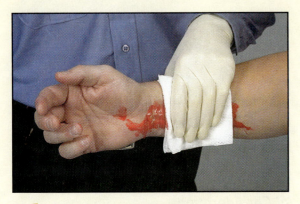

▲ **1.** Apply direct pressure to a bleeding wound with a gauze pad.

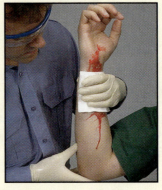

▲ **2.** Elevate a bleeding extremity above the level of the heart.

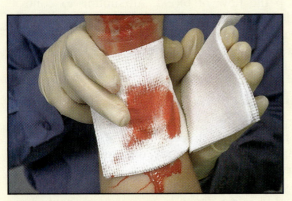

▲ **3.** If the wound continues to bleed, apply additional dressings over the first one.

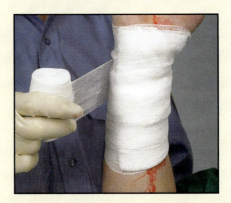

▲ **4.** Bandage the dressing in place.

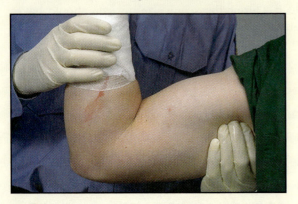

▲ **5.** If a wound to the arm continues to bleed, apply pressure to the brachial artery, or . . .

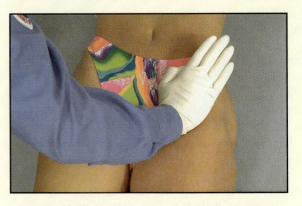

▲ . . . If a wound to the leg continues to bleed, apply pressure to the femoral artery.

- When you perform a rapid trauma exam during the focused history and physical exam, look for:
  - Pain, tenderness, swelling, or discoloration at the suspected injury site (Figure 21-4).
  - Bleeding from the mouth, rectum, vagina, or other orifice.
  - Bright red blood or dark, coffee-ground colored blood in vomitus.
  - Dark, tarry stools or stools with bright red blood.
  - Tender, rigid, and/or distended abdomen.
  - Other signs of hypovolemic (low-volume) shock. ✳

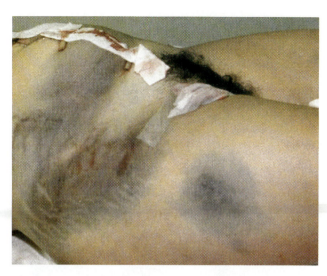

Figure 21-4 Bruising is one sign of internal bleeding.

Patient Care

Internal Bleeding

If you suspect internal bleeding in your patient, your emphasis should be on early recognition and early transport. Emergency care steps include the following:

1. **Take BSI precautions.**
2. **Maintain the patient's airway and breathing.** Provide artificial ventilations when necessary.
3. **Administer high-concentration oxygen.**
4. **Control any external bleeding.** Splint any painful, swollen, or deformed extremities.
5. **Provide immediate transport** for critical patients with signs and symptoms of shock. When one is available, patients should be transported to a trauma center or other hospital capable of handling such injuries. During transport, continually re-evaluate the critical patient with ongoing assessments every 5 minutes. ✳

SHOCK

The term "shock" is used interchangeably with the term "hypoperfusion," which more accurately describes the actual condition. Shock is essentially a result of inadequate or low (hypo-) perfusion of the body's cells and tissues caused by insufficient blood flow through the capillaries. This condition ultimately leads to death of the tissue. In cases of shock, peripheral perfusion is reduced due to inadequate circulating volume or heart (pump) failure. Patients with blood loss from internal or external bleeding are always at risk for shock.

The urgency in transporting patients suffering from shock is due to the fact that most injuries require surgical interventions to correct. The term "golden hour" has been used to describe the maximum time period between the time of injury and surgery. EMT-Bs should keep scene times to less than 10 minutes (unless extrication is required). This is referred to as the "platinum 10 minutes."

Patient Assessment

Shock

Follow these steps to assess for shock:

- During the initial assessment, evaluate the patient's mental status. A patient who is restless, anxious, has a "feeling of impending doom," or exhibits any altered mental status may be experiencing the early stages of shock. As you assess circulation, look for a weak, thready, or absent pulse in the distal extremities, which can be an indicator of decreased peripheral perfusion. Also, the skin may be pale, cool, and clammy.

- During the focused history and physical exam, complete a rapid trauma assessment, looking for any signs of further injury. Abnormal vital signs, such as increased pulse rate, with or without signs of external bleeding, may also indicate a patient at risk for shock. Also, a patient's breathing rate may increase and become labored, shallow, and irregular. Blood pressure may remain normal for some time; however, a late sign of shock is a decreasing blood pressure. Other signs to look for are dilated pupils, marked thirst, nausea or vomiting, and pallor with cyanosis (Figure 21-5). ✳

- Altered mental status
- Pale, cool, clammy skin
- Nausea and vomiting
- Vital signs changes:
  - Pulse—rapid, weak, thready
  - Respirations—increased, shallow, labored
  - Blood pressure—drops as a late, serious sign
- Other possible signs:
  - Thirst
  - Dilated pupils
  - Blue lips and nail beds

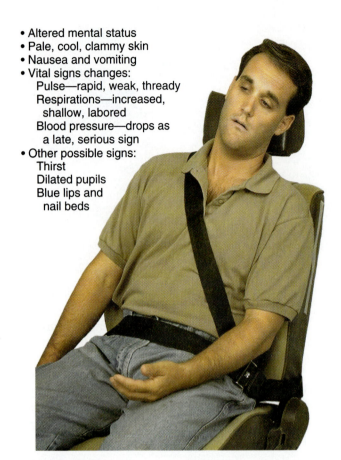

Figure 21-5 Signs and symptoms of shock.

LIFESPAN DEVELOPMENT

When infants and children under six are experiencing shock, capillary refill will be greater than 2 seconds in normal ambient air temperature. Unfortunately, however, infants and children can maintain (compensate) blood pressure until almost half of their blood volume is depleted. Therefore, if an infant or child's blood pressure is dropping, it is an ominous sign that the child may be close to death.

Patient Care

Shock

The steps for the emergency care of shock are similar to those for internal bleeding. Review Skill Summary 21-2 and the steps below:

1 **Take BSI precautions,** and use appropriate personal protective equipment.

2 **Maintain the airway and breathing.** Administer high-concentration oxygen through either a nonrebreather or bag-valve-mask assist.

3 **Control any external bleeding.**

4 **Elevate the lower extremities 8 to 12 inches,** if there are no suspected injuries to the spine, pelvis, or lower extremities.

5 **Splint all painful, swollen, or deformed extremities.** (Do not delay transport of high-priority patients.)

6 **Keep the patient warm.** Maintain body temperature.

Make an early transport decision, and transport the patient rapidly to an appropriate facility. ✳

Use of the PASG

While the use of a pneumatic antishock garment (PASG) for the treatment of shock has been controversial, its use is indicated in the presence of pelvic injuries or instability accompanied by shock (blood pressure, < 90 mmHg) and to control bleeding in massive soft-tissue injuries to the lower extremities. Medical experts agree that a PASG should not be used with thoracic trauma. Also, the garment is not recommended for shock caused by medical emergencies such as diabetic emergencies or a medical cardiac arrest. Apply the PASG in accordance with local medical direction and protocols. Remember to remove the patient's clothing before applying the garment to avoid pressure bruises on the skin.

Shock Management

Always take BSI precautions first.

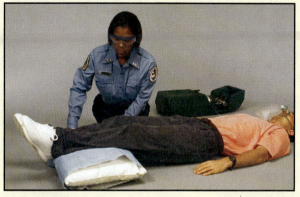

▲ **1.** Maintain an open airway, give high-concentration oxygen by nonrebreather mask, and control external bleeding. Assist ventilations and perform CPR as necessary.

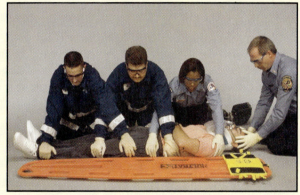

▲ **2.** Properly position the patient. If there is no serious injury, place the patient in a supine position with legs elevated 8 to 12 inches.

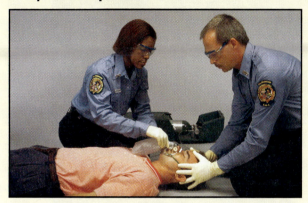

▲ **3.** If there is any possibility of serious injury to the head, neck, spine, chest, abdomen, pelvis, hip, or extremities, place the patient in a supine position with NO elevation of extremities.

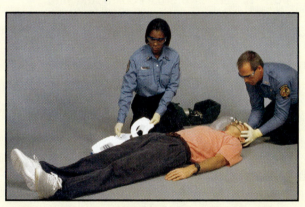

▲ **4.** Splinting of bone and joint injuries can help control shock but should be done en route. Meanwhile, placing the patient on a long backboard will have the effect of splinting the whole body.

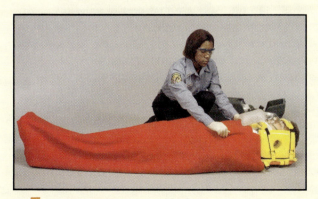

▲ **5.** Protect the patient from heat loss.

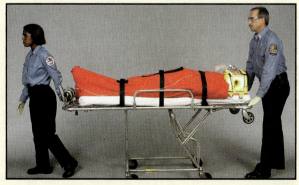

▲ **6.** Transport immediately.

Bleeding and Shock Emergencies

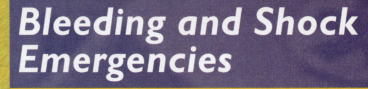

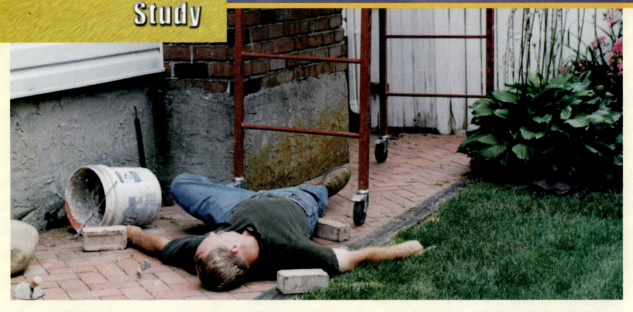

Dispatch: 12 Wilson Avenue   Fall   1317 hrs

Your ambulance has been dispatched for a fall at 12 Wilson Avenue. You respond to find an apparently safe scene where a man has fallen from a roof to the ground. As you continue to size-up the scene, you observe scaffolding alongside the single-level residential dwelling. A bucket on the scaffolding has been knocked over. You see the patient lying on the brick sidewalk below the scaffolding.

You and your crew don gloves before approaching the patient. Upon reaching the patient's side, you note that the man is conscious and responsive. One member of the crew maintains c-spine stabilization while you introduce yourself. The patient tells you that his name is Ken Malek. He appears oriented, is breathing adequately, and answers your questions. You listen with a stethoscope and hear equal breath sounds bilaterally. The patient complains of pain at the back of his head.

Mr Malek says that he slipped and fell from about halfway up the roof onto the scaffolding, then to the ground. He denies loss of consciousness, dizziness, or any other medical problems that could have caused the fall. You determine that there is a significant mechanism of injury and perform a rapid trauma assessment. Other than the swelling at the back of the head, the only other notable injury you find is some tenderness in the lower ribs on the right side. You check the patient's back before he is placed on the backboard and find

no additional injuries. The patient's vital signs are pulse 88 strong and regular; respirations 16 and adequate; blood pressure 118/72; pupils equal and reactive to light; and skin warm and moist.

The patient is placed into the ambulance and transportation begins for the 25-minute ride to the hospital. After verifying the oxygen delivery and patient's comfort, you perform a detailed assessment, which does not reveal further sign of injury. The bleeding remains controlled. There is some additional reddening around the area of the ribs. The patient denies past medical history and allergies. He ate lunch just before the fall. You repeat the vital signs to find the pulse 96 and regular but a bit weak; respirations 24 and adequate; blood pressure 110/68; pupils equal and reactive to light; and skin cool and moist.

You record these new vital signs next to the previous set and observe a difference. The patient may be beginning to show signs of shock. You had applied oxygen early due to the mechanism of injury. You maintain the patient's warmth, and notify the hospital of your findings. You repeat the vitals in 5 minutes and find that the pulse has increased to 106. You also note that the patient is becoming a bit anxious.

The hospital staff is awaiting your arrival. They quickly examine the patient and perform tests. They suspect internal bleeding and fast track the patient to the operating room.

CASE DISCUSSION

This patient fell from the roof of a single-story residence. In this case, it is important to note that he was halfway up the roof when he slipped. This could add to the potential for injury. The scaffolding may have played two roles in the injury. The first was to break the fall a bit. The second was to cause potential injury when the patient struck it on the way down. That the patient fell onto a brick sidewalk is also significant. Your observation of the mechanisms of injury are important when it comes to evaluating for potentially serious hidden injuries—as seen in this patient.

There was a 25 to 30 minute transport time on this call. The repeated evaluations helped to identify the deteriorating condition of the patient. Remember that decreasing blood pressure is a late sign of shock. In most cases, before the blood pressure drops, the patient will appear anxious. The pulse and respirations will rise, and the skin will become pale, cool, and sometimes moist.

This pattern contrasts to that in head injuries. In head injuries, with increasing pressure inside the skull, the blood pressure will rise while the pulse drops. This is the opposite of what happens to vital signs in shock. With head injuries, this change in vital signs is also a late finding.

It should be noted that a patient with a head injury who shows signs of shock (decreased blood pressure, increased pulse and respirations) usually has a hidden injury or bleeding in another area of the body. The skull is a closed container. Even if there were intracranial bleeding, there would not be enough space for the blood pooling to cause shock. This patient, with a closed head injury, is an ideal example. It is highly probable that the patient had an internal injury (such as a liver injury) which in turn caused the shock.

Name: Ken Malek
Age: 32
Chief Complaint: *"My head hurts"* (Fall)

ASSESSMENT INFORMATION	RELEVANCE TO THIS PATIENT
Mechanism of injury	• The height of the fall, the role of the scaffolding, and the surface landed on are all considerations in the mechanism of injury.
Physical assessment	• Spinal precautions were taken initially upon observing the MOI. • The scalp wound was noted initially but did not receive significant attention because it was not bleeding. • The tenderness around the ribs on the lower right side was quite significant (and possibly an indicator of the cause of the developing shock).
Patient history	• The patient denied events that could have caused the fall (loss of consciousness, dizziness, seizure). • His lack of past medical history supports this. If the patient had a history of seizures or diabetes, for example, you would want to spend more time evaluating possible causes of the fall.
Vital signs	• The vital signs initially seemed to be within normal limits. It is the change of vital signs over time (trending) which will reveal states of hypoperfusion (shock). • Remember that a drop in blood pressure is one of the last signs of shock.

SUMMARY

- There are two types of bleeding: external and internal.
- External bleeding may be arterial (bright red and spurting), venous (flowing), or capillary (oozing).
- Methods of controlling external bleeding include direct pressure, elevation, and pressure points.
- Air splints and the PASG are sometimes used for bleeding control and maintaining pressure on the wound.
- Rarely, if ever, is a tourniquet needed.
- Internal bleeding cannot be seen and is difficult to identify; such bleeding may be from trauma or medical causes.
- Signs and symptoms of internal bleeding include pain, tenderness, swelling, or discoloration to an area; bleeding from the mouth, rectum, vagina, or other body orifice; vomiting of blood or coffee ground-like material; tarry stools; and signs of shock.
- To care for internal bleeding, maintain airway and breathing, control any external bleeding, apply oxygen, maintain body temperature, and transport promptly.
- The terms "shock" and "hypoperfusion" are used interchangeably to describe a condition in which the body is unable to supply blood to the tissues.
- Trauma patients who are in shock require prompt transportation to a hospital because surgery is usually required to correct the internal injuries causing shock.
- Care for shock is identical to care for internal injuries.

REVIEW QUESTIONS

1. The three types of external bleeding include all of the following EXCEPT:
   a. lymphatic.
   b. arterial.
   c. venous.
   d. capillary.

2. The loss of _____ cc of blood would be considered serious in an adult patient.
   a. 1000
   b. 800
   c. 650
   d. 500

3. If a trauma patient is bleeding from the ears and nose, bleeding control should include:
   a. direct pressure and elevation.
   b. pressure points and diffuse pressure.
   c. a loose dressing to collect drainage.
   d. cold packs on the injury site.

REVIEW QUESTIONS *continued*

4. You suspect your patient has internal bleeding. Steps for emergency care include all of the following EXCEPT:

a. splinting any PSDEs.

b. administering oxygen.

c. taking BSI precautions.

d. using pressure points.

5. In pediatric patients, a sign of hypofusion is a capillary refill time of more than _____ seconds

a. 2

b. 5

c. 15

d. 30

WEB MEDIC

Visit Brady's *Essentials of Emergency Care* web site for direct web links. At **www.prenhall.com/limmer,** you will find information related to the following Chapter 21 topics:

- Leukemia
- Blood supplies
- Pneumatic antishock garment
- Red blood cells
- Hemophilia

*Correlates with the U.S. DOT
"EMT-Basic National Standard Curriculum"
Lesson 5-2"*

SOFT-TISSUE INJURIES

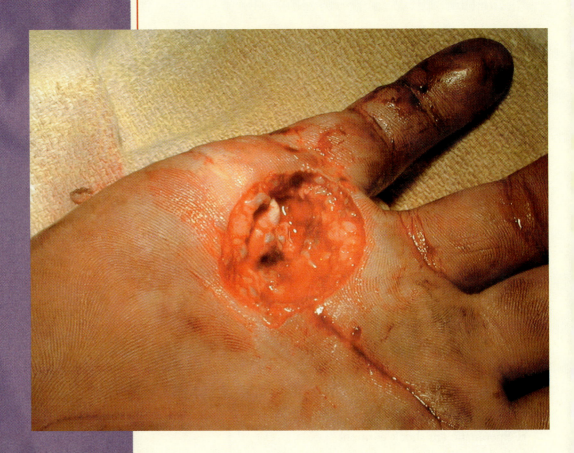

Soft-tissue injuries may range from minor scrapes and bruises to life-threatening injuries to the chest and abdomen. Such injuries are frequent calls for the EMT-B, and you are responsible for identifying and treating them skillfully.

One type of soft-tissue injury—burns—is the third leading cause of accidental death in the United States. Only motor-vehicle collisions and falls precede it. Approximately 12,000 people will die each year of a burn injury. Most people think burn injuries only affect the skin, but in fact burns often have an impact on other body systems.

CLOSED WOUNDS

A wound is caused by trauma, which disrupts the normal structure of the tissues, an organ, or a bone. Wounds are categorized as open or closed.

Closed wounds are beneath intact, or unbroken, skin. The three specific types of closed injuries are contusions, hematomas, and crush injuries. A **contusion,** or bruise, results when the epidermis remains unbroken; however, the cells and blood vessels contained within the dermis are injured, causing an accumulation of blood in surrounding tissues that is evidenced by discoloration (Figure 22-1). A contusion causes localized swelling and pain at the injury site.

A **hematoma** is also a collection of blood beneath the epidermis, but in larger amounts than in a simple contusion. Hematomas may also occur deep within the body cavity or, often catastrophically, within the layers of tissues surrounding the brain.

A **crush injury** results from a severe crushing force and may be serious, depending on its location and the underlying tissue or organ damage. Crush injuries are associated with internal injuries and shock (hypoperfusion).

Patient Care

Closed Wounds

Emergency care for a patient with closed wounds is as follows:

1. **Take BSI precautions.**
2. **Manage the patient's ABCs.** Apply high-concentration oxygen by nonrebreather mask.
3. **Provide care for internal bleeding and shock,** if there is any reason to suspect internal injuries.
4. **Splint extremities** that are painful, swollen, or deformed.

Continue to monitor the patient for the development of shock. Stay alert for the patient to vomit. Transport as soon as possible. ✳

OPEN WOUNDS

An **open wound** is any injury that damages the integrity of the skin. This break in the skin increases the chances for blood loss and the risk for infection.

Patient Assessment

Closed Wounds

Closed wounds may range from simple, small contusions to serious internal injuries. Assess for the following during your trauma assessments:

- Mechanism of injury
- Complaints of pain or tenderness
- Bruising or discoloration of the skin
- Swelling
- Deformity (this may include abnormal depressions in tissue, deformed extremities, or lack of symmetry in a body part). ✳

CORE CONCEPTS

In this chapter, you will learn about the following topics:

- Open vs. closed wounds
- Treatment of various types of open and closed wounds
- Care of specific injuries (amputations, impaled objects, neck wounds, chest injuries, burns)
- Principles of dressing and bandaging

✔ **Knowledge**

☐ 1. Provide care to a patient with a soft-tissue injury. (pp. 317, 320–323, 324, 327–333)

• Describe the emergency medical care of the patient with a closed soft-tissue injury. (p. 317)

• Describe the emergency medical care of the patient with an open soft-tissue injury. (pp. 317, 320–323, 324, 327–333)

✔ **Skills**

☐ 2. Demonstrate the steps in the care of open and closed soft-tissue injuries (chest injuries, abdominal injuries, burns, and amputations). (pp. 317, 320–323, 324, 327–333)

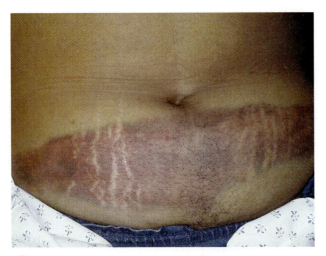

Figure 22-1 Contusions are the most common form of closed wound.

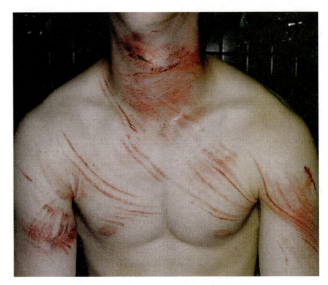

Figure 22-2 Abrasions and superficial lacerations.

An **abrasion** is a scrape (caused by friction), rubbing, or shearing of the outermost layer of the skin (Figure 22-2). Although an abrasion is considered a superficial injury, it can be extremely painful because it involves the nerve endings. In most cases, bleeding will be minimal and easily controlled. However, when a larger body surface area is injured, such as in the "road rash" that results when a motorcyclist falls off of a cycle, blood loss may be severe.

A **laceration** is a linear (regular) or stellate (irregular) tearing of the skin caused by sharp objects (Figure 22-3). The depth of a laceration may vary. Lacerations tend to bleed profusely, due to the severing of larger blood vessels.

An **avulsion** and an **amputation** are the ripping or tearing of skin and soft tissue that cause complete or incomplete detachment of a body part (Figure 22-4). Avulsions generally involve soft tissue only. Amputations involve bones as well. The amount of bleeding from these types of injuries can range from profuse (due to damage to large blood vessels) to negligible (due to retraction of the blood vessels).

A **penetration** or **puncture** wound is caused by a sharp object, such as a pencil or ice pick, being pushed into the soft tissues (Figures 22-5 and 22-6). External bleeding is usually minimal, but internal injury can be severe if the wound is located over a major blood vessel or organ. Apply a sterile dressing and be prepared to treat for shock if the puncture is to the torso or neck.

Figure 22-3 (A) Some lacerations have smooth edges. (B) Some lacerations have jagged edges.

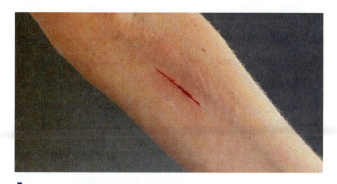

A

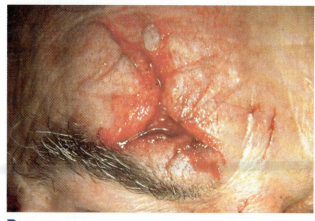

B

Figure 22-4 (A) Avulsed skin. (B) An amputation. (C) An x-ray of an amputation

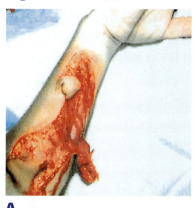

A

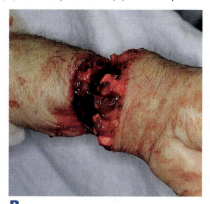

B

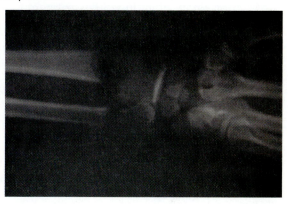

Figure 22-5 A penetrating puncture wound.

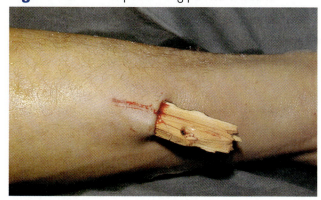

Figure 22-6 A perforating puncture wound.

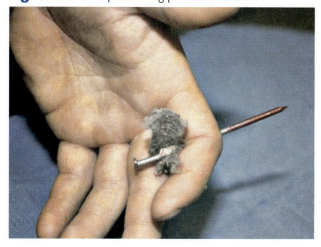

Patient Assessment

Open Wounds

There are many types of open wounds. Assessment of these wounds involves exposing the wound and identifying serious injuries, life threats, and the type of wound. For example, at the appropriate point in your assessment:

- Assess open wounds for bleeding severity
- Assess wounds for the following special conditions:

  - Amputations or avulsions that will require care of a body part
  - Open wounds to the chest or neck that may require an occlusive dressing
  - Open wounds to the abdomen that may have caused an evisceration of abdominal organs ✱

Patient Care

Open Wounds

Provide emergency care for a patient's open wounds as follows.

1. **Expose the wound.** Clothing that covers a soft-tissue injury must be lifted, cut, or split away. For some articles of clothing, this is best done with scissors or a seam cutter. Do not attempt to remove clothing in the usual manner. To do so may aggravate existing injuries and cause additional damage and pain.

2. **Clean the wound surface.** Do not try to pick out embedded particles and debris from the wound. Simply remove large pieces of foreign matter from its surface. When possible, use a piece of sterile dressing to brush away large debris from the surface. Do not spend much time cleaning the wound. Control of bleeding is the priority.

3. **Control bleeding.** Start with direct pressure or direct pressure and elevation. When necessary, use a pressure point. Remember, a tourniquet is used only as a last resort.

4. **Treat for shock.** For all serious wounds, provide care for shock, including the administration of high-concentration oxygen.

5. **Prevent further contamination.** Use a sterile dressing, if possible. When none is available, use the cleanest cloth material at the scene.

6. **Bandage the dressing in place, after bleeding has been controlled.** If an extremity is involved, check for a distal pulse to be sure circulation has not been interrupted by the application of a tight bandage. With the exception of a pressure dressing, bleeding must be controlled before bandaging is started. Periodically recheck the bandage to make certain that bleeding has not restarted.

7. **Keep the patient lying still.** Any movement will increase the patient's circulation and could restart bleeding.

8. **Reassure the patient.** This will help ease the patient's emotional response and perhaps lower pulse rate and blood pressure. In some cases, this may help to reduce the bleeding rate, too. A patient who feels reassured will usually be more willing to lie still, reducing the chances of restarting controlled bleeding. ✱

Patient Care

Penetrating Chest Injuries

The chest provides a closed, airtight system for respiration. When chest injuries occur, air may leak from the wound and disrupt respiration (Figure 22-7). When treating penetrating chest injuries, use an occlusive dressing to prevent air from entering the chest, which could cause a pneumothorax. Leave one side or corner of the dressing unsecured to allow air to escape as the patient exhales in order to prevent a tension pneumothorax (Figure 22-8). Administer oxygen and, if no spine injury is suspected, place the patient in a position of comfort. ✱

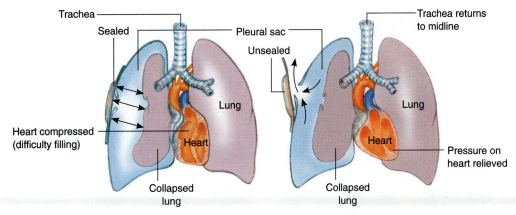

Sealing wound can cause increase in pressure within thoracic (chest) cavity.

If patient's condition declines after sealing puncture wound, open the seal immediately.

Figure 22-7 Open chest wound with punctured lung.

On inspiration, dressing seals wound, preventing air entry.

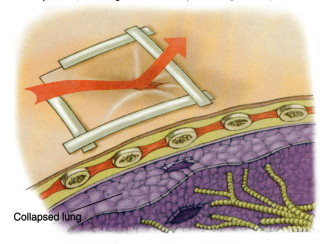

Expiration allows trapped air to escape through untaped section of dressing.

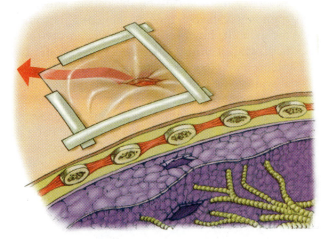

Figure 22-8 Creating a flutter valve to allow air to escape from the chest cavity.

Patient Care

Evisceration

When abdominal injuries result in an evisceration (an organ or part of an organ protruding through a wound opening), do not touch or attempt to push the organ back into the abdominal cavity. Cover the exposed organ(s) with a sterile dressing, which is moistened with saline, or an occlusive dressing large enough to cover all of the protruding organs. Avoid using an absorbent material, since it may adhere to the organs. However, an airtight dressing is not essential, unless you suspect the path of injury extends into the chest.

Keep the dressing in place with a large bandage or clean sheet to protect the site and prevent heat loss (Figure 22-9). If there is no suspected spinal injury, transport the patient with the hips and knees flexed to decrease tension on the abdominal muscles. ✳

Patient Care

Impaled Objects

Manually secure impaled objects in place to prevent movement that could cause further damage. Expose the area and control any bleeding with direct pressure around the wound edges. Stabilize the object with bulky dressings and secure in place (Figure 22-10). ✳

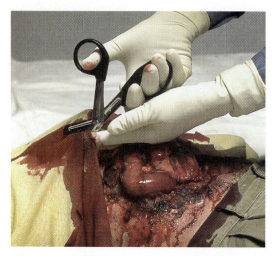

Figure 22-9A Cut away clothing from wound.

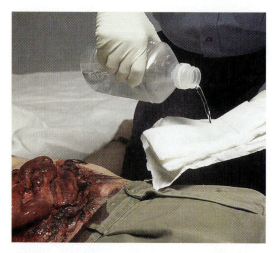

Figure 22-9B Soak a dressing with sterile saline.

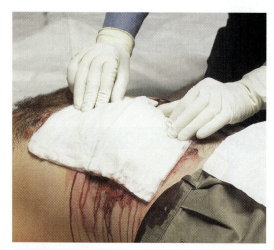

Figure 22-9C Place the moist dressing over the wound.

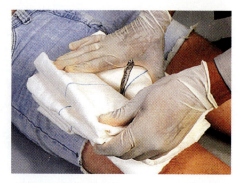

Figure 22-10A Expose the wound and control bleeding.

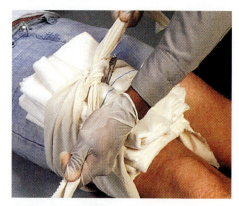

Figure 22-10B Stabilize the impaled object.

Patient Care

Amputations

Amputations create situations in which the EMT-B must care for not only the patient but also for the detached body part. However, always focus emergency medical care on the patient rather than expending valuable time looking for the amputated part. If, however, the amputated part is located, wrap it in dry, sterile dressings. Some EMS systems recommend moistening the dressing material with saline solution; check with medical direction to determine your local protocols.

After wrapping the body part in dressings, wrap or bag it in plastic. Label it with the date, the time the part was wrapped, and the patient's name. Then place it into a cooler or other suitable container on top of an ice pack or ice. Never place a body part directly on the ice pack or ice since this will freeze the body part. Do not use dry ice as it will burn the flesh. Never place the tissue in water as this will lead to tissue damage. If possible, transport the body part with the patient. If you are unable to locate the body part in time, transport the patient immediately and make arrangements to have the body part, if it is found, transported to the same hospital.

If your patient has an avulsion that is hanging by a small amount of tissue, do not complete the amputation. Instead, immobilize the part to prevent further injury. ✳

Patient Care

Open Wounds to the Neck

Because major blood vessels are located in the neck, a large open wound to the neck is susceptible not only to life-threatening bleeding but also to an air embolism. An **air embolism,** or bubble, can travel by veins to the heart and cause abnormal functioning of the heart, including cardiac arrest. Arterial bleeding from the neck is a grave sign. Venous bleeding may be profuse. Focus your care of the patient on establishing an adequate airway and breathing. Apply direct pressure with an occlusive dressing. Avoid pressing over the carotid artery (Skill Summary 22-1). ✳

BURN INJURIES

As you know, the skin is made up of three layers: the **epidermis** (outermost), the **dermis** (middle), and **subcutaneous** (deepest). Its thickness may range from one cell to several layers, and it serves multiple functions. The skin provides a barrier against infection and protection from pathogens, such as bacteria or other harmful agents found in the environment. It insulates and protects underlying structures and body organs from injury. It aids in the regulation of body temperature, and it provides for sensation transmission (hot, cold, pain, and touch). The skin also aids in elimination of some of the body's wastes, and it contains fluids necessary to the proper functioning of other organs and systems. Any or all of these functions can be impaired or destroyed by a burn injury.

Classifying Burn Injuries

During the scene size-up and in a more detailed evaluation during the focused history and physical exam, the first step in assessing a burn injury is to classify it according to the depth of injury to the skin. Burns are classified as superficial, partial-thickness, or full-thickness burns (Figure 22-11).

A **superficial burn,** or first-degree burn, is a painful injury that involves the epidermis. It is caused

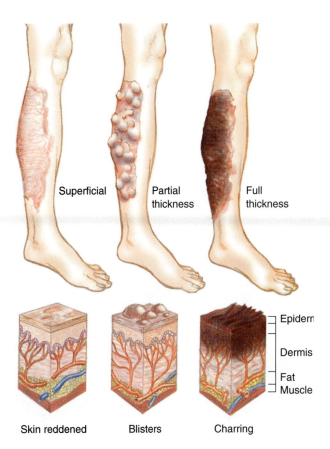

Figure 22-11 Burns are classified by depth.

by a flame, scald, or the sun. The skin will be dry and appear pink to red. In some cases, there may be a slight swelling but an absence of blisters. A superficial burn may take several days to heal.

A **partial-thickness burn,** or second-degree burn, involves not only the epidermis, but also portions of the dermis. Partial-thickness burns are caused by contact with a flame or flash, hot liquids or hot solid objects, chemical substances, or the sun. The skin may appear white to cherry red, moist, and mottled. Partial-thickness burns are characterized by blisters, a result of damage to the blood vessels, which causes plasma and tissue fluid to rise to the top layer of the skin. Because nerve endings are damaged, partial-thickness burns will cause intense pain. They will usually heal on their own in two to four weeks. However, if a large skin surface area or depth is involved, specialized interventions may be required.

A **full-thickness burn,** or third-degree burn, damages the entire dermis and can extend beyond it to the subcutaneous layer and into the muscle, bone, or organs below. Full-thickness burns are a result of contact with extreme heat sources. The skin will become dry, hard, tough, and leathery and may appear white-waxy to dark brown or black charred. Most full-thickness burns are not very painful since nerve

Open Neck Wound— Occlusive Dressing

Always take take BSI precautions first.

The dressing must be heavy plastic, sized to be 2 inches larger in diameter than the wound site. Note that for demonstration purposes, the patient is shown in an upright position.

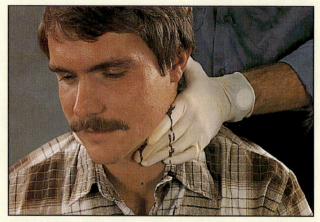

▲ **1.** Do not delay! Place your gloved palm over the wound to control bleeding.

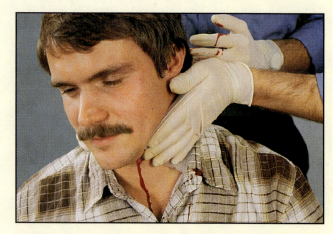

▲ **2.** Place an occlusive dressing over the wound site.

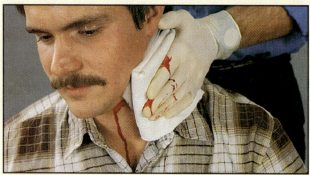

▲ **3.** Then place another dressing over the occlusive roll of gauze one. (A roll of gauze can be placed between the trachea and the dressing to help keep pressure off the airway.)

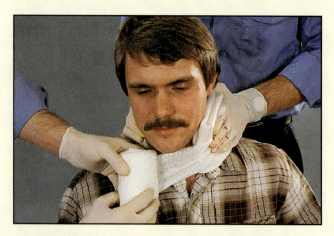

▲ **4.** Start a figure eight, bringing the bandage over the dressing and end the figure eight by crossing over the shoulder.

ending destruction is complete. However, most full-thickness burns are accompanied by partial-thickness burns, which can cause intense pain. Full-thickness burns usually require specialized surgical intervention and skin grafting. The length of the healing process depends on the size of the injured area and can take anywhere from two months to years. Scarring may be extensive, depending on the extent of the burn.

Determining Severity of Burn Injuries

In addition to classifying a burn during the focused history and physical exam, you also need to determine the burn's severity. The severity of a burn is dependent upon the percentage of **body surface area (BSA)** involved, the burn's location, the depth of the burn, and the patient's age and other preexisting medical conditions. Determining the source agent, or cause, of the burn is also helpful.

To quickly identify the amount of burned skin surface, you can use the **Rule of Nines** (Figure 22-12). Using this method, specific body surface areas are assigned percentages to determine the amount of BSA involved in the burn. The Rule of Nines is not only helpful in estimating a burn's severity, but also

enables you to appropriately triage, or categorize, the patient and alert the receiving facility about the severity of the patient's condition.

The location of a burn injury is a major factor in determining burn severity (Figure 22-13). Burns to the face are considered critical because of their potential to cause respiratory compromise and eye injuries. Burns to the hands and feet are critical because they can lead

LIFESPAN DEVELOPMENT

The body proportions of infants and children differ from those of adults, so the BSA percentages assigned to a child's body regions also differ. Since a child's head is much larger in relationship to the rest of the body, the child's head is counted as 18% of the entire body surface. The chest and abdomen are counted as 18%, the entire back as 18%, each upper extremity as 9%, each lower extremity as 14%, and the genital region as 1%.

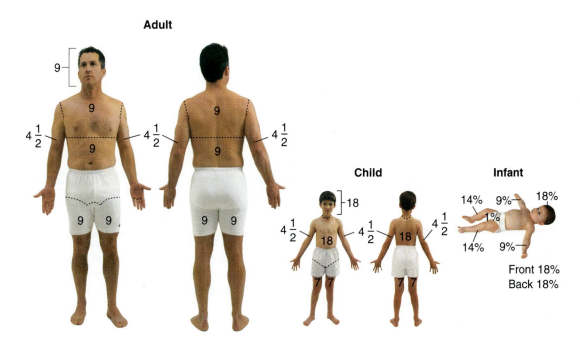

Figure 22-12   The Rule of Nines.

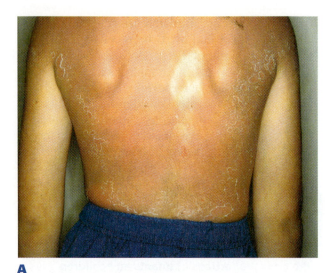

A

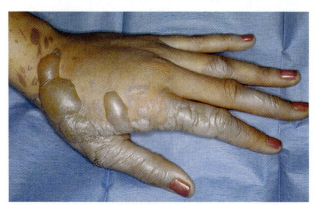

B

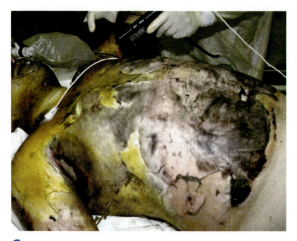

C

Figure 22-13 (A) A superficial burn, (B) a partial-thickness burn, and (C) a full-thickness burn.

to loss of function. Genital or groin region burn injuries can compromise genitourinary function and increase the chances for infection.

Circumferential burns encircle a particular body area, such as an arm, a leg, or the chest. The constriction or swelling of tissue over the joints of the extremities caused by circumferential burns can lead to circulatory compromise and nerve damage. Burns that encircle the chest may impede respiratory function by limiting chest expansion.

As an EMT-B, you know that a minor burn in a healthy adult can turn out to be a severe burn for a patient with preexisting medical conditions, such as diabetes. A patient with an existing respiratory illness or condition may be adversely affected if there is further respiratory compromise from a burn injury. A patient with an existing cardiovascular problem may have increased complications from a burn injury and the resulting fluid loss.

The source, or agent, that causes a burn is also important in determining burn severity. See Table 22-1 for a summary.

Table 22-1   Agents and Sources of Burns

Agents	Sources
Thermal	Flame; radiation; excessive heat from fire, steam, hot liquids, and hot objects
Chemicals	Various acids, bases, caustics
Electricity	AC current, DC current, lightning
Radiation	Nuclear sources; intense light sources, ultraviolet light (includes sunlight)

LIFESPAN DEVELOPMENT

The classification of burn-injury severity differs for children under five years old. Any full- or partial-thickness burn greater than 20%, or any burn involving hands, feet, face, or genitalia is considered a critical burn. Any partial-thickness burn of 10% to 20% is considered a moderate burn. Any partial-thickness burn less than 10% is considered a minor burn.

In order for you to provide optimal emergency medical care, to make early transport decisions, and to give an accurate receiving facility report, it is imperative for you to be able to classify the severity of a burn injury. Table 22-2 summarizes critical, moderate, and minor burn injuries.

Patient Care

Burn Injuries

Specific treatment for burn injuries may depend on your local medical direction, protocols, and practices. Always check your local area's specific treatment guidelines.

The two major goals in the treatment of burn injuries are to stop the burning process and to prevent further injury or contamination. Emergency care steps are as follows:

Table 22-2   Classifying Severity of Burns

Critical Burn Injuries

- Any burn injury complicated by respiratory tract injuries or other accompanying major traumatic injury (soft tissue or bone)
- Full-thickness or partial-thickness burns involving the face, hands, feet, genitalia, or respiratory tract
- Any full-thickness burn covering 10% or more BSA
- Any partial-thickness burn covering 30% or more BSA
- Burn injuries complicated by painful, swollen, deformed extremities
- Moderate burns in children less than 5 years old or adults older than 55
- Any burn that encircles a body part, such as an arm, a leg, or the chest

Moderate Burn Injuries

- Full-thickness burns covering 2% to 10% BSA, excluding the face, hands, feet, genitalia, or respiratory tract
- Partial-thickness burns with 15% to 30% BSA involvement
- Superficial burns greater than 50% BSA

Minor Burn Injuries

- Full-thickness burns involving less than 2% BSA
- Partial-thickness burns involving less than 15% BSA

1 **Protect yourself.** If you are not trained to enter a scene or cannot make it safe, then wait for additional specially trained and equipped resources to arrive.

2 **Stop the burning process.** Because burns may continue to injure the skin even after the burn source is removed, "cool" the burn with water or saline for the first 10 minutes after the injury. If the burn injury is thermal, wetting down the burn area will aid in stopping the burning process. If the burn source is a semisolid or liquid (tar, grease, or oil), cool the burn to stop the burning process. Do not attempt to remove the substance, since this could cause further tissue damage.

Try to remove any smoldering clothing, which still will be emitting heat, and any jewelry, whose metal retains heat. If any clothing remains adhered to the patient, cut around the area. **Do not** try to remove the adhered portion, since this may cause further damage to soft tissues.

3 **Perform an initial assessment and treatment.** After taking BSI precautions, assess the patient for any indications that the airway may be injured or compromised, such as sooty deposits in the mouth or nose, singed facial or nose hairs, signs of smoke inhalation, or any facial burns (Figure 22-14). Assessing the airway is of prime importance, since the first reaction when one is frightened or startled and in a confined space in which there is an explosion or fire is to deeply inhale. In such a situation, the air is superheated and has an adverse effect on the airway and respiratory function. Provide high-concentration oxygen via a nonrebreather mask or BVM assist. Remember that a patient's airway may swell as a result of a burn injury. So continually monitor the airway for closure.

Since most burns do not bleed, if profuse bleeding is evident, look for other causes or injuries and treat the patient for any signs or symptoms of shock.

4 **Perform a focused history and physical exam, and reassess the mechanism of injury.** During the rapid trauma assessment, evaluate the burn injury by assessing its depth, BSA percentage, and severity. Once you have stopped the burning process, cover the wounds with dry, sterile dressings or a burn sheet to prevent further injury or contamination.

5 **Perform an ongoing assessment.** Repeat the initial assessment, retake vital signs, and check interventions. En route to the hospital, complete the ongoing assessment every 5 minutes for unstable patients and every 15 for stable patients. Continually evaluate the airway especially when there are burns to the face. ✳

PRECEPTOR PEARL

Tell new EMT-Bs that continual use of a wet or moist dressing may cause hypothermia in the burn patient because the burned area is no longer capable of heat regulation. However, for partial- or full-thickness burns of 10% or less BSA, some EMS systems recommend use of moist, saline-soaked dressings to decrease the patient's pain. Always check with medical direction regarding the use of wet or moist dressings.

When using dry, sterile dressings, avoid using any material that shreds or leaves particles, since these can cause further contamination of the burn area. Never apply any type of ointments, lotions, or antiseptics to burn injuries since they can lead to heat retention. Never attempt to break or drain blisters, since this action may cause further contamination and fluid loss.

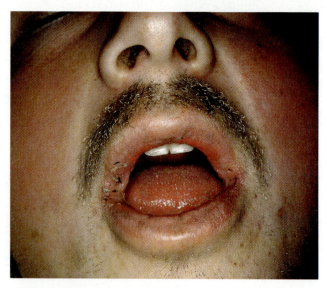

Figure 22-14 A singed mustache and burns to the tip of the tongue signal danger of airway burns or burns to the eyes.

Care for Thermal Burns

Always take BSI precautions first.

STOP THE BURNING PROCESS!

1. Flame—Wet down, smother, then remove clothing.
   Semisolid (grease, tar, wax)—Cool with water … do not remove substance.
2. Ensure an open airway. Assess breathing.
3. Look for airway injury: soot deposits, burnt nasal hair, and facial burns.
4. Complete the initial assessment.
5. Treat for shock. Provide a high concentration of oxygen. Treat serious injuries.
6. Evaluate burns — Depth
   Rule of Nines or Rule of Palm
   Severity

   Decide if special transport is needed.
   Remove clothing, if necessary.

| | Tissue Burned | | | | | |
Type of Burn	First Layer of Skin	Second Layer of Skin	Tissue below Skin	Color Changes	Pain	Blisters
Superficial	Yes	No	No	Red	Yes	No
Partial-Thickness	Yes	Yes	No	Deep red	Yes	Yes
Full-Thickness	Yes	Yes	Yes	Charred black or white	Yes/No	Yes/No

7. Do not clear debris from the wound.
8. Wrap with dry, sterile dressing.
9A. Burns to hands or toes—Remove rings or jewelry that may constrict with swelling. Separate digits with sterile gauze pads.
9B. Burns to the eyes—Do not open eyelids, if burned. Be certain burn is thermal, not chemical. Apply sterile gauze pads to both eyes to prevent sympathetic movement of injured eye if only one eye is burned. If burn is chemical, flush eyes for 20 minutes en route to hospital.

FOLLOW LOCAL BURN CENTER PROTOCOL, AND TRANSPORT ALL BURN PATIENTS AS SOON AS POSSIBLE.

Thermal Burns

Skill Summary 22-2 outlines the emergency care of a patient with thermal burns. ✳

Patient Care

Chemical Burns

Chemical burns require immediate care because the longer a chemical is in contact with the skin, the more severe a burn becomes. Use the following steps to treat chemical burn injuries (Figure 22-15):

1. **Protect yourself first.** Chemical burns are often the result of a hazardous material incident that you may not be trained to handle.

2. **Wear gloves and eye protection.** In cases where there is a danger of greater exposure to a chemical, you may need to wear an impervious (fluid-proof) gown to prevent further contamination.

3. **Stop the burning process.** Most chemical burns can be flushed with copious amounts of water. However, always be sure that the chemical may be diluted with water; some chemicals when mixed with water may produce combustion. Minimize further wound contamination by ensuring that the fluid used to flush the burn flows away from rather than towards any uninjured areas. Remove all clothing, jewelry, and shoes.

4. **Brush off dry chemicals,** such as lime, before flushing with water.

5. **Continue to flush** for at least 20 minutes while en route to the hospital.

After flushing, cover the injured area with a sterile dressing, treat for shock, keep the patient warm, and transport. ✳

Patient Care

Electrical Burns

Electrical burns—including those caused by electrical current and lightning—can cause severe damage not only to soft tissue, but to the entire body as well (Figure 22-16). Because electricity always seeks the path of least resistance to "ground," any tissues or organs in the energy flow from entrance to exit are suspect for injury. Since the body, especially the heart, produces its own electrical energy from chemical reactions, an outside electrical current can disturb or destroy these functions causing heart "rhythm" disturbances (dysrhythmia) or cardiac arrest. Because of the extremely hazardous nature of electricity, scene safety is an important consideration.

Follow these guidelines for emergency medical care:

- Never attempt to remove a patient from an electrical source unless trained and equipped to do so.

- Never touch a victim still in contact with the electrical source.

- Always assess for the burn's entrance and exit wounds. All tissue between these wounds, even if not readily visible, may be injured. Treat entrance and exit injuries the same as you would for thermal burns.

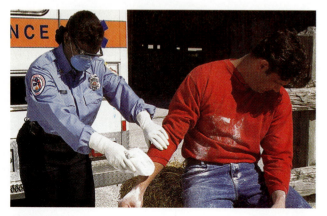
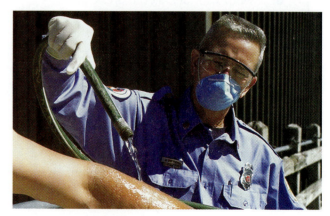

Figure 22-15 For a chemical burn, (A) brush away dry powders, and then (B) flood the area with water.

- Monitor the patient for respiratory and cardiac arrest. Use the automated external defibrillator (AED), if necessary.

- Assess the patient for muscle tenderness, which may or may not be accompanied by muscle twitching or seizure activity.

- Transport the patient as soon as possible. Most electrical burn injuries will have a slow onset, and underlying tissue or organ damage may not be readily apparent. ✳

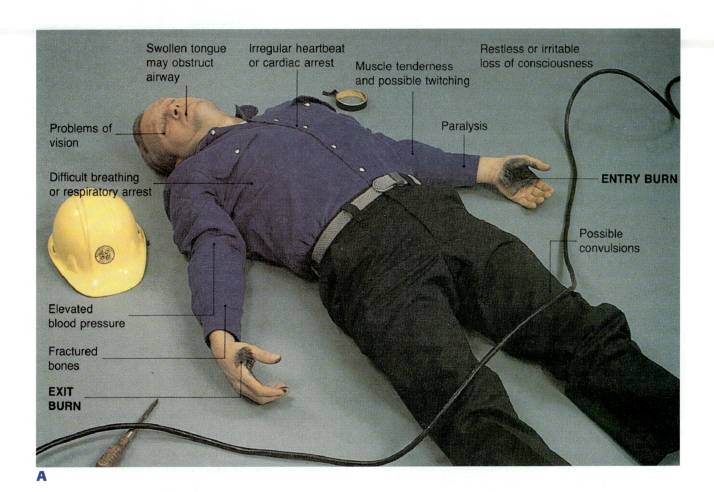

Swollen tongue may obstruct airway

Irregular heartbeat or cardiac arrest

Muscle tenderness and possible twitching

Restless or irritable loss of consciousness

Problems of vision

Paralysis

Difficult breathing or respiratory arrest

ENTRY BURN

Possible convulsions

Elevated blood pressure

Fractured bones

EXIT BURN

A

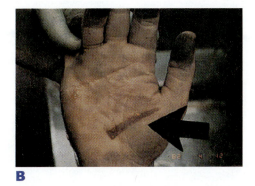

B

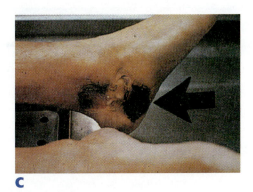

C

Figure 22-16 (A) Injuries due to electricity. (B) Electrical burn, contact with source. (C) Electrical burn, exit wound.

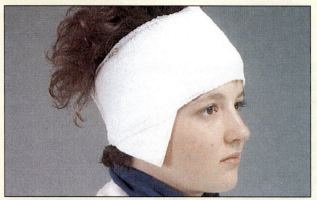

FOREHEAD (NO SKULL INJURY) OR EAR Place dressing and secure with self-adherent roller bandage.

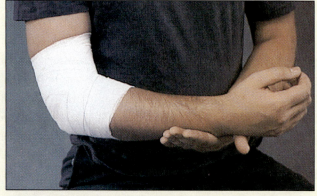

ELBOW OR KNEE Place dressing and secure with cravat or roller bandage. Apply roller bandage in figure-eight pattern.

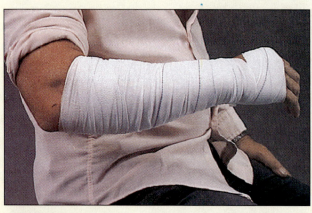

FOREARM OR LEG Place dressing and secure with roller bandage, distal to proximal. Better protection is offered if palm or sole is wrapped. Note: Always leave fingertips or toes showing to assess circulation.

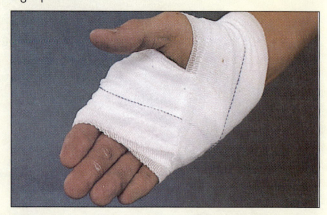

HAND Place dressing, wrap with roller bandage, and secure at wrist. When possible, bandage in position of function. Note: Always leave fingertips showing to assess circulation.

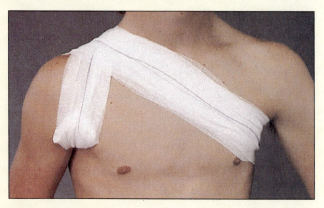

SHOULDER Place dressing and secure with figure-eight of cravat or roller dressing. Pad under knot if cravat is used.

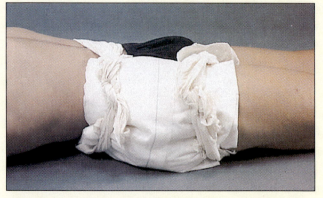

HIP Place bandage and large dressing to cover hip. Secure with first cravat around waist and second cravat around thigh on injured side.

Special Areas of Concern

Because the eyes, hands, and feet represent special areas of concern, use the following guidelines when treating burns to these areas.

- **Burns to the eyes.** Do not attempt to open burned eyelids. Assure that the burn is thermal, not chemical. Apply dry, sterile dressing to both eyes to prevent simultaneous movement. Flush chemical burns with water for at least 20 minutes while en route to the hospital. Flush from the medial to the lateral side of the eye to avoid injury to the opposite eye.

- **Burns of the hands and toes.** Remove all rings and jewelry since they retain heat and the swelling from the burn may cause them to be constrictive. Separate all digits with dry, sterile dressings to prevent the digits from adhering to each other.

Dressing and Bandaging

The purpose of dressings is to cover open wounds and prevent further contamination. Dressings must be sterile or clean in order to prevent infection. Most dressings will come in various sizes in commercially wrapped or prepared packages. Use will vary depending on specific injured body area.

Bandages hold or secure dressings in place. These also are available in various sizes. While a bandage should be secure enough to hold a dressing, it should not restrict circulation distal to the wound. Use will depend on the type and location of the injured body area. Skill Summary 22-3 summarizes various types of dressing and bandaging.

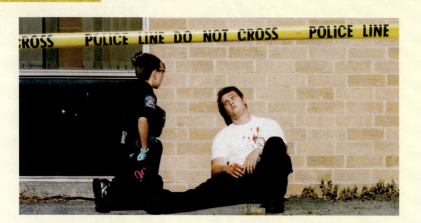

Dispatch: 2464 Kaiser Boulevard   **Man Down in Fight   1744 hrs**

Your ambulance is called to a fight in front of 2464 Kaiser Boulevard. You begin to drive to the scene and you are told by the dispatcher to stage at the corner of Kaiser and 22nd (two blocks away) until the police report the scene is secure.

Once the scene is reported to be secure, you enter in with caution. You observe the police questioning one man while another man is sitting on the ground with a laceration over his left eye. You speak to a police officer, who tells you that this was an apparent robbery. The perpetrator fled. The man being questioned was a witness. You put on gloves and protective eyewear and approach the patient.

Your initial observation is that the wound over the eye is only moderately bleeding, but the patient looks "bad." He tells you his name is Keith. He is slightly winded as he says his first name. Keith is 19 years old. During this initial conversation, he candidly tells you he was trying to buy heroin when he was robbed. He tells you that he got cut over his eye as he struggled against the man with the knife. Keith is oriented, but you are disturbed by his shortness of breath.

Keith's airway is clear. You cut off his T-shirt and find no wounds to his chest, but examination of his back reveals what appears to be a knife wound below his left shoulder blade an inch to the left of midline. His distress now makes a bit more sense. Your partner applies a three-sided occlusive dressing to the wound on the patient's back while you

listen to breath sounds. The sounds are diminished on the left side. You apply oxygen via a nonrebreather mask and begin plans for a priority transport of the patient. The rapid trauma assessment does not reveal further injuries. You observe the trachea in midline position. Vital signs are pulse 104 and weak, respirations 28 and labored, blood pressure 104/66, skin cool and moist, and pupils equal and reactive to light.

Keith is placed on the stretcher and moved to the ambulance. Three hospitals are within a 15-minute drive but only one of these is a trauma center, and you decide to transport the patient there. While in the ambulance, you perform a more detailed examination that does not reveal further injuries. You notify the hospital of the patent's condition and your ETA.

Reassessment of the patient's condition reveals a slight worsening of the respiratory distress, but Keith's breathing remains adequate. You verify that the oxygen is still flowing and reassess vital signs. His pulse is now 108 and weak, respirations 28 and labored, blood pressure 102/64, skin cool and moist, and pupils equal and reactive to light. Keith is beginning to get anxious and slightly combative as you arrive at the emergency department.

CASE DISCUSSION

This is a case where following both intuition and the assessment process paid off. The patient had an obvious wound in a visible spot.

Noting that the patient seemed short of breath, and noting the patient's young age at which lung conditions are not likely, further careful inspection in the initial assessment revealed a penetrating chest wound. This wound made the patient a high priority for transport and a candidate to be taken to a trauma center.

There were some interesting twists, such as the patient's admission that he was there to buy drugs. This had safety implications (this is an area where drugs are being sold) as well as the clinical implications of possibly having drugs in his system. If, in fact, the patient was taking heroin, that drug can be a powerful respiratory depressant that could worsen already serious injuries. Remember that even though police are on the scene, trouble can still erupt. At such a scene, always be alert for signs of danger such as developing unruly crowds, return of the perpetrator, or even the patient himself becoming increasingly violent or agitated.

Name: Keith Parks
Age: 19
Chief Complaint: Stab wound to chest/fight

ASSESSMENT INFORMATION	RELEVANCE TO THIS PATIENT
Dispatch information: "Fight"	Safety concerns should be paramount as you respond. The dispatcher acted appropriately in staging your ambulance away from (and out of sight of) the scene. Even once the police declare the scene "safe," you should still remain acutely aware of your surroundings and scan for dangers frequently.
Assessment: appearance of the patient	The patient looked "bad." You have likely seen both stable and unstable patients. Patients who are seriously ill or injured do sometimes look bad. If something isn't right, find out why. In this case, clinical intuition and good initial assessment led to the penetrating chest wound.
Assessment: the "chest" includes the back	Remember that wounds to the upper "back" are actually also to the upper chest—especially when it comes to penetrating injuries. If this was a gunshot with an exit wound in the chest, you would have to seal two open wounds.
Assessment: Drug use	• Heroin is a narcotic and will depress respirations. This is significant, especially in a patient with respiratory distress. • This information should also alert you to an increased potential for danger at the scene. • Beware when performing the assessment because many people inject heroin. The patient may have a hypodermic needle on his person, often reused or shared, which you would not want to be stuck with.
Assessment: midline trachea	One of the indicators of a worsening chest wound (a pneumothorax worsening to a tension pneumothorax) is the position of the trachea. If the trachea is shifted to one side (it will shift away from the damaged lung), it indicates a serious pressure increase within the chest.

SUMMARY

- Closed wounds are beneath intact or unbroken skin; open wounds damage the skin and sometimes the tissues below.

- There are several types of open wounds including abrasions, lacerations, amputations, avulsions, and penetrating wounds.

- Care for all open wounds includes exposing the injury, controlling bleeding, keeping the wound from becoming contaminated, dressing and bandaging the wound, and treating for shock as necessary.

- Burn injuries may be superficial, partial thickness, or full thickness depending on the depth of the burn.

- The Rule of Nines is a common method of determining the amount of body surface area burned.

- To care for burn injuries, be sure you are safe, then stop the burning process, if necessary. Watch for burns of the airway from flames or heated gases. Dress burns on the body with dry, sterile dressings.

- Burns to infants and children may be more severe than burns to adults due to fluid loss and body-surface considerations.

- Burns may also be caused by chemicals and radiation.

- Dressings are placed on a wound and should be sterile. Bandages hold dressings in place.

- Be sure to evaluate distal circulation after bandaging to be sure that it is not restricting circulation.

REVIEW QUESTIONS

1. A scrape, rubbing, or shearing of the outermost layer of skin is a(n):
   a. avulsion.
   b. abrasion.
   c. laceration.
   d. debridement.

2. With an evisceration, you should:
   a. push the protruding organ back into place.
   b. palpate the organ to determine if it is bleeding.
   c. cover the eviscerated organ with a saline-moistened sterile dressing.
   d. pack the exposed organ with ice packs.

3. You should handle an amputated body part by:
   a. placing it in a jar of water.
   b. placing it in a plastic bag with ice.
   c. wrapping it in dressing and putting it in a plastic bag on top of an ice pack or cooler.
   d. wrapping it in dressing and placing it beside the patient on the stretcher.

REVIEW QUESTIONS continued

4. The type of burn in which the patient presents with skin that is dry, hard, tough, and leathery and white-waxy to dark brown to black is a(n):

a. chemical burn.

b. partial-thickness burn.

c. superficial burn.

d. full-thickness burn.

5. Partial-thickness burn injuries covering what percentage of BSA should be considered critical?

a. 30 percent or more

b. 25 percent or more

c. 20 percent or more

d. 15 percent or more

WEB MEDIC

Visit Brady's *Essentials of Emergency Care* web site for direct web links. At **www.prenhall.com/limmer,** you will find information related to the following Chapter 22 topics:

- American Burn Association
- Crush injuries and crush syndrome
- Traumatic amputations
- Firearm injuries and fatalities
- Penetrating abdominal injuries

Chapter Twenty-Three

MUSCULOSKELETAL INJURIES

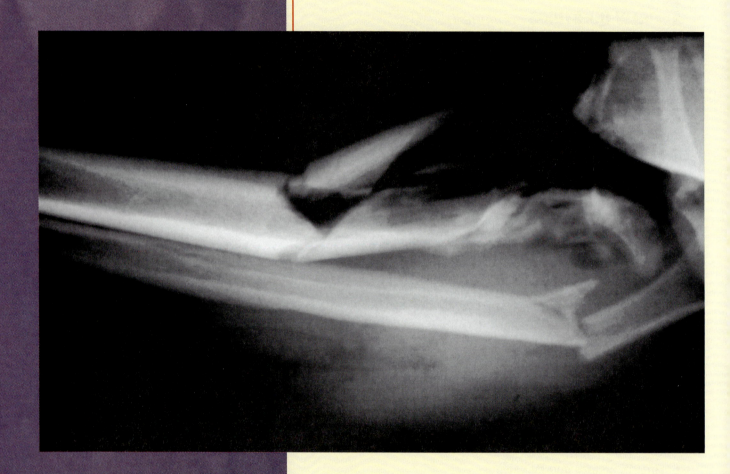

ESSENTIAL ELECTRONIC EXTRAS

CD ESSENTIALS

For preview and review of chapter material, see the student CD-ROM for

- Pretest
- Chapter quizzes
- Posttest

WEB ESSENTIALS

For additional review and enrichment, visit www.prenhall.com/limmer for

- Interactive student quizzes
- Links to online EMS resources
- Online case studies
- Audio glossary

njuries to the musculoskeletal system are very common in our fast-paced, action-oriented society. Injuries to muscles and bones can range from a low-priority injury in which the patient returns home from the hospital wearing a cast to an injury that can cause permanent disability or death. This chapter covers the spectrum of musculoskeletal injuries, with an emphasis on those injuries that can threaten a patient's life or limbs. Injuries to the bones of the head and chest are covered in other chapters of this book.

MUSCULOSKELETAL SYSTEM REVIEW

Some textbooks separate the musculoskeletal system into two body systems—the muscular system and the skeletal system. However, since both systems function to give the body its shape, provide for movement, and protect the body, they are often described as one complex system.

The Muscles

Muscles are classified into three types: skeletal, cardiac, and smooth muscles (Figure 23-1). The skeletal, or voluntary, muscles are under conscious control, which means you can direct them to move the body. **Voluntary muscles,** which are attached to the long bones, account for the bulk of the body mass. **Cardiac muscle** is comprised of specialized involuntary muscle cells that provide contraction and electrical stimulation of the heart. Smooth muscles, also known as **involuntary muscles,** control movement of materials through the gastrointestinal tract, lungs, blood vessels, and urinary system. For example, when constriction of the blood vessels is needed to compensate for blood loss, such as occurs in compensated shock, the smooth muscles see to it that the job gets done.

As an experienced EMT-B, you are familiar with the names of a number of the major muscles in the body. Muscles are usually named in reference to the bones they support and their insertion points on the bone. For example, one of the accessory muscles that moves the chest when a patient in respiratory distress attempts to breathe is the sternocleidomastoid muscle. This muscle is positioned from the sternum, over the clavicle, and inserts into the mastoid area of the skull, the bony area posterior to the ears on the lateral skull.

The Bones

Bones are classified with words that describe their appearance—long, short, flat, or irregular. The bones in the arms and legs are long bones. The majority of the short bones are in the hands and feet. The sternum, shoulder blades, and ribs are flat bones. The vertebrae are considered irregular-shaped bones. A bone is covered with a strong, white, fibrous membrane called **periosteum,** which contains the bone's blood supply and nerves. It is the periosteum that accounts for much of the bleeding and causes swelling of the soft tissue when a bone is injured.

There are two major divisions of the skeleton—axial and appendicular (Figure 23-2). The **axial** division includes the skull, spine, and ribs. The **appendicular** division includes the bones of the arms and legs, as well as the bones that comprise the joints that hold the limbs in place, such as the pelvis and the shoulder.

As an experienced EMT-B, you frequently refer to the bones by their medical names. Figure 23-3 provides a quick review of the body's major bone groupings.

CORE CONCEPTS

In this chapter, you will learn about the following topics:

- The major bones and regions of the musculoskeletal system
- How to identify open and closed extremity injuries
- The purposes and general procedures for splinting
- How to splint injured extremities

DOT OBJECTIVES

✔ **Attitude**

☐ **1.** Explain the rationale for splinting at the scene versus load and go. (p. 344)

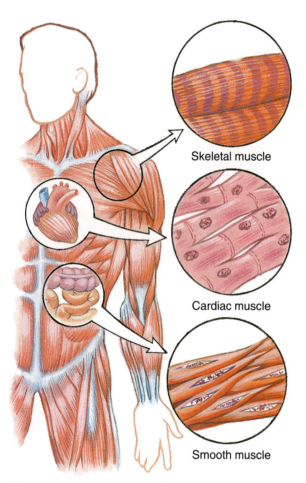

Figure 23-1 There are three types of muscles in the human body.

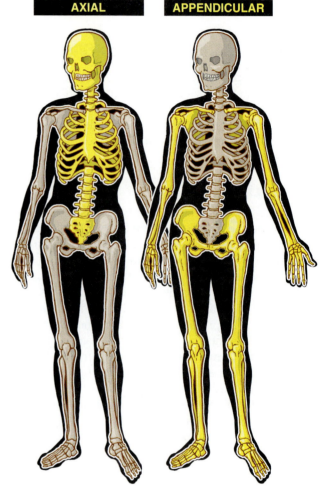

Figure 23-2 Two major division of the human skeleton: axial and appendicular.

LIFESPAN DEVELOPMENT

When fractures occur near the ends of long bones in children, they must be managed carefully. A bone's growth plates are located at the ends of the bone. A serious fracture in these locations can result in the permanent shortening of a limb.

■ **Skull.** The skull consists of the facial bones anteriorly and the **cranium** on the lateral, posterior, and superior sides. The upper jaw is the **maxilla;** the lower moveable jaw is the **mandible.** When we refer to the regions of the cranium, we refer to the top and sides as the **parietal,** the anterior sides as the **temporal,** the forehead as **frontal,** and the back as **occipital.**

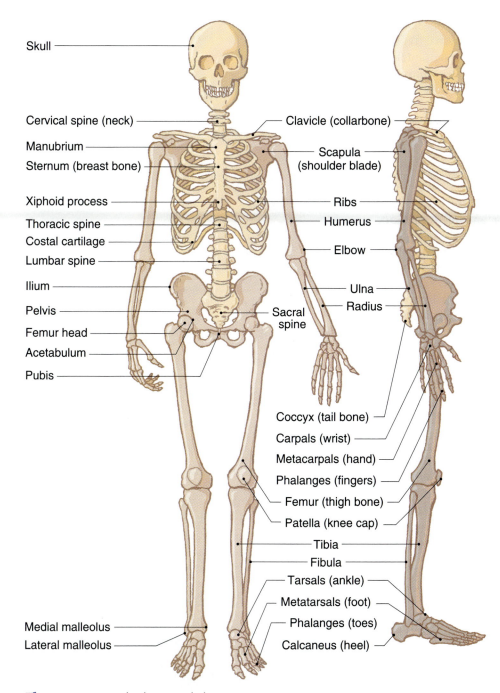

Skull

Cervical spine (neck)

Manubrium

Sternum (breast bone)

Xiphoid process

Thoracic spine

Costal cartilage

Lumbar spine

Ilium

Pelvis

Femur head

Acetabulum

Pubis

Clavicle (collarbone)

Scapula
(shoulder blade)

Ribs

Humerus

Elbow

Ulna

Radius

Sacral
spine

Coccyx (tail bone)

Carpals (wrist)

Metacarpals (hand)

Phalanges (fingers)

Femur (thigh bone)

Patella (knee cap)

Tibia

Fibula

Tarsals (ankle)

Metatarsals (foot)

Phalanges (toes)

Calcaneus (heel)

Medial malleolus

Lateral malleolus

Figure 23-3 The human skeleton.

- **Spinal column.** It consists of 33 vertebrae stacked one on top of another. The vertebrae are broken down into five divisions: the 7 cervical vertebrae found in the neck, the 12 thoracic vertebrae corresponding with the ribs and upper back, the 5 lumbar vertebrae in the lower back, the 5 fused sacral vertebrae that make up the posterior wall of the pelvis, and the 4 fused coccyx vertebrae, or tailbone.

- **Thorax.** The thorax, or chest, is made up of 12 pairs of ribs, the **sternum** (breast bone), and the

thoracic spine that surround and protect the heart, lungs, and great vessels. All 12 pairs of ribs attach to the spine in the back, yet only 10 pair attach to the sternum in the front. The two remaining bottom pairs are called "floating ribs." The sternum is a flat bone with three sections: the **manubrium,** or superior portion, the body, or center, and the **xiphoid process,** which is the inferior tip.

- **Pelvis.** This is a bowl-shaped structure composed of three major pairs of fused bones: the **ilium,** or major bone that your belt rests on laterally, the

ischium in the inferior posterior section, used as the attachment point for the traditional bipolar traction splint, and the **pubis** in the anterior, which protects the urinary bladder. The ilium joins with the sacral spine posteriorly to support the spinal column. The hip joints are formed laterally by the pelvic bones which create the socket called the **acetabulum** to which the ball-shaped head of the femur connects.

- **Upper extremities.** The upper extremities include your shoulder, which is made up of the **clavicle,** or collarbone, on the anterior surface, the **scapula,** or shoulder blade, in the posterior, and the **acromion,** the highest portion of the shoulder which with the clavicle forms the **acromioclavicular joint.** The arm consists of three bones which meet at the elbow: the humerus, or upper arm, the **radius** on the thumb side of the forearm, and the **ulna** on the pinky side of the forearm. The wrist bones are the **carpals;** the hand is made up of the **metacarpals,** and the fingers are the **phalanges.**

- **Lower extremities.** These include your leg which is made up of the **femur,** or thigh bone, the **tibia,** or long bone that forms the anterior surface of your lower leg, and the **fibula,** the thin bone on the lateral surface of your lower leg. The knee cap is called the **patella;** the bony prominence on the outside of the ankle is the lateral **malleolus;** the one on the inside of your ankle is the medial malleolus. The ankle joint itself is made up of the tarsal bones and the distal tibia and fibula; the foot includes the **tarsal** and **metatarsal** bones; and the toes, like the fingers, are called **phalanges.**

The connective tissue that helps to support the bones and muscles, especially where they join together, consists of cartilage, tendons, and ligaments. **Cartilage** is tough tissue that covers the joint ends of bones, as well as helps to form certain body parts such as the ear. **Tendons** are designed to connect the muscles to the bones. **Ligaments** act as fibrous elastic bands binding bones to bones (Figure 23-4).

For field purposes, EMT-Bs treat all **painful, swollen, deformed extremities (PSDE)** as if they were fractures by immobilizing them.

INJURIES TO THE MUSCULOSKELETAL SYSTEM

As you know, the EMT-B curriculum focuses on the assessment-based, or complaint-based, approach rather than the diagnosis-based approach used in the past. For example, in the past, if a patient complained of a painful, swollen, deformed extremity, we called the

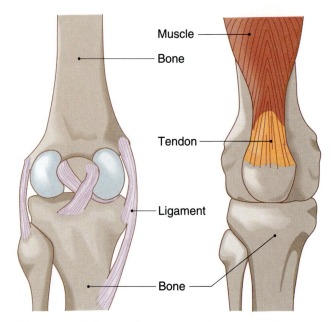

Figure 23-4   Tendons tie muscle to bone. Ligaments tie bone to bone.

injury either a "possible fracture" or an actual fracture if the extremity was severely angulated (bent) or if a bone was actually protruding. We also attempted to diagnose the injury. In fact, EMT texts of the past often showed x-ray pictures of various fractures that were named "greenstick," "oblique," "comminuted," or "transverse." Today's assessment-based approach uses the patient's complaint to name a musculoskeletal injury "a painful, swollen, deformed extremity (PSDE)." Since in the field the treatment for a fracture, dislocation, sprain, or strain is basically the same, there is no longer a need to distinguish among these injuries.

LIFESPAN DEVELOPMENT

Directing or twisting forces such as those that occur from tripping on a throw rug and falling onto a hard floor can cause a hip fracture. Elderly patients are more susceptible to this type of injury because of brittle bones or bones weakened by osteoporosis. Always be sure to evaluate the possibility that a syncopal episode or cardiac dysrhythmias may have caused the fall. It is also good advice to tell the family to not use throw rugs in an elderly person's home!

However, to ensure that you will understand the Emergency Department physician and other health professionals when they use medical terminology that refers to musculoskeletal injuries, some common terms follow for your review: A **fracture** is any break in a bone. It can be **angulated** (the broken bone is bent at an angle) and either open or closed (Figure 23-5). A **dislocation** is the disruption of the joint due to the tearing of the joint capsule and the soft tissue that surrounds it, such as occurs in a dislocated shoulder. It is important to note that many dislocations are accompanied by a nearby fracture. Since you do not have an x-ray or the ability to diagnose the injury in the field, treat dislocations as if they also have a fracture and immobilize them. A **sprain** is the stretching or tearing of muscles or ligaments. A **strain** is the stretching of muscle or tendon beyond its normal range of motion.

It is important for you to be able to differentiate between an open and a closed PSDE. The **open PSDE** has a laceration at the site of the injury, which is usually due to the bone breaking through the skin. In some instances, the bone may be protruding, but in others, the bone may pop back into place on its own. With a **closed PSDE,** there is no evidence that the bone ends have broken through the skin. To set a fracture, a physician first realigns the broken bone ends. This is called "reducing the fracture." At times, when you are attempting to move the bones of an angulated fracture into a splintable position, you may accidentally reduce it.

When treating a closed PSDE, it is important that you splint the injury where you find the patient by immobilizing the bone ends and two adjacent joints.

This will prevent the fracture from breaking through the skin and becoming an open fracture. Through gentle handling and splinting of closed fractures, EMT-Bs can help reduce the patient's pain, prevent lengthy hospital stays, and lower health care costs.

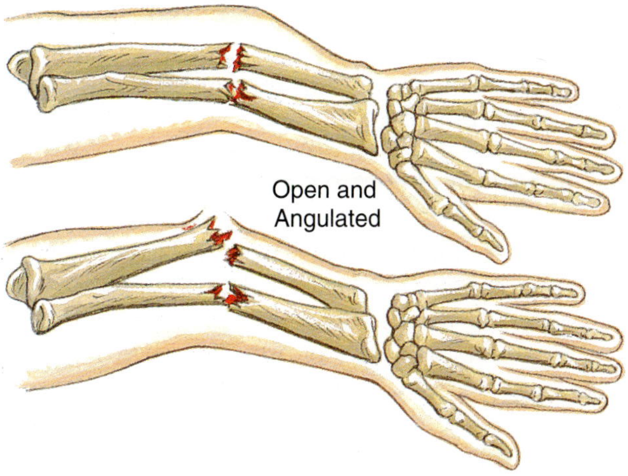

Patient Assessment

Musculoskeletal Injuries

First, make sure the scene is safe and that you will not become a victim of the same mechanism of injury as the patient. When assessing the musculoskeletal injury, expose it by removing at least part of the patient's clothing. Of course, the decision to expose an injury depends on weather conditions, the patient's degree of modesty, the severity of the injury, and patient refusal.

The signs and symptoms of a musculoskeletal injury include:

- Pain and tenderness
- Deformity or angulation
- Grating, or **crepitus,** which is the sound or feeling caused by broken bone ends rubbing together
- Swelling (Do not forget to remove the patient's jewelry before it needs to be cut off.)
- Bruising (**ecchymosis,** or large black-and-blue discoloration of the skin, which indicates an injury that is hours to days old)
- Exposed bone ends
- Joints locked into position
- Nerve or blood vessel compromise
- Inability to move the extremity ✴

Closed

Open and Angulated

Figure 23-5 Injuries to the bones may be open or closed and angulated (bent).

PRECEPTOR PEARL

Tell new EMT-Bs that they should not allow a grotesque PSDE to distract them from performing the initial and rapid trauma assessments and from making a priority decision. Also, remind them to always expose the injury. If an EMT-B fails to expose the injury prior to splinting, what he or she thought was a closed injury might actually be an open one and the protruding bone ends may grab a woman's stockings or skin-tight sportswear and pull them into the wound!

Patient Care

Musculosketal Injuries

Most fractures, though painful and disabling, are rarely fatal. To care for a patient with a musculoskeletal injury:

1 Take BSI precautions.

2 Perform the initial assessment. Attend to any life-threatening injuries quickly. Manually stabilize the trauma patient's cervical spine, assess the airway, assure that breathing is adequate, and administer oxygen. Perform a rapid trauma assessment, control severe bleeding, and manage shock.

3 Determine patient priority. For a high-priority patient, you may need to apply a long backboard for a total body splint rather than take time to splint individual fractures. Control any bleeding, apply sterile dressings if needed, and attempt to maintain body temperature.

If the patient is a low priority, apply individual splints, apply a cold pack to the injury site to minimize swelling, and elevate the splinted extremity.

Always be sure to assess and reassess the distal PMS (pulses, motor function, and sensation) before and after application of a splint. Document your findings on your prehospital care report (PCR). ✱

PRECEPTOR PEARL

Tell new EMT-Bs to remember: when a bone breaks, it bleeds. Therefore, a patient with multiple breaks can easily be in shock from significant blood loss. In the first two hours of an uncomplicated simple fracture of the tibia and fibula, a patient can lose a pint of blood. A fractured femur can cause a two-pint blood loss. A pelvic fracture can cause a three- to four-pint loss.

Splinting

The purpose of splinting is simply to immobilize the bone ends and the adjacent joints. Doing so minimizes the movement of the disrupted joints or broken bone ends, decreases the patient's pain, and helps to prevent any additional damage to nerves, arteries, veins, and muscles. A properly applied splint can prevent a closed fracture from becoming an open one, as well as minimize blood loss. In addition, splinting on a backboard prevents injury to the spinal cord and helps to prevent permanent paralysis.

When distal circulation is compromised, as in an angulated fracture or a cyanotic or pulseless limb, the lack of circulation causes oxygen-starved tissues to begin to die. Although the thought of realigning an extremity can be a frightening one, the experienced EMT-B knows that if the extremity is not realigned, a splint is often ineffective and can cause increased pain and possible further injury to the patient.

So, to realign a PSDE: while a partner places one hand above and one hand below the injury site, the first EMT-B grasps the distal extremity. The partner supports the site while the first EMT-B pulls gentle traction in the direction of the long bone axis of the extremity. If resistance is felt or if it appears as if the bone ends will come through the skin, stop realignment and splint in the position found. If no resistance is felt, maintain gentle traction until the extremity is splinted.

PRECEPTOR PEARL

Tell new EMT-Bs to always immobilize a stable patient in the spot where he or she is found. However, the actual extremity will need to be moved into a "splintable" position, which is straight enough to fit on a padded board. As the saying goes "immobilize them where they lie not as they lie."

Splinting Rules

Keep in mind these general rules of splinting:

- If the patient is unstable, do not waste time splinting. Care for life-threatening problems first. Then align the musculoskeletal injuries in anatomical position and immobilize the patient's entire body on a long spine board.

- The method of splinting is dictated by the patient's status and priority for transport. If the patient is a high priority for "load and go," choose a rapid method of splinting such as a long backboard (fastest method but only slightly better than no splinting) or the PASG for multiple-fractured legs. If the patient is a low priority, use a slower but more effective splinting method.

- If a patient must be rapidly removed from a car prior to splinting, try to stabilize the injured leg to the uninjured leg until you have the time to do the splinting.

- Before moving the injured extremity, expose it and control bleeding.

- Assess for and record distal PMS before and after splinting.

- To be effective a splint must immobilize the bone ends and two adjacent joints.

- If severe deformity exists or distal circulation is compromised, align long-bone injuries to anatomical position under gentle traction.

- Do not attempt to push protruding bones back into place. If they accidentally slip back into place during realignment, inform the Emergency Department staff and document this occurrence on your prehospital care report.

- Pad the voids between the body part and the splint to increase patient comfort and ensure proper immobilization. Many rigid splints do not conform to body curves and allow too much movement of the limb.

- The exception to the rules of splinting long bones is the femur, which is splinted using a traction splint.

Splinting Complications

Occasionally there are complications from splinting. Carefully observe for the following:

- *The EMT-B who forgets that the patient is high priority.* If the patient has a life-threatening problem, remember to expedite the splinting and concentrate on airway, breathing, and circulation problems.

- *A splint that is applied too tightly.* This can compress soft tissue and injure nerves, blood vessels, and muscles.

- *A splint that is applied too loosely.* This may allow too much movement and has the potential of converting a closed fracture into an open one or cause further soft-tissue damage.

- *A splinted extremity that is not realigned.* This can create further damage.

There are many types of splints for long bones such as rigid, formable, and traction splints. No matter what type of splint is used, the general procedures and rules remain the same. The procedure for immobilizing a long bone is shown in Skill Summary 23-1. The procedure for immobilizing a joint is shown in Skill Summary 23-2.

Splinting the Upper Extremities

Patients with a clavicle injury complain of pain in the shoulder, and you may observe a dropped shoulder (Figure 23-6). The patient is often found holding the injured arm against the chest. Sometimes a sharp blow to the shoulder blade injures the scapula. If, upon palpation of the entire shoulder, the head of the humerus is felt in front of the shoulder, this may indicate an anterior shoulder dislocation or fracture.

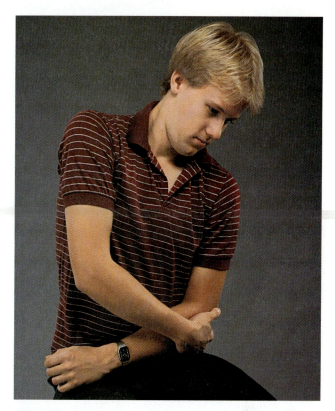

Figure 23-6   A fractured clavicle may present as a "dropped" shoulder.

If a dislocation or fracture occurs and the patient is found in this position, tie a blanket roll under the arm and around the body to give the patient something on which to rest the injured arm. Then apply a sling and swathe. Do not attempt to straighten or reduce any dislocations. Occasionally, some patients may pop their shoulder back into place. If this occurs, be sure to assess distal PMS, note the self-reduction on your PCR, and report it to the Emergency Department staff.

The sling and swathe is very useful for splinting a number of upper extremity PSDEs. The procedure for applying a sling and swathe is reviewed in Skill Summary 23-3 and also is shown as a means of splinting an injury to the humerus in Skill Summary 23-4. The sling and swathe can also be combined with the use of board splints, as shown in the care of the arm and elbow injuries (Skill Summary 23-5) and in the care of injuries to the forearm, wrist, and hand (Skill Summary 23-6).

PRECEPTOR PEARL

Tell new EMT-Bs that if a patient has a possible neck injury, never wrap a sling around the patient's neck.

Always take BSI precautions first.

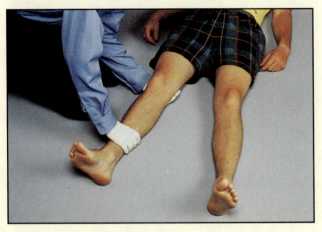

▲ **1.** Manually stabilize the limb.

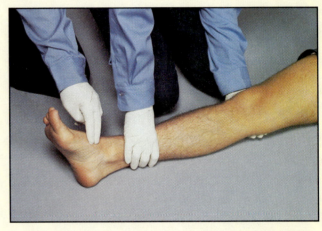

▲ **2.** Assess distal pulse, motor function, and sensation (PMS).

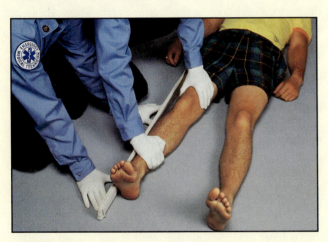

▲ **3.** Measure the splint. It should extend several inches beyond joints above and below the injury site.

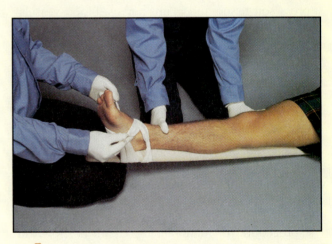

▲ **4.** Apply the splint and immobilize the joints above and below the injury site.

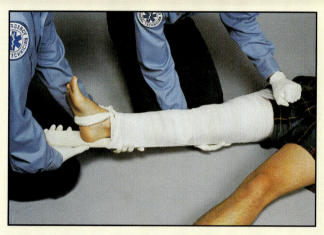

▲ **5.** Secure the entire injured extremity.

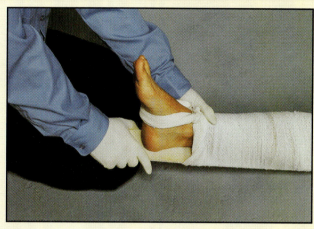

▲ **6.** Secure the foot in a position of function (as shown) . . .

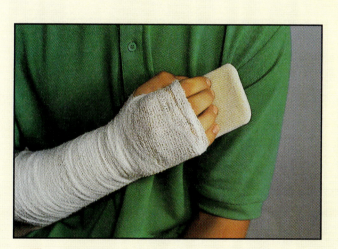

▲ **7.** . . . or if splinting an arm, secure the hand in a position of function with a roll of bandages.

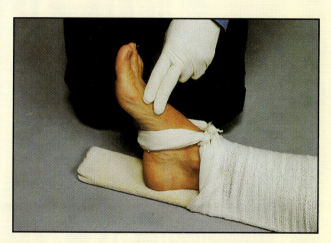

▲ **8.** Reassess distal pulse, motor function, and sensation (PMS).

Always take BSI precautions first.

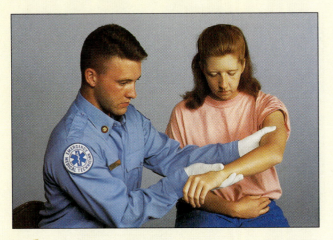

▲ **1.** Manually stabilize the limb.

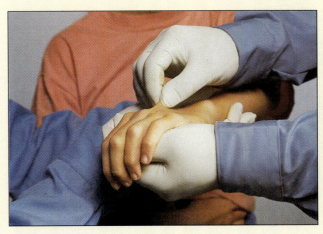

▲ **2.** Assess distal pulse, motor function, and sensation (PMS).

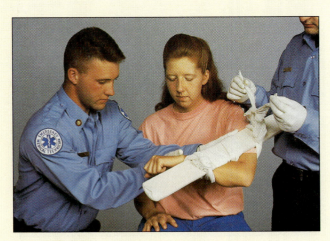

▲ **3.** Select proper splint material. Immobilize the site of injury and bones above and below it.

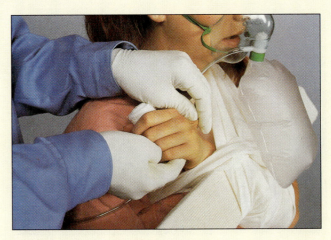

▲ **4.** Reassess distal pulse, motor function, and sensation (PMS).

Always take BSI precautions first.

A sling is a triangular bandage used to support the shoulder and arm. Once the patient's arm is placed in a sling, a swathe can be used to hold the arm against the side of the chest. Commercial slings are available. Velcro® straps may be used to form a swathe. Use whatever materials you have on hand, provided they will not cut into the patient.

NOTE: If the patient has a cervical-spine injury, do not tie a sling around his or her neck.

Always assess distal pulse, motor function, and sensation (PMS) both before and after immobilizing an extremity.

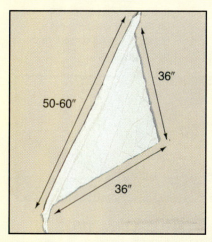

▲ **1.** The sling should be in the shape of a triangle.

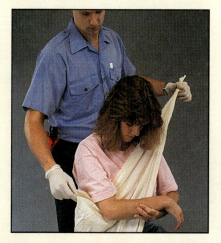

▲ **2.** Position the sling over the top of the patient's chest as shown. Fold the patient's injured arm across the chest.

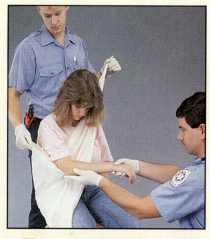

▲ **3.** If the patient cannot hold her arm, have someone assist until you tie the sling.

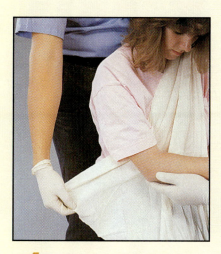

▲ **4.** Extend one point of the triangle behind the elbow on the injured side.

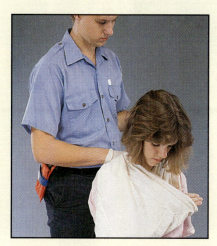

▲ **5.** Take the bottom point of the triangle and bring this end up over the patient's arm. When you are finished, take this point over the top of the patient's injured shoulder.

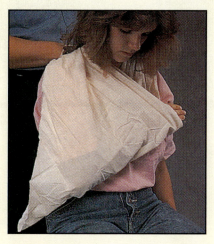

▲ **6.** Draw up the ends of the sling so that the patient's hand is about four inches above the elbow (exceptions are discussed later).

(continued)

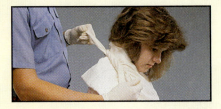

▲ **7.** Tie the two ends of the sling together, making sure that the knot does not press against the back of the patient's neck. The area may be padded with bulky dressings.

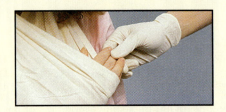

▲ **8.** Leave the patient's fingertips exposed to permit assessment of distal pulses, motor function, and sensation (PMS).

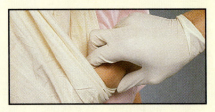

▲ **9.** Assess distal pulse, motor function, and sensation (PMS). If the pulse has been lost, take off the sling and reassess. Repeat the sling procedure if necessary.

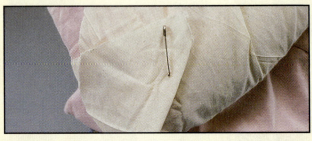

▲ **10a.** Take hold of the point of material at the patient's elbow and fold it forward, pinning it to the front of the sling. This forms a pocket for the patient's elbow.

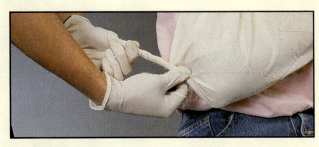

▲ **10b.** If you do not have a pin, twist the excess material and tie a knot in the point.

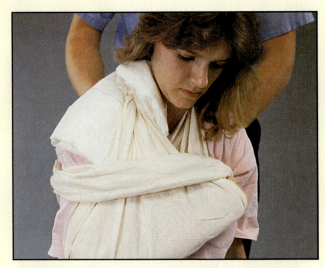

▲ **11.** Form a swathe from a second piece of triangular material. Tie it around the chest and the injured arm, over the sling. Do not place it over the patient's arm on the uninjured side.

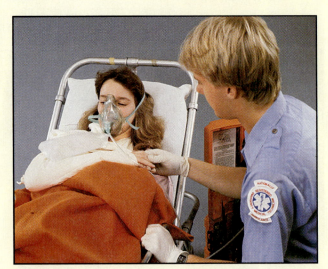

▲ **12.** Assess distal pulse, motor function, and sensation (PMS). Treat for shock, including administration of high-concentration oxygen. Take vital signs, and perform detailed and ongoing assessments as appropriate.

Injury to the Humerus— Soft Splinting

23-4

Variations for the Sling and Swathe

Always take BSI precautions first.

NOTE: Use rigid splints whenever possible to immobilize an injured humerus. However, depending on the size of the patient and equipment available, this may not be possible. Even with the use of rigid splints, a sling and swathe will be necessary to immobilize the elbow and shoulder (the adjacent joints).

You may have heard that the EMT-B was required to determine where on the injured extremity the suspected fracture was located (shaft, proximal or distal ends). This is unrealistic without the use of x-rays. Splinting of the humerus should be done with the goals of maximizing patient comfort and proper immobilization.

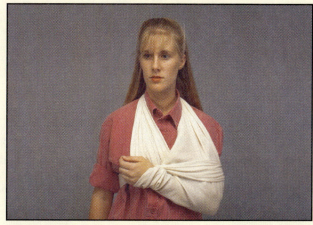

Variation 1 Apply a sling and swathe as shown. If you have only enough material for a swathe, you may bind the patient's upper arm to her body, taking great care not to cut off circulation to the forearm.

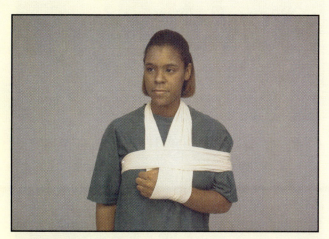

Variation 2 If you have only a short length of material to use as a sling, you may apply it so that it supports the wrist only.

WARNING: Before applying a sling and swathe to an injured humerus, check for distal PMS. If you do not feel a pulse and the patient has a closed fracture, attempt to straighten any slight angulation. Should straightening of the angulation fail to restore PMS, splint with a medium board splint, keeping the forearm extended. If there is no sign of PMS, you will have to attempt a second splinting. If this fails to restore distal PMS, transport immediately. Do not try to straighten angulation of the humerus if there are any signs of fracture or dislocation of the shoulder or elbow.

Elbow Injuries

Always take BSI precautions first.

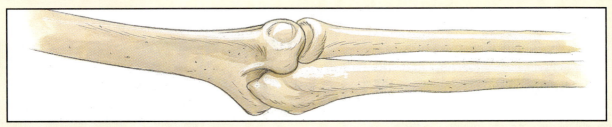

The elbow is a joint, not a bone. It is composed of the distal humerus and the proximal ulna and radius, forming a hinge joint. You will have to decide if the injury is truly to the elbow. Deformity and sensitivity will direct you to the injury site.

NOTE: Always assess distal pulse, motor function, and sensation (PMS) both before and after immobilizing an extremity.

CARE: If there is a distal pulse, the dislocated elbow should be immobilized in the position in which it is found. The joint has too many nerves and blood vessels to risk movement. When a distal pulse is absent, make one attempt to slightly reposition the limb after contacting medical direction. Do not force the limb into the anatomical position.

Elbow in or Returned to Bent Position

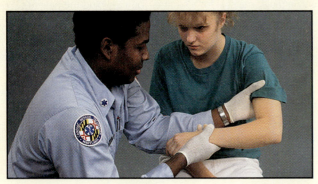

▲ **1.** Move limb only if necessary for splinting or if pulse is absent. Do not continue if you meet resistance or significantly increase the pain

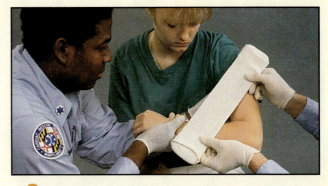

▲ **2.** Use a padded board splint that will extend 2 to 6 inches beyond the arm and wrist when placed diagonally.

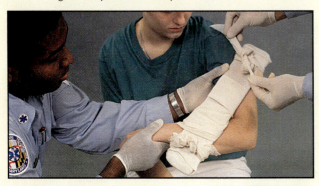

▲ **3.** Place the splint so it is just proximal to the elbow and to the wrist. Use cravats to secure to the forearm, then the arm.

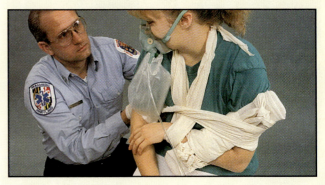

▲ **4.** Apply a wrist sling to support the limb. Keep the elbow exposed. Apply a swathe if possible.

Always take BSI precautions first.

Elbow in Straight Position

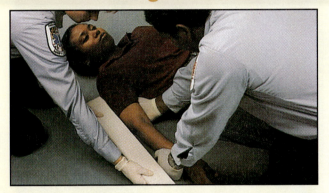

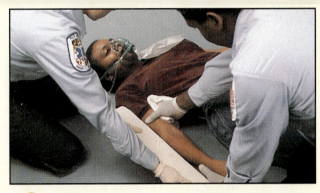

▲ **1.** Assess distal PMS.

▲ **2.** Use a padded board splint that extends from under the armpit to a point past the fingertips. Pad the armpit.

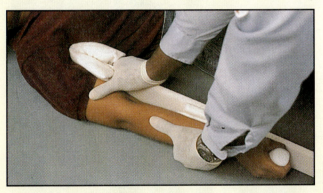

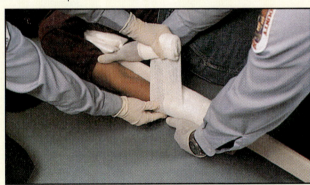

▲ **3.** Place a roll of bandages in the patient's hand to help maintain position of function. Place padded side of board against medial side of limb. Pad all voids.

▲ **4.** Secure the splint. Leave fingertips exposed.

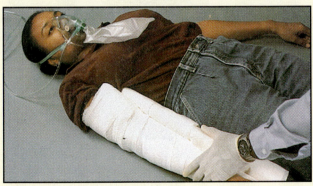

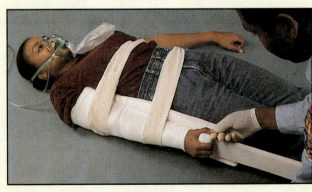

▲ **5.** Place pads between patient's side and splint.

▲ **6.** Secure the splinted limb to the patient's body with two cravats. Avoid placing them over the suspected injury site. Reassess distal PMS.

Always take BSI precautions first.

SIGNS:
- Forearm—deformity and tenderness. If only one bone is broken, deformity may be minor or absent.
- Wrist—deformity and tenderness.
- Hand—deformity and pain. Dislocated fingers are obvious.

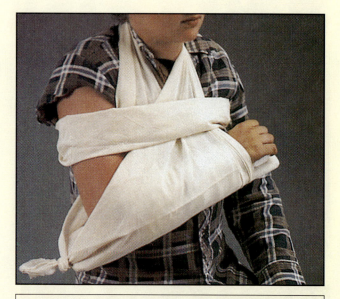

CARE: Injuries occurring to the forearm, wrist, or hand can be splinted using a padded rigid splint that extends from the elbow past the fingertips. The patient's elbow, forearm, wrist, and hand all need the support of the splint. Tension must be provided throughout the splinting. A roll of bandage should be placed in the hand to ensure a position of function. After rigid splinting, apply a sling and swathe.

NOTE: Always assess distal pulse, motor function, and sensation (PMS) before and after immobilizing an extremity.

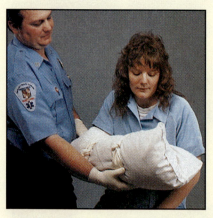
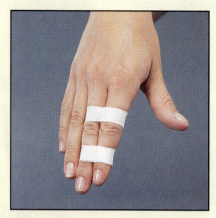
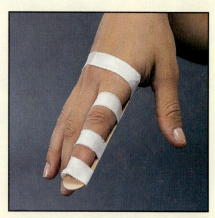

ALTERNATIVE CARE: Injuries to the hand and wrist can be cared for with soft splinting. Place a roll of bandage in the hand to maintain a position of function. Then tie the forearm, wrist, and hand into the fold of one pillow or between two pillows. An injured finger may be taped to an adjacent uninjured finger or splinted with a tongue depressor. Some emergency department physicians prefer that care be limited to a wrap of soft bandages. **NOTE: Do not try to "pop" dislocated fingers back into place.**

Splinting the Lower Extremities

Injuries to the pelvis can be very serious because of the potential for extreme blood loss and internal organ injury. The patient with a pelvic injury may complain of pain in the pelvis, hips, groin, or lower back. Often there is no deformity, but the mechanism of injury leads you to suspect a pelvic injury. The patient may have pain upon palpation of the iliac wings or the pubic bone or an unexplained pressure on the urinary bladder accompanied by a feeling of the need to urinate. The patient may be unable to lift the leg when supine, or the foot on the injured side may turn outward (lateral rotation). This rotation may also indicate a hip fracture.

It is difficult to distinguish between a fractured pelvis and a fracture of the upper femur. If in doubt, treat the patient for a pelvic fracture. Move the patient as little as possible and *never* log roll him. Straighten both of the patient's legs and place a folded blanket between them extending from the groin to the feet. Bind the legs and the blanket together with a series of cravats (Figure 23-7).

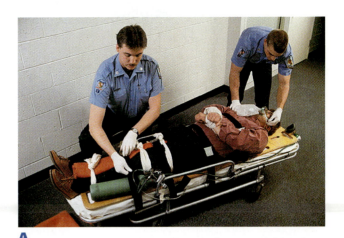

A

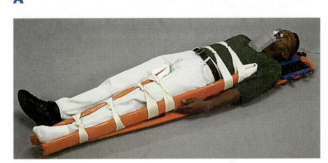

B

Figure 23-7 Immobilize a patient with a hip or pelvic injury (A) by binding the legs together, or (B) with a padded long board.

PRECEPTOR PEARL

Tell new EMT-Bs that when splinting multiple fractures, they should consider the "whole patient" before deciding on the immobilization device. If a patient is stable and has a fractured tibia and femur, a long board splint is appropriate. However, if the patient has signs and symptoms of shock or has sustained other multiple injuries, the use of the PASG is more appropriate, since both shock and the fracture can be treated at the same time.

Some EMS systems use the PASG for pelvic injuries, as well as to control shock and splint hip, femoral, and multiple-leg fractures. A PASG is strongly indicated for use with a pelvic fracture accompanied by hypotension (blood pressure below 90). If this is your EMS system's protocol, follow the application of the device shown in Skill Summary 23-7. A physician must order the removal of a PASG.

A hip dislocation (Figure 23-8) occurs when the head of the femur moves out of its socket. (It is difficult to tell the difference between a hip injury and a proximal femur injury.) Patients who have had a surgical hip replacement are at greater risk for a dislocation. In an anterior dislocation, the hip is flexed and the leg is externally rotated. In a posterior dislocation, the leg is dislocated inward, the hip is flexed, and the knee is bent. Often there is a lack of sensation in the limb due to injury to the sciatic nerve. This

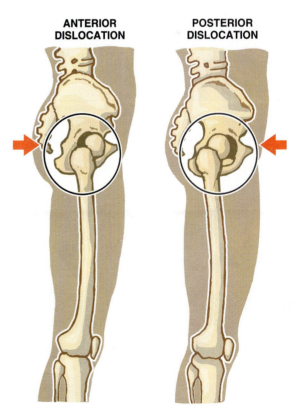

ANTERIOR DISLOCATION   POSTERIOR DISLOCATION

Figure 23-8 Anterior and posterior hip dislocation.

Always take BSI precautions first.

Follow local protocol regarding application and inflation of the anti-shock garment (also called MAST).

NOTE: In the photos below, the patient's clothing remains on for demonstration purposes only. For actual use of the PASG, the patient's clothing should be removed.

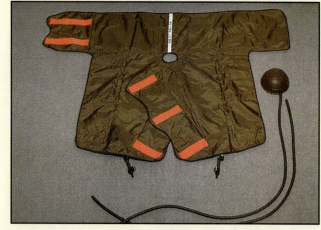

Pneumatic anti-shock garment and inflation pump.

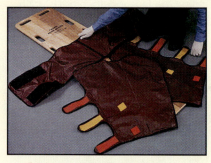

▲ **1.** Unfold the garment and lay it flat on a backboard. It should be smoothed of wrinkles.

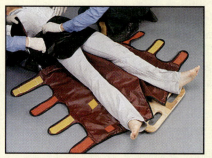

▲ **2.** Log roll the patient onto the garment, or slide it under the patient. The upper edge of the garment must be just below the rib cage.

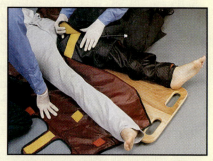

▲ **3.** Enclose the left leg, securing the Velcro® straps.

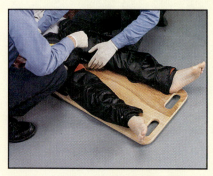

▲ **4.** Enclose the right leg, securing the Velcro® straps.

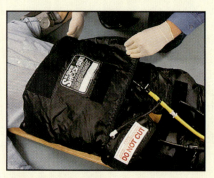

▲ **5.** Enclose the abdomen and pelvis, securing the Velcro® straps.

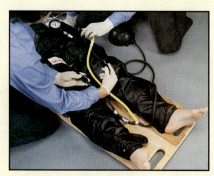

▲ **6.** Check the tubes leading to the compartments and the pump.

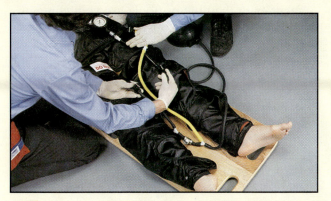

▲ **7.** Open the stopcocks to the legs and close the abdominal compartment stopcock.

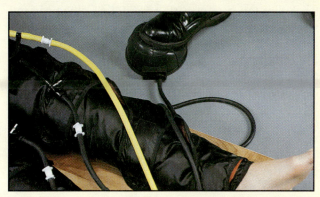

▲ **8.** Use the pump to inflate the lower compartments simultaneously. Inflate until the Velcro® makes a crackling noise.

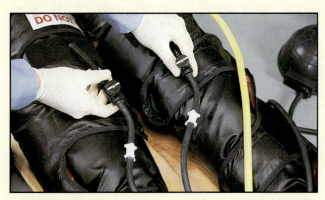

▲ **9.** Close the stopcocks.

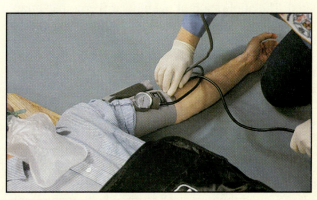

▲ **10.** Check the patient's blood pressure.

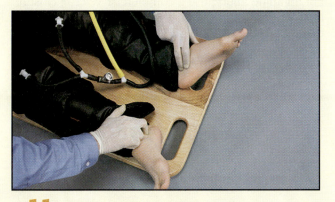

▲ **11.** Check both extremities for distal pulse.

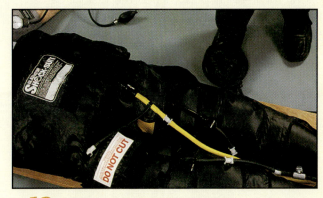

▲ **12.** If systolic BP is still below 90 mmHg, open the stopcock and inflate the abdominal compartment. Close the stopcock.

NOTE: Monitor and record vital signs every 5 minutes. If the garment loses pressure, add air as needed. Some protocols call for simultaneous inflation of all three compartments of the garment. Always follow local protocols. Some systems require on-line medical direction to inflate.

type of injury often occurs in a motor-vehicle collision when the occupant's knees strike the dash. A patient with a suspected hip dislocation may be splinted on a long backboard (as described for a pelvis injury), or a padded board that extends from the armpit to the foot can be placed between the patient's legs and secured with cravats.

Splint the patient with a PSDE that obviously involves the femur with a traction splint. The injured leg will often appear shortened due to the overriding of the bone ends, and the patient may have intense pain. The traction splint is needed because the large muscles surrounding the femur, the quadriceps, and hamstrings, go into spasm and literally can grind down the ends of the broken bone. This causes severe pain, additional soft-tissue injury, and bleeding. The traction counteracts the muscle spasms and reduces the pain.

There are two types of traction devices frequently used: the bipolar, with two poles, such as the Hare® or Fernotrac® traction splint, and the unipolar, with one pole, such as the Sager® traction splint. The unipolar units are less likely to lose traction when the patient is lifted. The application of the bipolar (Fernotrac®) traction splint is shown in Skill Summary 23-8. A variation of the traction splint is shown in Skill Summary 23-9. The unipolar (Sager®) device is shown in Skill Summary 23-10, and the Kendrick traction device is shown in Skill Summary 23-11.

If you suspect a fracture to the knee or tibia/fibula, do not use the traction splint. Apply the ankle hitch as shown in Skill Summary 23-12.

Knee injuries can be very complex. The patella can become displaced when the lower leg is twisted and can cause ligament damage. A knee dislocation occurs when the tibia itself is forced either anteriorly or posteriorly in relation to the distal femur. Always check for a distal pulse, since the dislocated knee joint can compress the popliteal artery and stop the major blood supply to the lower leg. If there is no pulse, contact medical direction for permission to gently move the leg anteriorly to allow for a pulse and transport the patient immediately. The splinting of a bent knee using a technique called "triangulation" with two long board splints is shown in Skill Summary 23-13, and the splinting of the straight knee is shown in Skill Summary 23-14.

Injuries to the tibia or fibula are very common. Sometimes they are very obvious due to the deformity accompanying them, while other times they are quite subtle and are only found on an x-ray in the Emergency Department (Figure 23-9). When the "shin" area of the tibia is broken, there is always the danger of mishandling the injury, turning a simple (closed) fracture into a compound (open) fracture.

If you reach down and touch your shin, you can feel that the bone is very close to the skin. When excessive patient movement turns a closed fracture into an open fracture, patient care increases dramatically as do medical costs and the chances of patient disability. Usually a closed fracture is x-rayed and set in a cast, and the patient does not even have to stay over in the hospital. An open fracture, on the other hand, requires surgical debridement and at least one night's hospital stay. This is why it is so important to limit the movement of a fracture prior to application of a splint. Injuries to the tibia or fibula are usually splinted with two boards as shown in Skill Summary 23-15. An air splint can also be used on a lower leg or straight arm as shown in Skill Summary 23-16.

Injuries to the ankle or foot can be splinted using a pillow splint (Figure 23-10). However, remember that a pillow does not immobilize the knee. Therefore, the patient must be placed on a stretcher with the knee strapped down in place. Keep the toes exposed so the patient's circulation can be monitored. For an ankle injury, use a commercial Velcro®-closure type splint with both a foot section and a leg section that extends above the knee.

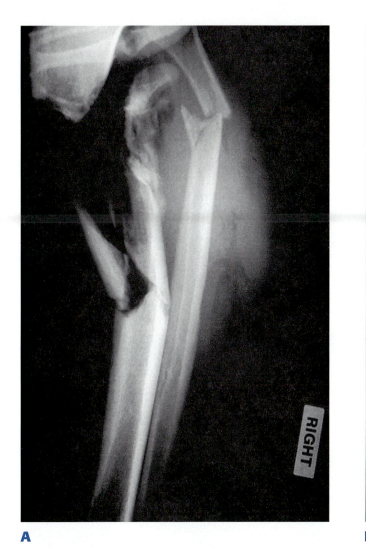

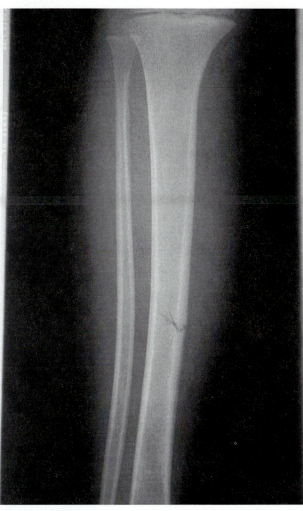

A

B

Figure 23-9 (A) Some fractures are severe and obvious during external exams, while (B) others are subtle and difficult to detect without an x-ray.

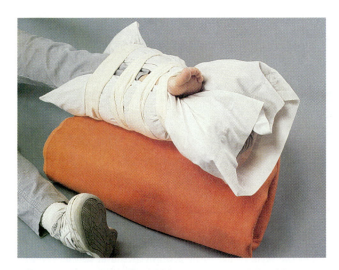

Figure 23-10 Pillow splint for an injured ankle.

Always take BSI precautions first.

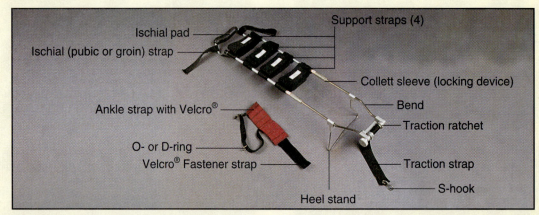

Ischial pad
Ischial (pubic or groin) strap
Support straps (4)
Collett sleeve (locking device)
Ankle strap with Velcro®
Bend
Traction ratchet
O- or D-ring
Velcro® Fastener strap
Traction strap
S-hook
Heel stand

The Fernotrac® traction splint

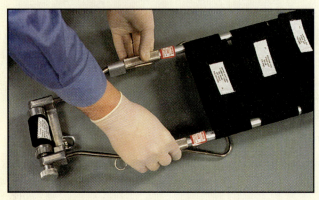

▲ **1.** Loosen the sleeve locking device.

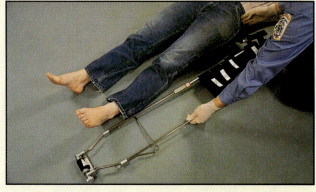

▲ **2.** Place next to uninjured leg—ischial pad next to iliac crest.

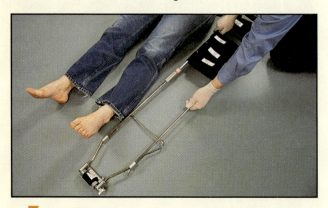

▲ **3.** Hold top and move bottom until bend is at heel.

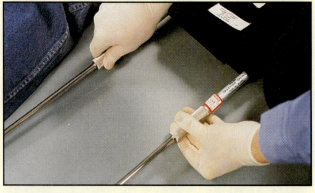

▲ **4.** Lock sleeve.

NOTE: Some splints currently in use are measured by placing the ring at the level of the bony prominence that can be felt in the middle of each buttock (ischial tuberosity). The distal end of the splint should be placed 8 to 10 inches beyond the foot. Also, remember to always assess distal pulse, motor function, and sensation (PMS) both before and after immobilizing or splinting an extremity.

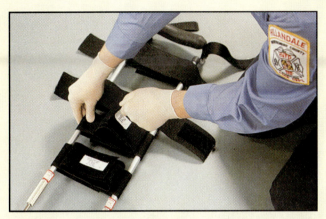

▲ **5.** Open support straps.

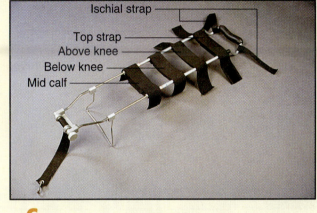

Ischial strap
Top strap
Above knee
Below knee
Mid calf

▲ **6.** Position straps under the splint in the areas shown on this photo.

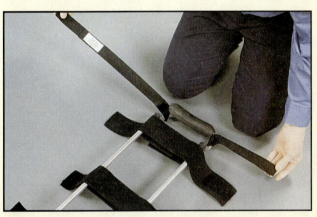

▲ **7.** Release ischial strap. Attached ends should be next to ischial pad.

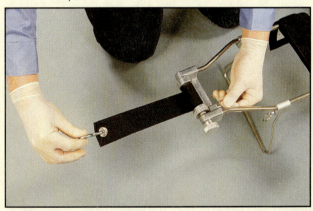

▲ **8.** Pull release ring on ratchet and . . .

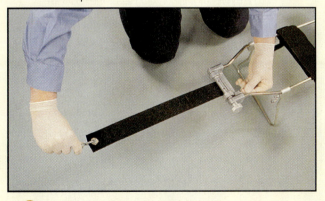

▲ **9.** . . . release the traction strap.

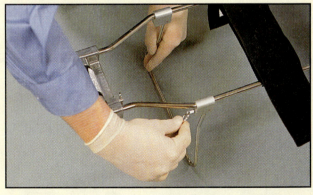

▲ **10.** Extend and position heel stand after splint is in position under patient.

NOTE: Traction splints vary depending on the manufacturer. Learn to use the equipment supplied in your area and keep up to date with new equipment as it is approved for use.

Always take BSI precautions first.

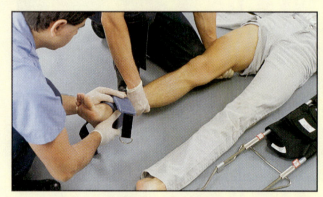

▲ **1.** Some systems attach the ankle hitch prior to applying manual traction (tension). EMT-B #1 applies the hitch while EMT-B #2 stabilizes the limb.

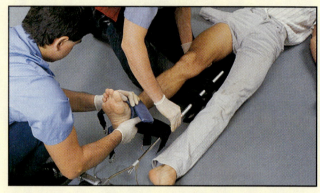

▲ **2a.** While EMT-B #1 applies manual traction (tension), EMT-B #2 positions the splint.

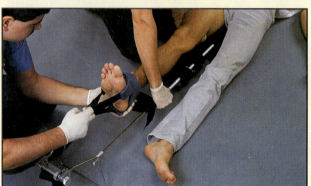

▲ **2b.** Some systems allow manual traction to be applied by grasping the D-ring and ankle.

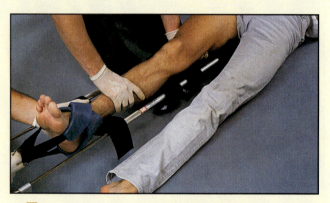

▲ **3.** EMT-B #1 maintains manual traction (tension) and lowers the limb onto the cradles of the splint.

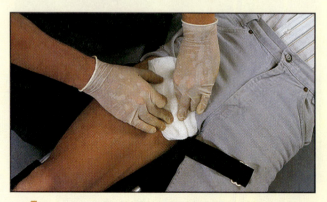

▲ **4.** While EMT-B #1 maintains manual traction, EMT-B #2 applies padding to the groin area before securing the ischial strap. Note: Some EMS systems do not apply padding in order to reduce slippage.

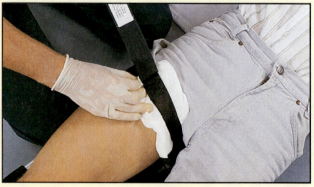

▲ **5.** EMT-B #2 secures the ischial strap, connects the ankle hitch to the windlass, tightens the ratchet to equal manual traction (tension), and secures the cradle straps.

NOTE: Always assess distal pulse, motor function, and sensation (PMS) before and after immobilizing or splinting an extremity.

Always take BSI precautions first.

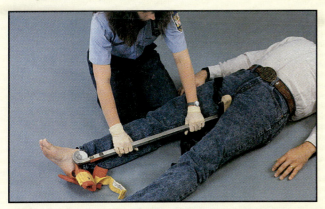

▲ **1.** Place the splint medially.

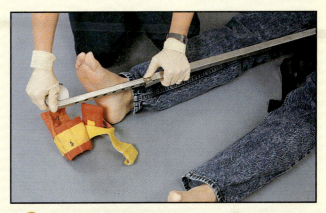

▲ **2.** Measure the length from the groin to 4 inches past heel. Unlock to slide.

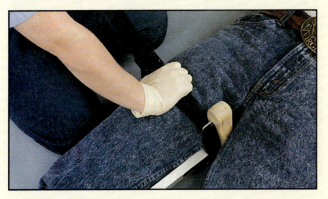

▲ **3.** Secure thigh strap.

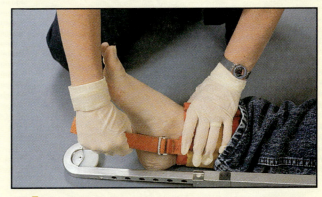

▲ **4.** Wrap ankle harness above ankle (malleoli) and secure under heel.

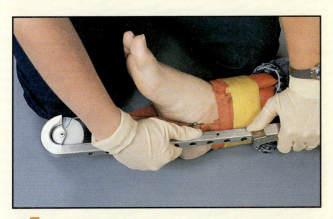

▲ **5.** Release lock and extend splint to achieve desired traction (in pounds on pulley wheel).

NOTE: Always assess distal pulse, motor function, and sensation (PMS) before and after immobilizing an extremity.

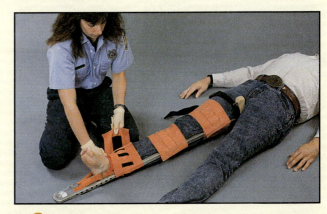

▲ **6.** Secure straps at thigh, lower thigh and knee, and lower leg. Strap ankles and feet together. Secure to spine board.

Always take BSI precautions first.

NOTE: Always assess distal pulse, motor function, and sensation both before and after immobilizing or splinting an extremity.

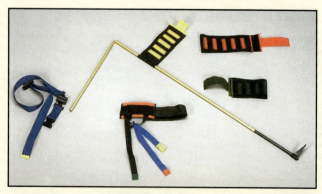

▲ Components of the Kendrick traction device.

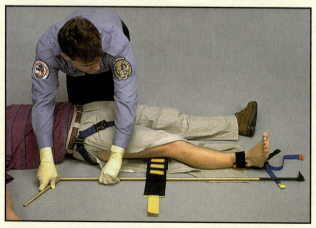

▲ **1.** Apply ankle hitch snugly just above the ankle.

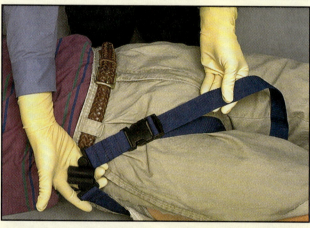

▲ **2.** Apply thigh strap with traction pole receptacle at belt line or pelvic crest.

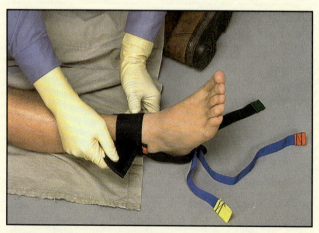

▲ **3.** Size pole so that one section extends beyond the patient's foot.

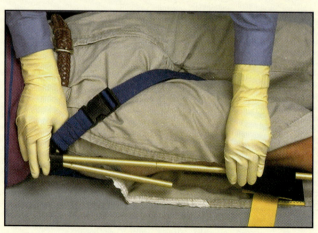

▲ **4.** Insert pole ends into traction pole receptacle.

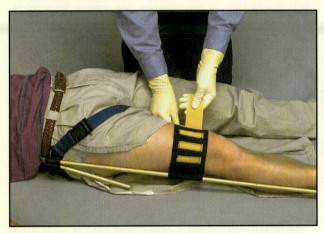

▲ **5.** Secure elastic strap around knee.

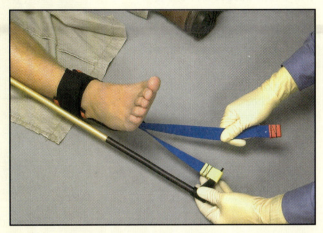

▲ **6.** Apply traction by pulling red tab.

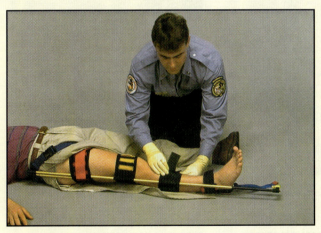

▲ **7.** Apply elastic straps over thigh and lower leg.

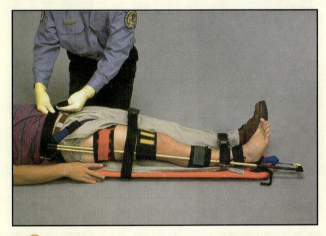

▲ **8.** Secure patient's torso and traction splint to long board for transport.

Always take BSI precautions first.

NOTE: Always assess distal pulse, motor function, and sensation (PMS) before and after immobilizing an extremity.

The ankle hitch can be used with a single padded board splint to immobilize injured knees and legs. It is made with a three-inch wide cravat.

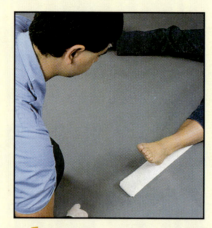

▲ **1.** Kneel at distal end of limb.

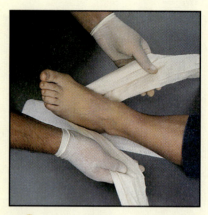

▲ **2.** Center cravat in arch.

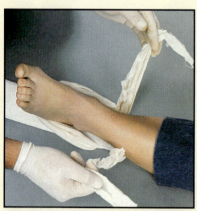

▲ **3.** Place cravat along sides of foot and cross cravat behind ankle.

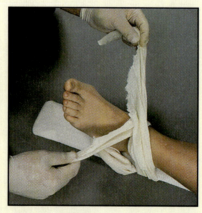

▲ **4.** Cross cravat ends over top of ankle.

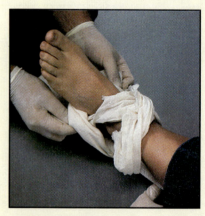

▲ **5.** A stirrup has been formed.

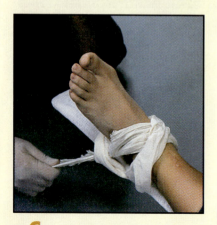

▲ **6.** Thread ends through stirrup.

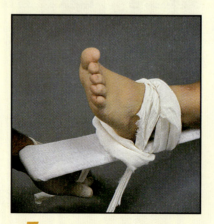

▲ **7.** Pull ends downward to tighten.

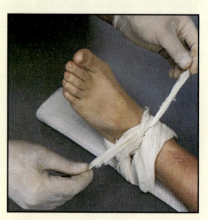

▲ **8.** Pull upward and tie over ankle wrap.

Knee Injuries—Bent Knee—Two-Splint Method

Always take BSI precautions first.

If there is distal PMS, or if the limb cannot be straightened without meeting resistance or causing severe pain, an injured knee should be splinted with the knee in the position in which it is found.

NOTE: Always assess distal pulse, motor function, and sensation (PMS) before and after immobilizing an extremity.

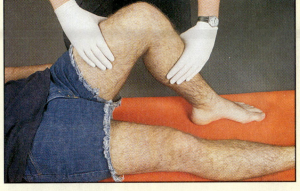

▲ **1.** Stabilize the knee above and below the injury site as shown.

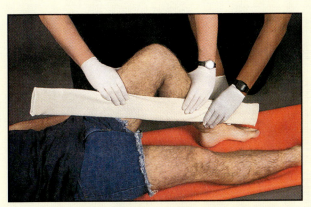

▲ **2.** Make sure the splints are equal and extend 6–12 inches beyond the mid thigh and mid calf.

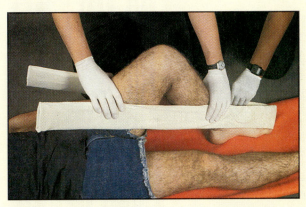

▲ **3.** Place padded side of splints next to extremity.

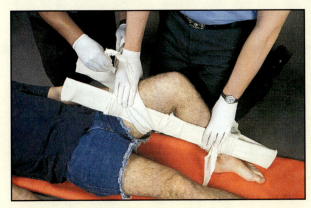

▲ **4.** Place a cravat through the knee void and tie the boards together.

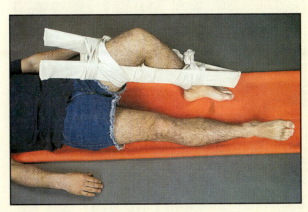

▲ **5.** Using a figure eight, secure one cravat to the ankle and the boards; secure the second cravat to the thigh and the boards.

Always take BSI precautions first.

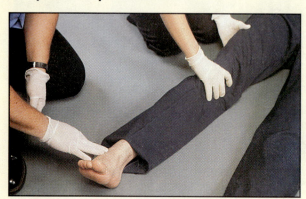

▲ **1.** Assess distal PMS.

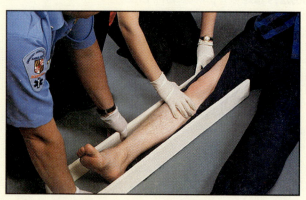

▲ **2.** Place padded board splints, medial from groin, lateral from iliac crest, both to 4 inches beyond foot.

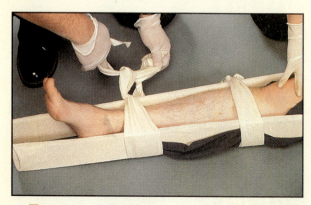

▲ **3.** Stabilize the limb and pad groin.

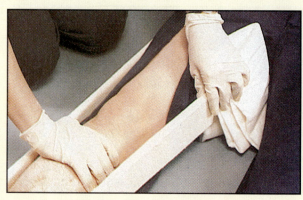

▲ **4.** Position splints.

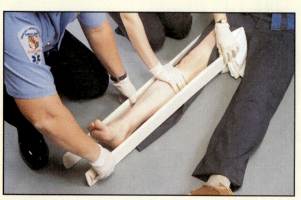

▲ **5.** Secure splints at thigh, above and below knee, and at mid calf. Pad voids.

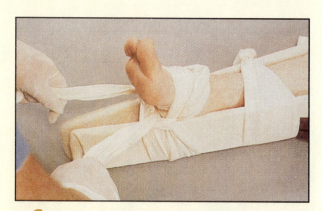

▲ **6.** Cross and tie two cravats at the ankle or hitch the ankle. Treat for shock and administer high-concentration oxygen.

NOTE: Always assess distal pulse, motor function, and sensation (PMS) before and after immobilizing an extremity.

Leg Injuries— Two-Splint Method

Always take BSI precautions first.

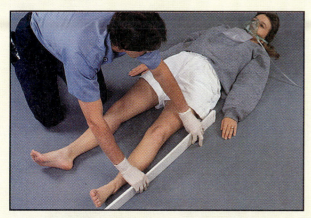

▲ **1.** Measure splint. It should extend above the knee and below the ankle.

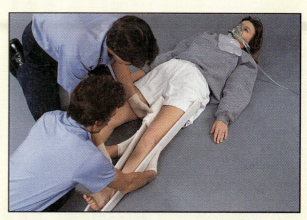

▲ **2.** Apply manual traction and place one splint medially and one laterally. Padding is toward the leg.

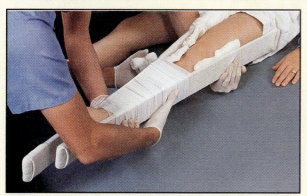

▲ **3.** Secure splints, padding voids.

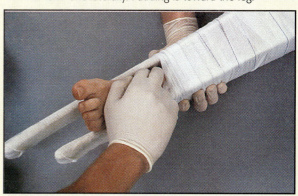

▲ **4.** Reassess distal PMS.

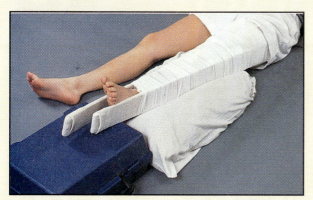

▲ **5.** Elevate, once immobilized.

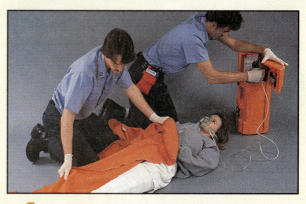

▲ **6.** Treat for shock and administer high-concentration oxygen. Transport on a long spine board.

NOTE: Always assess distal pulse, motor function, and sensation (PMS) before and after immobilizing an extremity.

Always take BSI precautions first.

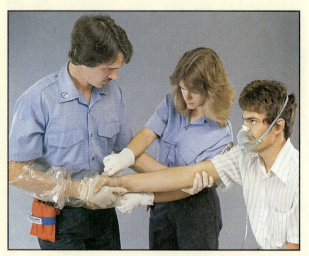

1. Slide the inflated splint up your forearm, well above the wrist. Use the same hand to grasp the hand of the patient's injured limb as though you were going to shake hands. Apply steady tension.

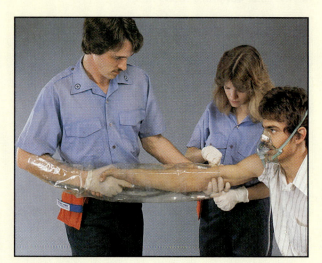

2. While you support patient's arm, your partner gently slides the splint over your hand and onto the patient's injured limb. The lower edge of the splint should be just above his knuckles. Make sure the splint is free of wrinkles.

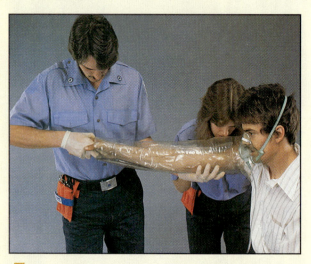

3. Continue to support the arm while your partner inflates the splint by mouth to a point where you can make a slight dent in the plastic when you press it with your thumb.

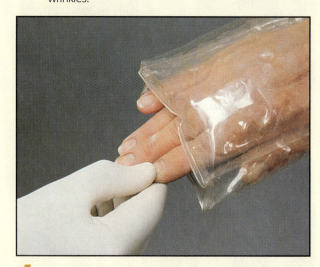

4. Continue to assess distal PMS.

WARNING: Air-inflated splints may leak. When applied in cold weather, an inflatable splint will expand when the patient is moved to a warmer place. Variations in pressure also occur if the patient is moved to a different altitude. Frequently monitor the pressure in the splint with your fingertip. Air-inflated splints may stick to the patient's skin in hot weather.

NOTE: Always assess distal pulse, motor function, and sensation (PMS) before and after immobilizing an extremity.

SUMMARY

- Although musculoskeletal injuries are usually not life threatening, if treated improperly, many of them can result in permanent disability.
- In the field, patients with painful, swollen, or deformed extremities should be treated as if they have a fracture.
- Proper splinting of a PSDE can prevent further damage to soft tissues, organs, nerves, and muscles, and also can keep a closed injury from becoming an open one.

- The signs and symptoms of a musculoskeletal injury include pain and tenderness, deformity or angulation, grating or crepitus, swelling, bruising or ecchymosis, exposed bone ends, joints locked into position, nerve or blood vessel compromise, and the inability to move the extremity.
- When caring for a PSDE, always check and record the distal PMS before and after splinting.

REVIEW QUESTIONS

1. The connective tissue that helps to support the bones and muscles, especially where they join together, consists of:
   a. cartilage, tendons, and ligaments.
   b. proximal, medial, and distal malleoli.
   c. axial and appendicular skeletons.
   d. voluntary, involuntary, and cardiac fibers.

2. A large black-and-blue discoloration of the skin that indicates an injury that is hours old is:
   a. psoriasis.
   b. impetigo.
   c. dermatitis.
   d. ecchymosis.

3. All of the following may result in splinting complications EXCEPT a(n):
   a. splinted extremity that is not aligned.
   b. splint that has been applied too loosely.
   c. emphasis on the PSDE rather than the ABCs.
   d. splint that has been applied too tightly.

4. In a _____, the head of the femur is out of its socket.
   a. dislocated hip   c. fractured femur
   b. dislocated tibia   d. fractured pelvis

5. For which type of injury should the patient NOT be log rolled?
   a. tibia
   b. pelvis
   c. cervical spine
   d. humerus

WEB MEDIC

Visit Brady's *Essentials of Emergency Care* web site for direct web links. At **www.prenhall.com/limmer,** you will find information related to the following Chapter 23 topics:

- Traction splinting
- Injuries to the pelvis
- Injuries to the knees
- Bone marrow
- Falls in the elderly

Chapter Twenty-Four

INJURIES TO THE HEAD AND SPINE

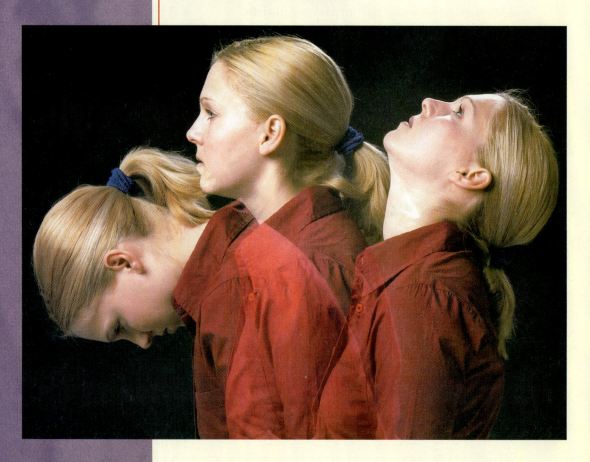

ESSENTIAL ELECTRONIC EXTRAS

CD ESSENTIALS

For preview and review of chapter material, see the student CD-ROM for

- Pretest
- Chapter quizzes
- Posttest

WEB ESSENTIALS

For additional review and enrichment, visit www.prenhall.com/limmer for

- Interactive student quizzes
- Links to online EMS resources
- Online case studies
- Audio glossary

Throughout this textbook, you can read, "Assess the airway" with the added caveat: "Keep in mind the possibility of an injury to the spine." Although not as common as less harmful bone injuries, a spine injury, if not handled appropriately, can result in permanent disability or death. Second only to proper assessment and emergency care for the patient's ABCs, proper assessment and care for head and spine injuries are your most important responsibilities as an EMT-B.

NERVOUS SYSTEM REVIEW

In order to understand injuries to the head and the spine, knowledge of the anatomy and physiology of the nervous system and skeleton is necessary.

Anatomically and physiologically, the nervous system (Figure 24-1) is divided into three sub-systems: the central nervous system (CNS), the peripheral nervous system, and the autonomic nervous system. The **central nervous system (CNS)** consists of the brain and spinal cord. The **peripheral nervous system** includes the pairs of nerves that enter and exit the spinal cord between each vertebra, all the branches of these nerves that are responsible for sensation and motion throughout the body, and the 12 pairs of cranial nerves that travel between the brain and structures of the head and neck without passing through the spinal cord.

The **autonomic nervous system** connects the brain and spinal cord to many organs including the heart, lungs, glands, muscles in the walls of hollow organs, and blood vessels in the skin. The autonomic system controls involuntary functions, or those we cannot consciously control, such as increasing or decreasing the rate and strength of heart contractions; constricting or dilating blood vessels in skeletal muscles, skin, and abdominal organs; changing bronchial diameter; contracting and relaxing the urinary bladder; and increasing or decreasing the secretion of saliva and digestive juices. The autonomic nervous system is also referred to as the "fight or flight" system, which, when the body is stressed, will allow you to run away or stay and fight something or someone who threatens you.

Messages of sensation—such as those of light, sound, touch, heat, and cold—are carried from the sense organs to the brain over a network of "sensory nerves." The brain then interprets the messages and sends back orders for action to the muscles over another network of nerves called "motor nerves." Motor nerves control voluntary movements such as walking or grasping.

As the motor nerves exit the brain and extend into the spinal cord, they cross over to the opposite side of the body. This is why an injury to the right side of the brain is exhibited by weakness or lack of sensation on the left side of the body. Since the cranial nerves exit the brain above this crossover, they control the same side of the body on which they are located.

CORE CONCEPTS

In this chapter, you will learn about the following topics:

- The mechanisms of head and spine injury

- How to stabilize the cervical spine

- The proper application of a cervical spine immobilization device for patients found in the standing, seated, or supine positions

- How and when to perform a rapid extrication

- Procedures for helmet removal

- Proper immobilization or removal of a child in a car seat

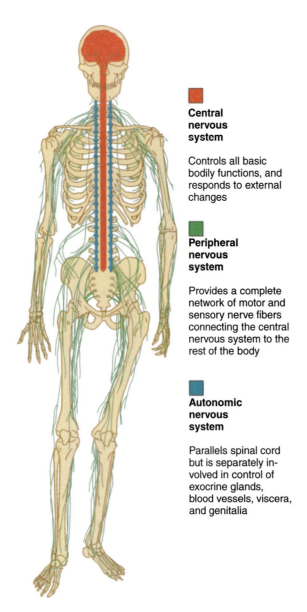

Central nervous system

Controls all basic bodily functions, and responds to external changes

Peripheral nervous system

Provides a complete network of motor and sensory nerve fibers connecting the central nervous system to the rest of the body

Autonomic nervous system

Parallels spinal cord but is separately involved in control of exocrine glands, blood vessels, viscera, and genitalia

Figure 24-1 Anatomy of the nervous system.

The Brain

The brain is the master organ of the body. It is the center of consciousness, self-awareness, and thought. It controls basic functions, including breathing and, to some degree, heart activity. Messages from all over the body are received by the brain, which decides how to respond to changing conditions both inside and outside the body. The brain sends messages to the muscles so that we can move or to a particular organ so that it will carry out a desired function.

The brain is divided into three major sections: the cerebrum, the cerebellum, and the brain stem. The **cerebrum** is the largest part of the brain. It contains the centers for hearing, seeing, touching, tasting, and smelling, which receive messages from the body's main sense organs. The cerebrum also sends messages to the muscles so that we can move. The **cerebellum** coordinates the body's muscle movements. If it is injured, control over the muscles is greatly disturbed. The **brain stem** connects the cerebrum with the spinal cord. Nerves on their way to and from the higher centers of the brain pass through the brain stem. The lowest part of the brain stem, the **medulla oblongata,** helps regulate vegetative functions such as breathing, digestion, and circulation.

The soft, spongy mass of tissue that makes up the brain is covered by three **meninges,** or membranes, which also cover the spinal cord. The outermost membrane is called the **dura mater,** the middle layer, the **arachnoid,** and the inner layer, the **pia.** Collections of blood (hematomas) around or within the brain are named in relationship to these membranes. You will read more about hematomas under brain injuries later in this chapter.

The brain and spinal cord are bathed in **cerebrospinal fluid (CSF).** When the continuity of the skull is broken due to a basilar (base of the skull) fracture, CSF may exit through the nose, ears, or throat. When a patient in an automobile collision tells you that he has hit his head on the dash and has a salty taste in his mouth, this is most likely due to CSF, which is high in salt content. For this fluid to exit the ears, it exits the brain through a tear in the meninges, passes through a ruptured eardrum, and then flows from the external ear, where this clear fluid mixes with blood.

The Spinal Cord

The spinal cord is a relay between most of the body and the brain. A large number of the messages to and from the brain are sent through the spinal cord. Damage to the cord can isolate a part of the body from the brain, and function of this part can be lost, possibly forever.

The spinal cord is also the center of **reflex** activity. Reflexes allow us to react quickly to such things as pain and excessive heat without orders sent by the brain. In a reflex action, sensory nerves flash a message to the spinal cord. In turn the spinal cord, acting as a relay center, flashes back a message to motor nerves in the muscle telling it to move at once—and it also sends another message to the brain about the original message.

The spinal cord is protected by the spine, 33 separate irregular-shaped bones called **vertebrae** which sit on top of one another (Figure 24-2). Each vertebra has a **spinous process,** which is one of the lumps you can palpate on a patient's back. Two **transverse processes** are located on the sides of

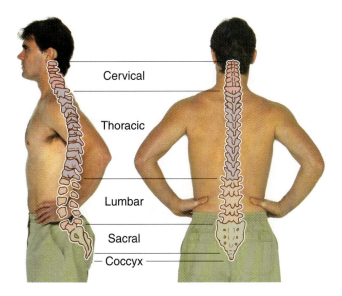

Figure 24-2 The divisions of the spinal column.

each vertebra. The body of the vertebra forms a channel approximately 15 mm in diameter. The spinal cord is about 10 mm in diameter. Between each vertebra is a fluid-filled cartilage disk which provides some cushioning of the bones and allows for flexibility of the spine.

The areas of the spine that are most often injured are those areas where the natural curvature of the spine changes its direction and those areas that are not supported by bone such as the ribs and pelvis. This is why cervical and lumbar injuries are very common.

The healing power of the brain and nerve tissue is limited. Once this tissue is damaged, to a certain extent, function is lost and cannot be restored. As an EMT-B your initial care can often prevent additional damage to the brain, spinal cord, and major nerves of the body.

INJURIES TO THE HEAD

Skull Injuries

Skull injuries include fractures to the cranium and facial bones. Severe injuries to the skull can also injure the brain. Skull injuries can be either open or closed. The words "open" and "closed" refer to the skull bones. When the bones of the cranium are fractured, and the scalp overlying the fracture is lacerated, the patient has an open head injury. In other cases, there may be a laceration of the scalp; however, if the cranium is intact, or free of fractures, the term "closed head injury" is used. In practice, it may not be possible for the EMT-B to determine if a head injury is open or closed. It is safest for you to assume that there may be an open head injury beneath any laceration of the scalp.

Brain Injuries

Brain injuries are classified as direct or indirect. **Direct injuries** occur when the brain is lacerated, punctured, or bruised by the broken bones of the skull, by bone fragments, or by foreign objects. **Indirect injuries** to the brain can be the result of closed injuries to the skull and certain types of open skull injuries. In other words, the impact of the injury to the skull is transferred to the brain.

Like any other mass of tissue, the brain swells when it is injured. This swelling is serious since there is little room for the brain to expand within the rigid skull. Swelling makes it more difficult for blood to get to the brain. This leads to lowered oxygen levels and increased carbon dioxide levels in brain tissue. The presence of high carbon dioxide levels further increases the swelling.

Indirect injuries to the brain include **concussions** and contusions. When a person strikes his or her head in a fall, or is struck by a blunt object, a certain amount of the force is transferred through the skull to the brain, sometimes causing a concussion. A concussion may be so mild that the patient is unaware of the injury. Usually there is no detectable damage to the brain and the patient may or may not lose consciousness. Most patients who sustain a concussion will feel a little "groggy" after receiving a blow to the head and usually develop headaches. The patient with a concussion may experience a period of altered mental status, but if there is a loss of consciousness, it usually is brief and it does not tend to reoccur. Witnesses of auto collisions often describe the victim who sustains a concussion as a person who "just sat there staring off into space for a few minutes." Some short-term memory loss concerning the events that surrounded the collision is fairly common. Long-term memory loss associated with concussion is rare. Memory loss, whether short- or long-term, is called **amnesia.**

A contusion, or a bruise of the brain, can occur when the force of a blow to the head is great enough to rupture small blood vessels found on the surface of, or deep within, the brain. Since there is little space in which the brain can move before it strikes the walls of the cranial cavity, a contusion often appears on the side of the brain opposite the point of impact to the skull. A contusion is usually caused by an **acceleration/deceleration** injury in which the brain hits the one side of the cranial cavity on acceleration, bounces off the opposite side on deceleration, and then rebounds to strike the first side of the cranial cavity again. Bruising of the brain on the same side as the skull injury is called a **coup.** Bruising that occurs on the side opposite the injury is called **contrecoup.**

The inside of the skull has many sharp, bony ridges that can lacerate a moving brain. The brain can also be lacerated by a penetrating or perforating wound to the cranium. Not only is there the problem of direct injury, but there also may be severe indirect injury due to hematoma formation. For example, a subdural hematoma would be a collection of blood below the dura, yet outside the brain tissue itself.

The brain is supplied with a rich supply of blood through four major arteries, two vertebral arteries, which travel through the spine, and two carotid arteries. An acute blockage to any one of these four arteries can have a catastrophic effect on the brain. One very important artery is the **middle meningeal artery.** Since this artery is located in a very thin area of the skull above the ear, it is easily damaged. When severed, it causes a hematoma in the **epidural space** (outside the dura and inside the skull). A patient with

an epidural hematoma is usually knocked unconscious, then proceeds to regain consciousness (this period is referred to as a "lucid interval"); and then consciousness begins to decrease again in the next few minutes to hour.

PRECEPTOR PEARL

Tell new EMT-Bs that an epidural hematoma is often associated with severe blows to the temporal regions of the head. If they recognize an epidural hematoma in its early stages and promptly transport the patient to a trauma center, it can make the difference between life and death. Tell them to be aggressive if they suspect an epidural hematoma may be developing.

The brain's venous flow is very close to the surface. When the brain is bruised, lacerated, or punctured, blood from ruptured vessels can flow between the brain and its meninges (Figure 24-3). When a hematoma develops in the subdural space, this is often due to venous bleeding and has very

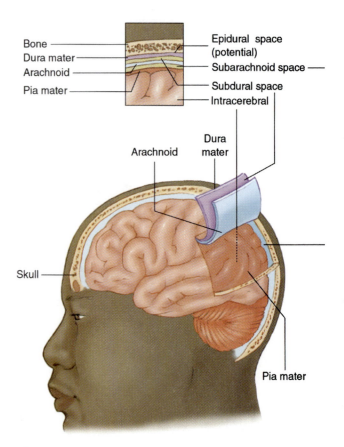

Figure 24-3 Meninges (covering layers) of the brain.

serious ramifications. Often, this bleeding is a slow venous flow. Even when the bleeding stops, the hematoma will continue to grow in size as it absorbs tissue fluids. Since there is no room for expansion in the skull, severe pressure can be placed on the brain. Death can occur if vital brain centers are damaged. This type of hematoma may occur rapidly or over a prolonged period of time.

An intracerebral hematoma occurs when blood pools within the brain itself, pushing tissues against the bones of the cranium. This can develop into a fatal injury in minutes to hours depending on the area of the brain that is damaged and the extent of bleeding. When the brain is injured and begins to bleed or swell, intracerebral pressure (ICP) rises.

When assessing for signs and symptoms of injury to the skull or brain, also be alert for the strong possibility of cervical-spine injury as well.

Patient Assessment

Head Injury

Unless accompanied by an open head injury, a penetrating injury, a CSF leak, or a hematoma, a skull fracture is generally not considered critical. Brain injuries that result in increased intracranial pressure (ICP) and a hematoma are very serious. Consider the possibility of a skull fracture or brain injury whenever you note any of these signs or symptoms:

- Confusion, disorientation, deteriorating mental status, unresponsiveness.

- Short-term memory loss, in which the patient keeps asking the same questions over and over again.

- Personality changes ranging from irritable to irrational behavior.

- Depressions or deformity of the skull, large swellings ("goose eggs"), or anything that looks unusual about the shape of the cranium.

- Severe pain or swelling at the site of a head injury. Pain may range from a headache to severe discomfort. Do not palpate the injury site with your fingertips since this could push bone fragments into the brain.

- Deep laceration or severe bruise to the scalp or forehead. Do not probe into the wound or separate the wound opening to determine wound depth.

- Visible bone fragments and perhaps bits of brain tissue. These are the most obvious signs of skull fracture, but the majority of skull fractures do not produce these signs.

- Bleeding from the ears and/or the nose.

- CSF flowing from the ears and/or the nose.

- "Battle's sign," a bruise or swelling behind the ear. This is a late sign of a basilar (base of skull) fracture.

- Impaired hearing, ringing in the ears.

- Equilibrium problems in which the patient is unable to stand still with the eyes closed or stumbles when attempting to walk. (Do not test for this.)

- "Raccoon's eyes," black eyes, or discoloration of the soft tissues under and around both eyes. This is usually a delayed finding indicating a basilar skull fracture.

- One eye that appears to be sunken.

- Blurred or multiple-image vision in one or both eyes.

- Deteriorating vital signs.

- Irregular-breathing patterns such as Cheyne Stokes (increasing rate of respirations followed by periods of apnea).

- Cushing's syndrome, the combination of an increased blood pressure and a decreased pulse rate.

- Unequal pupils that may not react to light. This is a late sign caused by compression of the cranial nerve that controls pupil constriction (Figure 24-4).

- Increased or decreased temperature, a late sign that indicates damage to temperature-regulating centers in the brain.

- Forceful or projectile vomiting.

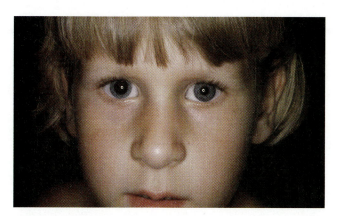

Figure 24-4 Unequal pupils

- Neurological posturing when painful stimulus is applied, such as flexing the arms and wrists and extending the legs and feet (called "decorticate posture"), or extending the arms with the shoulders rotated inward and the wrists flexed, legs extended (called "decerebrate posture"). These postures may also be assumed spontaneously, without painful stimulus.
- Paralysis on one side of the body (hemiplegia).
- Mechanism of injury, such as starring of windshield or deformity of helmet. ✴

LIFESPAN DEVELOPMENT

Shock is rarely a sign of head injury, except in infants. This is due to their proportionately larger heads and the still unfused soft spots, or anterior fontanelles, which close up at around 18 months. There simply is not enough room in the adult skull to permit enough bleeding (over 25% to 30% of the blood volume) into the head to cause shock. In an adult, if a head injury is accompanied by shock, look for indications of blood loss at some other place on the body.

Neurological Assessment/The Glasgow Coma Scale

All patients who sustain head injury or suspected brain damage must be continually and carefully monitored and reassessed during transport. Always be prepared for the patient to vomit or have a seizure. The early signs of deterioration are subtle changes in mental status that can be easily overlooked if you fail to look for them. What you observe and report to the Emergency Department staff can have a great bearing on their initial actions.

Many EMT-Bs use the **Glasgow Coma Scale (GCS)** in addition to AVPU for ongoing neurological assessment and triage (Table 24-1). For a patient with a GCS of 8 or less, some systems would immediately triage directly to the trauma center if they are within 30 minutes transport time. You should become familiar with the GCS if it is used in your EMS system. When using this scale, remember to consider the following:

- Note if there are eye injuries or injuries to the face that prevent the patient from opening the eyes. If the injuries are more than minor ones, do not ask the patient to open his or her eyes.
- Spontaneous eye opening means that the patient can open his or her eyes without your help. If the patient's eyes are closed, then you should say, "Open your eyes" to see if the patient will obey this command. Try a normal level of voice. If this fails, shout the command. Should the patient's eyes remain closed, apply an accepted painful stimulus (e.g., pinch a toe, scratch the palm or sole, rub the sternum).

Table 24-1 The Glasgow Coma Scale

Eye Opening Response	Spontaneous	4
	To voice	3
	To pain	2
	None	1
Best Verbal Response	Oriented	5
	Confused	4
	Inappropriate words (e.g., curses)	3
	Incomprehensible sounds (mumbles, moans, groans)	2
	None	1
Best Motor Response	Obeys command	6
	Localizes pain	5
	Withdraws (pain)	4
	Flexion (pain)	3
	Extension (pain)	2
	None	1
	TOTAL	3–15

- When evaluating the patient's verbal responses, use the following criteria:
  - **Oriented.** The patient, once aroused, can tell you who he is, where he is, and he can name the correct day of the week. A person who can answer all three of these questions appropriately is said to be alert on the AVPU scale.
  - **Confused.** The patient cannot answer the above questions, but he can speak in phrases and sentences.
  - **Inappropriate words.** The patient says or shouts a word or several words at a time. Usually this requires physical stimulation. The words do not fit the situation or a particular question. Often, the patient curses.
  - **Incomprehensible sounds.** The patient responds with mumbling, moans, or groans.
  - **No verbal response.** Repeated stimulation, verbal and physical, does not cause the patient to speak or make any sounds.

- The following are the criteria used to evaluate motor response:
  - **Obeys command.** The patient must be able to understand your instruction and carry it out. For example, you can ask (when appropriate) for the patient to hold up two fingers.
  - **Localizes pain.** Should the patient fail to respond to your commands, apply pressure to one of the nail beds for 5 seconds or firm pressure to the sternum. Note if the patient attempts to remove your hand. Do not apply pressure over an injury site. Do not apply pressure to the sternum if the patient is experiencing difficulty breathing.
  - **Withdraws.** Draws back after painful stimulation. Note the elbow flexing, the patient moving slowly, the appearance of stiffness, the patient holding his forearm and hand against the body, or the limbs on one side of the body appearing to be paralyzed (hemiplegic position).
  - **Posturing.** Occurs after painful stimulation. Note extending legs and arms, apparent stiffness with moving, and any internal rotation of the shoulder and forearm.

Patient Care

Head Injury

Emergency care of a patient with a head injury is as follows:

1. **Take BSI precautions.**

2. **Open the airway.** Assume a cervical-spine injury and use the jaw-thrust maneuver to open the airway.

3. **Maintain an open airway.** Monitor the conscious patient for changes in breathing. For the unconscious patient, insert an oropharyngeal airway without hyperextending the neck. Provide resuscitative measures if needed.

4. **Immobilize the spine.** Apply a rigid collar, immobilize the neck and spine, and evaluate the method of extrication, either normal or rapid (Figure 24-5).

5. **Be prepared for vomiting.** Have your suction unit ready. It may be necessary to flip the long backboard on its side, which allows the patient's airway to drain if vomiting occurs.

6. **Administer oxygen** via nonrebreather mask and evaluate the need for positive pressure ventilations. This is critical should there be any brain damage. If the patient shows definite signs of a brain injury (i.e., increased blood pressure and decreased pulse, combined with an altered mental status and a blown pupil), hyperventilate with oxygen-assisted ventilations (bag-valve-mask device or positive pressure) at the rate of 16–20 per minute, rather than the usual 12 ventilations per minute. This will help reduce brain-tissue swelling by lowering carbon dioxide levels and raising oxygen levels. It should be noted that use of hyperventilation is controversial as it has been shown to increase intracranial pressure. Check with your medical director for your local protocol.

7. **Control bleeding.** Do not apply pressure if the injury site shows bone fragments, depression of the bone, or if the brain is exposed. Do not attempt to stop the flow of blood or cerebrospinal fluid from the ears or the nose. If the skull is fractured, you may increase intracranial pressure and may also increase the risk of infection. Use a loose gauze dressing.

8. **Dress and bandage open wounds.** Stabilize any penetrating objects. Do not remove any objects or bone fragments.

9. **Keep the patient at rest.** This can be an important factor, since excessive movement can increase intracranial pressure.

10. **Perform an ongoing assessment.** Monitor vital signs every 5 minutes en route to the hospital. Talk to the conscious patient, providing emotional support. Ask questions so that the patient will have to concentrate. This will also help you detect changes in the patient's mental status. ✳

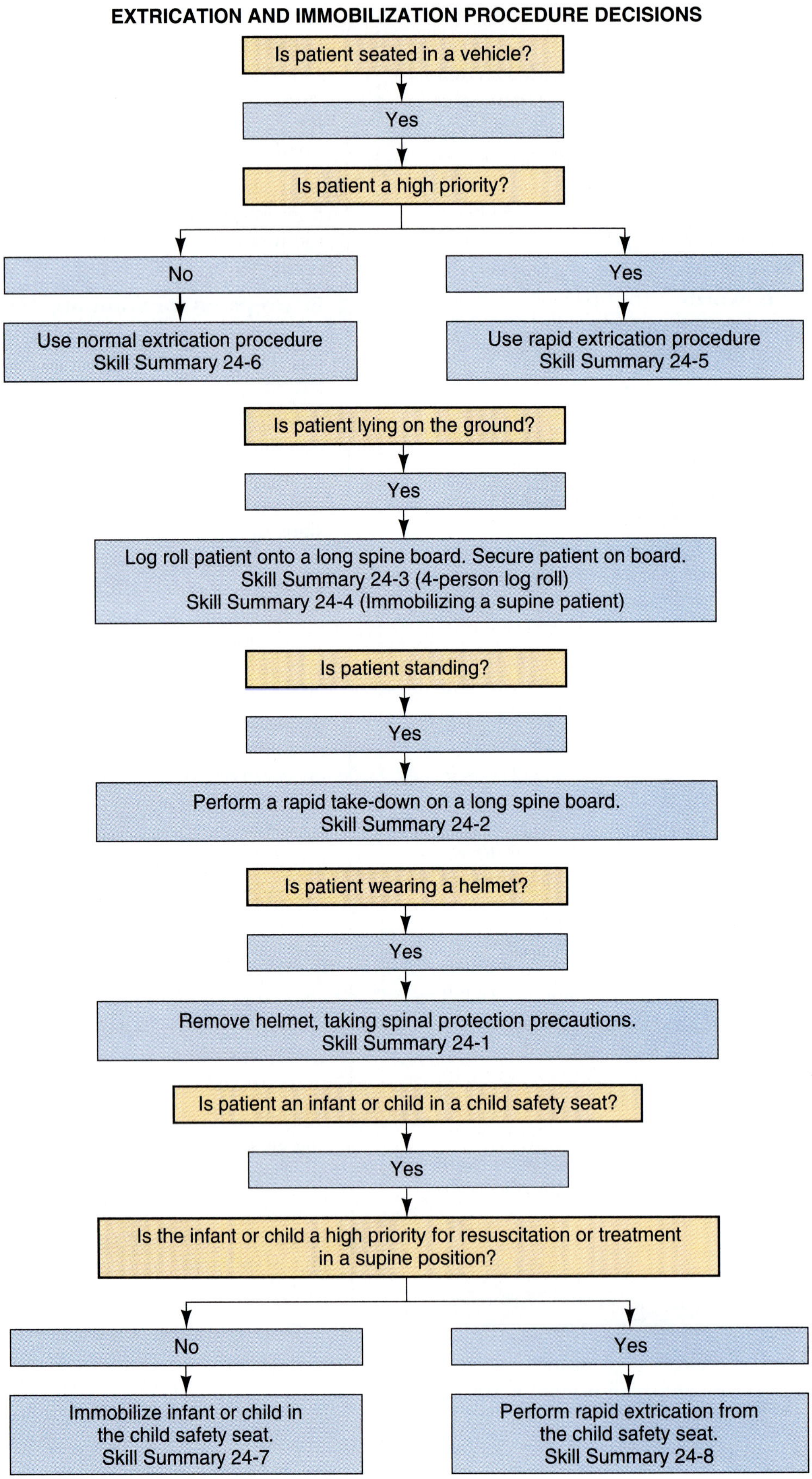

EXTRICATION AND IMMOBILIZATION PROCEDURE DECISIONS

Is patient seated in a vehicle?

Yes

Is patient a high priority?

No → Use normal extrication procedure
Skill Summary 24-6

Yes → Use rapid extrication procedure
Skill Summary 24-5

Is patient lying on the ground?

Yes

Log roll patient onto a long spine board. Secure patient on board.
Skill Summary 24-3 (4-person log roll)
Skill Summary 24-4 (Immobilizing a supine patient)

Is patient standing?

Yes

Perform a rapid take-down on a long spine board.
Skill Summary 24-2

Is patient wearing a helmet?

Yes

Remove helmet, taking spinal protection precautions.
Skill Summary 24-1

Is patient an infant or child in a child safety seat?

Yes

Is the infant or child a high priority for resuscitation or treatment
in a supine position?

No → Immobilize infant or child in
the child safety seat.
Skill Summary 24-7

Yes → Perform rapid extrication from
the child safety seat.
Skill Summary 24-8

Figure 24-5 Choose appropriate extrication and immobilization procedures.

If you are unsure of the severity of the patient's injuries and there is evidence of cervical-spine injury, or if the head-injured patient is unconscious, apply a rigid cervical, or extrication, collar and position the patient on a long spine board. Elevate the head of the spine board slightly if there is no evidence of shock. This full-body immobilization will allow you to rotate the patient on the board into a lateral position so that blood and mucus can drain freely. It also prevents vomitus from causing an airway obstruction. Some patients will vomit without warning. Many vomit without first experiencing nausea. If other injuries prevent such positioning, constant monitoring and frequent suctioning are necessary.

INJURIES TO THE SPINE

Injuries to the spine must always be considered whenever there is trauma to any part of the body. Do not overlook the possibility of spine injury when dealing with head, chest, abdominal, or pelvic injuries. Even injuries to the upper and lower extremities caused by intense impact can produce spinal injury. You must always do an initial assessment and rapid trauma exam and then determine the priority of the patient. Failure to complete the patient assessment and to determine the most appropriate immobilization method could lead to further injuries. In the field, always "uptriage" or overtreat patients with potential spine injuries because the costs in terms of pain, suffering, disability, and dollars soar when a spine-injured patient is not immobilized.

Injuries to the spinal column include: fractures, with and without bone displacement; dislocations; ligament sprains; and disk injury, including compression. When the disk fluid leaks out, this is referred to as a "herniated," or ruptured, disk. Since the vertebrae are supported by a series of muscles and ligaments, if the spine is hyperflexed or hyperextended, it is possible to injure a muscle or ligament allowing the vertebrae to dislocate or move out of alignment. When this happens, it is possible to stretch, tear, or compress the spinal cord.

Most voluntary motor messages from the brain travel down the spinal cord to peripheral nerves. A pair of peripheral nerves exit between each pair of vertebra. These control sensory and motor functions of the body. When the spinal cord is damaged, it can render the peripheral nerves below the injury inoperable. A cervical-spine injury can cause **quadriplegia,** or inability to move all four extremities, whereas a lumbar or thoracic injury can cause **paraplegia,** or inability to move the lower extremities.

The vertebral column may be injured without damage to the spinal cord or spinal nerves. For example, a fractured coccyx is below the level of the spinal cord.

Ligament sprains are relatively simple injuries. However, when displaced fractures and dislocations occur, the cord, disk, and spinal nerves may be severely injured. Serious contusions and lacerations, accompanied by pressure-producing swelling, can take place. The entire column can become unstable, leading to cord compression that may produce paralysis or death.

Some parts of the spine are more susceptible to injury than others. Because it is somewhat supported by the attached ribs, the thoracic segment of the spine is not usually damaged except by the most violent accidents or by gunshot wounds. The pelvic-sacral spine attachment helps to protect the sacrum in the same way. The cervical and lumbar vertebrae are susceptible to injury because they are not supported by other bony structures. When treating a suspected spine injury, immobilize the entire spine, not just a section of it.

The experienced EMT-B knows to maintain a high degree of suspicion for spine injury when finding any of the following:

- Motor-vehicle collision (especially with "starring" of the windshield)
- Significant traumatic or soft-tissue injuries above the level of the clavicles
- Cervical-spine tenderness to palpation after any form of trauma
- Neck pain after any form of trauma
- Moderate or high-speed "MVCs"
- Pedestrian hit by a vehicle
- Falls from heights
- Blunt injury to the spine or above the clavicles
- Penetrating trauma to the head, neck, or torso
- Diving-related injuries
- Hanging
- Any trauma patient with an altered mental status
- Any trauma patient with significant painful, distracting injuries that limit ability to quantify neck pain or tenderness

PRECEPTOR PEARL

Tell new EMT-Bs that there is a simple rule they can follow: If the mechanism of injury exerts great force on the upper body or if there is any soft-tissue damage to the head, face, or neck due to trauma (from being thrown against a dashboard, for example), then assume that there is a cervical-spine injury. Any blunt trauma above the clavicles may damage the cervical spine. Clearing the spine in the field is still very controversial and requires additional training, protocols, and medical direction.

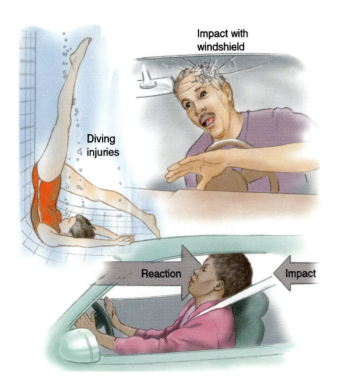

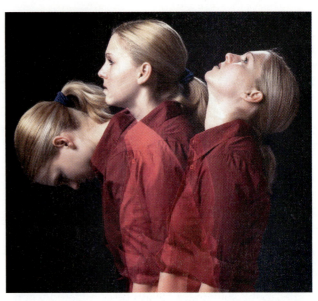

Figure 24-6 Mechanisms of injury to the upper body

Figure 24-7 Usually whiplash is caused by a poorly adjusted or absent head rest during a rear-end collision.

The spine is most often injured by **compression** or excessive **flexion, extension,** or **rotation** (Figure 24-6). An excessive pull on the spine, such as that which occurs in a hanging, is called a **distraction injury.** Years ago rescuers were taught to pull traction on the neck of an injured patient sitting in an automobile, which actually had the potential to cause further injury. Now, EMT-Bs are taught to manually stabilize the head and neck or, basically, to hold them still.

The adult skull weighs more than 17 pounds, and it rests on a very small area of the cervical spine, somewhat like a pumpkin on a broom handle. Because of this weight and positioning, when two vehicles collide, for example, the occupant's head can whip quickly back and forth. Although the vehicle decelerates abruptly, the occupant's head continues to travel in the direction and at the same rate of speed at which the vehicle was traveling, even if the body is held by safety restraints. This head movement usually exceeds the neck's normal range of motion, causing injury that can be severe (Figure 24-7).

A fall also can produce spine injury if the victim strikes an object or other hard surface. The force generated during a fall may be enough to fracture, crush, or dislocate vertebrae.

Today more and more people are participating in sports of all kinds: in-line skating, bicycling, surfing, rock climbing, and others too numerous to mention. Many sports accidents can cause spine injury. A sledding, snowmobiling, or skiing accident

may hurl a person into a tree or other fixed object, twisting or compressing the spinal column. There may be no PSDE, or signs of injury may be hidden by bulky clothing. As a result, improper care may be rendered as a patient with a possible spine injury is placed on a stretcher without adequate examination and immobilization.

LIFESPAN DEVELOPMENT

When immobilizing a 6-year-old or younger child, you should pad behind the shoulder blades. This will help compensate for the size of a child's relatively large head as compared to the rest of his or her body. With extra padding, the child's neck will drop into a flexed position.

Fractured spines in elderly patients are often caused by falls. Elderly patients may also experience spontaneous fractures of brittle bones, which in turn cause falls and possible spinal injury.

Diving accidents often produce injury to the cervical spine. When the diver strikes the diving board, the side or bottom of the pool, or an underwater object, the head can be severely forced beyond its normal limits of motion. Cervical vertebrae may be fractured or dislocated, ligaments may be severely sprained, and the spinal cord may be compressed or otherwise traumatized in the cervical region and at other spots along its length.

Football and other contact sports can cause accidents severe enough to produce spine injury. Spear tackling, using the head, has been outlawed in grade schools and high schools for a number of years due to the incidence of cervical compression fractures. Whenever an injury involves player contact or falling to the ground, be on the alert for spine injury.

Patient Assessment

Spine Injury

Signs and symptoms of a possible spine injury are listed below. However, always assume that an unconscious trauma patient has a spine injury and take spinal precautions. Whenever you are in doubt with any patient, assume spine injuries.

- **Paralysis, pain with or without movement, and tenderness anywhere along the spine.** These are reliable indicators of possible spine injury in the conscious patient. If they are present, manually stabilize the patient before proceeding with assessment. If immediate immobilization is not possible, use extreme care in handling the patient. In the field, it is not possible to rule out spine injury, even when the patient has no pain and is able to move the limbs. The mechanism of injury alone may be the deciding factor to immobilize.

  - **Pain without movement.** The pain is not always constant and may occur anywhere from the top of the head to the buttocks. Pain in the leg is common for certain types of injury to the lower spinal cord and vertebral column. Other painful injuries can mask this symptom of spine injury.

  - **Pain with movement.** The patient normally tries to lie perfectly still to prevent pain on movement. You should not request the patient to move just to determine if pain is present. However, if the patient complains of pain in the neck or back with voluntary movements, suspect spine injury. Pain with

movement in apparently uninjured shoulders and legs is another good indicator of possible spine injury.

  - **Tenderness.** Gentle palpation of the injury site, when accessible, may reveal point tenderness.

- **Impaired breathing.** Neck injury can impair nerve function to the chest muscles. Watch the patient breathe. If there is only a slight movement of the abdomen, with little or no movement of the chest, it is safe to assume that the patient is breathing with the diaphragm alone. The nerve that controls the diaphragm is located high in the cervical area and is often unharmed, but the intercostal nerves that control the chest muscles are often damaged in cervical and thoracic injuries.

- **Deformity.** Removing clothing to check the back for deformity is not recommended. Obvious spine deformities are rare. However, if you note a gap between the spinous processes (bony extensions) of the vertebrae or if you can feel a broken spinous process, suspect serious spine injuries. It is also possible to feel tight muscles in spasm.

- **Priapism.** A nonemotionally justified, persistent erection of the penis is a reliable sign of spinal cord injury affecting nerves to the external genitalia.

- **Posturing.** In some cases of spine injury, motor nerve pathways to the muscles that extend the arm can be interrupted, but those that lead to the muscles that bend the elbow and lift the arm remain functional. The patient may be found on his or her back with the arms extended above the head, which may indicate a cervical-spine injury. Arms flexed across the chest or extended along the sides with wrists flexed also signal spine injury.

- **Incontinence,** or loss of bowel or bladder control.

- **Nerve impairment to the extremities.** The patient may have loss of use, weakness, numbness, or tingling in the upper or lower extremities.

- **Paralysis of the extremities.** This is probably the most reliable sign of a spine injury in a conscious patient.

- **Severe spinal shock**. This may occur even when there are no indications of external or internal bleeding. It can be caused by the failure of the nervous system to control the diameter of blood vessels (neurogenic shock).

> Remember that the pulse rate may be normal because the message to "speed up" the heart may never have reached the heart due to the spine injury. ✱

When assessing the responsive spine-injured patient, be sure to ask questions about the mechanism of injury. Question the patient to determine if there is any pain in the back or neck and determine if he or she is able to move and feel a light touch on all four extremities. If the patient describes a feeling of "pins and needles" in the legs, this is a positive sign of a potential spine injury. Observe for contusions, lacerations, punctures, penetrations, swelling, and deformities to the neck and back. Check by palpating for tenderness or muscle spasm in the neck and back. Also compare the strength of the arms by a simple hand grip and the legs by asking the patient to push against your hands.

If the patient is unresponsive, do not spend time attempting to exclude a spine injury. Obtain information from others at the scene to determine information relevant to the mechanism of injury or the patient's mental status prior to your arrival on scene. Immobilize the patient if a mechanism of spine injury exists.

PRECEPTOR PEARL

Tell new EMT-Bs that if there is a potential mechanism for a spine injury, treat for one by immobilizing the patient. Also, always assess and document the neurological function in all four extremities before and after immobilizing the spine.

Patient Care

Spine Injury

Regardless of where in the neck or back an apparent spine injury is located, emergency care is the same. First take BSI precautions and perform an initial assessment and rapid trauma exam. Determine the patient's priority since this affects how he or she will be immobilized.

Then, for all patients with a possible spine injury and for all accident victims when there is doubt as to the extent of injury, you should:

1. **Continue to manually stabilize the head and neck.** Apply an extrication or rigid cervical collar. Continue to maintain manual stabilization until the patient is completely immobilized.

2. **Assess pulse, motor function, and sensation (PMS)** in all four extremities, if the patient is responsive.

3. **Administer oxygen via nonrebreather mask,** and evaluate the need for positive pressure ventilations. This is critical should there be any cord damage. If the patient shows signs of shock, edema to the cord may impair oxygen delivery to the cord. When this occurs, cellular death can take place.

4. **Immobilize the patient.** Based on the patient's priority, apply the appropriate spinal immobilization device at the appropriate speed (Figure 24-8).

5. **Reassess PMS in four extremities,** if the patient is responsive. ✱

Immobilization Issues

Patients Found with a Helmet On

Helmets are worn in many sporting events, such as hockey, football, and skiing, and by most motorcycle riders. A sporting helmet is typically open on the front and provides easier access to the patient's airway than does a motorcycle helmet, which has a shield and usually a full-face section that is not removable. Facial-, neck-, and spine-injury care and airway management may call for the removal of the helmet.

A helmet should not prevent you from reaching the patient's mouth or nose if resuscitation efforts are needed. Protection shields can be lifted and face

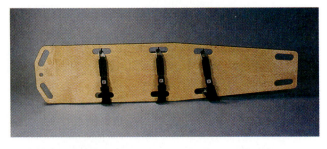

Figure 24-8 Long backboard with quick-hook straps.

guards can be cut away. If a face guard is to be cut, one EMT-B must steady the patient's head and neck with manual stabilization. The other EMT should snap off the guard or unscrew it.

Do not attempt to remove a helmet if doing so causes increased pain or if the helmet proves difficult to remove, unless there is a possible airway obstruction or ventilatory assistance must be provided. The indications for leaving the helmet in place include the following:

- The helmet has a snug fit that provides little or no movement of the patient's head within the helmet.
- There are absolutely no impending airway or breathing problems nor any reason to ventilate the patient.
- Removal would cause further injury to the patient.
- Proper spinal immobilization can be done with the helmet in place.
- There is no interference with the EMT-B's ability to assess and reassess the patient's airway.

It is important to note that if an injured football player is wearing shoulder pads, you should either remove the pads or pad behind the head to make up for the fact that the shoulders are off the ground. This will prevent the head from falling into a hyperextended position when the helmet is removed and the head is slowly lowered to the ground. When a helmet must be removed, it is a two-rescuer procedure (Skill Summary 24-1).

> ## PRECEPTOR PEARL
>
> Tell new EMT-Bs that many EMS providers put the controversy of helmet removal vs. nonremoval into the following perspective: If your child's neck was injured in a football accident, would you want the trainer and the EMT-B to work together to remove the helmet at the scene or would you prefer that this be left to the emergency department staff, who probably will not have the assistance of the trainer or the benefit of frequent practice in the helmet-removal technique?

Tips for Applying a Cervical Collar

Cervical-spine immobilization devices, or extrication collars, have come a long way since the early days of EMS. Originally, ambulance personnel would borrow soft collars from the hospital's emergency department. Unfortunately most early ambulance personnel did not realize that soft collars were put on patients whose X-rays determined that they had no fracture or dislocation. These soft collars were applied by the ED staff merely to remind patients not to move their necks so muscle strain could heal. The patients who had actual fractures were admitted and placed in traction. Thus, soft collars or "neck warmers" have no place in prehospital care.

The collars of today are rigid and are designed to limit flexion, extension, and lateral movement when combined with an immobilization device such as a long backboard or a vest-style device. Even though there have been marked improvements in collars, there is still no collar that completely eliminates movement of the spine. For this reason, when applying a collar, always maintain manual stabilization of the neck and head in a neutral position in alignment with the rest of the body. The latest devices are designed to be adjustable so one collar can fit a variety of sizes.

Do not stop after applying a cervical collar! Always continue to hold the neck and head until a short or long backboard is applied to the patient.

Since the sizing of a collar depends upon the brand, make sure you are familiar with the collar application procedure for collars used by your EMS service. Make certain that you assess the patient's neck prior to placing the collar. Take special care to look at the neck for tracheal deviation, distended jugular veins, and injuries prior to covering it. Ensure that the collar neck is not so tight that it obstructs the patient's breathing or the opening of the airway.

Make sure the collar is the right size for the patient. A large patient may not require a large collar; whereas, a small patient with a long neck may need the largest collar. The front width of the collar should fit between the point of the chin to the chest at the suprasternal (jugular) notch. Once in place, the collar should rest on the clavicles and support the lower jaw.

> ## PRECEPTOR PEARL
>
> Tell new EMT-Bs to remember: airway maintenance always takes the highest priority. Therefore, if you cannot perform a jaw-thrust maneuver and are unable to adequately ventilate your patient because the cervical collar is obstructing your ability to open the airway, then remove the collar. In this case, you will need to manually stabilize the patient while doing a two-handed jaw-thrust to open the airway. A second EMT-B will need to ventilate the patient with a bag-valve-mask device unless the patient has an endotracheal tube in place.

Helmet Removal from Injured Patient

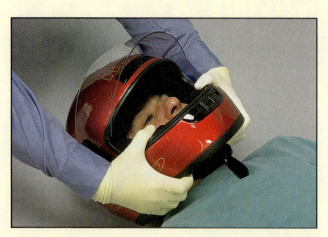

▲ **1.** EMT-B #1 is positioned at the top of the patient's head and maintains manual stabilization. Two hands hold the helmet stable while the fingertips hold the lower jaw.

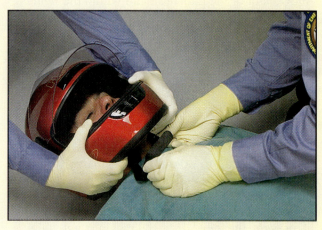

▲ **2.** A second EMT-B opens, cuts, or removes the chin strap.

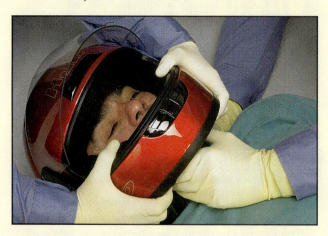

▲ **3.** EMT-B #2 then places one hand on the patient's mandible and, using the other hand, reaches in behind the neck and applies stabilization at the occipital region. Using the combination of the hand in front of the chin and the hand behind the neck, this EMT-B should be able to hold the head very securely. If the patient has glasses on, they should be removed now, prior to removal of the helmet.

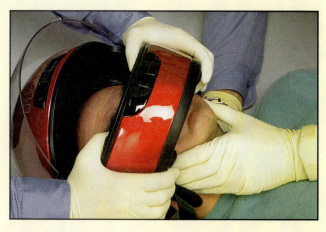

▲ **4.** EMT-B #1 can now release manual stabilization and slowly remove the helmet. The lower sides, or ear cups, of the helmet will have to be gently pulled out to clear the ears.

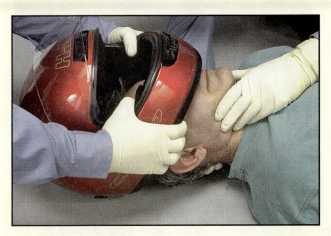

▲ **5.** The helmet should come off straight without tilting it backward. A full-face helmet may need to be tilted just enough for the chin guard to clear the nose. EMT-B #2 must support and prevent the head from moving as the helmet is removed.

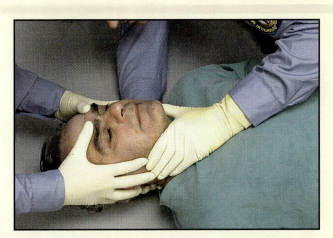

▲ **6.** EMT-B #1, after removing the helmet, re-establishes manual stabilization and maintains an open airway by using the jaw-thrust maneuver.

Helmet Removal—Alternative Method

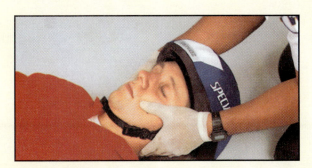

▲ **1.** EMT-B #1 applies manual stabilization with the patient's neck in a neutral position.

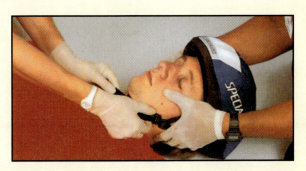

▲ **2.** EMT-B #2 then removes the chin strap.

(continued)

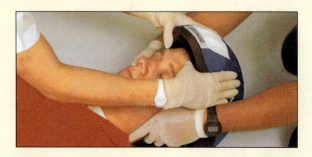

▲ **3.** EMT-B #2 removes the helmet, pulling out on each side to clear the ears.

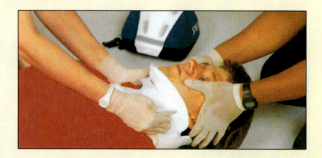

▲ **4.** EMT-B #1 maintains manual stabilization as EMT-B #2 applies a cervical collar.

NOTE: If the patient has shoulder pads and you are removing a football helmet, remember to remove the shoulder pads or pad behind the head to keep it aligned with the padded shoulders. With either helmet-removal method, manual stabilization must be maintained until the patient is secured to a long backboard with full immobilization of the head and neck.

When applying a collar be sure to remove the patient's necklaces and large earrings. Also keep the head in the anatomical position when applying manual stabilization and the collar. Be certain to keep the patient's hair out of the way, maintain manual stabilization while the collar is secured, and continue to manually immobilize the head and neck until the patient is secured to a short or long backboard.

If a collar does not fit, try using a rolled towel and tape to secure the head to the board after the torso is immobilized. An improperly fitting collar can cause more harm than good. So have a full set of various sizes.

Tips for Dealing with the Standing Patient

When you approach a vehicle and see the tell-tale sign of a spider-cracked windshield, this is evidence that whoever sat behind that windshield will need full spinal immobilization. Sometimes, such a patient will be up and walking around at the collision scene. It can be very dangerous to have such a patient sit or lie down on the long backboard. Therefore, use a backboard to carefully, but rapidly, take the patient down to the supine position without compromising the spine.

A rapid takedown of a standing patient allows immobilization of the patient in the position found (Skill Summary 24-2). Note that it requires attention to the procedure and to the patient. Be sure to keep the patient informed of what you are doing. Patients are startled when they are lowered backward, and they will tense up and grab for something to keep from falling. Patients who are intoxicated, combative, or dizzy make the procedure even more challenging. To perform this procedure, be sure to have the proper equipment (a set of collars, a long backboard, and straps) and at least three EMTs.

Tips for Applying a Long Backboard

The following tips will help you round out your knowledge of the application of the devices used for immobilization of the supine patient:

- Log roll the patient to apply the long backboard (Skill Summaries 24-3 and 24-4). This procedure must be done carefully, keeping the patient's spine aligned. Whenever a move is done involving neck stabilization, the EMT-B holding the neck calls for the move (i.e., we will turn on three. One. . . two. . . three. . .).

- When a patient is secured to a long backboard, the order of straps goes from chest to foot. A backboard with Velcro® straps or quick-hook clip straps makes the job easier. Secure the head last, using three-inch hypoallergenic adhesive tape. The tape offers support, especially if the patient and board are to be tilted to allow for drainage.

However, blood on the patient's skin and hair may make using tape impractical. You should learn to use cravats or Kling® as a backup method. Do not tape or tie the cravats across the patient's eyes.

- When immobilizing a child six years old or younger, it is necessary to provide padding beneath the shoulder blades to compensate for the child's proportionally large head.

- Additional immobilization for the head and neck can be provided with light foam-filled sandbags, a commercial head-immobilization device (Ferno Washington head immobilizer, Bashaw CID, or the Laerdal Head Bed), or a blanket roll. If used, apply these after securing the patient's body to the long backboard but before securing the head with tape.

- If you are treating a full-term pregnant patient, after immobilizing her on the backboard, prop the board on its side (right side up, left side down) to minimize the uterus compressing the vena cava, which can cause hypotension and dizziness.

- Unless the backboard has specific directions for straps intended to criss-cross the shoulder/chest area, it is best to strap across the upper chest including the arms, the pelvis excluding the hands, and the thighs. If the patient needs to be vertical in order to carry him or her through a narrow hallway, up a basement stairwell, or into a small elevator, make sure the chest strap is secure under the axilla (arm pits) and tight on the thighs to prevent shifting on the board.

- If your service transports to a helicopter, make sure that your selected backboard will fit inside it. Depending on the helicopter loading configuration, there are some restrictions on the size or taper of the long backboard. Be sure you are aware of this configuration in advance.

- For a water-rescue or diving injury, various specialty backboards, such as the Miller board, are designed to float up beneath the patient and utilize Velcro® closures for ease of application.

LIFESPAN DEVELOPMENT

If you do not carry a pediatric-size long spine immobilization device, then practice immobilizing a child using adult equipment and plenty of towels or blankets for padding. EMT-Bs are usually very good at improvising. However, in this case, your first improvisation should be in the classroom so you respond quickly in the field!

Rapid Takedown of a Standing Patient

Always take BSI precautions first.

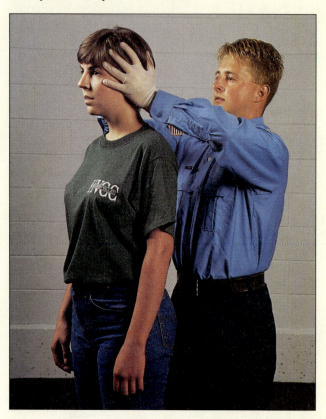

▲ **1.** Position your tallest crew member (EMT-B #1) behind the patient to hold manual in-line stabilization of the head and neck. This rescuer's hands will not leave the patient's head until entire procedure is completed and the patient's head is secured to the long backboard.

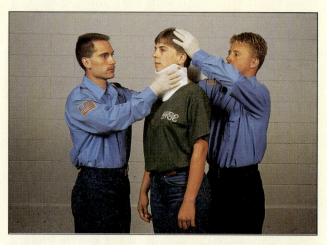

▲ **2.** EMT-B #2 applies a properly sized cervical collar to the patient. EMT-B #1 continues manual stabilization (collar does not replace manual stabilization).

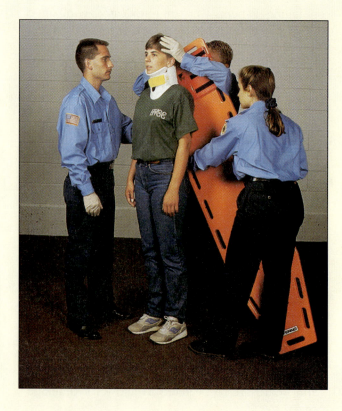

▲ **3.** EMT-B #1 continues manual stabilization as EMT-B #2 and EMT #3 position a long backboard behind the patient, being careful not to disturb EMT-B #1's manual stabilization of patient's head. It will help if EMT-B #1 spreads elbows to give EMT-B #3 more room to maneuver the backboard. EMT-B #2 assists with the positioning.

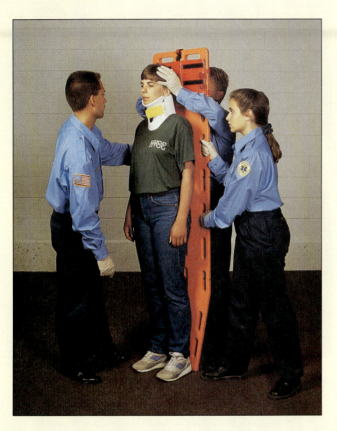

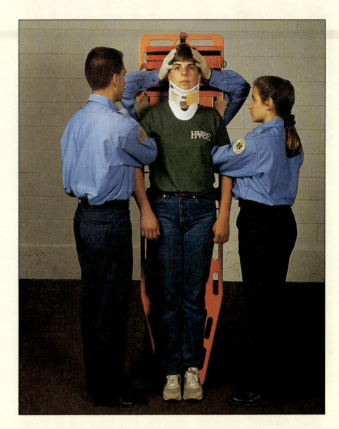

▲ **4.** EMT-B #1 continues manual stabilization. EMT-B #2 looks at the backboard from the front of the patient and does any necessary repositioning to be sure it is centered behind the patient.

▲ **5.** EMT-B #1 continues manual stabilization. EMT-B #2 and EMT-B #3 reach with arm that is nearest patient under patient's armpits and grasp the backboard. (Once the board is tilted down, the patient will actually be temporarily suspended by armpits.) To keep patient's arms secure, they use other hands to grasp patient's arms just above elbow and hold them against the patient's body.

(continued)

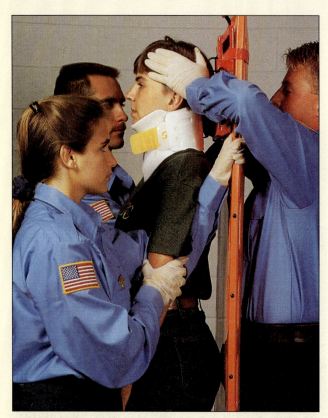

▲ **6.** EMT-B #2 and EMT-B #3, when reaching under patient's armpits, must grasp a hand-hold on the backboard at patient's armpit level or higher.

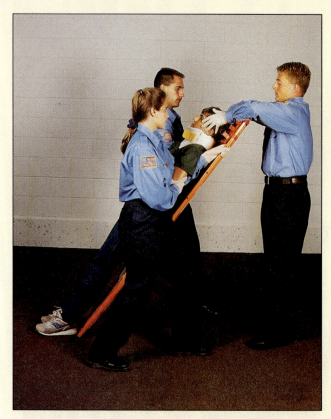

▲ **7.** EMT-B #1 continues manual stabilization. EMT-B #2 and EMT-B #3 maintain their grasp on the spine board and patient. EMT-B #1 explains to patient what is going to happen, then gives signal to begin slowly lowering board and patient to the ground. EMT-B #1 walks backward and crouches, keeping with the board as it is lowered. As patient is lowered, EMT-B #1 must allow patient's head to slowly move back to the neutral position against the board. EMT-B #1 must accomplish all this without holding back or slowing the lowering of the board. EMT-B #1 may need to rotate somewhat so that once the board is almost flat he is holding the head down on the board. Once patient's head comes in contact with the board, it must not be allowed to leave the board, to avoid flexing the neck. Two rescuers are needed to control the board while it is being lowered so that it moves slowly and evenly on both sides. They should also move into a squatting position as they lower the board to avoid injuring their backs.

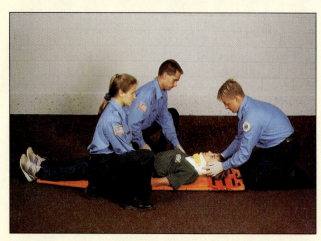

EMT-B #1 continues manual in-line stabilization throughout the procedure.

NOTE: This procedure is designed for 3 rescuers. It is not recommended with fewer rescuers. A two-person crew may need an additional rescuer or bystander to help position the backboard behind the patient.

Always take BSI precautions first.

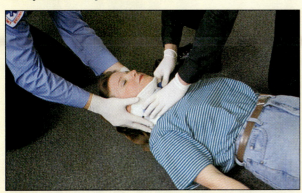

▲ **1.** Stabilize the patient's head and apply a rigid cervical collar.

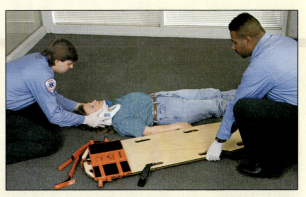

▲ **2.** Place the backboard parallel to the patient.

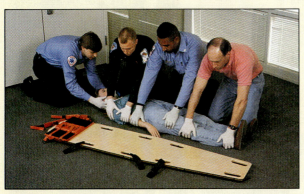

▲ **3.** Three rescuers will kneel at the patient's side opposite the board, leaving room to roll the patient toward them. Place one rescuer at the shoulder, one at the waist, and one at the knee. One EMT-B will continue to stabilize the head. The rescuers will reach across the patient and take proper hand placement before the roll.

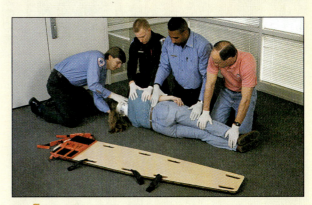

▲ **4.** The EMT-B at the head and neck will direct the others to roll the patient as a unit.

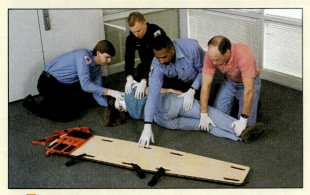

▲ **5.** The EMT-B at the patient's waist will grip the spine board and pull it into position against the patient. (This can be done by a fifth rescuer.)

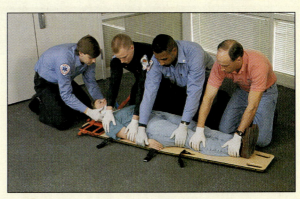

▲ **6.** Roll the patient onto the backboard.

Always take BSI precautions first.

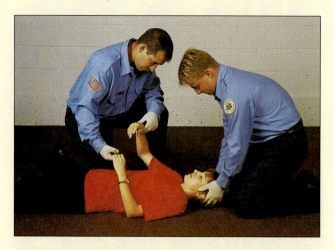

▲ **1.** Place head in neutral, in-line position and maintain manual stabilization of the head. Assess distal pulses, motor function, and sensation (PMS).

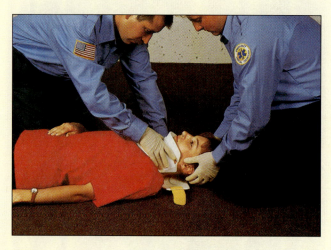

▲ **2.** Apply the appropriate size cervical collar.

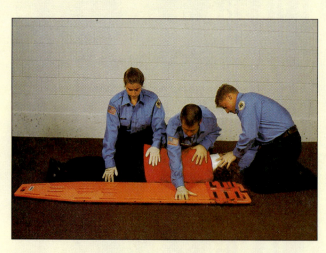

▲ **3.** Position the immobilization device. Check the patient's back and buttocks.

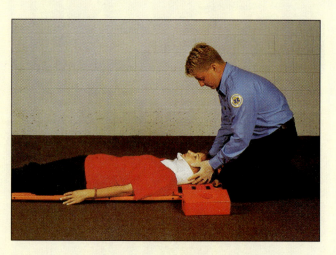

▲ **4.** Move the patient onto the device without compromising the integrity of the spine. (Apply padding to voids between torso and board as necessary.)

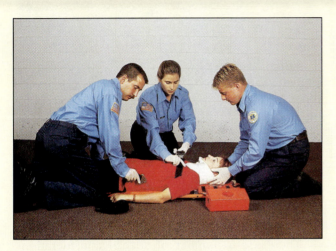

▲ **5.** Immobilize the patient's torso to the backboard.

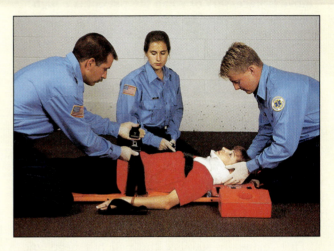

▲ **6.** Secure the torso straps.

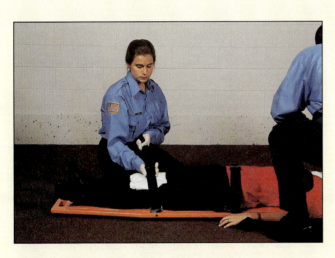

▲ **7.** Secure the patient's legs to backboard.

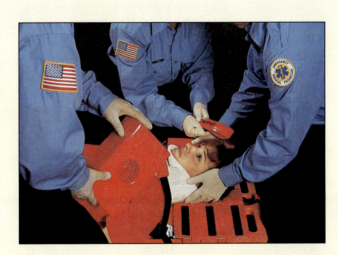

▲ **8.** Pad and immobilize the patient's head. Reassess distal pulses, motor function, and sensation (PMS).

Tips for Immobilizing a Seated Patient

When a patient is found in the sitting position, decide if he or she is a high or low priority. For a high-priority patient, use the rapid extrication technique (Skill Summary 24-5).

If the patient is stable and a low priority, use the normal procedure for spinal immobilization (Skill Summary 24-6). In such situations, when time is not of the essence, secure the patient to a short backboard or extrication device that will immobilize the head, neck, and torso until the patient can be transferred to a long backboard or other full-body immobilization device.

First, manually stabilize the patient's head and neck and quickly assess PMS to all four extremities. Next apply a rigid cervical collar. Then secure the patient to the short backboard or extrication device.

The short backboard is just a shortened version of a long backboard. This original extrication device has been used for many years and although still often used, it is used less frequently now, not because of loss of popularity among users, but due to narrow bucket seats in cars.

Today's automobiles have fewer bench-type seats and more bucket-type seats whose contoured backs do not accommodate a flat board. Also, the conventional short backboard is often too wide and too high to be used effectively in a small car. In these cases, a vest-style extrication device, a flexible piece of equipment, is useful for immobilizing patients with possible cervical-spine injury. It can be used when the patient is found in a bucket seat, in a short compact car seat, in a seat with a contoured back, or in a confined space. It is also useful when the short backboard cannot be inserted into a car because of obstructions. A number of commercial vest-style extrication devices such as the Kendrick Extrication Device (KED), Kansas backboard, XP-1, and the LSP Vest are available. Use the devices approved by your EMS system.

Whether you are applying a short backboard or a flexible extrication device, a particular sequence must be followed. You must secure the torso first and the head last. This approach offers greater stability throughout the strapping process and may help prevent compression of the cervical spine. If the patient has suffered abdominal injuries or displays diaphragmatic breathing that prevents adequate securing of the torso, the torso straps must still be used, but care must be taken to prevent interfering with the patient's breathing.

There are a number of special considerations when applying a short backboard to the patient.

- Any assessment or reassessment of the back, scapulae, arms, or clavicles must be done before the device is placed against the patient.
- The EMT-B applying the board must angle it to fit between the arms of the rescuer who is stabilizing the head from behind the patient—without striking or jarring.
- You must push a backboard as far down into the seat as possible. If you do not, the board may shift and the patient's cervical spine may compress during application. To provide full cervical support, the top of the board should be level with the top of the patient's head. The uppermost holes must be level with the patient's shoulders. The base of the board should not extend past the coccyx.
- Never place a chin cup or chin strap on the patient. Such devices may prevent the patient from opening the mouth if he or she has to vomit.
- When applying the first strap to secure the torso, do not apply the strap too tightly. This could aggravate existing abdominal injury or limit respirations for the patient with diaphragmatic breathing.

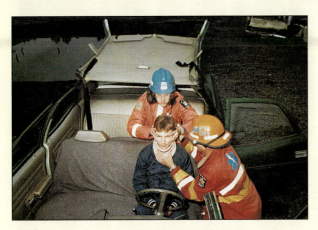

▲ **1.** Manually stabilize the patient's head and neck. Have a second EMT-B apply a cervical collar.

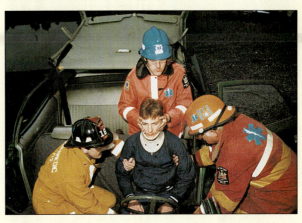

▲ **2.** At the direction of the EMT-B stabilizing the head and neck, two EMT-Bs each lift the patient by his armpits and buttocks/thighs, just high enough for a bystander or additional rescuer to slide a long backboard between the patient and the vehicle seat.

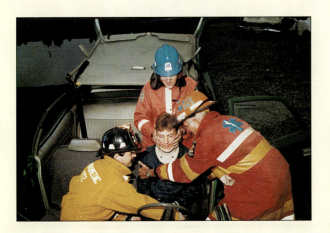

▲ **3.** The EMT-Bs reposition their hands so the EMT-B on the front seat inside the vehicle holds the patient's legs and pelvis, while the EMT-B outside the vehicle holds the upper chest and arms.

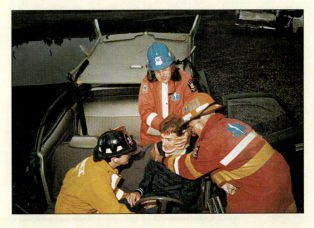

▲ **4.** At the direction of the EMT-B holding the head and neck, carefully turn the patient a quarter turn so his back is facing the side door of the vehicle.

NOTE: In the photos, the roof of the vehicle has been removed to allow for easier illustration of the positions of the EMT-Bs. In most cases, this procedure will be done and should be practiced with the roof intact.

(continued)

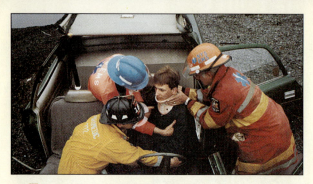

▲ **5.** The EMT-B who was holding the pelvis temporarily holds the chest so the EMT-B who was holding the chest can take over head and neck stabilization. The EMT-B in the back seat can then reach over the seat and assist with the chest, and the EMT-B inside on the front seat can move his hands back to the pelvis.

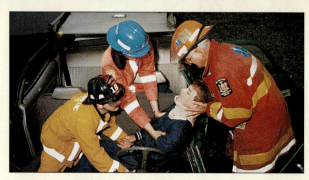

▲ **6.** At the direction of the EMT-B at the head and neck, gently lower the patient to the spineboard. NOTE: Sometimes it may be necessary to move the patient inside the vehicle a few inches so there is ample room to lay him down without touching the upper door opening.

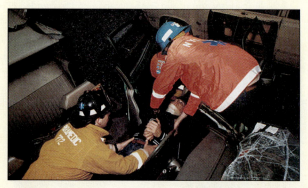

▲ **7.** As a bystander or additional rescuer holds the end of the backboard, the EMT-Bs slide the patient to the head end of the board.

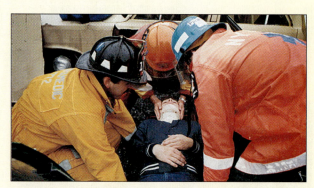

▲ **8.** Quickly apply straps to the patient's chest, pelvis, and legs and remove the patient to a stretcher or the ground, under the direction of the EMT-B stabilizing the head and neck. NOTE: Since the patient's head is not yet fully immobilized (it is only being manually held stable by the EMT-B and collar). DO NOT walk more than a few steps with the patient. Once on stable ground or on the stretcher, apply a head immobilizer or blanket roll and wide tape.

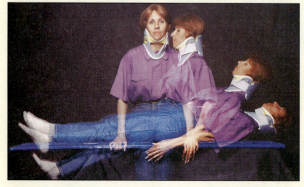

▲ As you move the patient from a sitting to a supine position, her spine must not bend, twist, or get jolted. Handle her very gently, and make sure you have enough assistance to perform the move correctly.

NOTE: The rapid extrication procedure is only for critical or unstable high-priority patients who must be moved in less time than would be required to apply a short backboard or extrication vest inside the vehicle before moving the patient to the long backboard. The normal extrication procedure is shown in Skill Summary 24-6.

Spinal Immobilization of a Seated Patient—Using a KED

Always take BSI precautions first.

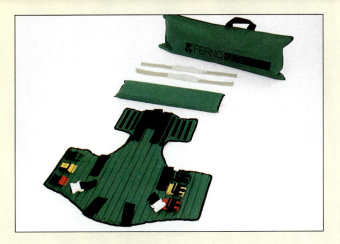

▲ **1.** Select the immobilization device.

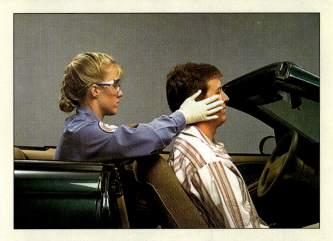

▲ **2.** Manually stabilize patient's head in a neutral, in-line position.

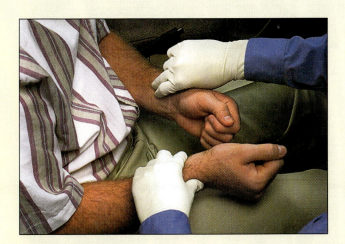

▲ **3.** Assess distal pulses, motor function, and sensation (PMS).

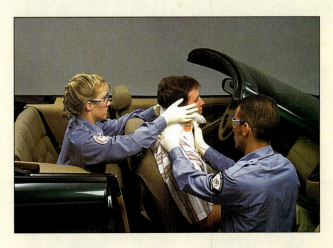

▲ **4.** Apply appropriately sized rigid extrication collar.

(continued)

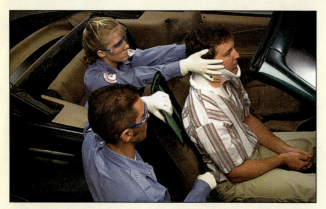

▲ **5.** Position the immobilization device behind the patient.

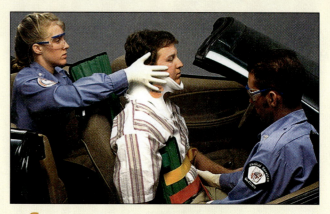

▲ **6.** Secure the device to the patient's torso.

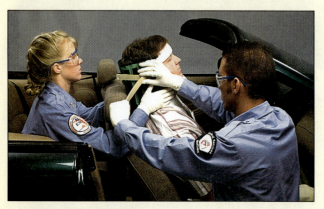

▲ **7.** Evaluate and pad behind patient's head as necessary. Secure the patient's head to the device.

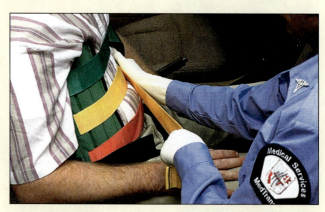

▲ **8.** Evaluate and adjust straps. They must be tight enough so the device does not move up, down, left, or right excessively, but not so tight as to restrict patient's breathing.

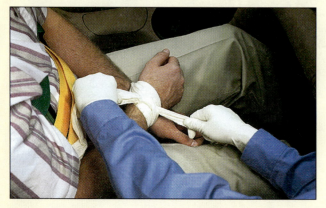

▲ **9.** As needed, secure the patient's wrists and legs.

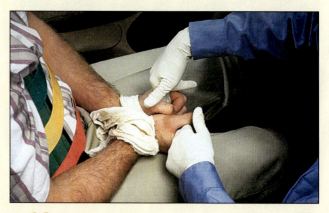

▲ **10.** Reassess PMS, and transfer the patient to the long backboard.

- Some short backboards have buckles with release mechanisms that can be accidentally loosened during patient transfer. This is true of "quick-release" buckles, which should be taped closed after the final adjustment of the straps.

- Do not pad between collar and board unless it is needed. To do so will create a pivot point that may cause the hyperextension of the cervical spine when the head is secured. Instead, padding should be placed at the occipital region, but only pad enough to fill any void. This will help keep the head in a neutral position. Often if the shoulders are rolled back to the board, the head will also come back to the board, which eliminates the need for padding.

- The placement of straps for the short backboard is somewhat complex (Figure 24-9). Most services carry these devices as a last-call backup for a collision involving numerous patients. Make sure you occasionally review the application of this device so you will be comfortable using it.

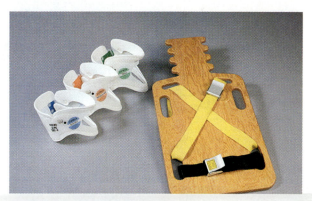

Figure 24-9   Short backboard.

PRECEPTOR PEARL

Tell new EMT-Bs never to use excessive padding behind the head because once the patient is removed from the vehicle, he or she will be placed in a supine position. At that point, the shoulders will fall back, but the head, if it is excessively padded, will not. This will place the patient's head in a position of flexion rather than the desired neutral position.

LIFESPAN DEVELOPMENT

Spinal immobilization of pediatric patients can be another challenge for EMT-Bs. Try to use the skills you learned for immobilizing an adult patient with a child. Practice adapting adult equipment to the child patient in the classroom to gain the needed experience prior to treating a child in the field.

When a child is found in an intact child-restraint seat, he or she can be immobilized right in the seat (Skill Summary 24-7) or rapidly extricated from the seat as shown in Skill Summary 24-8. The key decision point is that if a child would have to be in a supine position in order to be treated, then the patient must be rapidly extricated from the seat. This makes it easier to resuscitate the patient. When attempting to lay the seat back in a supine position, the patient's legs would be raised, which creates abdominal pressure on the diaphragm and restricts ventilation.

Immobilizing in a Child Safety Seat

Always take BSI precautions first.

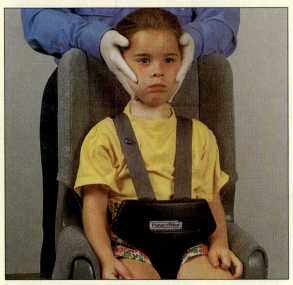

▲ **1.** EMT-B #1 stabilizes the car seat in upright position and applies manual head/neck stabilization.

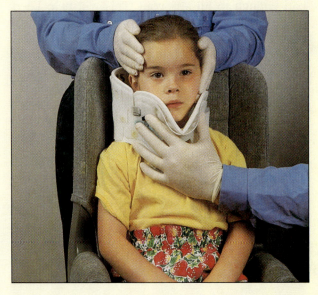

. . . as EMT-B #2 prepares equipment, and then applies cervical collar or improvises with rolled hand towel for the newborn or infant.

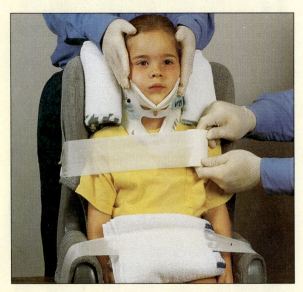

▲ **2.** As EMT-B #1 maintains manual head/neck stabilization, EMT-B #2 places small blanket or towel on child's lap, and then straps or uses wide tape to secure pelvis and chest area to seat.

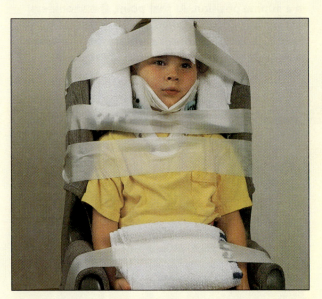

▲ **3.** EMT-B #2 places a towel roll on both sides of head to fill voids, tapes forehead in place, and then tapes across collar or maxilla. (Avoid taping the chin, which would place pressure on the child's neck.) EMT-B #1 maintains manual head/neck stabilization as the patient and seat are carried to the ambulance and strapped onto stretcher with stretcher head raised.

Rapid Extrication from a Child Safety Seat

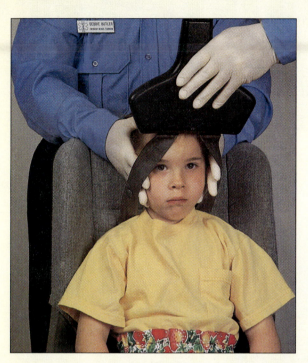

▲ **1.** EMT-B #1 stabilizes the car seat in an upright position, applies manual head/neck stabilization as EMT-B #2 prepares equipment, then loosens or cuts the seat straps and raises the front guard.

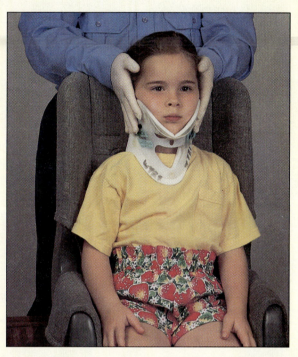

▲ **2.** The cervical collar is applied to the patient as EMT-B #1 maintains manual stabilization of the head and neck.

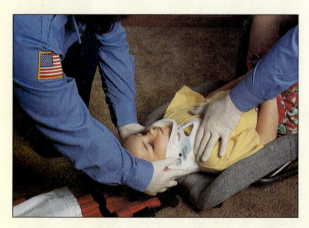

▲ **3.** As EMT-B #1 maintains manual head/neck stabilization, EMT-B #2 places child safety seat on the center of the backboard and slowly tilts it into supine position. EMT-Bs are careful not to let the child slide out of the chair. For the child with a large head, place a towel under the area where shoulders will eventually be placed on the board to prevent head from tilting forward.

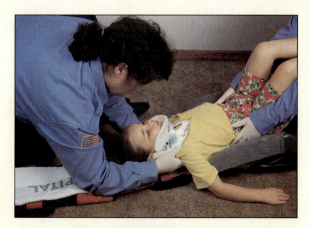

▲ **4a.** EMT-B #1 maintains manual head/neck stabilization and calls for a coordinated long axis move onto backboard.

(continued)

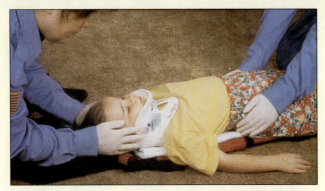

▲ **4b.** EMT-B #1 maintains manual head/neck stabilization as the move onto the backboard is completed. The child's shoulders should be over the folded towel.

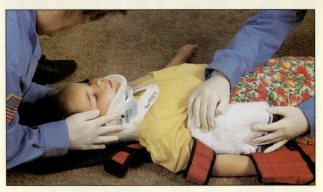

▲ **5.** EMT-B #1 maintains manual head/neck stabilization as EMT-B #2 places rolled towels or blankets on both sides of the patient.

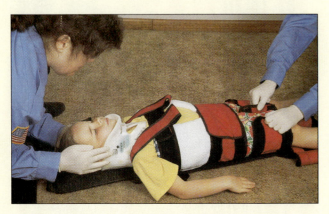

▲ **6.** EMT-B #1 maintains manual stabilization as EMT-B #2 straps or tapes the patient to board at level of upper chest, pelvis, and lower legs. DO NOT STRAP ACROSS ABDOMEN.

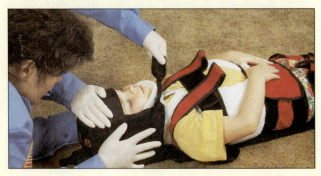

▲ **7.** EMT-B #1 maintains manual head/neck stabilization as EMT-B #2 places rolled towels on both sides of head, then tapes head securely in place across forehead and maxilla or cervical collar. DO NOT TAPE ACROSS CHIN TO AVOID PRESSURE ON NECK.

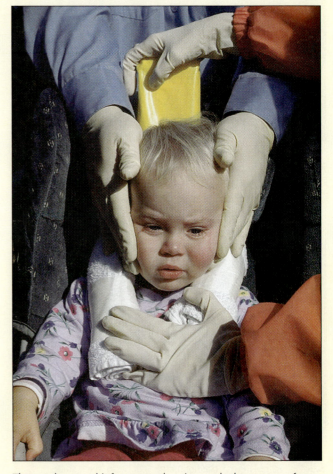

The newborn and infant procedure is exactly the same as for a child, except that an armboard is inserted behind the child in Step Two. If the infant is very small, the armboard may actually be used as the spine board.

Head Injuries

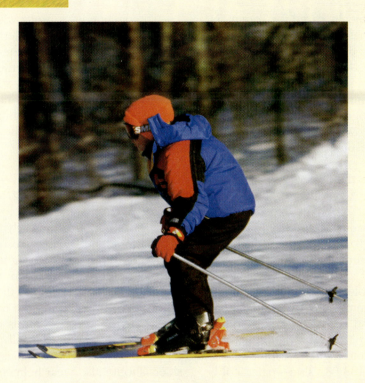

Your ambulance is dispatched to a local ski mountain's first-aid room to meet the ski patrol, which is treating a child who was injured while skiing. You pull into the loading dock at the entryway to the side of the ski lodge. Here you are met by one of the patrollers. As you quickly load your first-in bag and oxygen onto the stretcher, he tells you that the patient is already immobilized on a long backboard. Upon entering the first-aid room, you observe no dangers. However, the room is a very busy place since the lifts have just closed and a number of skiers were injured on their last run of the day.

The patient is a young boy. His father has just arrived in the first-aid room. The child is unconscious and has already been immobilized on a long backboard. A rigid cervical collar is in place. The child is receiving oxygen by a non-rebreather mask. All of his clothing has been removed, except for his underpants. Although the child has clearly sustained a contusion to the right frontal area of the skull, you also note a large amount of bleeding from lacerations in the same area of the skull. Your general impression is that of an elementary-school-aged male with an injury to the front of his head who is unconscious. This is enough for you to assign him a high priority for transport.

The patient's friend witnessed the incident and, although very excited, he is able to explain what happened. "We were on our last run of the day racing down the double-diamond trail when Tommy turned around to look for me. All of a sudden, he flew off the trail into a tree. Tommy thinks ski helmets are weird, so he wasn't wearing one. As soon as he hit the tree, his head started to bleed really bad. He was awake for a few minutes, but really confused. He said he had a killer headache and kept asking for his dad. I popped off my skis and started waving for someone to send the ski patrol. It seemed like it took forever for help to come, but I guess it was only a couple of minutes."

(continued)

The patroller who initially cared for Tommy is present. She tells you that the patient's ABCs presented no immediate life threat. However, she was concerned about his head and the possibility of a neck injury. So when more help arrived, the patrollers immobilized Tommy and took him down to the lodge on the toboggan. He was never alert. The initial mental status was verbal, but it diminished to painful by the time they arrived at the first-aid room.

Quickly you update the father. You then obtain a SAMPLE history. According to the father, Tommy has no medical problems except an allergy to penicillin. In a calm, professional manner, you tell the father that Tommy needs to be transported to the nearest trauma center. Due to poor weather conditions and a low cloud cover, helicopter assist is unavailable.

Before loading Tommy into the ambulance, you conduct your own assessment, observing proper BSI precautions. Tommy's vital signs are as follows: pulse—56 and regular; respirations—26 and shallow; BP—188/98; skin—pale, cold, and moist; pupils—unequal with a right pupil that is slightly larger than the left and sluggish to react to light. Although the lacerations have stopped bleeding, Tommy has a hematoma on the right temporal area of his skull. He responds to painful stimuli by withdrawal, and there is no indication of paralysis from a spine injury. He has equal lung sounds bilaterally and his pulse oximeter reading is 95 percent. No other injuries appear to be present.

After transferring the patient and backboard to your stretcher, you set up the portable oxygen and administer it at 15 liters per minute. You then request a paramedic intercept en route to the trauma center. The father tells you that he will follow in his personal vehicle. You then ask one of the patrollers to give him directions and to advise him not to keep pace with the ambulance, which could result in yet another injury.

During transport, you perform an ongoing assessment. Because the patient is critical, you retake the vital signs every 5 minutes . En route, the paramedic meets your ambulance and, after a momentary stop, you assist her in applying the ECG monitor, starting an IV line, and initiating endotracheal intubation.

The paramedic consults with medical direction and decides to assist the patient's ventilations with the BVM. She also reports the following information to medical direction: the MOI, assessment findings, the altered mental status followed by a lucid interval and then a rapidly deteriorating mental status, treatments administered, and your estimated time of arrival at the hospital.

CASE DISCUSSION

The patient is experiencing a possible epidural hematoma from a severe blow to the temporal area of the skull. Your early recognition of this "classic epidural" hematoma injury—and subsequent rapid transport to a trauma center— can be life saving for this patient. An epidural hematoma is usually due to an injury to the middle meningeal artery, which runs along the temporal area of the skull. This area of the skull is very thin and easily injured. That is why baseball players wear a batter's helmet to cover the sides of their heads. All skiers should also wear helmets, but unfortunately this is not the case. As a result, many skiers continue to be injured seriously when they lose control and run into a tower, tree, or another skier.

In this case, Tommy struck the side of his head on a tree and was initially unconscious. This was followed by a period of altered consciousness in which he was verbally responsive. He then proceeded to deteriorate rapidly. Such rapid deterioration usually occurs when the middle meningeal artery pumps lots of blood into the space outside the dura, creating a rapidly forming hematoma. Ultimately, if the hematoma is not evacuated in a hospital, it will cause brain herniation, often leading to death.

With rapid recognition of the problem and rapid transport to the appropriate facility to care for serious head trauma, this patient has a fighting chance for survival. The EMT-B increased the odds in the patient's favor by calling for a paramedic intercept.

In some areas of the country, once it is clear that a head injury is causing rising intracranial pressure, the decision may be made by medical direction or by local protocols to hyperventilate the patient. In Tommy's case, medical direction encouraged the paramedic to intubate the patient and then to assist Tommy's ventilations to a rate of 20 times a minute.

Name: Tommy Youngblood
Age: 10
Chief Complaint: Unconscious from striking his head at a high rate of speed

ASSESSMENT INFORMATION	RELEVANCE TO THIS PATIENT
MOI	• The story of how the accident happened is extremely important in determining the severity of the injury. The MOI, for example, indicates a strong possibility of an accompanying spine injury.
Mental Status	• The documented deteriorating changes in the mental status help the EMT-B to prioritize the patient for rapid transport.
SAMPLE History	• A history of a penicillin allergy is important to pass along to the hospital for subsequent care. It will not be an immediate concern for the EMT-B in the prehospital phase of care.
Vital Signs	• The slow pulse, rising BP, altered mental status combined with the MOI, and unequal pupils all paint a picture of rising intracranial pressure and a very seriously injured patient.
Physical Examination	• The EMT-B identifies a hematoma over the temporal area of the skull. • The lacerations have stopped bleeding, although they initially bled a lot. This is because the face is very vascular. • The pale and cold skin indicates poor perfusion. The patient is probably slightly hypothermic from lying in the snow.
Medications	• The patient does not take any medications nor will medical direction order any meds, aside from oxygen, for the EMT-Basic to administer.
Other Considerations	• Depending upon distance and time to the trauma center, a helicopter assist might be appropriate. However, in this case the helicopter was grounded due to a low cloud ceiling. Depending upon Tommy's prognosis, it might be appropriate to discuss the purchase of a ski helmet.

SUMMARY

- After proper assessment and care for the patient's ABCs, proper assessment and care for head and spine injuries are the EMT-B's most important responsibilities.
- Always assume a head or spine injury whenever there is a mechanism of injury of sufficient force or an injury to the head, neck, or upper body.
- If there is a head injury, suspect a brain injury as well as a spine injury.
- Provide high-concentration oxygen, immobilize, and transport the patient.

- When caring for a spine-injured patient, manually stabilize the head and neck and apply a cervical collar.
- Manual stabilization should be continued until the patient is fully immobilized on a long backboard.
- Always monitor and document any changes in the mental status of a head- or spine-injured patient.

REVIEW QUESTIONS

1. When the brain is lacerated, punctured, or bruised by broken bones of the skull, bone fragments, or foreign objects, it is referred to as a(n):
   a. transfer injury.
   b. indirect injury.
   c. direct injury.
   d. referred injury.

2. A pooling of blood within the membranes of a brain is a(n):
   a. concussion.
   b. hematoma.
   c. amenorhaer.
   d. epstaxis.

3. A late sign of a basilar (base of skull) fracture is:
   a. "raccoon's eyes."
   b. Farrell's syndrome.
   c. "Battle's sign."
   d. Cushing's syndrome.

4. The Glasgow Coma Scale measures a patient's:
   a. olfactory response.
   b. memory.
   c. eye opening, verbal, and motor responses.
   d. verbal acuity.

5. You are treating a patient who has been involved in a motorcycle collision. His helmet is cracked in two, and he is unresponsive. He has a blown pupil on the left side and little-to-no response to painful stimuli. What treatment, though controversial, is probably indicated for this patient?
   a. hyperventilation
   b. oropharyngeal airway
   c. epinephrine
   d. oral glucose

WEB MEDIC

Visit Brady's *Essentials of Emergency Care* web site for direct web links. At **www.prenhall.com/limmer,** you will find information related to the following Chapter 24 topics:
- Bicycle-related head injuries
- Brain injuries
- Shaken baby syndrome
- Migraine headaches
- Back pain

Correlates with the U.S. DOT "EMT-Basic National Standard Curriculum" Lesson 6-1

INFANTS AND CHILDREN

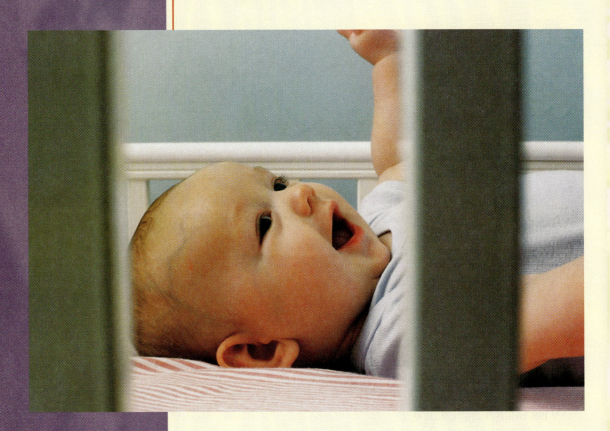

ESSENTIAL ELECTRONIC EXTRAS

CD ESSENTIALS

For preview and review of chapter material, see the student CD-ROM for

- Pretest
- Chapter quizzes
- Posttest

WEB ESSENTIALS

For additional review and enrichment, visit www.prenhall.com/limmer for

- Interactive student quizzes
- Links to online EMS resources
- Online case studies
- Audio glossary

In the past, the quality of out-of-hospital care of children was less than desirable. Two principal factors led to this outcome: inadequate coverage of the topic in EMT courses and EMS providers' lack of understanding of the growth and development patterns of healthy children. Both factors hindered the EMT-B's ability to deal with the emotional and physical needs of injured or ill children. In addition, most EMS personnel, like the majority of other people, consider children to be "special" and tend to become emotionally involved in the care of these patients.

Being extra attentive to children's needs just because they are children is understandable, but this extra attention should not overshadow your major goals: proper assessment and emergency medical care. To accomplish these goals, EMT-Bs need to be able to manage not only the assessment and care of young children, but also the tumultuous feelings that accompany them.

NOTE: At this time, you may wish to review material on pediatric patients in Chapter 10.

PEDIATRIC RESPIRATORY EMERGENCIES

Maintaining an Open Airway

To properly open the airway and to align the spine, it is important to place the child's head and neck in a neutral position. Use the folded-towel technique and perform a head-tilt chin-lift if there is no trauma, or a jaw-thrust maneuver with spinal stabilization if trauma is suspected.

Be prepared to suction the child's airway with a properly sized catheter, but avoid stimulating the gag reflex in the back of the throat. Stimulating the back of the throat can cause vomiting or slowing of the heart rate.

Children often have considerable amounts of secretions, which can block the narrow airways and require suctioning. Never suction for more than 15 seconds (which is roughly equal to the amount of time you can hold your own breath), and ventilate the inadequately breathing patient before and after suctioning.

Foreign Body Airway Obstruction

If you suspect a pediatric patient's airway is blocked by a foreign body, follow the most current American Heart Association (AHA) guidelines. Briefly:

- **Conscious child with good air exchange who is choking.** Encourage the patient to continue to cough, and monitor closely. Relief of the obstruction should be attempted only if the cough is or becomes ineffective (loss of sound), if there is increased respiratory difficulty accompanied by stridor, or if the patient loses consciousness.

- **Conscious child with poor to no air exchange.** Perform abdominal thrusts until effective or until the patient loses consciousness.

- **Unconscious child with poor to no air exchange.** Establish unresponsiveness, open the airway, and attempt to ventilate; if unsuccessful, reposition the airway and attempt to ventilate again. Then give up to five abdominal thrusts, followed by a tongue-jaw lift. If you see the object, perform a finger sweep to remove it. Repeat these steps, starting with opening the airway, until help arrives or as you begin transport and en route to the hospital.

- **Conscious infant with poor to no air exchange.** Perform a series of five back blows and five chest thrusts until effective or until the patient loses consciousness (Figure 25-1).

- **Unconscious infant with poor to no air exchange.** Establish unresponsiveness, open the airway, and attempt to ventilate; if unsuccessful, reposition the airway and attempt to ventilate again. Give up to five back blows and five chest thrusts. Perform a tongue-jaw lift and, if you can see the object, perform a finger sweep to remove

CORE CONCEPTS

In this chapter, you will learn about the following topics:

- Pediatric respiratory emergencies

- Other pediatric medical emergencies

- Pediatric trauma

DOT OBJECTIVES

✔ **Knowledge**

☐ **1.** Assess and provide care to an ill or injured infant or child with:
- Respiratory distress (pp. 413–415)
- Shock (hypoperfusion) (pp. 416–417)
- Cardiac arrest (p. 414)
- Seizures (pp. 418–419)
- Trauma (pp. 415–418)

✔ **Attitude**

☐ **2.** Explain the rationale for having knowledge and skills appropriate for managing infant and child patients. (p. 411)

☐ **3.** Understand the provider's own response (emotional) to caring for infants and children. (p. 421)

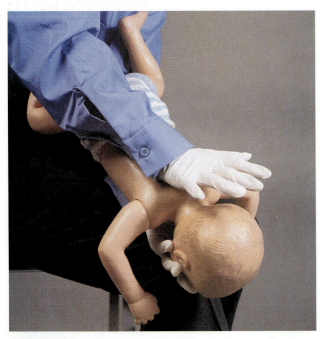

A Back blows

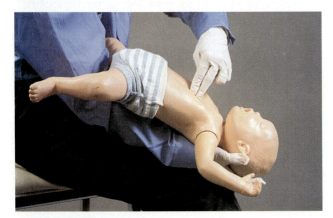

B Chest Thrusts

Figure 25-1 For a complete airway obstruction in an infant, alternate (A) back blows and (B) chest thrusts.

it. Repeat these steps in order, starting with opening the airway, until help arrives or as you begin transport and en route to the hospital.

Never perform "blind" finger sweeps in the mouth of an infant or child. Look in the mouth for an obstruction and use your fingers only to remove an object you can actually see.

Oral Airway Insertion

Because of its larger size, the tongue of an infant or child is likely to fall back into and block the airway. If this occurs when the patient is unconscious, does not have a gag reflex, and you have to ventilate for a prolonged period of time, you may insert an oropharyngeal (oral) airway to prevent the tongue from blocking the airway.

To insert the airway, use a tongue depressor or gloved finger to push the tongue down against the floor of the mouth while placing the properly sized airway straight into the pharynx. Unlike the procedure for adults, do not "flip" the airway over the tongue, since this may damage the uvula or soft palate or cause bleeding in a young child (Figure 25-2).

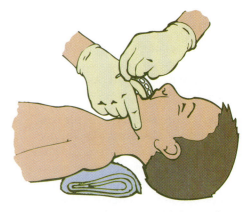

Figure 25-2 In an infant or child, the oral airway is inserted with the tip pointing toward the tongue and throat, which is the same position it will be in after insertion.

Respiratory Problems

Patient Assessment

Respiratory Distress

As you begin to assess a child in respiratory distress, ask yourself, "Is the child alert and calm?" Children in respiratory distress (Figure 25-3) usually are not. Then ask yourself, "Is the child agitated or sleepy?" **Hypoxemia** (too little oxygen in the blood) can make a child agitated. **Hypercarbia** (too much carbon dioxide in the blood) can make a child sleepy. Hypoxemia is more common in children.

Ask the patient's parents or other adults who were present at the onset of the emergency whether the child might have put a foreign body into his or her mouth. Common examples of such objects are pieces of hot dogs, peanuts, grapes, and toys. If there is reason to believe the child has a foreign body in his or her airway, use the techniques described earlier to expel the item. If, on the other hand, the history indicates the child has an illness as the cause of breathing difficulty, do not use back blows or chest thrusts.

Next evaluate the patient's skin color by asking a parent to remove the shirt so you can examine the skin and look for chest wall movement. Severe hypoxemia can cause cyanosis, and poor perfusion can cause mottling of the skin. Pallor or a grayish hue can indicate severe hypoxemia, which signals impending respiratory collapse.

Next, assess the respiratory rate by comparing it to normal rates. Is the rate elevated for the child's age? Increased respiratory effort is always an indicator of some level of airway compromise.

The signs of increased respiratory effort include:

- **Nasal flaring.** The dilation of the child's nares in an attempt to decrease airway resistance and increase air flow.

- **Stridor.** A high-pitched crowing sound usually heard upon inspiration that indicates obstruction of the upper airway.

- **Retractions.** Visible movements of the muscles, especially supraclavicular (above the clavicles), intercostal (between the ribs), and subcostal (along the lower margin of the ribs) that assist the movement of the rib cage in breathing.

- **Wheezing.** An audible sound heard over the chest during the expiratory phase of breathing which indicates obstruction of the lower airway.

- **Grunting.** Heard in infants, especially newborns with immature lungs, upon exhalation when air is pushed against a closed glottis to keep the lower airways open.

Next ask yourself, "Is the child flaccid or agitated by my approach?" A flaccid child is seriously ill and may be close to respiratory arrest. An agitated child may be hypoxemic.

Finally, to complete your assessment, feel for air movement at the nose. Minimal air movement indicates depression of respiratory efforts. Check the child's peripheral perfusion for delayed capillary refill, an indicator of severe hypoxemia and hypoventilation. ✳

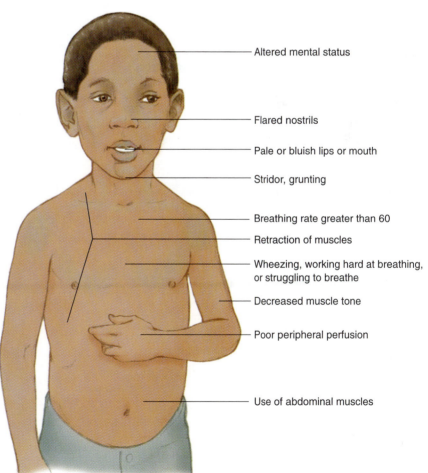

Figure 25-3   Signs of respiratory distress.

- Altered mental status
- Flared nostrils
- Pale or bluish lips or mouth
- Stridor, grunting
- Breathing rate greater than 60
- Retraction of muscles
- Wheezing, working hard at breathing, or struggling to breathe
- Decreased muscle tone
- Poor peripheral perfusion
- Use of abdominal muscles

Patient Care

Respiratory Distress

Emergency care for the child in respiratory distress must begin immediately with proper airway management, suctioning, administration of 100% oxygen (humidified if available) by mask, and evaluation of the need for ventilatory assistance with a BVM. ✱

A child in respiratory distress can quickly slide down a slippery slope that degenerates from respiratory distress to respiratory failure, then from ventilatory failure to respiratory arrest, and finally to cardiac arrest. Respiratory failure is oxygenation difficulty severe enough to cause obvious physical tiring, with increased ventilatory effort and rate. When a patient can no longer compensate and becomes physically exhausted, he or she deteriorates into severe hypoxia.

Pre-respiratory arrest signs include cyanosis, which degenerates to a grayish hue to the skin. **Bradycardia,** or slowness of the heart manifested in a pulse rate usually under 60 beats per minute (or 80 in a younger child), is a sign that signals severe hypoxemia and acidosis. Any child with respiratory distress and bradycardia should receive immediate ventilations with a BVM and 100% oxygen.

Children do not generally die from primary cardiac causes; the few exceptions are due to congenital heart defects. However, children can suffer primary respiratory arrests that result in cardiac arrests.

Children and infants go into cardiac arrest less often than adults and for different reasons. Whereas most adults arrest because of cardiac problems, children arrest because of respiratory problems. Unlike adults, children rarely go into ventricular fibrillation. In the rare case in which a child under 8 does go into cardiac arrest, AEDs capable of delivering the appropriate electric shock are now available for this size child. In most instances, however, the key to resuscitating a child in cardiac arrest is to maintain an open airway and provide effective ventilation.

The steps in assessment and management of an infant or child in cardiac arrest are summarized in Table 25-1.

Providing Supplemental Oxygen and Ventilations

High-concentration oxygen should be administered to all pediatric patients in respiratory distress, with inadequate respirations, or with possible hypoperfusion. Hypoxia is the underlying reason for many of the most serious pediatric medical problems. Inadequate oxygen immediately affects the heart and the brain, as evidenced by a slowed heart rate and an altered mental status.

Since infants through preschoolers are often afraid of an oxygen mask, try a "blow-by" technique. That is, have a parent hold the mask 2 inches from the child's face so the oxygen will pass over it and be inhaled. Some children respond well when

---

PRECEPTOR PEARL

Tell new EMT-Bs that pediatric-care experts emphasize that the priority of children in respiratory distress is "AAA," not just "ABC." In other words, if you manage the patient's airway and oxygenate, circulation improvement will follow!

Table 25-1   CPR for Infants and Children

	Child	Infant
Age	1–8 years	birth–1 year
Each Ventilation	1 to 1½ seconds	1 to 1½ seconds
Pulse Check Location	carotid artery	brachial artery
Compression Depth	1 to 1½ inches (approx. ⅓ to ½ the depth of the chest)	½ to 1 inch (newborn ⅓ the depth of the chest)
Compression Rate	100/minute	at least 100/minute (newborn 120/minute)
Compressions to ventilations ratio (one or two rescuers)	5:1	5:1 (newborn 3:1)

the tubing is pushed through the bottom of a paper cup or plastic comic character cup. Hand the cup to the child, who will instinctively explore it and hold it near the face, which accomplishes the desired result.

It may become necessary to ventilate a child, to assist a child's ventilations, or to actually resuscitate the nonbreathing child. Guidelines for ventilating the infant and the child are shown in Table 25-2. It is essential that you be well practiced in the use of the pediatric-sized pocket masks and a BVM using the correct face mask size. Follow these guidelines when ventilating the infant or child patient:

- Avoid breathing too hard through the pocket face mask or using excessive bag pressure and volume. Use only enough to make the patient's chest rise.
- Use properly sized face masks to assure a good mask seal.
- Do not use flow-restricted, oxygen-powered ventilation devices since they are contraindicated in infants and children.
- If ventilation is not successful in raising the patient's chest, perform the procedures for clearing an obstructed airway. Then try to ventilate again.
- Do not use a pop-off valve on any size BVM. If your service has one of these valves, replace the BVM with a new one.

PEDIATRIC TRAUMA

Childhood injury is the principal childhood public health problem in the United States today, causing more deaths than all childhood diseases combined and contributing greatly to childhood disability. Nearly half of all pediatric trauma deaths result from motor vehicle crashes, followed by drowning, burns, firearms, and falls. Blunt trauma exceeds penetrating trauma in children by four or more to one. Because of their curiosity, children are often injured investigating their environment. Their constant explorations lead to a range of injuries from accidental falls, things falling on them, burns, entrapment, and crushing to sporting and recreational activities and other mechanisms of injury.

Injury Patterns

Because of their anatomical and physiological differences, children's injury patterns differ from those of adults. During motor-vehicle collisions, unrestrained child passengers tend to sustain head and neck injuries, while restrained passengers tend to sustain abdominal and lower-spine injuries. Head, spine, and abdominal injuries are common when children are struck by an automobile while riding a bicycle. The child who has been struck by a vehicle may present with the combination of head, chest/abdominal, and lower extremity injuries. Other common injuries include diving injuries with associated head and spine injuries. Sports activities also account for a considerable number of musculoskeletal injuries to children.

Head Injuries

Head injuries are very common in children, along with injuries to the organs in the chest and abdomen. Common signs and symptoms of head injury include

Table 25-2 Artificial Ventilation and Clearing the Airway

	Child over 8	Child 1 to 8	Infant
Age	8 years and older	1–8 years	birth–1 year
Initial ventilation	1½ to 2 seconds	1 to 1½ seconds	1 to 1½ seconds
Ventilation rate	12 breaths/minute	20 breaths/minute	20 breaths/minute
Obstructed airway—conscious	abdominal thrusts	abdominal thrusts	alternate 5 back blows with 5 chest thrusts
Obstructed airway—unconscious	5 abdominal thrusts, finger sweep, ventilate	5 abdominal thrusts, remove visible objects, ventilate	5 back blows, 5 chest thrusts, remove visible objects, ventilate

nausea and vomiting. One of the problems that can result from a head injury is hypoxia from airway obstruction caused by the tongue falling to the back of the throat in an unresponsive child.

When managing a child with a head injury, be sure to keep the airway open with a jaw-thrust maneuver, administer high-concentration oxygen, ventilate as appropriate, and immobilize the head and spine. Do not use sandbags to stabilize the head. If you need to turn the patient and the board to protect the patient's airway, the weight of the sandbags could tip the child's head to one side, compromising your efforts to keep the spine aligned.

Abdominal Injuries

Since the muscles that surround the abdominal cavity are not very strong or well developed in children, internal organs can be and frequently are injured. This type of injury may be difficult to pin down because the child cries constantly or because of the lack of external wounds. Maintain a high index of suspicion for abdominal injuries and treat the patient with a significant mechanism of injury for shock (hypoperfusion). Keep in mind that children under stress or in severe pain frequently swallow air, leading to gastric distention which can interfere with the patient's efforts to breathe or your attempts to ventilate.

Shock (Hypoperfusion)

Trauma is a major cause of shock, or hypoperfusion, in children (Figure 25-4). (Shock, or hypoperfusion, is the inadequate circulation of blood and oxygen throughout the body.) The circulating blood volume in a healthy child is approximately 8% of the total body weight; an adult's is 6% to 7%. Despite the higher proportion of blood volume in the child, the total volume is much less because of the child's size. An infant typically has 340 cc of blood, a toddler 1,300 cc, and a school-age child 1,900 cc.

Dehydration from diarrhea is the leading cause of childhood death in the world. Both diarrhea and vomiting can cause dehydration and may lead to life-threatening hypoperfusion. The younger the child, the

more quickly dehydration can occur. Therefore, if an infant or toddler has a history of diarrhea and vomiting for more than a day, this is cause for concern.

The most important thing to understand about hypoperfusion in infants and children is that their bodies are able to compensate for it for a long time. Then the compensating mechanisms suddenly fail and decompensated hypoperfusion develops very rapidly. Children do not turn the corner from compensated to decompensated hypoperfusion, with an accompanying drop in systolic blood pressure until they have lost about 30% of their blood volume. This is because they have excellent vasoconstriction, which helps maintain their blood pressure.

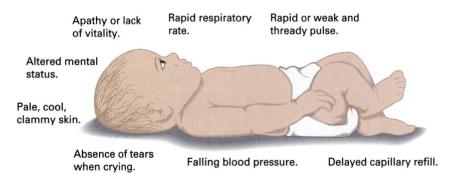

Figure 25-4 Signs of shock in an infant or child.

Apathy or lack of vitality.

Rapid respiratory rate.

Rapid or weak and thready pulse.

Altered mental status.

Pale, cool, clammy skin.

Absence of tears when crying.

Falling blood pressure.

Delayed capillary refill.

Patient Assessment

Hypoperfusion

Because of the broader range and greater variability in children's vital signs, and the fact that these signs do not change significantly until moments before circulation fails, they are not the best indicators of whether or not a child is hypoperfusing. Assessment should be based on clinical signs of inadequate tissue perfusion. These signs develop as the body attempts to compensate for the decreased circulating blood volume by shunting blood from the peripheral tissues to core organs.

The early signs of hypoperfusion are:

- Tachycardia
- Tachypnea
- Delayed capillary refill time
- Mottling

The late signs are:

- Marked tachycardia
- Markedly delayed tachypnea
- Marked capillary refill time
- Peripheral cyanosis
- Hypotension ✱

PRECEPTOR PEARL

Remind new EMT-Bs that the key indicators of inadequate perfusion and severe shock in a child are weak or absent peripheral pulses as compared to central pulses and/or delayed capillary refill.

The goal of the treatment for hypoperfusion is to maintain perfusion to the core organs (i.e., brain, heart, lungs, kidneys, liver) for as long as possible. The definitive treatment, regardless of the cause, is restoration of adequate circulation. For most pediatric patients this means replacing the blood or fluid that has been lost, and in some instances, surgical control of bleeding.

Patient Care

Hypoperfusion

The keys to improving the survival rate of pediatric trauma patients include the following:

- Rapid airway management with a jaw-thrust, if you suspect trauma.
- Oxygenation by way of a nonrebreather mask.

- Evaluation of the need to ventilate with a BVM.
- Immobilization of the spine.
- Maintaining body heat.
- Elevation of the legs.
- Immediate transport to the hospital.
- ALS backup, if available ✱

In some EMS systems, the PASG may be used for the treatment of shock. If used, it must fit the patient. Never place the infant in one leg of an adult garment. Do not inflate the abdominal section since it may compromise breathing. A PASG may be indicated for the pediatric trauma patient with signs of severe hypoperfusion and pelvic instability.

Nonaccidental Pediatric Trauma (Child Abuse)

Authorities agree that the incidence of trauma caused by child abuse is unknown. There is no question that many cases go unrecognized and unreported. Between 60% and 65% of reported abuse is categorized as physical. Current estimates are that there may be as many as 2,000 abuse-related deaths per year in the United States alone.

Since infants often develop the chronic abdominal pain of infancy called colic, they often undergo periods of irritability and incessant crying. These children are often at risk for child abuse from "shaken baby syndrome," pinching, and forced bottle feeding. Other children at risk of physical or psychological injury include those with learning disorders, seizures, feeding difficulties, chronic respiratory complaints, and developmental delays. Since these children often require constant special care and attention, their parents or other caretakers sometimes run out of patience and turn to abuse as a way of dealing with their frustration.

After completing your initial assessment and focused physical exam on a child you suspect may have been physically abused, compare your findings to information the parent or caretaker supplied. In some cases, a parent or caretaker will actually describe a history of injuries he or she has inflicted on the child; such a parent or caretaker is begging for help. In other situations, there is a remarkable absence of any history that would pinpoint the cause of the injury. Such unexplained events should trigger a heightened degree of suspicion on your part. At times, parents' explanations of the cause of their child's injury differ. These conflicting histories should be documented in "quotes" on the prehospital care report (PCR).

The location of an injury may also heighten your degree of suspicion. Anatomical sites for accidental injuries include the shins, hips, knees, lower arms, back, forehead, and under the chin. Inflicted wound sites are most often on the upper arms, torso, upper legs, side of the face, ears, neck, genitalia, and buttocks.

When a child exhibits bruises in various stages of healing, especially in the inflicted wound areas listed above, consider the possibility of abuse. Bruises undergo recognizable stages of healing. In the first 24 hours after a bruise is sustained, the color will be red or reddish blue. Over the next 1 to 4 days the wound will turn dark blue or purple color. Over the next 5 to 10 days, the area turns green to yellow green to brown. By 1 to 3 weeks the bruise should disappear.

Specific patterns are created on the skin from rope burns, scalds, cigarette burns, dipping injuries, a belt or paddle, pinching, and slaps. Learn to recognize these patterns.

Serious central nervous system damage without any evidence of external trauma is often the result of forcible shaking of a child. The shaking shears veins in the skull causing internal bleeding and altered mental status.

In addition to physical abuse, children are also subjected to emotional abuse, neglect, and sexual abuse. Remember that child abuse is a crime and your goal in the treatment of children who have been abused is to ensure their safety. Never accuse anyone of hurting a child, since you cannot be absolutely sure who the perpetrator was and the person in charge may react to accusations by refusing to allow you to treat the child. Treat the child and recognize that gaining the parent's permission to do so will enable you to transport the child to the Emergency Department where the facts can be sorted out by the proper authorities.

PRECEPTOR PEARL

Tell new EMT-Bs that the Emergency Department physician is required to report cases of child abuse. Therefore, they should complete the PCR with factual information that they observed about the child's home environment, the condition of the home, the reaction of the parents or other caretakers, the child's hygiene, and general interaction of all family members involved, and call it to the attention of the physician.

In many states, EMT-Bs are required to report suspicions of child abuse. Learn the laws of your state concerning the reporting of child abuse.

Injury Prevention

EMT-Bs can do their part in reducing injuries to children by becoming role models in their community and advocates for injury prevention. Many injuries are predictable or preventable. Examples of causes to promote in your community include:

- **Use of protective equipment.** Encourage the use of helmets for bicycling and helmets plus knee and elbow pads for skate boarding, in-line skating, and riding on scooters.
- **Playground safety.** Clean up the glass in the community playground.
- **Use of child safety restraints.** Do you always use an infant seat or seat belts? Do you always place your children in the back seat of the car?
- **Water safety.** Encourage diving into swimming pools feet first to test the water's depth, which can significantly reduce the number of spine injuries. Install fences around swimming pools, and always provide adult supervision of children around water. Ensure that children wear personal floatation devices when near the water or boating. Teach children to swim.
- **Avoid bus mishaps.** A knapsack worn on a child's back for books and papers will help decrease the possibility that he or she will drop them under the school bus and try to retrieve them.
- **Burn prevention.** Use smoke and carbon monoxide detectors, and encourage fire prevention education. Keep children away from wires and stoves. Adjust hot water heater (120 degrees or less).
- **Poisons.** Properly label and store poisons.
- **Guns.** Unload guns in the home and lock them in a safe place out of children's reach. Lock ammunition in a separate location.
- **Prevent falls.** Encourage use of window gates on high-rise buildings.

PEDIATRIC MEDICAL EMERGENCIES

Seizures

High fever, epilepsy, infections, poisoning, hypoglycemia, trauma (including head trauma), or decreased levels of oxygen can bring on seizures. Some seizures in children are of unknown cause. They may be brief or prolonged and are rarely life-threatening in children who have them frequently. However, EMT-Bs should consider childhood seizures potentially life-threatening, including those caused by fever.

Interview the patient or family member to determine if the child has a history of seizures. If so, ask about the child's normal seizure pattern and whether or not the child takes any anti-seizure medication. You should be able to describe the current seizure for the ED physician, as this may help determine the cause.

Emergency care of a seizure includes airway management, suctioning, administering 100% oxygen and ventilations as needed, maintaining body heat, monitoring vital signs, and transport. Position the child on the side if no possibility of spine injury exists. Since children's temperatures fluctuate widely over short periods, it is rarely necessary to cool a child. If local protocols direct you to do so, cool a febrile child by removing the child's clothing and sponging the child with tepid water. Carefully monitor the child for shivering, since overcooling can result in hypothermia. The significance of fever varies with age. Even the slightest fever in a newborn may be indicative of a life-threatening infection. A fever in an older child may not be as significant.

Poisoning

Children are often poisoned accidentally by ingestion of household products or medications. Poisons can quickly depress the respiratory system and cause respiratory arrest or life-threatening conditions of the circulatory and nervous systems. The airway and gastrointestinal tract can be burned by corrosive substances ingested or vomited. Some types of poisonings not often associated with adults but common to children are:

- **Aspirin.** Watch for hyperventilation, vomiting, and sweating. The skin may feel hot. Severe cases cause seizures, coma, and shock.

- **Acetaminophen.** Many non-prescription medications contain this compound, which can cause nausea, vomiting, and abdominal pain.

- **Lead.** Poisoning is caused by ingestion of lead (frequently in the form of paint chips) leading to chronic build-up of lead in the body. The child may experience nausea with abdominal pain and vomiting, muscle cramps, headache, muscle weakness, and irritability.

- **Cyanide.** In sufficient quantities, apple seeds and the kernels in apricot and peach pits cause the release of cyanide in the body.

- **Petroleum products.** The child's vomit or cough will have a distinctive distillate odor (e.g., gasoline, kerosene, heating fuel).

The management of a poisoning involves airway management and oxygen administration; medical direction may be contacted for additional advice. Activated charcoal, as discussed in Chapter 17, should be given only with the permission of the ED physician.

Croup and Epiglottitis

Croup is a viral illness that causes inflammation of the larynx, trachea, and bronchi. Tissues of the upper airway become swollen and restrict the passage of air. It is typically an illness of children 6 months to 4 years of age. It often gets worse at night following an upper respiratory infection. The child will have a mild fever, some hoarseness that develops into a loud "seal bark" cough, and signs of respiratory distress. Patients may also have nasal flaring, retraction of the muscles between the ribs, tugging at the throat, difficulty breathing, restlessness, and cyanosis.

Emergency care includes administering humidified oxygen and placing the patient in a position of comfort. Cool night air is helpful to the patient because it reduces the edema in the airway tissues.

Epiglottitis is most commonly caused by a bacterial infection that produces swelling of the epiglottis and partial airway obstruction. The typical patient is between 3 and 7 years old. Because children are now vaccinated against the bacterium most likely to cause epiglottitis (*H influenzae*), this uncommon disease has become extremely rare in children.

Children with epiglottitis present with a sudden onset of high fever and painful swallowing that causes drooling as the patient attempts to avoid swallowing. The patient often assumes the "tripod" position, sitting upright and leaning forward with the chin thrust outward in a sniffing position, and opens the mouth widely to maintain an open airway.

Epiglottitis can be life-threatening, and all effort should be taken to prevent further aggravation of the patient. Prepare for immediate transport and provide "blow-by" humidified oxygen. Monitor closely to ensure that the respiratory distress does not degenerate to respiratory failure or arrest. Advise the hospital of the patient's condition so they can prepare for the patient's arrival.

Do not place anything in the child's mouth, including a thermometer, tongue blade, or oral airway. To do so may set off spasms of the larynx and swelling of tissues in the upper airway, causing total obstruction.

Sudden Infant Death Syndrome

Every year in the United States, from 6,500 to 7,500 babies die from **sudden infant death syndrome (SIDS),** which is the unexplained death during sleep of an apparently healthy baby in its first year of life. The peak incidence of SIDS is between 2 and 3 months of age. It is rarely seen in infants older than 6 months. The greatest incidence occurs during the winter months, and there is often a history of a viral illness that was noted one to two weeks prior to the incident. Infants who were premature and who are small for gestational age are at a greater risk for SIDS, as are infants who underwent a stressful delivery that resulted in birth asphyxia, birth trauma, and central nervous system impairment. The incidence of SIDS has decreased about 50% in countries that have promoted campaigns to put infants to sleep on their backs ("back to sleep" campaigns).

It is believed that when asleep, the typical SIDS patient will show periods of cardiac slowdown and temporary cessation of breathing known as **sleep apnea.** Eventually, the infant will stop breathing and will not start again on his or her own. The condition is most commonly discovered in the early morning when the parents attempt to wake the baby.

It is not up to you to diagnose SIDS. When you find a child in respiratory or cardiac arrest, you should treat the child as you would any other patient. Unless there is rigor mortis, severe dependent lividity, decomposition, an obvious mortal injury, decapitation, or an advanced directive, provide resuscitation and let the pronouncement of death come from the hospital.

Ensure that the parents receive emotional support and that they believe that everything possible is being done for the child at the scene and during transport. Parents who lose a child to SIDS often suffer intense guilt feelings from the moment they find the child. Never speak with a suspicious or accusatory tone, as this may add to their guilt feelings.

Meningitis

Meningitis, which is caused by either a bacterial or a viral infection, is an inflammation of the **meninges,** the three layers of membranes that cover the brain and spinal cord. It is more common in children than adults. The patient presents with a high fever, lethargy, irritability, headache, stiff neck, and a sensitivity to light. The child may have an accompanying rash. In infants, the fontanels may be bulging, unless the child is dehydrated. Any movement may be painful, and seizures may occur.

Emergency care of these patients involves managing the ABCs and the symptoms to make the patient more comfortable. Since meningitis is a true emergency, transport the patient to the hospital as soon as possible.

Since meningitis is a communicable disease, make sure you take BSI precautions; avoid oral secretions by using a mask. If you are exposed to meningitis, check with your service's infection-control liaison to receive appropriate evaluation and care.

Dealing with Special Needs

Over the years, medical care has improved significantly, allowing many children who would formerly have died to live. Oftentimes, however, these children have special needs that must be met. Children with special needs include premature infants with lung disease and children with heart disease, neurological disease, chronic diseases, or altered function from birth (Figure 25-5).

Often these children are able to live at home with their parents and with the aid of various medical devices. When things go wrong, EMT-Bs are called to respond and often they must deal with complicated medical technologies such as tracheostomy tubes, artificial ventilators, central IV lines, gastrostomy and gastric feeding tubes, and shunts. The children's parents will be familiar with the devices and will be a useful resource to you.

Tracheostomy Tubes

Children who have been placed on a ventilator for a prolonged period often have a tracheostomy tube in place. The tube is placed in the trachea and is designed to create an open airway. The typical complications include obstruction, bleeding from or around the tube, an air leak around the tube, an infection, or a dislodged tube. Emergency care consists of assuring an open airway, suctioning the tube, allowing the child to remain in a position of comfort, and transporting to the hospital.

Home Artificial Ventilators

More and more ventilators are being placed in the home for use by special-needs patients. Often, parents face mechanical problems accompanying the use of these devices that lead to a call for EMS. Emer-

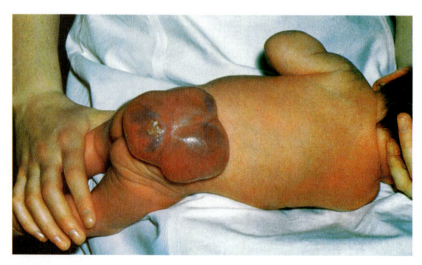

Figure 25-5   Child with spina bifida.

gency care includes maintaining an open airway, artificially ventilating with a BVM and oxygen, and then transporting to the hospital. Some communities are also prepared for power outages and arrange for emergency power for patients on home ventilators.

Central Intravenous Lines

Unlike peripheral IV lines (IVs in the arms, legs, or external jugular vein), central IV lines may be left in place for long-term use. Used for medication administration, a central IV line is placed with its tip close to the heart. Possible complications of central lines include infection, bleeding, clotting, or a cracked line. Emergency care includes applying pressure, if there is bleeding, and transporting the patient.

Gastrostomy Tubes and Gastric Feeding

A gastrostomy tube is placed through the abdominal wall directly into the stomach. The tube is used to feed a patient who cannot eat anything by mouth. Emergency care includes being alert for altered mental status in a diabetic patient. When unable to eat, diabetic children can quickly become hypoglycemic. Emergency care includes assuring an open airway, suctioning as needed, providing oxygen, and transporting the patient in either a sitting position or lying on the right side with head elevated to reduce risk of aspiration.

Shunts

Patients who have excess cerebrospinal fluid (CSF) in the brain often have a drainage device called a **shunt** inserted. Shunts drain fluid from the brain to the abdominal cavity. Should there be a malfunction of a shunt or an infection, pressure inside the skull will rise, causing headache, vomiting, and/or an altered mental status. These patients are prone to respiratory arrest. Emergency care includes maintaining an open airway, ventilating with a BVM and high-concentration oxygen, and transporting.

EMOTIONAL RESPONSE OF THE FAMILY AND EMT-B

Parents may react in many ways when confronted with a sudden illness or injury of a child. Their first reaction may be one of denial or shock. Some parents will react by crying, screaming, or becoming angry. Another reaction is self-blame and guilt. In all instances, be calm, reassuring, and supportive. Use simple language to explain what has happened and what is being done to and for the patient.

If the parents are able, use them to help you provide care and talk to their child (Figure 25-6). The most effective method may be to have the parent

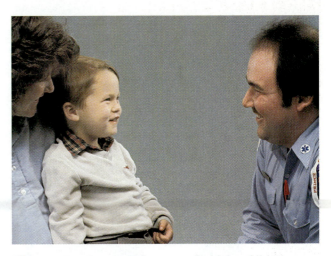

Figure 25-6   Have the parent hold the child in a position of comfort to involve the parent as well as to soothe the child.

hold the child in a position of comfort in the lap, if appropriate, during assessment and treatment. Offer as much emotional support as possible to the parent. However, avoid allowing communication with the parent to distract you from patient care. Also remember that some adolescents may not want their parents to hear their responses to your questions.

It is well known that pediatric calls can be among the most stressful for EMT-Bs, even when they are uneventful. EMT-Bs who have children often identify patients with their own children. Other EMT-Bs have no experience with children and feel anxious about talking to and treating them. However, the skills of communicating and treating pediatric patients can be learned and applied. Sometimes the EMT-B who starts out knowing nothing about children turns out to have a real knack for dealing with them. Most of the emergency care of children consists of applying what you have learned about the care of adult patients and combining it with knowledge of key differences in the developmental characteristics and the anatomy and physiology of children.

Often the most serious stresses an EMT-B faces result from pediatric calls that involve a critically ill, critically injured, or abused child. Calls involving an accidental death of a child or an MCI with numerous children are very stressful. Such calls are, fortunately, rare and can be prepared for with additional training.

When you have had an experience like this, talk with other EMT-Bs. Many believe that unless you resolve the impact of stressful events, the problems created may compound and could lead to "burnout." You may wish to contact your local critical incident stress debriefing (CISD) team for assistance after these incidents.

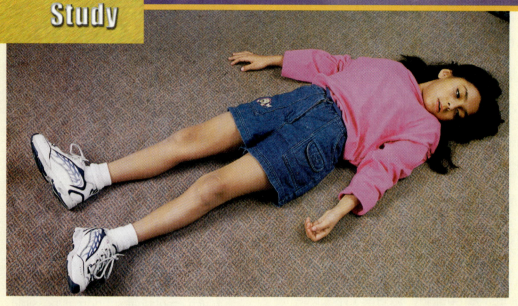

Dispatch: 83 Barlow Street   Convulsion   1642 hrs

Your ambulance is dispatched to a 6-year-old girl having a "convulsion." You have difficulty finding the scene initially because few houses on that street have house numbers. Finally, an anxious man flags down your ambulance. He confirms that he called EMS. Your driver now parks the ambulance as you take a closer look for potential hazards. Since this call is for a sick child, you know that adults can become distraught and do things they wouldn't otherwise consider.

The man identifies himself as Ted Bankhart, the father of the patient. He says his 6-year-old daughter Melissa just had a convulsion a few minutes ago. When you ask whether the little girl hit her head or sustained any other injury before the incident, he tells you she was playing on the floor and did not sustain any injury that he knows of. As you continue into the house, you look for out-of-control adults or potentially menacing pets, but see none. You find a child lying on her back on the living room floor. Her mother, Sarah Bankhart, is holding the girl's hand and is crying. The child looks flushed and unresponsive, but you observe chest movement from the other side of the room.

You introduce yourself to the patient's mother and open the patient's airway with a head-tilt chin-lift. This relieves the snoring sound you heard. When you look, listen, and feel for breathing, you see adequate chest rise at a rate that would be fast for an adult, but not a 6-year old. Melissa's radial pulse is rapid and strong, and her skin is flushed and sweaty. There is no sign of bleeding. She moans slightly when her mother calls her name. You assign this patient a high priority because of her altered mental status.

Her mother is able to tell you that Melissa was playing on the floor when she suddenly stiffened and then began thrashing around. Your careful questioning reveals that the patient's movements during the seizure involved all four extremities and lasted less than a minute, although it seemed longer to her mother. After the seizure, Melissa wouldn't respond to anyone and the father called EMS. .

With a calm, empathetic manner of questioning, you are able to learn from Mrs. Bankhart that the patient is 6 years old. She has never had any similar incidents and has no history of diabetes, seizures or other medical problems. Melissa takes no medications and did not have access to adult medications. She has not had a fever and is allergic to amoxicillin.

Your physical exam of the patient reveals no bleeding from the mouth, no lacerations to the tongue, and no signs of injury elsewhere. During the exam, you note urinary incontinence. The patient has a pulse of 116, BP 98/70, respirations 24 and full, skin pale and flushed, pupils equal and reactive to light, and a mental status responsive to voice by moaning.

As you apply high-concentration oxygen by pediatric nonrebreather mask to Melissa, you explain to her parents that their daughter probably had a seizure that needs further evaluation at a hospital. They quickly agree to have you transport her.

During the 20-minute trip, Melissa begins to wake up, opening her eyes and asking what happened. By the time you transfer her care at the emergency department, she is becoming oriented to her surroundings and is looking much better.

CASE DISCUSSION

Seizures are a relatively common reason for EMS calls. Although they can be frightening, seizures in themselves are not life-threatening as long as they are not prolonged or repeated in rapid succession.

When these events occur in children, the usual anxiety associated with seizures is compounded by the fear in parents that their child is in grave danger.

Seizure disorders often begin in childhood between the ages of 2 and 14. It is important that the EMT-B obtain information about the onset and progression of the seizure, including which extremities were involved and how long the episode lasted. This information is valuable to the other health care providers who will take care of the patient after you leave.

Anxious parents can be difficult to deal with under these circumstances, but it is important you include them in your management of the patient. A calm, empathetic demeanor will often make parents feel less anxious and more cooperative.

Name: Melissa Bankhart
Age: 6
Chief Complaint: Convulsion

ASSESSMENT INFORMATION	RELEVANCE TO THIS PATIENT
History of the present illness	• The loss of consciousness and involvement of all four extremities make this a generalized seizure. • The time the seizure lasted is important to rule out status epilepticus (prolonged or repeated seizures without return of consciousness). • The lack of access to adult medications makes poisoning less likely as a cause of the problem.
SAMPLE history	• The lack of a noticeable fever makes a febrile seizure unlikely. • The lack of a history of diabetes suggests this seizure is not the result of hypoglycemia. • The lack of a history of seizures suggests this is the onset of a new problem.
Physical examination	• Bleeding from the mouth caused by lacerations to the tongue is not uncommon in these cases. • It is important to look for injuries that might have been sustained during the seizure. • Urinary incontinence is common.
Other considerations	• Airway maintenance and high-concentration oxygen are important elements of the treatment. • A patient who has had a seizure typically takes 20 to 30 minutes to wake up and become oriented. • The care of a 6 year old must include one or both parents if they are present.

SUMMARY

- Airway management is the keystone of success in treating critically injured and ill children.
- Children compensate for blood loss long before they suddenly start to deteriorate.
- Epiglottitis is now a disease primarily of adults, not of children.
- The cause of SIDS is still a mystery, but its incidence can be reduced by encouraging parents to put their infants to sleep on their backs.
- Children with advanced medical devices and children dependent on technology like respirators should receive the same attention to ABCs that other patients receive.

REVIEW QUESTIONS

1. The proper ratio of chest compressions to breaths for an infant in cardiac arrest is:

   a. 5:1.

   b. 5:2.

   c. 15:1.

   d. 15:2.

2. When providing artificial ventilation to a 2-year-old child, ventilate at a rate of _____ breaths per minute.

   a. 20

   b. 40

   c. 60

   d. 80

3. When clearing the obstructed airway of an unconscious child over 8 years old, perform in sequence:

   a. 5 back blows, 1 chest compression, ventilation.

   b. 5 abdominal thrusts, finger sweep, ventilation.

   c. 5 abdominal thrusts, tongue-jaw lift, ventilation.

   d. 5 back blows, 5 chest thrusts, finger sweep, ventilation.

4. One of the key indicators of inadequate perfusion and severe shock in a child is:
   a. weak or absent peripheral pulses.
   b. accelerated capillary refill.
   c. weak central pulses.
   d. diarrhea.

5. Common causes of seizure in pediatric patients include:
   a. infection and epilepsy.
   b. hypoglycemia.
   c. high fever and head trauma.
   d. all of the above.

WEB MEDIC

Visit Brady's *Essentials of Emergency Care* web site for direct web links. At **www.prenhall.com/limmer,** you will find information related to the following Chapter 25 topics:

- Child abuse
- The National Safe Kids Campaign
- SIDS
- Childhood injury
- Missing children

Chapter Twenty-Six

Correlates with the U.S. DOT "EMT-Basic National Standard Curriculum" Lesson 7-1

AMBULANCE OPERATIONS

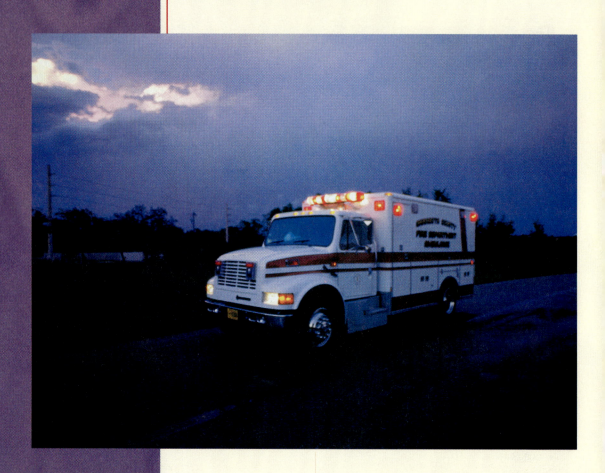

ESSENTIAL ELECTRONIC EXTRAS

CD ESSENTIALS

For preview and review of chapter material, see the student CD-ROM for

- Pretest
- Chapter quizzes
- Posttest

WEB ESSENTIALS

For additional review and enrichment, visit www.prenhall.com/limmer for

- Interactive student quizzes
- Links to online EMS resources
- Online case studies
- Audio glossary

This chapter covers the "nuts and bolts" of an ambulance call. Your nonmedical operational responsibilities as an EMT-B may differ, depending on the type of service that you work for. However, most of your duties will fall into one of the five phases of an ambulance call: preparation, responding, transferring the patient to the ambulance, transporting to and arrival at the hospital, and terminating the call.

AMBULANCE OPERATIONS

Ambulance Equipment

The modern ambulance has come a long way from the "body wagons" used to transport the dead in medieval times. The ambulance is far more than just a vehicle for transporting a patient to the hospital. Today's ambulance is well-equipped and efficiently organized. Anyone who has been in this profession for 25 or more years can tell you that until the late 1960s hearses were traditionally used as ambulances because they were the only vehicles in which a person could be transported lying down.

It is likely that hearses would still be the vehicle of choice if it were not for the 1966 white paper, "Accidental Death and Disability: The Neglected Disease of Modern Society." This paper called for vehicles that were better suited to the purpose of transporting the sick or injured to hospitals. Not long after, the U.S. Department of Transportation issued the modern ambulance specifications known as the KKK 1822(A), which are currently in their fourth (D) revision. These specs called for Type I (pickup truck with a box back), Type II (van), and Type III (van front with a box back)—vehicles we all use today (Figure 26-1).

However, due to the extra equipment placed on ambulances in the 1990s for specialty rescue operations and ALS, the gross vehicle weight was easily exceeded. This paved the way for the medium-duty truck chassis (maximum gross vehicle weight 21,000 to 24,000 pounds) that is built for rugged durability and has large storage and work areas (Figure 26-1D). As patient-care needs continue to expand and OSHA mandates evolve, the standards for ambulances will continue to change.

No matter what your region's vehicle is called, and even though it is especially designed and constructed, an ambulance is just another vehicle if it does not have the proper equipment for patient care and transportation.

Initial Assessment Bags

To decrease your scene time, carry the "right stuff" to the patient's side and package your supplies and equipment in a user-friendly manner. Portable kits or first-in bags come in all shapes, sizes, and designs. When setting up a first-in kit, keep in mind the steps of the initial assessment, focused medical history, and rapid trauma exam, which dictate the specific equipment needed at the patient's side in order to expedite care. In order to ensure proper care, your initial-assessment bag should include:

- **Head and neck stabilization and mental status check**—set of rigid cervical collars
- **Airway**—oral and nasal airways, suction unit and Yankauers, and personal protective equipment including BSI supplies
- **Breathing**—adult and pediatric stethoscopes, BVM, oxygen tank and regulator, pocket face mask with one-way valve, oxygen tubing, nonrebreather masks, and optionally a pulse oximeter with adult and pediatric finger probes

CORE CONCEPTS

In this chapter, you will learn about the following topics:

- The equipment carried on an ambulance and the importance of shift checks

- The basics of most states' emergency driving laws and regulations

- The proper operation of an emergency vehicle

- The proper transfer of a patient to the emergency department staff

- The usefulness of aeromedical evacuation in communities where it is an available transportation option

- **Circulation**—sphygmomanometer kit with separate cuffs for average-size and obese adults as well as infant and child sizes; bandages and dressings; occlusive dressings.

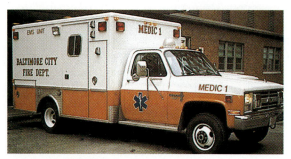

A Type I ambulance.

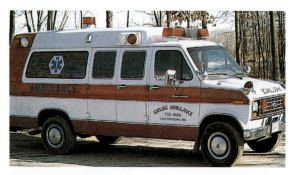

B Type II ambulance.

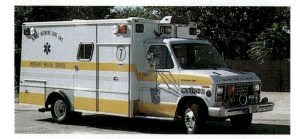

C Type III ambulance.

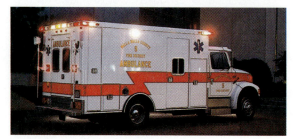

D Medium-duty ambulance.

Figure 26-1 Ambulance types.

- **Exposure**—scissors to expose, as necessary, and a blanket to deal with exposure. Optionally, carry patient information cards, a disposable thermometer, a hypothermia thermometer that goes down to at least 82°F, and a penlight.

PRECEPTOR PEARL

The new EMT-B must realize that the most modern, well-equipped ambulance is not worth the room it takes in the garage if it is not ready to respond. A state of readiness results from a planned preventive maintenance program, periodic servicing of the vehicle, and taking the daily shift checks very seriously.

Depending on the nature of the call, an AED and backboard with straps may be needed at the patient's side. Typical emergency care equipment and supplies carried on a modern ambulance are shown in Figure 26-2.

LIFESPAN DEVELOPMENT

Many ambulances carry sanitized, soft, or padded, brightly colored toys or stuffed animals to give to patients who are toddlers. Often local community service groups or commercial organizations are willing to purchase and donate these toys for this purpose. It is helpful to have the toy to break the ice with the child and make it easier to obtain important assessment information from the child. Also in some instances, the parents may be the injured patient(s) and the toy can be helpful to temporarily amuse the young child. Just remember—when you give the child a toy to play with, it becomes theirs and you should not expect it back!

It is always a good idea to carry extra blankets and pillows for elderly patients who are often cold and may need to be propped up into a more comfortable position for transport.

Supplies: Infection Control, Patient Comfort, Protection

- ❐ 2 pillows
- ❐ 4 pillow cases
- ❐ 2 spare sheets
- ❐ 4 blankets
- ❐ 6 disposable emesis bags or basins
- ❐ 2 boxes of facial tissues
- ❐ 1 disposable bed pan, urinal, and toilet paper
- ❐ 1 package of drinking cups
- ❐ 1 package of wet wipes
- ❐ 4 liters of sterile water or saline
- ❐ 4 soft restraining devices
- ❐ 3 large and 3 small red biohazard bags
- ❐ 3 large yellow bags
- ❐ 1 EPA-registered intermediate-level disinfectant
- ❐ 1 EPA-registered low-level disinfectant (e.g., Lysol®)
- ❐ 1 empty plastic spray bottle with a line at the 1:100 level
- ❐ 1 plastic bottle of water
- ❐ 1 plastic bottle of bleach
- ❐ 6 eye shields
- ❐ 1 large sharps container for vehicle
- ❐ 1 drug box sharps container for ALS unit
- ❐ 1 box (S/M/L) disposable gloves
- ❐ 6 disposable form-fitting masks in each size
- ❐ 6 disposable HEPA or N-95 masks fitted for crew

Equipment: Patient Transfer

- ❐ 1 wheeled ambulance stretcher
- ❐ 1 Reeves stretcher
- ❐ 1 folding stair chair
- ❐ 1 scoop, or orthopedic, stretcher
- ❐ 1 Stokes, or basket, stretcher accessible on a rescue truck or supervisory vehicle
- ❐ 1 child safety seat for transporting infants and toddlers
- ❐ 1 air mattress or EVAC® full body splint (optional)

Equipment: Airways, Ventilation, Resuscitation, Suction, O₂ Therapy

- ❐ OPAs in sizes suitable for adults, children, and infants
- ❐ soft rubber NPAs in sizes 14 to 30
- ❐ 2 child-size, manually operated, self-filling, BVM with reservoir (disposable preferred)
- ❐ 2 adult-size, manually operated, self-filling, BVM unit with reservoir (disposable preferred)

- ❐ clear masks with air cushion (various sizes)
- ❐ 2 pocket face masks with one-way valves and disposable filters
- ❐ 2 commercially available jaw blocks
- ❐ 1 fixed oxygen delivery system. A typical installation consists of a minimum 3,000-liter reservoir, a two-stage regulator, and the necessary yokes, reducing valve, non-gravity-type flowmeter, and humidifier (for infants and children).
- ❐ 2 portable oxygen delivery systems that have a capacity of at least 350 liters. The system should have a regulator capable of delivering at least 15 liters of oxygen per minute. Many ambulances are equipped with multiple-function regulators, which can be used for liter flow oxygen, suctioning, and positive pressure ventilation as well as a demand valve.
- ❐ 2 spare D, E, or jumbo D oxygen cylinders (preferably aluminum) with a current hydrostat test date seal imprinted in the tank
- ❐ 6 adult-size and 4 pediatric-size nonrebreather masks
- ❐ 6 adult-size and 4 pediatric-size nasal cannulas
- ❐ 1 automatic transport ventilator (optional)
- ❐ 1 plastic cartoon cup for administering blow-by oxygen to a child
- ❐ 1 fixed suction system that can provide an air flow of over 30 liters per minute at the end of the delivery tube. A vacuum of at least 300 mmHg should be reached within four seconds after the suction tube is clamped. The installed system should have a large-diameter, nonkinking tube fitted with a rigid tip.
- ❐ 1 spare, nonbreakable, disposable suction bottle, and a container of water for rinsing the suction tubes
- ❐ an assortment of sterile catheters
- ❐ 1 portable suction unit fitted with a nonkinking tube and a large-bore Yankauer tip
- ❐ 3 spare rigid-tip Yankauers
- ❐ 1 portable pulse oximeter unit (optional)

Supplies and Equipment: Immobilization of PSDEs

- ❐ 1 traction splint (e.g., Sager, Hare, or Kendrick)
- ❐ 2 padded 3″ × 54″ splints
- ❐ 2 padded 3″ × 36″ splints
- ❐ 2 padded 3″ × 15″ splints
- ❐ a variety of splints (air-inflatable splints, vacuum splints, wire ladder splints, cardboard splints, soft rubberized splints with aluminum stays and Velcro® fasteners, padded aluminum [SAM] splints, and splints that are inflated with cryogenic [cold] gas)

Figure 26-2 Typical BLS ambulance equipment *(continued)*

- ☐ 12 tongue depressors for broken fingers
- ☐ 12 triangular bandages
- ☐ 6 rolls of Kling® or self-adhering roller bandage
- ☐ 6 chemical cold packs
- ☐ 2 long spine boards (with speed clips or Velcro® straps)
- ☐ 3 sets of rigid cervical collars in short/medium/tall/no-neck adult & child
- ☐ 2 KEDs, XP1s, Kansas boards, or LSP boards
- ☐ 6 web straps, 9′ × 2″ with aircraft-style buckles or D-rings
- ☐ 2 head immobilizers (e.g,, Headbed, Bashaw CID, Ferno)

Supplies: Wound Care and Shock (Hypoperfusion)

- ☐ 24 sterile 4″ × 4″ gauze pads
- ☐ 6 combine dressings, 5″ × 9″
- ☐ 2 sterile multi-trauma 10″ × 30″ dressings
- ☐ 6 Kling® bandages in 4″ and 6″ widths
- ☐ 6 occlusive dressings (Vaseline® gauze)
- ☐ aluminum foil (sterilized in separate package)
- ☐ 2 sterile burn sheets or burn kit
- ☐ adhesive strip bandages for minor wound care
- ☐ 6 rolls of 1″ and 3″ hypoallergenic adhesive tape
- ☐ 12 large safety pins
- ☐ 1 pair bandage scissors
- ☐ 1 pair PASG
- ☐ 2 aluminum blankets (survival blankets)

Supplies for Emergency Childbirth

- ☐ 1 pair of surgical gloves
- ☐ 4 umbilical cord clamps or umbilical tape
- ☐ 1 rubber bulb syringe, 3 oz
- ☐ 12 gauze pads, 4″ × 4″
- ☐ 4 pairs of sterile disposable gloves
- ☐ 5 hand towels
- ☐ 2 baby receiving blankets
- ☐ 1 infant swaddler
- ☐ 4 sanitary napkins
- ☐ 2 large plastic bags
- ☐ 2 stockinette infant caps
- ☐ 2 surgical gowns
- ☐ 2 surgical caps
- ☐ 2 surgical masks
- ☐ 2 pairs of goggles or eye shields

Supplies and Equipment: Treatment of Poisoning and Altered Mental Status

- ☐ drinking water
- ☐ activated charcoal
- ☐ paper drinking cups
- ☐ equipment for irrigating a patient's eyes with sterile water
- ☐ constriction bands for snakebites
- ☐ instant glucose paste

Equipment: Safety and Miscellaneous

- ☐ *North American Emergency Response Guidebook*
- ☐ 1 pair binoculars
- ☐ 1 clipboard and prehospital care reports (PCRs)
- ☐ 1 ring cutter
- ☐ 25 assessment cards
- ☐ 1 portable radio
- ☐ 6 MCI management logs
- ☐ 50 triage tags and destination logs
- ☐ 1 each command vests (EMS Command, Triage, Treatment, Transport, Staging)
- ☐ 4 tarps in red, green, black, and yellow for MCI field treatment areas
- ☐ 6 disposable Tyvek® jumpsuits (optional)
- ☐ 6 flares
- ☐ 2–4 traffic cones (optional)
- ☐ 1 pair of jumper cables
- ☐ set of turnout gear for each crew member: coat, helmet, goggles, gloves
- ☐ 1 large floodlight/spotlight
- ☐ concentrated Gatorade®, a cooler, and cups for a rehabilitation sector (optional)
- ☐ self-contained breathing apparatus (optional)
- ☐ 2 spring-loaded center punches
- ☐ 1 Glas-Master™ or flat-head axe
- ☐ 1 small sledge hammer, prybar, or Biel™ tool
- ☐ 2 wheel chocks
- ☐ 100 feet of utility rope
- ☐ 2 stuffed animals for pediatric patients
- ☐ PFDs for each crew member
- ☐ water rope throw bag (optional)

Figure 26-2 *(continued)*

Ambulance Inspection: Engine Off	Ambulance Inspection: Engine On Outside Quarters
❐ Inspect the body of the vehicle.	*Set the emergency brake, put the transmission in "park," and have your partner chock the wheels before undertaking the following steps:*
❐ Inspect the wheels and tires for damage or proper inflation and wear. Don't forget to inspect the inside rear tires.	❐ Check the dash-mounted indicators.
❐ Inspect, adjust, and clean the windows and mirrors.	❐ Check dash-mounted gauges.
❐ Check the doors, latches, and locks.	❐ Depress the brake pedal and note if pedal travel seems correct or excessive.
❐ Inspect the cooling system. Allow the engine to cool first!	❐ Check air pressure as needed.
❐ Check all other fluid levels.	❐ Test the parking brake.
❐ Check the battery fluid level. If the battery is the sealed type, determine its condition by checking the indicator port.	❐ Turn the steering wheel from side to side.
❐ Inspect the interior surfaces and upholstery for damage and cleanliness.	❐ Check the operation of the windshield wipers and washers.
❐ Check the windows for operation and cleanliness.	❐ Turn on the vehicle's warning lights and check each flashing and revolving light.
❐ Test the horn and siren.	❐ Turn on the other vehicle lights and walk around the ambulance checking the headlights (high and low beams), turn signals, four-way flashers, brake lights, side- and rear-scene illumination lights, and box-marker lights.
❐ Check the safety belts and ensure that the latches and retractor mechanisms work.	
❐ Adjust the seat for comfort and optimum steering wheel and pedal operation.	❐ Check the operation of the heating and air-conditioning equipment.
❐ Check the fuel level.	❐ Operate the communications equipment. Test portable as well as the fixed radios and any radio-telephone communications.
	❐ Check the back-up alarm if you have one.

Figure 26-3 Ambulance inspection checklist.

Ambulance Inspection

As soon as you report for duty, speak with the crew members who are leaving. Determine whether or not they experienced any problems with the ambulance or its equipment during their shift. Make a thorough bumper-to-bumper inspection of the ambulance. Use the checklist provided by your service to do this. Examples of mechanical items to check include those in Figure 26-3.

Shut off the engine and complete your inspection by checking the patient compartment and all exterior cabinets (Figure 26-4). Look for damage to the interior surfaces and upholstery. Be certain that any needed decontamination has been completed and that the compartment is clean. Check treatment supplies and rescue equipment. See that an item-by-item inspection of everything carried on the ambulance is done.

Not only should items be identified during the ambulance inspection, but they also should be checked for completeness, condition, and operation. The pressure of oxygen cylinders should be checked. Air splints should be inflated and examined for leaks. Oxygen and ventilation equipment should be tested for proper operation. Rescue tools should be examined for rust and dirt that may prevent them from

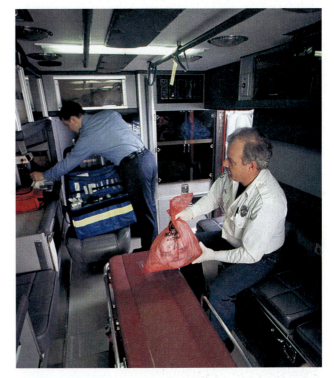

Figure 26-4 Checking the patient compartment in the ambulance.

working properly. Battery-powered devices should be operated to ensure that the batteries have a proper charge. Some equipment, such as the AED, may require additional testing.

When you are finished with your inspection of the ambulance and its equipment, complete the inspection report. Correct any deficiencies and replace missing items. Notify your supervisor of any deficiencies that cannot be immediately corrected.

Finally, clean the unit, if necessary, for infection control and appearance. Maintaining the ambulance's appearance enhances your service's image in the public's eye. If you take pride in your work, show it by taking pride in the appearance of your ambulance.

Emergency Medical Dispatcher

Many cities and communication centers have implemented training and certification based upon the medical priority card system, which originated in 1979 through the leadership of Jeffrey Clawson, M.D. The responsibilities of an **emergency medical dispatcher (EMD)** include:

- Interrogating callers and prioritizing the calls using a medically driven card system
- Providing medical pre-arrival instructions to callers and information to crews
- Dispatching and coordinating EMS resources
- Coordinating with other public safety agencies

The communication center should have central access such as enhanced 911 with 24-hour availability. When answering a call for help, the EMD must obtain as much information as possible about the situation in order to assist the responding crew. The essential information is the nature of the call and location. The questions the EMD will ask to obtain the dispatch information are:

- **"What is the exact location of the patient?"** The EMD must ask for the house or building number and the apartment number, if any. It is important to ask the street name with the direction designator (e.g., north, east), the nearest cross street, the name of the development or subdivision, and the exact location of the emergency.
- **"What is your call-back number? Stay on the line. Do not hang up until I (the EMD) tell you to."** In life-threatening situations, after the units have been dispatched, the EMD will offer instruction to the caller that the caller or others on scene should follow until the units arrive. The call-back number is also important should there be any question about the location. For example, several streets within a community may have the same name but a different direction designator, such as North Main or South Main.

- **"What is the problem or nature of the call?"** This helps the EMD understand the caller's perception of the chief complaint. It also helps the EMD decide which line of questioning to continue with and, according to medical response protocols, the priority of the response to send.
- **"How old is the patient?"** This information will allow the EMS crew to be prepared with the pediatric kit if the patient is a child. Further, if pre-arrival CPR instructions are given, it is necessary to determine if the patient is an infant, child, or adult.
- **"What is the patient's sex?"** This is asked if it is not already obvious by the caller's voice, or the caller is not the patient.
- **"Is the patient conscious?"** An unconscious patient elicits the highest priority response.
- **"Is the patient breathing?"** If the patient is conscious and breathing, the EMD often asks many additional questions relative to the chief complaint. This is done to determine the appropriate level of response, for example first responders, paramedics, or ambulance responding COLD or ALPHA (at normal driving speed)—or HOT or CHARLIE or DELTA (an emergency, lights-and-siren mode). If the patient is not breathing, or the caller is not sure, the EMD dispatches the maximum response and begins the appropriate pre-arrival instructions for a nonbreathing patient, which may also involve telephone directions for CPR if the patient is pulseless.

In addition, in trauma calls the EMD asks for the number of patients and about the severity of the injuries, as well as the name of the caller and details of any other special problems.

An EMD might dispatch an ambulance to the location of an injured person in this way:

> "MEDCOM to Ambulance 621 and Medic 620, respond priority DELTA with Engine 10 to a 40-year-old unconscious male who fell from the roof of a house. The location is 165 Central Parkway, with Bridge Street on the cross. Time now is 1645 hours."

The EMD will repeat the message to minimize any question about its content and to assure that the ambulance and medic receive the call.

Driving the Ambulance

No textbook can teach you how to drive an ambulance, nor can you become a good ambulance operator through experience alone. If you will be driving an ambulance, even occasionally, attend an emergency-vehicle-operator course that has both classroom and driving practice.

In the course, you will learn how a vehicle operates, how it behaves on different types of roads, the proper use of audible and visual warning devices, and laws regarding the operation of emergency vehicles. You will learn how to prevent collisions by staying alert for problems caused by other motorists, changing road conditions, and hazards. You will then spend time behind the wheel as you are coached by an experienced ambulance driving instructor. On the driving range, you will learn how to use the vehicle's mirrors properly and to judge the vehicle's size, how to change lanes quickly and safely, how to recover from skids, and how to back up and park the vehicle.

To be a safe ambulance operator, you must:

- **Be physically fit.** You should not have any impairment that prevents you from turning the steering wheel, operating the gearshift, or depressing the floor pedals. Nor should you have any medical condition that might disable you while driving, such as a heart condition or epilepsy.
- **Be mentally fit and have your emotions under control.**
- **Be able to perform under stress.**
- **Have a positive attitude.** Take pride in your driving ability, without becoming an overly confident risk taker.
- **Be tolerant of other drivers.** Always keep in mind that people react differently when they see an emergency vehicle. Accept and tolerate the bad habits of other drivers without flying into a rage.
- **Never drive while under the influence of drugs or alcohol.**
- **Never drive with a suspended license.**
- **Always wear your glasses or contact lenses if required for driving.**
- **Evaluate your ability to drive.** Consider the effects of personal stress, illness, fatigue, or sleepiness.

Driving Laws

Every state has statutes that regulate the operation of emergency vehicles. Although the provisions may vary, the intent of the laws is essentially the same. Emergency-vehicle operators are generally granted certain exemptions with regard to speed, parking, passage through traffic signals, and direction of travel. However, the laws also clearly state: If an emergency-vehicle operator does not drive with due regard for the safety of others, he or she must be prepared to pay the consequences for his or her actions—consequences such as tickets, lawsuits, or even time in jail.

Following are some points usually included in typical state laws that regulate the operation of ambulances. Be sure to review the actual laws in your state.

- An ambulance operator must have a valid driver's license and may be required to complete a training program.

- Privileges granted under the law to the operators of ambulances apply when the vehicle is responding to an emergency or is involved in the emergency transport of a sick or injured person. When the ambulance is not on an emergency call, the laws that apply to the operation of nonemergency vehicles also apply to the ambulance.
- Even though certain privileges are granted during an emergency, they do not provide immunity to the operator in cases of reckless driving or disregard for the safety of others.
- Privileges granted under the law to the operators of ambulances apply only if the operator uses warning devices in the manner prescribed by law.
- The emergency-vehicle operator may park the vehicle anywhere, as long as it does not damage personal property or endanger lives.
- The emergency-vehicle operator may proceed past red stop signals, flashing red stop signals, and stop signs. Some states require that operators come to a full stop, and then proceed with caution. Other states require only that an operator slow down and proceed with caution.
- The emergency-vehicle operator may exceed the posted speed limit as long as life and property are not endangered.
- The emergency-vehicle operator may pass other vehicles in designated no-passing zones after properly signaling, ensuring that the way is clear, and taking precautions to avoid endangering life and property. This does not include passing a school bus with the red lights blinking. Wait for the driver to clear the children and to turn off the red lights.
- With proper caution and signals, the emergency-vehicle operator may disregard regulations that govern direction of travel.

Should you ever become involved in an ambulance collision (Figure 26-5), the laws will be interpreted by the court based upon two key issues: Did you use due regard for the safety of all others? Was it

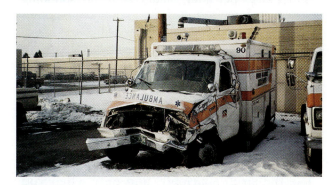

FIGURE 26-5 An ambulance that was involved in a collision.

a true emergency? The requirement of due regard actually sets a higher standard for drivers of emergency vehicles than for the rest of the driving public.

Most states reserve emergency operation for a **true emergency**—a call in which the best information you have is that there is a possibility of loss of life or limb. A dispatch to a "collision" will usually get an emergency response. However, once you arrive and find that your patient has a minor injury, the call is no longer a true emergency. A lights-and-siren, high-speed response to the hospital in such a situation would be ruled illegal in most states.

The Siren

Ambulance operators sometimes become so obsessed with the idea that sirens and flashing lights will clear the roads that they overlook hazards and take chances. Audible and visual warning devices do serve a purpose; however, safe emergency-vehicle operation can be achieved only when the proper use of warning devices is coupled with sound emergency and defensive driving practices. It is important to note that studies have shown that most other drivers do not see or hear your ambulance until it is within 50 to 100 feet of their vehicle.

The siren is the most commonly used audible warning device. It is also the most abused. Consider the effects that sirens have on motorists, your patients, and ambulance operators:

- Motorists are less inclined to yield to ambulances when sirens are continually sounded.
- Many feel that the right-of-way privileges granted to ambulances by law are being abused when sirens are sounded.
- The continuous sound of a siren may cause a sick or injured patient to suffer increased fear and anxiety, worsening the patient's condition.
- Ambulance operators themselves are affected by the continuous sound of a siren.

Tests have shown that inexperienced ambulance operators tend to increase their driving speeds from 10 to 15 miles per hour while continually sounding the siren. In some reported cases, operators using a siren were unable to negotiate curves that they easily could pass through when not sounding the siren. Sirens can also affect your ability to hear other traffic.

Many states have laws that regulate the use of audible warning signals, and where there are no such statutes, ambulance organizations usually create their own standard operating procedures (SOPs). If your service does not have guidelines, the following suggestions may be helpful:

- **Use the siren sparingly, and only when you must.** Some states require the use of the siren at all times when the ambulance is responding in the emergency mode. Other states require it only when the operator is exercising any of the exemptions discussed above.

- **Never assume that all motorists will hear your signal.** Buildings, trees, and dense shrubbery may block siren sounds. Soundproofing keeps outside noises from entering vehicles. Radios, tape, or CD systems also decrease the likelihood that your siren will be heard.

- **Always assume that some motorists will hear your siren and ignore it.**

- **Be prepared for the panic and erratic maneuvers of other drivers when they hear your siren.**

- **Do not pull up close to a vehicle and then sound your siren.** Such action may cause the driver to jam on the brakes so quickly that you will be unable to stop in time. Use the horn when you are close to a vehicle ahead.

- **Never use a siren to scare someone.**

Emergency Lights

Whenever the ambulance is on the road, night or day, turn on the headlights to increase its visibility. In some states, the headlights of all vehicles must be turned on whenever the windshield wipers are being used. In most states it is illegal to drive at night with one headlight out, so alternating flashing headlights should be used only if they are secondary head lamps.

Probably the most useful light is the one in the center of the cowling on the front vehicle hood. This is easily seen in the rearview mirror of another vehicle and will get a driver's attention even if your siren fails to do so. Lights on the front bumper or in the grille are usually mounted too low to be effective warning signals. The large lights found in the upper, outermost corners of the patient compartment, or module, should blink in tandem, or unison, rather than wigwagging or alternating. This helps the driver of a vehicle that is approaching from a distance to identify the size of your ambulance.

There is a good deal of controversy over the use of strobes on ambulances. When planning the lighting package, refer to the latest research. Presently, researchers suggest combining single-beam bulbs and strobes rather than using either type of lighting system alone. When the ambulance is in the emergency response mode—either responding to the scene or responding to the hospital with a critical or unstable patient—all the emergency lights should be used (Figure 26-6). The vehicle should be easily seen from 360 degrees.

Four-way Flashers and Directional Signals

The four-way flashers and directional signals should not be used as emergency lights. This practice is very

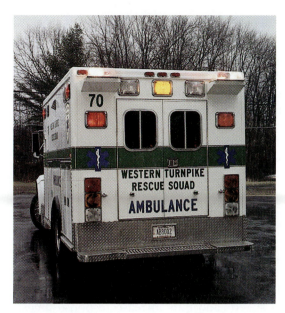

Figure 26-6 Yellow lights on the rear of the ambulance.

confusing to the driving public, as well as illegal in some states. Drivers expect a vehicle using four-way flashers to be traveling at a very slow rate of speed. Additionally, the flashers disrupt the function of the directional signals. In some communities, fire department ambulances returning to the station after calls still use their emergency lights. This "tradition" was established when firefighters rode on the back step of the vehicle. The lights were kept on to alert the public of their presence. According to OSHA regulations, it is now illegal to build a fire truck with a back step for personnel. Avoid the practice of keeping emergency lights on when returning to station to prevent confusing the public.

Effects of Speed

When visibility is poor or when the road surface is slippery, drive slowly. Although your major concern is getting the patient to the hospital as quickly as you can, excessive speed increases the probability of a collision. Speed also increases the ambulance's stopping distance, which reduces your chance of avoiding a hazardous situation.

Stopping distance is dependent on a variety of factors including the speed at which the vehicle is traveling, the vehicle's condition, road conditions, and the alertness of the operator. **Stopping distance** is the total of the reaction distance and the braking distance. **Reaction distance** is the number of feet the vehicle travels from the moment that the operator decides to stop until his or her foot applies pressure to the brake pedal. **Braking distance** is the number of feet the vehicle travels from the start of the braking action until the vehicle comes to a complete stop.

Learn the stopping distances for a light truck, which is comparable to a typical Type I, II, or III ambulance (10,000 to 12,000 gross vehicle weight). As you would expect, the medium-duty vehicles (21,000 to 24,000 gross vehicle weight) will have longer stopping distances. **Perception distance** is the number of feet the vehicle travels while the operator recognizes the hazard and decides how to react. Perception distance does, of course, add to stopping distance but is usually not included in stopping distance estimates because it varies with the individual.

What effect does speed have on an ambulance run? Consider a 5-mile trip from an emergency scene to a hospital. Assuming that you will not have to stop or slow down, at 60 miles per hour you will be able to cover 5 miles in 5 minutes. At 50 miles per hour it will take 6 minutes to reach the hospital. At 60 miles per hour the ambulance will travel 426 feet before the operator can bring the vehicle to a complete stop once he or she reacts to a dangerous situation; whereas, at 50 miles per hour the operator will be able to stop the ambulance in 280 feet. Clearly, the one minute gained in response time is not worth the risk of collision brought about by the 52% increase in stopping distance.

Driving Defensively

The ambulance operator must practice defensive driving at all times. Limit your perception distance by staying aware and alert and by scanning the road, your mirrors, and your speed every 5 seconds to maintain continual focus on your driving and the environment. Reaction distance can be decreased by recognizing potential hazards and instinctively "covering the brake"; if the potential hazard becomes an actual hazard, braking can be accomplished quickly. You can also decrease braking distance by maintaining a reasonable and prudent speed for the conditions as well as by driving a safe vehicle that is frequently checked and adequately maintained.

Now, compare a nondefensive and a defensive operator in a potentially hazardous situation. Assume that both drivers are experienced drivers and are in good physical and emotional condition, that the ambulance brakes have been well maintained, and that weather and road conditions are ideal.

A nondefensive operator is driving down a suburban street approaching three children playing ball close to the street, a potentially hazardous situation. Expecting the children to watch out for the ambulance, he does not take any special precautions. Typically, this nondefensive operator has his right foot on the accelerator while driving. When the potential hazard turns into an actual one, he must move the right foot from the accelerator onto the brake pedal. The ambulance is traveling 30 miles per hour as it approaches the children. Suddenly, when one of the children chases the ball into the street, the operator recognizes the hazard and decides to apply the brake. While he is reacting, the ambulance continues to travel 33 feet until the brakes are applied. At this point, the braking distance begins and the ambulance travels 67 additional feet before coming to a complete stop. The total stopping distance is 100 feet. To get an accurate picture of this distance, use a tape measure and chalk to mark off 100 feet on a street.

Consider a defensive ambulance operator who habitually "covers the brake" in potentially dangerous traffic situations. As soon as she sees the children playing and recognizes a potential hazard, she moves her foot from the accelerator to cover the brake, almost a reflex action. Like the nondefensive one, the defensive operator is traveling at 30 miles per hour when she first sees the children. When the child runs into the street, she is ready to brake. The ambulance would travel 9 feet until the brake is depressed, but covering the brake gives her an additional benefit. Taking the foot off the accelerator slightly reduces the speed, bringing reaction distance down to about 8 feet. For the same reason, braking distance is reduced to about 66 feet. So the total stopping distance is 74 feet. This defensive driver, by being alert and covering the brake, saves 26 feet, which in this case could be just enough to save the child's life.

Escorts and Multiple Vehicles

When the police provide an escort for an ambulance, additional hazards may be created. Too often, an inexperienced ambulance operator follows the escort vehicle too closely and is unable to stop when it makes an emergency stop. Also, the inexperienced operator might assume that other drivers know that a vehicle is following the escort. In fact, other drivers do not and often pull out in front of the ambulance just after the escort vehicle passes.

Multiple-vehicle responses can be as dangerous as escorted responses, especially when responding vehicles travel in the same direction close together. In multiple-vehicle responses, when two vehicles approach the same intersection at the same time, not only may they fail to yield to each other, but other drivers may yield for the first vehicle only, not the second one. Extreme caution must be taken when approaching intersections.

Situations That Affect Response to a Call

A study conducted in New York State, based on 18 years of ambulance collisions, shows that the typical ambulance collision happens on a dry road (60%), in clear weather (55%), during daylight hours (67%), and in an intersection (72%). During this 18-year period, 5,782 ambulance collisions involving 7,267 injuries and 48 fatalities took place.

An ambulance response can be affected by any of the following factors:

- **Day of the week.** Weekdays are usually the days of heaviest traffic because people are commuting to and from work. On weekends, traffic increases around urban and suburban shopping centers. Superhighways and interstate roads may be crowded on Friday and Sunday evenings. In resort areas, weekend traffic may be heavier than weekday traffic.
- **Time of day.** Traffic over major arteries tends to be heavy in all directions during commuter hours. At these times, ambulance operators can expect gridlocked intersections, packed roads, and crawling vehicles regardless of the direction in which they must travel.
- **Weather.** Adverse weather conditions reduce driving speeds and thus increase response times. A heavy snowfall can temporarily prevent any response at all. Always lengthen your following distance whenever there is decreased road grip due to inclement weather.
- **Road construction.** Road construction and road maintenance activities can seriously impede traffic flow. So pay attention to road construction in your district and plan responses accordingly.
- **Railroad crossings.** There are more than a quarter of a million grade railroad crossings in the United States. Communities where they occur should consider placing emergency response systems on both sides of the tracks to ensure emergency responses are not delayed.
- **Bridges and tunnels.** In general, the traffic over bridges and through tunnels slows during rush hours. When a collision occurs, the flow of vehicles, including emergency ones, may stop altogether.
- **Schools and school buses.** An ambulance's response time is also affected by reduced speed limits during school hours. An emergency vehicle should never pass a stopped school bus that has its lights flashing. Instead, wait for the school bus driver to turn off the bus's lights as a signal for you to proceed. Also, the operator of every emergency vehicle should slow down when approaching a school or playground.

When it appears that an ambulance will be delayed in reaching a sick or injured person because of these or other factors, consider taking an alternative route or requesting the response of another ambulance or first response unit. Always plan for times when changing conditions affect response. Obtain detailed maps of your service area. On the maps, indicate usually troublesome traffic spots such as schools, bridges, tunnels, railroad crossings, and heavily congested areas. Also indicate temporary problems such as road and building construction sites and long- and short-term detours. Using another color, indicate alternative routes to areas where normal routes are often blocked. Indicate snow routes, and so on. Hang one map in your quarters and place another map in the ambulance. If you follow these procedures, you will be able to select alternative routes that will get you to your destination quickly and safely.

Parking the Ambulance

Usually there is no problem parking the ambulance at the location of a sick or injured person. The unit may be parked at a curb or in a driveway. However, the parking task is not as easy at the scene of a collision (Skill Summary 26-1). The only way to ensure the safety of an ambulance at the scene of a vehicle collision is to park it completely off the roadway on a service road, shoulder, or driveway and utilize flares for traffic control.

PRECEPTOR PEARL

Studies have shown that red revolving beacons attract intoxicated or tired drivers. Remind new EMT-Bs to consider pulling off the road, turning off headlights, and using just amber rear sealed beam blinkers that blink in tandem or unison to identify the size of their vehicles.

There are two schools of thought about positioning an ambulance or other emergency vehicle on a road leading to a collision site. Some argue that the ambulance should be located beyond the wreckage (relative to the direction of traffic flow) to prevent it from being struck by oncoming traffic. Others favor placing the ambulance at the edge of the danger zone between the wreckage and approaching vehicles. The unit's warning lights will help alert oncoming traffic to the hazard ahead, although this does not reduce the need for other warning devices. Side beacons can be used for scene lighting. Once the ambulance is parked, set its emergency brake.

Transferring the Patient

Transfer of the Patient to the Ambulance

On most ambulance calls you will be able to reach a sick or injured person without difficulty, assess the patient's condition, carry out emergency-care procedures, and then transfer the patient to the ambulance. The patient's condition, the structure in which the patient is located, and the pathway over which you will carry the patient all affect your choice of a method for moving him or her.

Usually you need do little more than place the patient on a stretcher and move it a short distance to the ambulance. However, the process can become more complicated if you suspect the patient may have spine injuries. In this case, full spinal immobilization on a long backboard must be done prior to placing the patient on the stretcher. If a traction splint has been applied to a tall patient, you need to make sure the patient is loaded properly to avoid slamming the door on the splint. You may need to place a patient with a traction splint into the ambulance feet first. In this case, if the patient also needs oxygen or suction, use the portable oxygen and suction units since the permanent units are usually on the front wall of the compartment and will not reach the rear of the ambulance.

Transferring the patient to the ambulance is accomplished in the following steps:

- Selecting the proper patient-carrying device
- Packaging the patient for transfer
- Moving the patient to the ambulance
- Loading the patient onto the ambulance

You may wish to turn to Chapter 5 at this time to review techniques for lifting and moving patients.

En Route to the Hospital

In most areas of the country, it is the responsibility of the EMT-B to contact and report to the hospital while en route. The report should include the following information:

- Hospital identification
- Ambulance designation
- Brief description of the chief complaint and patient status or priority
- Facts learned during history-taking
- Facts learned during the physical exam and while taking vital signs
- Your assessment of injuries or medical problems (what you suspect)
- Emergency care provided thus far
- Your estimated time of arrival (ETA) at the medical facility

Arrival at the Emergency Department

Definitive emergency care cannot be delivered by a single individual; it must come from a well-educated and competent team of EMDs, EMT-Bs, EMT-Ps, RNs, MDs, administrators, and allied health personnel. Although the responsibilities of team members may vary, each one has an important role. Failure of any team member to do his or her job may mean the difference between rehabilitation and disability, a short-term or long-term hospital stay, even life or death to the victim of a sudden illness or injury. It is critical

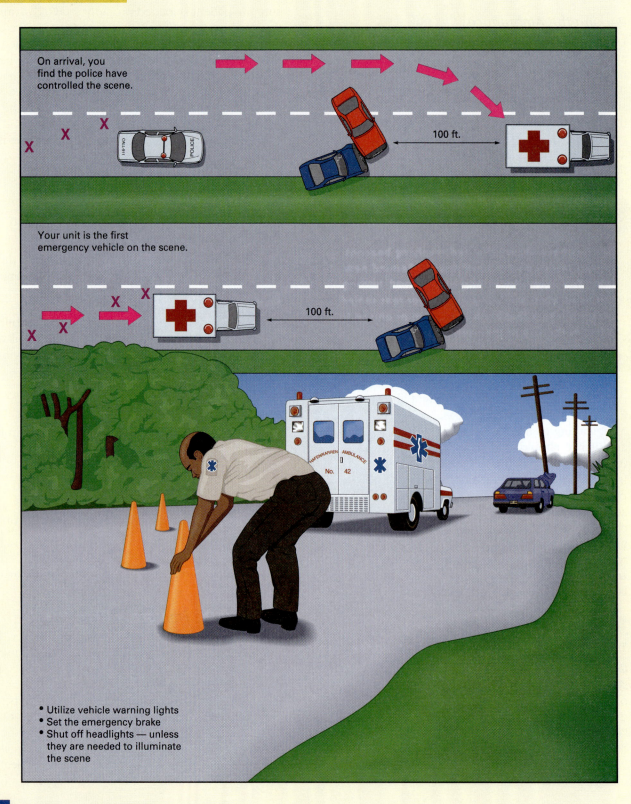

On arrival, you find the police have controlled the scene.

100 ft.

Your unit is the first emergency vehicle on the scene.

100 ft.

- Utilize vehicle warning lights
- Set the emergency brake
- Shut off headlights — unless they are needed to illuminate the scene

that all personnel responsible for some facet of life support and emergency care strive to provide optimum service at all times and in complete harmony with other persons within the system. Brief as it may be, the transfer is a crucial step during which your primary concern must be the continuation of patient-care activities.

It is usually the emergency department nurse to whom the EMT-B most directly relates, through both the ambulance-hospital communication and face-to-face contact upon arrival at the hospital.

PRECEPTOR PEARL

Tell new EMT-Bs that under no circumstances should they ever simply wheel a nonemergency patient into a hospital, place him or her in a bed, and leave! This is an important point. Unless the EMT-B transfers care of the patient directly to a member of the hospital staff, the EMT-B may be open to a charge of abandonment.

Keep in mind that staff members may be treating other seriously ill and injured persons, so suppress any urge to demand attention for your patient. Simply continue emergency care measures until someone can assume responsibility for the patient. When properly directed, transfer the patient to a hospital stretcher.

Verbal and Written Reports

Upon arrival at the hospital emergency department (ED), provide a verbal report to the emergency department personnel at your patient's bedside. Although similar to the radio report transmitted en route, this report stresses any changes you have observed in the patient's condition.

All EMT-Bs should participate in the early emergency department care of sick and injured persons. Even when the emergency department staff has taken over completely, it is often beneficial for you to remain in the area to be of assistance. This action promotes better patient care and also fosters improved communication and understanding between EMT-Bs and emergency department personnel. Working with the ED staff gives you the opportunity to learn more about definitive care procedures and, in turn, the ED staff gains respect for your abilities. Regrettably, this interaction may not be possible in an EMS system with a high volume of calls since it is more important for you to quickly prepare the ambulance for another call.

Remember that your job is not over until the paperwork is complete. Using your assessment card or notes and any additional changes you have observed in the patient's condition, you can now find a "quiet" spot and complete your prehospital care report (PCR). It should include all assessment and history findings, interventions, and any other pertinent information about the call.

The minimum data set includes the following information:

- Chief complaint
- Level of responsiveness in the AVPU format
- Systolic blood pressure for all patients older than 3 years
- Skin perfusion or capillary refill for patients less than 6 years old
- Skin color and temperature
- Pulse rate
- Respiratory rate and effort

In addition, the PCR should have the following administrative information: time incident was reported, time your unit was notified, time of arrival at patient, time your unit left the scene, time of arrival at the hospital, and the time of transfer of care.

Be sure to complete all the boxes on the PCR form and avoid stray marks, especially if your form is scanned into a computer. The narrative section of the form should describe your observations only. Pertinent negatives, such as the lack of chest or abdominal pain, the lack of shortness of breath, or the lack of an altered mental status are important patient observations to document. If you use abbreviations on the PCR, make sure they are standardized ones used by the medical profession and not "made up" ones. Spell the terms correctly and look up the spelling if necessary. Be sure to record the time and findings for every reassessment.

PRECEPTOR PEARL

Remember that the principle of medical documentation is: "If you didn't write it down, you didn't do it!" Stress this point when working with new EMT-Bs.

Since personal, sensitive information is written on the PCR, it is your responsibility to maintain confidentiality. Follow your state laws pertaining to confidentiality and the procedure for distribution of PCR copies in your region. Before handing in the PCR at the hospital, review it with your crew to make sure it is an accurate reflection of what was done and to ensure there is nothing on the form that might embarrass you.

If you make an error while writing out the PCR, you should draw only a single, straight line through the error and place your initials at the side of the correction.

If a patient's valuables or other personal effects were entrusted to your care, transfer them to a responsible emergency department staff member. Some services have policies that involve obtaining a written receipt from emergency department personnel to protect the service from a charge of theft.

Terminating the Call

An ambulance run is not over until the personnel and equipment that comprise the prehospital emergency care delivery system are ready for the next response. This final phase of activity includes more than just changing the stretcher linen and cleaning the ambulance. A number of tasks must be accomplished at the hospital, during the return to quarters, and after arrival at the station.

At the Hospital

While still at the hospital, follow engineering controls and housekeeping procedures to ready yourself, your crew, and the ambulance for the next response.

En Route and at Quarters

To ensure a safe return to quarters, follow the same safety guidelines that are used while en route to a hospital. Defensive driving must be a full-time effort. Radio the EMD that you are returning to quarters and that you are available (or not available) for service. Refuel the ambulance per service policy.

When you return to quarters, a number of activities must be completed before the ambulance can be placed in service and before it is ready for another call. The emphasis on protection from infectious diseases should not be underestimated; you need to take every precaution in order to protect yourself. It is essential that you follow your service's exposure control plan in accordance with OSHA regulations.

AEROMEDICAL EVACUATION

In some circumstances, it is best for the patient to be transported by a helicopter or fixed-wing aircraft (Figure 26-7). These services are not available in all parts of the United States. Therefore, it is important for you to know your local capabilities for air transport, when and whom to call, and what types of mission they will accept. Some programs do interhospital transfers only, while others do the complete range

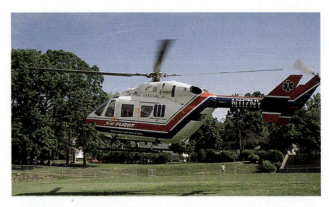

Figure 26-7 Patients are sometimes transported by air rescue helicopter.

of missions from scene extrications to backcountry search-and-rescue operations.

Air rescue may be required for either operational or medical reasons. Operational reasons for using a helicopter include:

- Ground transportation to the appropriate critical care facility exceeds 30 minutes.
- The helicopter can be airborne with a proper crew and at the scene faster than an ambulance can transport the patient(s) to the nearest hospital.
- Extrication time at the scene is estimated to exceed 20 minutes.
- Ground transportation could be hazardous to the patient. Possible reasons are weather conditions and confirmed spinal-cord injury.
- A multiple-casualty incident threatens to overload local capabilities.
- Difficult access situations exist, such as wilderness rescue, access or egress impeded at the scene by road conditions, weather, traffic, or search-and-rescue situations.
- A patient needs a higher level of ALS care than your agency can provide.

Medical reasons for using a helicopter include those in which the patient's condition is a "life- or limb-threatening" situation. A patient is high priority for rapid transport if he or she was injured in a collision in which evidence of any one of the following high-energy conditions exists or your physical examination reveals any of the following abnormal vital signs or findings:

- Fall of 15 feet or more
- Patient struck by a vehicle moving at 20 mph or faster
- Patient ejected from a vehicle
- Vehicle rollover with unrestrained passengers
- High-speed crash with 20 inches or more front-end deformity

- Deformity of 15 inches or more into passenger compartment
- Patient survived motor-vehicle collision during which a death occurred in the same vehicle
- Glasgow Coma scale of 13 or less
- Trauma score of 14 or less
- Sustained pulse rate of 120 per minute or more for an adult
- Head trauma with altered mental status, hemiplegia
- Penetrating injuries of head, neck, chest, abdomen, or groin
- Chest trauma with signs and symptoms of respiratory distress
- Two or more proximal long-bone fractures
- Amputations requiring reimplantation
- Facial burns, airway burns, burns of 15% body surface area or greater
- Interhospital transfer of a critical patient
- Transport to a hyperbaric chamber

NOTE: Cardiac-arrest patients are usually not transported by helicopter unless they are hypothermic. As always, follow your local protocols.

Calling for a Helicopter

If your patient's situation meets local criteria for helicopter utilization, make sure you call for it as soon as possible so no time is lost in response. Contact the helicopter access point in your region and be prepared to give them the following information: your name and callback number, your agency name, nature of the situation, exact location of the incident including crossroads and major landmarks, exact location of a safe landing zone (LZ), communications frequency, and whom to contact as the helicopter approaches the scene.

Setting Up a Landing Zone

A landing zone, or LZ, is approximately an area of 100 feet by 100 feet, depending on the actual ship that is used in your region. To measure 100 feet walk out approximately 30 large paces (Figure 26-8). The LZ should be clear of wires, towers, vehicles, people,

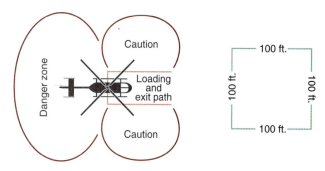

Figure 26-8 The air rescue helicopter landing zone.

and loose objects. It must be on firm ground with less than an eight-degree slope. In the LZ, keep emergency red lights on, but turn off any white or blue lights, which may obstruct the pilot's view. Do not allow traffic or smoking within 100 feet of the LZ. Place a flare on the upwind side of the LZ. Once the LZ is set and the helicopter is nearby, the LZ Officer should report the following to the pilot:

- Description of the LZ relationship to terrain (for example, in the valley, on top of the hill)
- Description of major landmarks near the LZ (such as rivers, factories, water towers, major highways)
- Estimate of the distance between the LZ and the nearest town (examples: LZ is located at the South Colonie High School soccer field; there are wires to the north and west side of the LZ, there are no other obstructions; the wind is out of the southeast)

Approaching a Helicopter

Standing nearby a "hot" or running helicopter can be extremely dangerous. Never approach a helicopter that has landed until the pilot or co-pilot has waved you to approach. Then it is important that you carefully approach from a safe zone. Never go near the tail rotor since it spins so fast that you cannot see it spinning. Skill Summary 26-2 on the next page provides helpful information that could save your life.

Danger Areas Around Helicopters

26-2

▲ **1.** The area around the tail rotor is extremely dangerous. A spinning rotor cannot be seen.

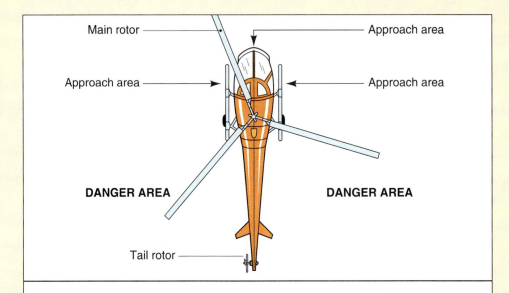

Main rotor

Approach area

Approach area

Approach area

DANGER AREA

DANGER AREA

Tail rotor

▲ **2.** A sudden gust of wind can cause the main rotor of a helicopter to dip to a point as close as four feet from the ground. Always approach a helicopter in a crouch when the rotor is moving. However, do so only with the approval of the pilot.

Approach crouched

Ground

▲ **3.** Approach the aircraft from the downhill side when a helicopter is parked on a hillside.

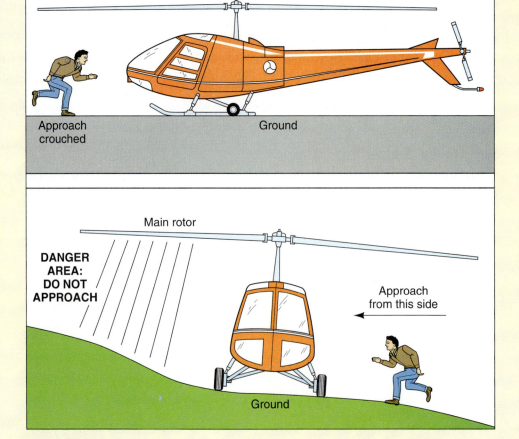

Main rotor

DANGER AREA: DO NOT APPROACH

Approach from this side

Ground

SUMMARY

- Understand the importance of inspecting the ambulance each shift and always keeping it ready for a response.
- Become keenly aware of the laws, rules, and regulations for driving an emergency vehicle in your state.
- Always respond to a dispatch in as safe a manner as possible, keeping in mind the principles of good defensive driving.
- When driving the ambulance, remember that motorists may not always hear your siren, see your emergency light, or have a clue about how to react to your vehicle.

- The call is not complete until the patient is properly transferred to the emergency department staff, the PCR is completed, and the ambulance is properly cleaned and resupplied.
- Know when and how to call for aeromedical evacuation.
- Know how to set up a landing zone and the proper way to approach the aircraft if instructed to do so by the flight crew.

REVIEW QUESTIONS

1. A Type II ambulance is a:
   a. van.
   b. pickup truck.
   c. van front with a box back.
   d. pickup truck with a box back.

2. A safe ambulance driver is one who:
   a. tolerates the bad habits of other drivers.
   b. is physically, mentally, and emotionally fit.
   c. is able to perform under stress.
   d. all of the above.

3. When extrication time at the emergency scene is estimated to be more than _____ minutes, consider air rescue.
   a. 5   b. 10   c. 20   d. 30

4. Which one of the following is NOT included in the radio report given while en route to the hospital?
   a. ambulance identifier
   b. patient's chief complaint
   c. patient's insurance company
   d. results of patient assessment

5. Approach a helicoptor from the _____ side when it is parked on a slope or hillside.
   a. downhill   c. front
   b. uphill   d. back

WEB MEDIC

Visit Brady's *Essentials of Emergency Care* web site for direct web links. At **www.prenhall.com/limmer,** you will find information related to the following Chapter 26 topics:
- NHTSA ambulance specs
- Ambulance collisions
- National Academy for Professional Driving
- National Academy of Emergency Medical Dispatch
- National Safety Council CEVO II Course
- National Association of Flight Paramedics

Correlates with the U.S. DOT "EMT-Basic National Standard Curriculum" Lesson 7-2

GAINING ACCESS AND RESCUE

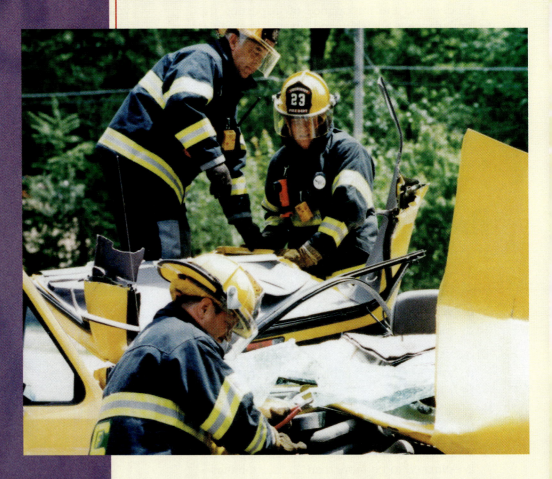

ESSENTIAL ELECTRONIC EXTRAS

CD ESSENTIALS

For preview and review of chapter material, see the student CD-ROM for

- Pretest
- Chapter quizzes
- Posttest

WEB ESSENTIALS

For additional review and enrichment, visit www.prenhall.com/limmer for

- Interactive student quizzes
- Links to online EMS resources
- Online case studies
- Audio glossary

As an EMT-B, you usually gain access to your patients without much trouble. However, in situations where this is not possible or safe, you will need to request specialized assistance. As an EMT-B, you are usually not responsible for extrication and rescue, but you should understand how it is done, how it may affect the patient, and when you may safely begin emergency medical care.

EMT-B'S ROLE AT AN EXTRICATION

In some communities, there are at least 10 types of special operations teams available. Each "special op" requires a significant amount of additional training over and above an EMT-B course. Examples of special operations include: vehicle rescue, water rescue, ice rescue, high-angle rescue, hazardous-materials response, trench rescue, dive rescue, back country or wilderness rescue, farm rescue, and confined-space rescue. Training in each of these specialties is often a function of the types of emergency responses in your community. If there is a gorge in the middle of town, there often is a high-angle team. Likewise if there is a river with low-head dams running through your district, a water-rescue team would be appropriate.

Extrication is the process by which entrapped patients are rescued from vehicles and other devices, buildings, tunnels, and other dangerous environments. The 10 fundamental phases of the extrication process are:

1. Prepare for the rescue.
2. Size up the situation.
3. Recognize and manage hazards.
4. Stabilize the vehicle or structure prior to entering.
5. Gain access to the patient.
6. Perform an initial patient assessment and a focused trauma exam.
7. Disentangle the patient.
8. Immobilize and extricate the patient.
9. Provide ongoing assessment, triage, treatment, and transport.
10. Terminate the rescue.

Every step of this process needs to have medical input from the EMT-B, who acts as an advocate for the patient's medical needs with the Incident Commander, the Triage Sector Officer, and the Rescue Sector Officer. Safety is your highest priority. You need to minimize the potential for injury to yourself and other rescuers, as well as avoid additional injury to your patient. Although you may never have personally provided the disentanglement, since this is most often done by a fire department rescue squad in many communities, it is important for you to understand the process so you can keep your patient informed and anticipate any dangerous steps in the extrication action plan.

Since extrication of a patient from a vehicle is the most common type of rescue across the United States, the next few pages focus on your role in this procedure. This chapter discusses phases 2, 3, 4, and

CORE CONCEPTS

In this chapter, you will learn about the following topics:

- Extrication and the 10 fundamental phases of the extrication process
- The role of the EMT-B at an extrication
- How to size-up and recognize potential hazards at the rescue scene
- What personal protective equipment should be worn at the rescue scene
- How to determine the need for extrication
- The importance of safety equipment at a rescue scene
- How to stabilize a vehicle and gain access to the patient
- Examples of typical disentanglement action plans used at a vehicle rescue

5 of the process, as well as the approach rescue teams should take for phase 7. Phases 1, 6, 8, and 9 have already been addressed in other chapters.

SIZING UP THE SITUATION

It is important to have a keen eye as you arrive on the scene of a collision. Your first task is to evaluate hazards and calculate the need for additional assistance. That assistance may be BLS or ALS backup, police, fire, power company, or specialty rescue response. Quickly determine how many patients are involved, their priority, and the mechanisms of injury. If you think additional ambulances will be needed, call for them immediately. You can always cancel your request for ambulances if later you determine they are not needed.

Then "read" the collision vehicle. Develop a plan of action based on your knowledge of rescue operations and each patient's status. Determine the extent of entrapment and the means of egress for each patient. As soon as possible, evaluate the patients as high or low priority. Remember that a high-priority patient has only a "golden hour"—the time the injury occurred to the time internal bleeding can be controlled in surgery at the hospital.

A low-priority patient can wait for rescue personnel to force open doors, remove the roof, or displace the front end of the vehicle. For a low-priority patient, there is time to do a short-board or vest-type immobilization and careful transfer to the stretcher using the long backboard. However, if the patient is high priority, it may make more sense to use the rapid extrication technique, either for a vertical removal through the opened roof or for a horizontal removal through a doorway. The principles of spinal immobilization remain the same, but the requirements for speed of removal will dictate the specific technique you use.

During scene size-up, check to see if the vehicle is equipped with air bags. A car with an air bag has a large, rectangular steering wheel hub. Airbags are sometimes placed in the glove compartment area for front seat passengers, while new cars have side-impact air bags. Special steps should be followed if the air bag has not deployed. (See "Displacing the Front End" later in this chapter.)

If an air bag has deployed, observers may have noticed "smoke" inside the vehicle during deployment. The "smoke" is actually dust from the cornstarch or talcum used to lubricate the bag, as well as the seal and particles from within the bag. The powder may contain sodium hydroxide, which can irritate the skin. For this reason, it is important to wear protective gloves and eyewear when you gain access to the passenger compartment and to protect patients from getting additional dust in their eyes or wounds. Air-bag manufacturers recommend that you move the inflated bag to examine the steering wheel because damage to the wheel may indicate that the patient has a serious chest injury.

RECOGNIZING AND MANAGING HAZARDS

In some rural areas, fire departments have no rescue capabilities, so ambulance services are called upon to carry out vehicle rescue. In areas where rescue and fire units are available, the ambulance may nevertheless arrive on scene first. Time and lives can be saved if you are able to recognize and initiate hazard management at least until personnel with more expertise arrive.

Hazards at a collision scene can range from nuisances such as broken glass and debris, a slippery road, inclement weather, or darkness to severe threats to safety such as downed wires, spilled fuel, or fire. Also during size-up, watch out for loaded bumpers. Most cars are equipped with 5-mph bumpers designed to absorb low-speed front- and rear-end collision damage. If the bumpers were involved in the collision, you may notice that the bumper shock absorber system is compressed, or "loaded." Some rescue teams are trained to unload the shock absorber or to chain it to prevent an uncontrolled release.

PRECEPTOR PEARL

Remind new EMT-Bs that traffic and spectators can become hazards if they are not controlled. A number of EMT-Bs have been killed at the scene of collisions by drivers who were watching the collision rather than the EMT-B crossing the street.

Safeguarding Yourself

Collision-related hazards must be managed, if not eliminated, before any attempt is made to reach injured persons in damaged vehicles.

Collision sites can be dangerous workplaces. Jagged edges, flying glass, and fire are only a few of the hazards you may need to deal with. Remember that you are no good to your patient and crew if you become a patient yourself. It is vital that you take the time to properly protect yourself prior to engaging in any rescue activities. The unsafe act that contributes most to collision scene injuries is failure to wear protective gear during rescue operations.

A careless attitude toward personal safety and a lack of skill in tool use are human factors that can increase your potential for injury at a collision site. Physical problems that impede strenuous effort include:

- Unsafe and improper acts
- Failure to eliminate or control hazards
- Failure to select the proper tool for the task
- Using unsafe tools
- Failure to recognize mechanisms of injury and unsafe surroundings
- Lifting heavy objects improperly
- Deactivating safety devices designed to prevent injury
- Failure to wear highly visible outer clothing, especially when exposed to highway traffic

Figure 27-1 shows an EMT-B dressed for collision scene operations. Unfortunately, many services still allow their personnel to work around broken glass and the sharp metal of a collision in short-sleeve shirts or nylon jackets! This is a dangerous practice. Any personnel allowed to work in the "inner circle" of a collision scene (the area immediately around and including the vehicle) should wear full protective gear to avoid being injured. Appropriate gear for a rescue operation includes: headgear, eye protection, hand protection, and body protection. Remember the value of protective gear. Get your own if your service does not provide it (most states require it on ambulances), and use it!

Good head protection is essential. Trendy baseball caps, uniform hats, and wool watch caps do little except protect against sunlight, identify the wearer as a member of an emergency service, or keep the head warm. Also, plastic "bump caps" worn by butchers and warehouse workers do not provide adequate protection.

The rescue helmet offers adequate protection. The best rescue helmets do not have the firefighter helmet rear brim, which can be awkward in tight spaces, although many EMT-Bs prefer and use fire-

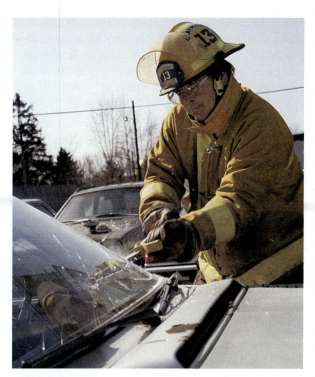

Figure 27-1 Dress for vehicle rescue.

fighter helmets. All helmets should be brightly colored, with reflective stripes and lettering, to make the wearer visible both day and night. They also should display the "Star of Life" on each side to identify the wearer as an EMS provider. Your level of training should also be indicated in order to facilitate management of a scene involving both EMS and rescue units.

Eye protection is vital. Hinged plastic helmet shields do not provide adequate protection; flying particles can strike the eyes from underneath or from the side. Wear safety goggles with a soft vinyl frame that conforms to the face and indirect venting to keep them fog-free. Or choose safety glasses with large lenses and side shields. These types of eyewear will also suffice for infection-control eye protection.

Optimal hand protection should also be available to you. Wear disposable gloves underneath either firefighter gloves or leather gloves. Firefighter gloves will protect your hands from a variety of sharp, hot, cold, and dangerous surfaces. They are bulky, but they can be worn in most rescue situations. If dexterity is impeded by firefighter gloves, wear intermediate-weight leather gloves. Fabric garden or work gloves are too thin to offer adequate protection.

Protection for your body is also necessary. Never wear light shirts or nylon jackets inside the inner circle because they do little to protect you from jagged metal, broken glass, or flash fires. Wear either a short or mid-length OSHA-approved turnout coat to protect your body. Use a heavy-duty EMS or rescue jacket to protect you from inclement weather and minor injury. Bright colors and reflective material help make your jacket more visible. To protect your lower body, wear either turnout pants with cuffs wide enough to pull over work shoes or fire-resistant trousers or jumpsuits. Also consider wearing steel-toe work shoes with extended tops to protect your ankles.

Safeguarding the Patient

It is your responsibility to ensure that further injuries are not inflicted on your patients during the rescue operations. The following items can be used to protect patients from heat, cold, flying particles, and other hazards:

- An aluminized rescue blanket offers protection from weather and, to a degree, from flying particles. A paper blanket does not afford this protection; it merely restricts the patient's view of the approaching glass or metal.
- A lightweight, vinyl-coated paper tarpaulin can protect from weather.
- A wool blanket protects the patient from cold. Cover the wool blanket with an aluminized blanket or a salvage cover whenever glass is being broken near a patient, since glass particles are almost impossible to remove from wool blankets.
- Short and long wood spine boards shield a patient from contact with tools and debris.
- Hard hats, safety goggles, industrial hearing protectors, disposable dust masks, and thermal masks (in cold weather—and unless the patient is on oxygen) protect a patient's head, eyes, ears, and respiratory passages.

LIFESPAN DEVELOPMENT

Often, whether people are traveling across town or across the state, they do not wear heavy coats while in their cars. Of course they never would expect to become involved in a major collision and require EMS and rescue services!

When assessing and managing patients who have been involved in a car crash, be sure to keep them warm. Exposing patients to the wind or inclement weather during a lengthy extrication can make their conditions worsen. The best rule of thumb is that if you need a heavy coat, so will patients. Cover them up with blankets while you wait for the rescue team to complete the disentanglement.

Managing Traffic Hazards

Collisions almost always produce traffic problems. Often the wreckage blocks several lanes. Even if it does not, backups are caused when nosy drivers slow down to "rubberneck." Rescuers, firefighters, and police usually handle traffic control, but your ambulance may be the only responding unit or you may arrive ahead of other emergency service units.

Obviously, personal safety, rescue, and emergency care have priority. Because traffic is a natural predator of the EMT-B, an ambulance crew should still initiate basic traffic control, channeling vehicles past the scene. Your ambulance warning lights will serve as the first form of traffic control; however, you should position other warning devices as soon as possible. Bad weather, darkness, vegetation, and curved or hilly roadways may prevent approaching motorists from seeing your ambulance.

Controlling Spectators

Spectators do more than just create problems for passing motorists. If allowed to wander freely, they will close in on the wreckage to get a better view. They may get so close that they interfere with rescue and emergency care efforts. Rescue squads, police, and fire units have personnel and equipment for crowd control; ambulances usually do not. However, you can usually initiate some crowd-control measures. If local policies permit it, ask for assistance from one or more responsible-looking bystanders. Ask them to keep the spectators away from the danger zone. Give them a roll of barricade tape if you have one. But remember not to put the recruited personnel in unsafe positions such as near spilled fuel or an unstable vehicle.

Electrical Utility Hazards

Electricity poses many dangers at vehicle collision scenes. When there is an electrical hazard, establish a danger zone and a safe zone. The danger zone should be entered only by individuals responsible for controlling the hazard, such as power company personnel or a specialty rescue crew. The safe zone should be sufficiently far away to assure that an arcing or moving wire could not possibly injure any of the rescue personnel or bystanders.

Keep the following safety points in mind, as they may save your life someday:

- High voltages are not as uncommon on roadside utility poles as people often think.
- In some areas, wood poles support conductors of as much as 500,000 volts.
- Assume that the entire area is extremely dangerous. Conductors may have touched and energized

any part of the system, including electrical, telephone, cable television, and other wires supported by the utility pole; guy wires; ground wires; the pole itself; the ground surrounding the pole; and nearby guardrails and fences.

■ Assume that severed or displaced conductors may be energizing every conductor and wire at the highest voltage present. Dead wires may be re-energized at any moment. Energized conductors may arc to the ground.

■ Ordinary protective clothing does not protect against electrocution.

A broken utility pole with wires down is very dangerous (Figure 27-2). You cannot work safely in the area until a power company representative assures you that the power is off and the scene is safe. If you discover that a utility pole is broken and wires are down, park the ambulance outside the danger zone. Before exiting the ambulance, be sure that no portion of the vehicle, including the radio antenna, is contacting any sagging wires. Discourage occupants of the collision vehicle from leaving the wreckage, and use perimeter tape to set off a large safety zone. Keep bystanders outside the safety zone and prohibit traffic flow through the danger zone until the police can take over this responsibility. Determine the number of the nearest pole you can safely approach, and ask your dispatcher to advise the power company of the pole number and location. Stand in a safe place until the power company cuts the wires or disconnects the power.

Be especially careful when approaching a collision located in a dark area, such as a rural roadside at night. As you walk from the ambulance, sweep the area ahead of you to each side and overhead

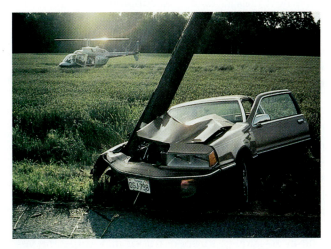

Figure 27-2 Damaged utility pole with wires down.

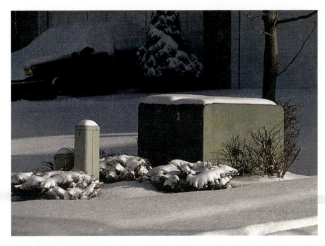

Figure 27-3 A pad-mounted transformer, if damaged, poses a serious threat

with the beam of a powerful hand light. An energized conductor may be dangling just at head level. If you discover that a wire is down, leave the area immediately and notify the power company. Even if wires are intact, a broken utility pole is still dangerous. Conductors supporting the pole can break at any time, dropping pole and wires onto the scene. Pad-mounted transformers and underground cables instead of utility poles and overhead wires supply electricity in many areas. When an aboveground transformer is struck and damaged, it poses a threat of electrocution (Figure 27-3). A vehicle may be energized by such a transformer.

Sometimes, especially in wet weather, a phenomenon known as **ground gradient** may provide your first clue that a wire is down. Voltage is greatest at the point where a conductor touches the ground, then diminishes as distance from the point of contact increases. That distance may be several inches or many feet. Being able to recognize and respond properly to energized ground can save your life. Stop your approach immediately if you feel a tingling sensation in your legs and lower torso. This sensation means that you are on energized ground. Current is entering one foot, passing through your lower body, and exiting through your other foot. If you continue on, you could be electrocuted! Turn 180 degrees and take one of two escape measures: bend one knee, grasp the foot of that leg with one hand, and hop to a safe place on one foot; or shuffle away from the danger area with both feet together, allowing no break in contact between your two feet or between your feet and the ground. Either technique helps prevent your body from completing a circuit with the energized ground.

Vehicle Fire Hazards

Extinguishing a vehicle fire is the responsibility of firefighters, who are trained and equipped for the job. When you find a vehicle on fire, always request their assistance. Never assume that someone else has called the fire department. A fire engine should always stand by at a vehicle rescue.

If you have been trained in the use of an extinguisher, there are some measures that you can take before fire units arrive (Figure 27-4). For small fires, a 15- or 20-pound class A:B:C dry chemical fire extinguisher can extinguish virtually anything that may be burning in a vehicle, including upholstery, fuel, and electrical components. Only burning magnesium and other flammable metals cannot be extinguished by an A:B:C extinguisher. Before attempting to put out a fire, always put on a full set of protective gear.

Many rescue units routinely disable the electrical system of every collision vehicle by cutting a battery cable. This was a reasonable practice years ago when vehicles had more combustible materials and when wiring did not have self-extinguishing insulation. Today, however, the situation is different. Unless gasoline is pooled under a vehicle or undeployed air bags need to be disabled, cutting the battery out of the electrical system not only may be a waste of time, it may actually hinder the rescue operation.

Remember that many cars have electrically powered door locks, windows, and seat-adjustment mechanisms. Having the option of lowering a window rather than breaking it eliminates the likelihood of spraying the vehicle's occupants with glass. Being able to operate door locks may eliminate the need to force doors open. Also, if you are able to operate a powered seat, you can create space in front of an injured driver.

If there is reason to disrupt the electrical system, disconnect the ground cable from the battery. In this way, you will not be likely to produce a spark that can drop onto spilled fuel or ignite battery gases. Such a spark can be created when the positive cable is pulled away from the battery terminal or when a tool touches a metal component while in contact with the positive terminal or cable.

STABILIZING THE VEHICLE

Unstable collision vehicles pose a hazard to rescuers and patients alike. Rescuers often fail to stabilize collision vehicles because they appear to be stable. Rather than risking serious injury, consider any collision vehicle unstable and act accordingly. If safe to do so, signal to the occupants to reassure them that help is on its way and begin to get an idea of their conditions.

A vehicle may be found on its wheels, on its roof, or on its side. A collision vehicle that is upright on four inflated tires looks stable. However, it is easily rocked up and down, side to side, and back and forth as rescuers climb into and over it. These motions can seriously aggravate the occupants' injuries.

If you have access to the inside of the vehicle, make sure the engine is turned off, the gearshift is in park, the keys are removed from the ignition, and the parking brake is set. Use three **step chocks** (cribbing)—one on each side and a third under the front or back of the vehicle—to stabilize a vehicle on its wheels. Then deflate all the tires. Simply pull the valve stems from their casing with pliers. Then tell a police officer what you have done so investigators will not think that the tires are flat as a result of the collision.

Equipment needed to accomplish vehicle stabilization and gaining access is listed in Table 27-1. If your ambulance is not equipped with step chocks, a degree of stabilization can be accomplished by placing wheel chocks or 2 × 4 cribbing in front of and behind two tires on the same side.

If a car has rolled over several times and has come to rest on its wheels, the roof may be crushed, which prevents access through the windows. The roof may need to be raised with heavy-duty jacks before doors can be opened or the roof removed.

When a vehicle is on its side, there is a tendency for spectators to push it back onto its wheels. They fail to realize that this movement may injure, or more severely injure, occupants of the vehicle. Instead, the vehicle should be stabilized on its side, using ropes, hi-lift jacks, and/or cribbing. Do not attempt to gain access before this is accomplished. While a car on its side may appear stable, simply climbing onto one side in an attempt to open a door may cause the vehicle to drop onto its roof or wheels. Moreover, you can be trapped under the vehicle when it topples.

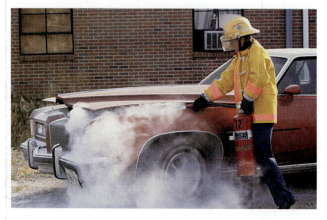

Figure 27-4 Extinguishing a fire in the engine compartment when the car hood is partially open.

Table 27-1 Supplies and Equipment for Vehicle Stabilization and Gaining Access

Quantity	Item
10	2″ × 4″ × 18″ cribbing
10	4″ × 4″ × 18″ cribbing
4	step chocks
6	wood wedges
2	vehicle wheel chocks
100 feet	nylon 1/2″ utility rope
2	Hi-lift heavy-duty jacks
1	"Door-and-window kit" with hand tools such as . . .
1	pair battery pliers
1	12″ adjustable wrench
1	3-pound or 4-pound drilling hammer
1	spring-loaded center punch
1	hacksaw with spare blades
1	10″ locking-type pliers
1	10″ water-pump pliers
	several 12″ to 15″ flat pry bars
1	8″ flat blade screwdriver
1	12″ flat blade screwdriver
1	spray container of power steering fluid as lubricant
1	flat-head ax
1	Glas-Master™ windshield saw
1	combination forcible entry tool such as a Halligan or a Biel™ tool
500 feet	perimeter tape

Position a safety guide at each end of the vehicle to "feel" the movement of the vehicle and quickly warn the rescuers placing cribbing, jacks, or ropes to get back if the vehicle begins to tip over. Some services will deploy two ropes looped around the same wheel in both directions so that personnel can temporarily hold the vehicle stable while jacks and/or cribbing are placed. The objective is to increase the number of contacts with the ground to make the vehicle on its side more stable, as shown in Skill Summary 27-1.

There are many ways to stabilize a vehicle on its side—through sheer manpower or through the use of hydraulic rams and pneumatic jacks. If your ambulance is equipped with stabilization equipment,

you should attend a formal vehicle rescue course that includes basic stabilization procedures, taught by a qualified instructor.

PRECEPTOR PEARL

Tell new EMT-Bs that when placing cribbing, they should never kneel down. Always squat down, staying on both feet so you can quickly move away from the vehicle if necessary.

Once a vehicle is stabilized, if a door must be opened, tie it in the fully open position before you try to crawl inside. If the ambulance does not carry stabilization devices, or if you are not trained in their use, wait for a rescue squad to arrive before you try to enter the vehicle.

If the vehicle is resting on its roof, roof posts are intact, and the vehicle appears stable, it may be tempting to immediately try to reach the occupants through window or door openings. However, if the posts collapse, as is often the case when the windshield integrity has been broken, the vehicle may come crashing down and injure the EMT-B who is attempting the rescue. You must wait to gain access until the rescue crew has stabilized the vehicle. This is usually accomplished by building a box crib with 4 × 4s under the vehicle. If the vehicle is tilted with the engine (its heaviest part) on the ground and the trunk in the air, you can try using two step chocks upside down under the trunk.

If the roof is crushed against the body of the vehicle, the vehicle is stable, but it is impossible to gain access through a window, door, or the roof. However, it may be possible to cut through the floor pan and either crawl inside, if the opening is big enough or if the EMT-B is small enough, or to reach through the opening to touch and offer emotional support to the occupants until rescue personnel can lift or open the vehicle.

GAINING ACCESS TO THE PATIENT

As an EMT-B, your responsibility is not the rescue of the vehicle but the rescue of the patient. Usually you will assume that the occupant of a collision vehicle has sustained life-threatening injuries. At least one EMT-B needs to gain quick access to the patient, even while rescuers are working to gain a more wide-open access, create exitways, and disentangle the occupant.

Always take BSI precautions first.

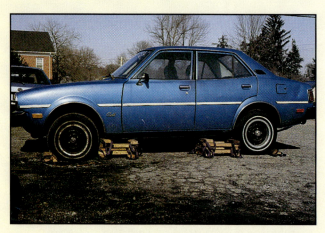

▲ **1.** You can stabilize a car on its wheels can by placing cribbing under the rocker panels to minimize rescuer-produced movements that may be harmful to the occupants. Deflate the vehicle's tires for maximum stability.

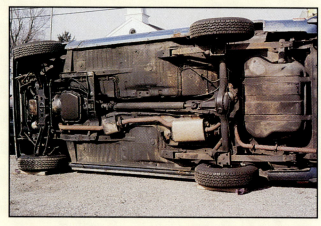

▲ **2.** You can stabilize a car on its side by placing cribbing under the wheels, moving the car to the vertical position, and then . . .

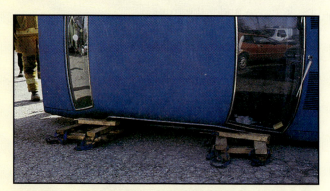

▲ **3.** . . . placing cribbing under the A- and C- posts. Stabilizing in this manner allows EMTs to pull the roof down to expose the entire interior of the car.

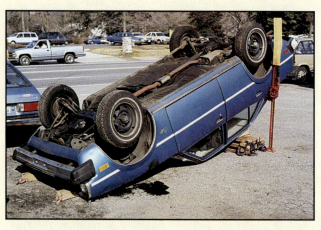

▲ **4.** You can stabilize an overturned car by placing jacks and/or cribbing under the trunk, under the hood, or at both locations, depending on the position of the vehicle.

After the vehicle is stable enough for you to approach it safely, check to see if a door can be opened or a window rolled down in the usual way. (*Try Before You Pry!*) Failing this, you may need to break a window to gain access even while the rescue crew is dismantling the vehicle for extrication of the occupants.

All automotive glass is one of two types: laminated or tempered. Windshields and some side and rear van and truck windows are laminated safety glass: two sheets of plate glass bonded to a sheet of tough plastic, like a glass-and-plastic sandwich. Most passenger-car side and rear windows are tempered glass. They are very resilient, but when they do break, rather than shattering into sharp fragments, they break into small rounded pieces.

Try to gain access through a side or rear window as far away as possible from the occupants. Use a spring-loaded center punch against a lower corner to break the glass. Punch out fingerholds in the top of the window and use your gloved fingers to pull fragments away from the window.

A flathead ax is usually required to break through a windshield. However, it can also be done very quickly using a Glas-Master™ saw (Figure 27-5). A windshield is usually not broken to gain access, but the rescue squad may need to remove it if they plan to displace the dash or steering column or remove the roof. Before the windshield is broken, if possible, cover passengers with aluminized rescue blankets or tarps.

Once an entry point is gained, at least one properly dressed EMT-B should crawl inside the vehicle and begin an initial assessment and focused trauma exam as well as manual cervical stabilization. Do not forget to explain to the patient what is going on and provide emotional support by reassuring him or her that everything possible is being done.

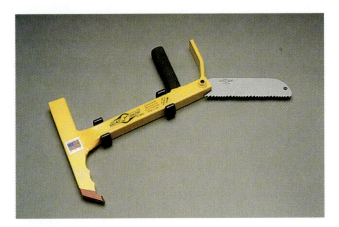

Figure 27-5 A saw such as the Glas-Master™ can aid in windshield removal.

Disentanglement Action Plan

In most instances, EMS personnel will not be directly involved in the disentanglement other than staying inside the vehicle and acting as the patient's advocate. The action plan that may be used by rescue personnel to free the trapped patient is a three-step procedure that can be carried out by fire, rescue, and EMS personnel with the appropriate equipment. The three steps are: removing the roof, removing doors and roof posts, and displacing the front end.

This procedure is uncomplicated, requires minimal special equipment, and is not vehicle specific; that is, it can be used on virtually any car or truck. Therefore EMS personnel can be trained in a brief course and the ambulance compartments need not be overloaded with rescue equipment.

Must this entire three-part procedure be used for all extrication operations and always be performed in the same order? Not necessarily! In some cases, it may be necessary only to force a door open to reach a single patient and create an exitway for his or her removal. In other cases, it may be prudent to open doors before disposing of the roof. In still other situations, there may not be a need to displace the front end of a collision vehicle.

Remember, the main purpose of your understanding of extrication procedures is so you can integrate them with your patient-care plan.

Removing the Roof

For more than 20 years, emergency service personnel have been trained to carry out a progression of procedures to reach the occupants of a wrecked vehicle: First try the doors. If that fails, unlock and unlatch the doors by nondestructive or destructive means. When all else fails, gain access through window openings.

This multi-part procedure is time-consuming and requires a number of tools. A quicker and far more efficient procedure is to dispose of the roof of a collision vehicle as soon as hazards have been controlled and the vehicle is stable. Removing the roof makes the entire interior of the vehicle accessible. EMS personnel can stand beside or climb into the vehicle and pursue emergency care efforts while rescuers carry out disentanglement procedures. In addition, removing the roof creates a large exitway through which an occupant can be quickly removed when he or she has a life-threatening injury or when fire or another hazard is threatening the operation. It also provides fresh air and helps cool the patient when heat is a problem.

Skill Summary 27-2 illustrates the procedure for folding a collision vehicle's roof back like the roof of a convertible. While this is the most commonly used procedure, it is not the only way to dispose of a roof. A roof can be folded forward after cutting both C- and B-posts (rear and middle posts), folded to either side after cutting the posts of the opposite side, or removed altogether after severing all of the roof posts. If you lack a hydraulic rescue tool, you can accomplish all of these procedures with a hacksaw and a spray container of lubricant.

Removing Doors and Roof Posts

When rapid vertical extrication through the open roof is not indicated, the next step is to open doors and remove roof posts. The benefits of this step are that EMS personnel can kneel beside the vehicle while carrying out patient care and immobilization procedures, and the immobilized patients can be easily rotated onto long backboards. Skill Summary 27-3 shows a rescue team using a hydraulic rescue tool to open doors that cannot be unlatched and pulled open in the usual manner, as when doors are damaged or locks and latches jammed.

Displacing the Front End

Most vehicle rescue training courses include procedures for displacing or removing seats, dash assemblies, steering wheels, steering columns, and pedals. A quicker and more efficient way to disentangle an injured driver and/or passenger from these mechanisms of entrapment is to displace the entire front end of the vehicle. While the task sounds difficult, it is not. Skill Summary 27-4 illustrates the procedure for displacing the front end of a passenger car with a combination hydraulic rescue tool. A dash displacement can also be accomplished with heavy-duty jacks and hacksaws.

If the steering wheel hub is large and rectangular, the car probably has an air bag or bags (the passenger-side bag is in the area of the glove compartment). If the bags have not deployed, they are not likely to deploy now unless extrication involves displacing the dash or steering wheel. If such displacement is to be done, air bag manufacturers recommend that you avoid placing your body or objects against an air bag module or in its path of deployment. Follow this recommendation before you disconnect the battery cables. Air bag manufacturers strongly advise against displacement or cutting the steering column until the air bag system has been fully deactivated, cutting or drilling into an air bag module, or applying heat in the area of the steering wheel hub.

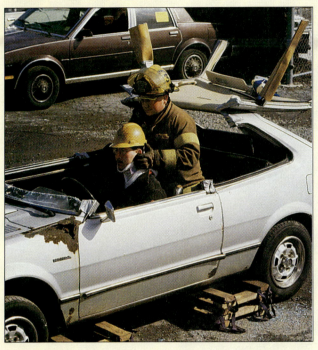

▲ **1.** The traditional procedure is to sever the A- and B-posts, cut through the roof rails just ahead of the C-posts, and fold the roof back like the roof of a convertible. It is necessary either to remove or to cut the windshield, depending on the need for working space.

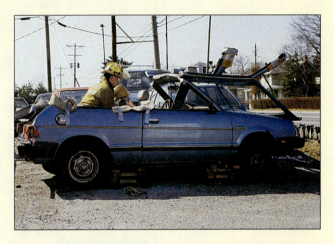

▲ **2.** Folding the roof forward can be accomplished quickly when the C-posts are narrow. The roof is hinged either on top or on the bottom of the windshield, depending on the need for working space.

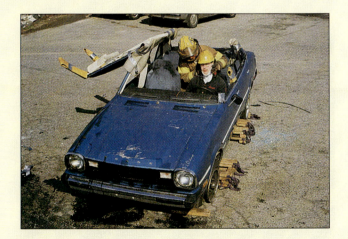

▲ **3.** When a car has only one occupant, the roof can be folded to one side after severing the A-, B-, and C-posts of the opposite side.

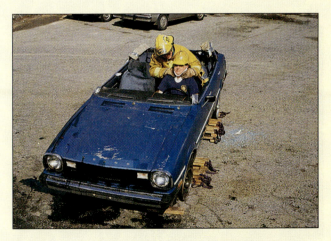

▲ **4.** When a car has narrow C-posts, removing the roof altogether provides maximum working space.

Displacing Doors and
Roof Posts of a Car

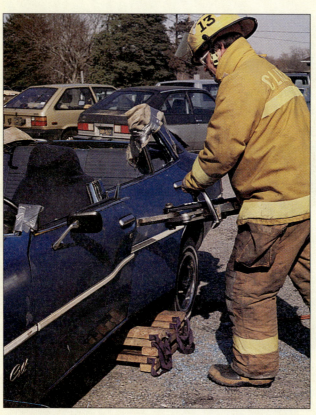

▲ **1.** A collision vehicle's doors can be opened quickly with a hydraulic rescue tool. Doors can be opened at the latch or by breaking the hinges.

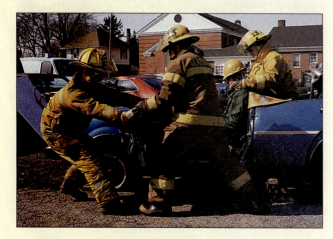

▲ **2.** Once the front door has been opened, it can be moved beyond the normal range of motion by simply pushing on it. Seldom is there a need for removing a front door.

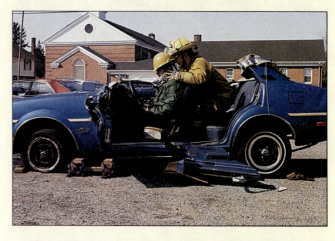

▲ **3.** When the front doors of a four-door car have been opened at the latch side, the roof post and rear door can be pulled down simultaneously to expose the entire side of the vehicle.

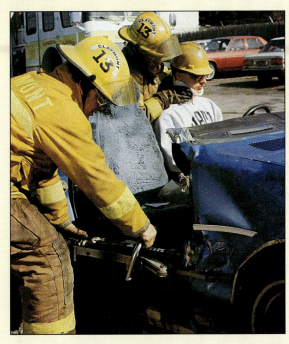

▲ **1.** Relief cuts are made at the junction of the A-post with the rocker panel, and in the A-post between the door hinges.

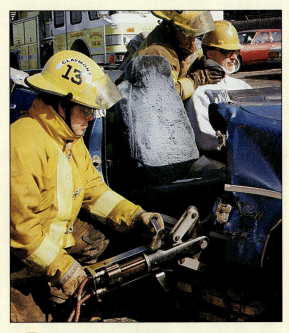

▲ **3.** The combination hydraulic tool can be used in the spreading mode to displace the front end.

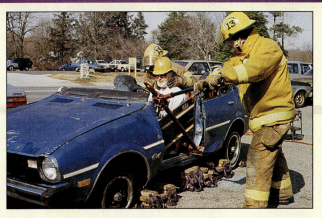

▲ **2.** Heavy-duty jacks can be used to pivot the front end of the vehicle away from the relief cuts.

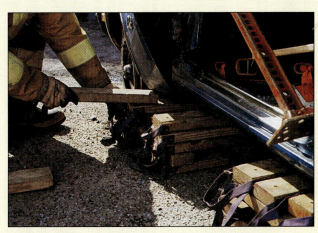

▲ **4.** Displacing the front end will tend to lift the vehicle from the cribs. Cribbing must be added to the front cribs to prevent destabilization.

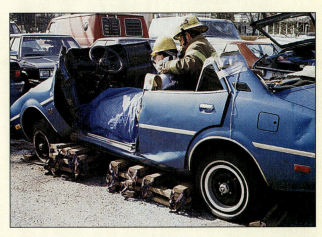

▲ **5.** Displacing the front end creates working space by moving a number of mechanisms of entrapment away from the front seat occupants.

SUMMARY

- Understand the process of vehicular extrication so you can keep the patient informed and anticipate any dangerous steps in the extrication action plan.

- Realize the importance of personal protective equipment for the rescuers as well as for the patient during an extrication.

- Learn to become keenly aware of the potential hazards to the rescuers, the patient, and bystanders at the rescue scene.

- Understand that your role as an EMT-B in an extrication is to rescue the patient, and not the vehicle.

REVIEW QUESTIONS

1. The _____ offers adequate protection for the EMT-B at the scene of the collision.
   a. firefighter helmet.
   b. plastic bump cap.
   c. wool watch cap.
   d. baseball cap.

2. A phenomenon, especially common in wet weather, that may provide the first clue that a power line has been downed at the scene of a collision is a(n):
   a. aura.
   b. ground gradient.
   c. reboot.
   d. Bainbridge effect.

3. Gear that provides adequate protection at a rescue scene with jagged metal, broken glass, and flash fires includes all of the following EXCEPT:
   a. hinged plastic helmet shield.
   b. turnout pants with wide cuffs.
   c. high-top, steel-toe work shoes.
   d. latex gloves under leather gloves.

4. When there is an electrical hazard on scene, the safe zone should be:
   a. as close to the nearest utility pole as possible.
   b. far enough away so arcing cannot injure anyone.
   c. established only by power company personnel.
   d. at least 10 feet from ground gradient.

5. Once a vehicle involved in a collision is stable, the EMT-B should attempt to gain access to the patient first by:

a. removing a door or the roof of the car.

b. breaking a window close to the patient.

c. trying to open a door or roll down a window.

d. using a flathead ax to break the windshield

WEBMEDIC

Visit Brady's *Essentials of Emergency Care* web site for direct web links. At **www.prenhall.com/limmer,** you will find information related to the following Chapter 27 topics:

- NFPA standards on protective gear
- Air bags
- Vehicle stabilization
- Fire extinguishers
- Vehicle extrications

Chapter Twenty-Eight

SPECIAL OPERATIONS

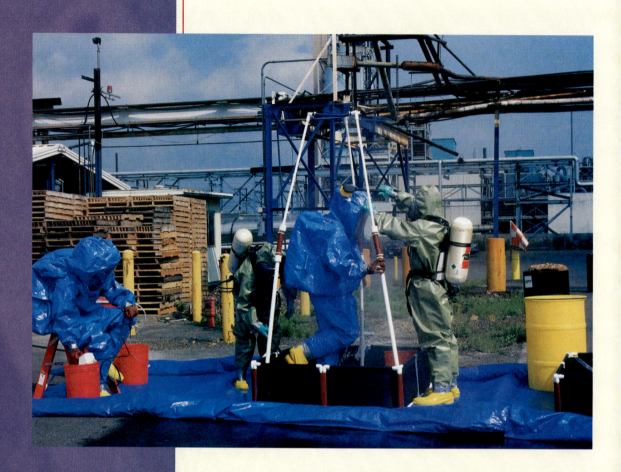

ESSENTIAL ELECTRONIC EXTRAS

CD ESSENTIALS

For preview and review of chapter material, see the student CD-ROM for

- Pretest
- Chapter quizzes
- Posttest

WEB ESSENTIALS

For additional review and enrichment, visit www.prenhall.com/limmer for

- Interactive student quizzes
- Links to online EMS resources
- Online case studies
- Audio glossary

As an EMT-B, you will respond to emergencies that require the involvement and cooperation of a large number of EMS and other specialized personnel. Such incidents may involve hazardous materials or the challenge of multiple patients. Most communities have detailed plans for such emergencies. Your responsibility is to be familiar with those plans and the roles EMS, fire, law enforcement, and other agencies play.

MANAGING THE MULTIPLE-CASUALTY INCIDENT

A **multiple-casualty incident,** or **MCI,** is an event that places a great demand on EMS resources (equipment and personnel) (Figure 28-1). A situation that involves more than one patient or requires an ambulance response of three or more vehicles is generally referred to as an MCI. However, the definition of an MCI differs from community to community and is based upon the resources that are available at any given moment.

A large-scale disaster can easily tax, if not overwhelm, a single agency. One way to minimize the operating difficulties of a large-scale MCI or disaster is for every EMT-B in the agency to become familiar with the local disaster plan. A **disaster plan** is a predetermined set of instructions that tells a community's various emergency responders what to do in specific emergencies. While no disaster plan can address every problem that could arise, there are several features common to every good disaster plan. A good disaster plan should be:

- Written to address the events that are conceivable for a particular location
- Well publicized so each emergency responder is familiar with the plan and how it is to be put into operation
- Realistic and based upon the actual availability of resources
- Rehearsed frequently to get all the "bugs" out. This is best done as an extension of what EMT-Bs do every day. That is why many services declare a medical MCI for incidents requiring three or more ambulances and major collisions.

Components of an Incident Management System

An **incident management system (IMS)** has been developed to assist with the control, direction, and coordination of emergency response resources. IMS has nine key components:

- Strong visible command
- Common terminology
- Modular organization based upon incident needs
- Comprehensive resource management
- Manageable span of control
- Assurance of personnel safety and accountability
- Integrated communications
- Unified command
- Consolidated action plans using goals and objectives

CORE CONCEPTS

In this chapter, you will learn about the following topics:

- The components of an incident management system as they apply to EMS

- The roles of the triage, treatment, and transport sector officers

- How to use triage tags and prioritize patients at an MCI

- The role of EMS personnel at a hazardous materials incident

- The levels of training specified by OSHA for responders to hazardous materials incidents

- Substance identification at a hazardous materials incident

- The differences between the NFPA 704 and DOT U.N. classifications for placarding hazardous materials at fixed locations and in transit

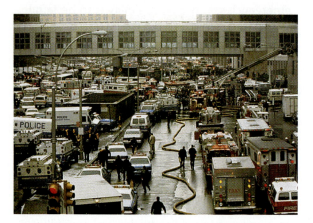

Figure 28-1 A multiple-casualty incident.

When integrated, these components provide the basis for an effective operation. There is an essential need for common terminology in any emergency management system, which will potentially involve multiple agencies from different disciplines. Plain English always works best! Instead of trying to remember that the EMS Commander is unit 615 or car 2 or ambulance 7, simply refer to the individual by the name of the position: "EMS Command." This also facilitates transfer of command to supervisory personnel who may arrive later in the incident and assume command. The person in EMS Command should wear a clearly identifiable, bright-colored vest for easy identification, as should each of the sector officers.

At each incident, IMS organizational structure develops in a modular fashion. Since the development of the organization is top down, there is always at least an **incident commander (IC)** identified at any incident. If the incident's needs dictate, the IC may delegate additional responsibilities to other personnel.

Management of communications at an incident requires integrated communications. An integrated communications plan includes standardized procedures, use of clear instruction with common terminology, two-way confirmation that messages are received, and status reports to update the IC on assignments that were delegated. Radio frequencies should be set up in advance to ensure that all arriving units have common frequencies and that these are tactical and command frequencies that can be used at the incident.

There are two methods of command: singular and unified. **Singular command** is used when all resources are specifically under the jurisdiction and control of one agency. In many communities, EMS is managed by fire services. Accordingly, singular command is often used at fire and rescue incidents. However, if police agencies have major involvement, if there is a separate EMS provider, or if other agencies are involved, **unified command** is more appropriate (Figure 28-2).

In most communities, unified command is the best way to manage resources since incidents tend to grow more complex and the right agency must take the lead at the appropriate time, with command officers from all agencies cooperating. In a unified command system, all agencies involved contribute to the command process by establishing a consolidated action plan. Complex incidents may require written action plans that cover all strategic goals, all tactical objectives, and support activities for the incident's entire operational period. A unified command structure is best achieved by setting up one command post instead of separate ones for police, fire, and EMS.

Another important component of IMS is span of control. A manageable span of control spells out the number of subordinates that one supervisor can manage effectively. The desired range is three to seven, with five being optimum. It is very easy to lose track of your crew members at an incident if they are not assigned to smaller units.

IMS also designates incident facilities such as the **command post,** which is where each agency representative, the communications center, and the center of all planning and incident operations direction are located. Many communities utilize a **mobile command center,** which is a vehicle with desk space, maps, multiple radio frequencies, and enough room for the command officers from each agency. **Staging areas** are designated facilities designed to keep the scene from being clogged with equipment, vehicles, and personnel, yet keeping them within a few minutes of the incident so they can respond as directed.

Comprehensive resource management is attained by maximizing resource use, consolidating control of large numbers of ambulances, and reducing the communications load. Knowledge of the status of personnel and vehicles is critical to effective resource management.

IMS Functional Areas

IMS has five major functional areas, or sections: command, operations, planning, logistics, and finance. In

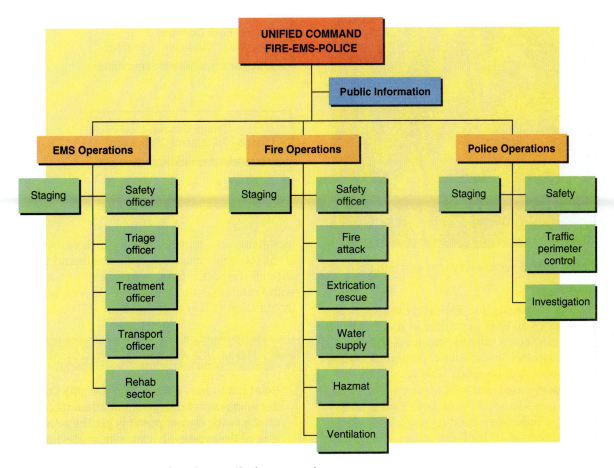

Figure 28-2 An organization chart for a unified command system.

a major incident, each of the five may be a different person's responsibility; in a smaller incident these functional areas may be combined.

The **command section** is always staffed no matter what the size of the incident. The incident commander has overall responsibility for managing. The IC's responsibilities include assessing incident priorities, determining the strategic goals and tactical objectives, developing an incident action plan and the appropriate organizational structure, managing incident resources, ensuring personnel safety, coordinating activities of outside agencies, and authorizing release of information. With this long list of responsibilities, it is easy to see the need for delegation and establishment of various sector officers.

The **operations section** is responsible for all tactical operations at an incident, including those with which you are most familiar—patient care, firefighting, and hostage negotiations. The **planning section** is responsible for the collection, evaluation, dissemination, and use of information about the development of the incident and the status of resources. This includes situation status, resource status, and documentation and demobilization units, as well as technical specialists.

The **logistics section** is responsible for providing facilities, services, and materials for the incident. This includes the communications unit, medical unit, food unit, service branch, supply unit, facilities unit, and ground support units. The **finance section** is responsible for all costs and financial considerations at an extensive incident. This includes the time, procurement, compensations, claim, and cost units.

EMS Command at an MCI

In a primarily EMS incident, the **EMS Command,** or Medical Command as some agencies refer to it, would often be the first crew leader on the first arriving EMS unit. The senior EMT-B's first responsibility includes confirming the incident by radio to the dispatcher. The EMS command describes the nature of the emergency, its exact location, and the best estimate of the number of patients. This crucial information is used by the dispatcher to send additional resources to the scene. The radio report also includes a request for any special resources that the EMT-Bs feel may be necessary.

Additional responsibilities of EMS command include sizing up resources and the need for additional

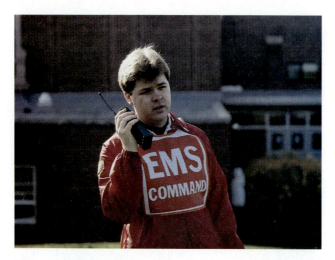

Figure 28-3 EMS command with a vest and radio.

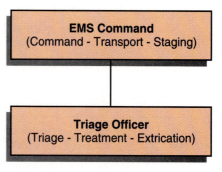

Figure 28-4 An organization chart for a smaller incident.

EMS response, managing the EMS response, coordinating activities of all EMS personnel at the incident, designating EMS sector officers, ensuring the safety of all EMS personnel, establishing communications contacts, and notifying hospitals. The EMS Commander dons the designated vest so that all units arriving on the scene can identify him or her (Figure 28-3). The EMS Commander may need to establish a Command Post and remain at that location. If a Command Post is already established, the EMS crew chief becomes the EMS representative at the Command Post. He or she works cooperatively with police and fire service commanders in the Command Post. The EMS sectors that are established as needed include:

- Staging sector
- Triage sector
- Treatment sector
- Transport sector
- Extrication sector (may be a fire-rescue responsibility)
- Mobile command center

At small incidents, it may only be necessary to designate command and the triage sector (Figure 28-4). At medium-sized incidents, command, triage, treatment, and transport may be designated (Figure 28-5). At larger incidents, EMS Command may designate all the sector officers and have an aide to assist with communications, a safety officer, and a public-information officer (Figure 28-6).

Safety Officer and Staging Sector

When it becomes necessary, EMS Command may choose to designate a safety officer and a staging sector officer. The **EMS Safety Officer** is responsible for ensuring scene safety for all EMS personnel. This officer pays close attention to details that EMS Command may not have the time to focus on, such as whether or not personnel are identified adequately or wearing the appropriate protective gear for the incident. The safety officer determines if personnel are about to encounter dangerous situations and takes responsibility for assuring compliance with OSHA

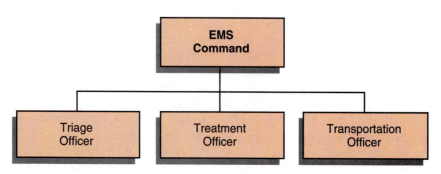

Figure 28-5 An organization chart for a medium-sized incident.

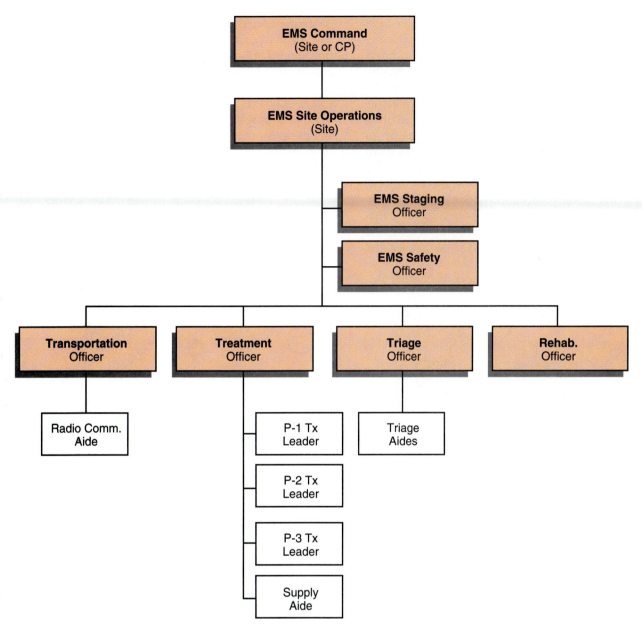

Figure 28-6 An organization chart for a major incident.

regulations for the appropriate level of infection control follow-up for the incident.

The **EMS Staging Sector Officer** is responsible for establishing an assembly point and mobilization area for personnel and vehicles, releasing resources to the incident as requested by the transport sector officer, and ensuring that the physiological needs of the personnel are being met. After an ambulance transports a patient to the hospital, it usually returns to the staging sector.

The Triage Sector

The **Triage Sector Officer** is responsible for establishing triage procedures as dictated by incident type. For easy identification, the triage officer dons the appropriate vest (Figure 28-7). The first triage cut is

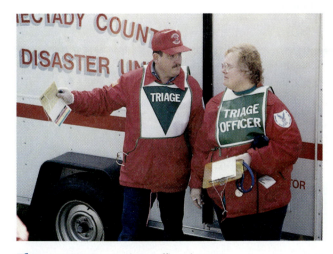

Figure 28-7 A triage officer in vest.

done rapidly by using a bullhorn, PA system, or loud voice to direct all patients capable of walking (Priority 3) to move to a particular location. This action has a two-fold purpose. It quickly identifies those individuals who have an open airway and adequate circulation, and it physically separates them from patients who need more care. In some cases, triage involves extrication of trapped patients; in other cases, it involves corralling all patients in order to funnel them to the treatment sector for medical evaluation.

When extrication is needed or patients are entrapped, the triage officer must work very closely with the **Extrication Sector Officer** to assure that the patients are removed from the wreckage in the correct order. In instances in which patients are piled on top of one another, it may be necessary to remove a low-priority patient in order to access a higher pri-

ority patient. The triage officer is responsible for coordinating personnel and equipment usage and can appoint triage support personnel as needed to aid in the movement of patients to treatment and/or transportation sectors. Usually patients are immobilized on backboards if necessary and carried by "runners" to the appropriate treatment sector. Extensive treatment does not take place at the incident site because it is in a hazard zone and rescue and initial treatment of other patients could be impeded.

Triage is a French word which means "to sort." If you are assigned to work in the triage sector, you will need to do an initial triage and apply a **triage tag** to each patient (Figures 28-8 and 28-9). Different localities use different tagging systems. It is important that you know and understand the system used in your area. Because many MCIs are multiple-agency

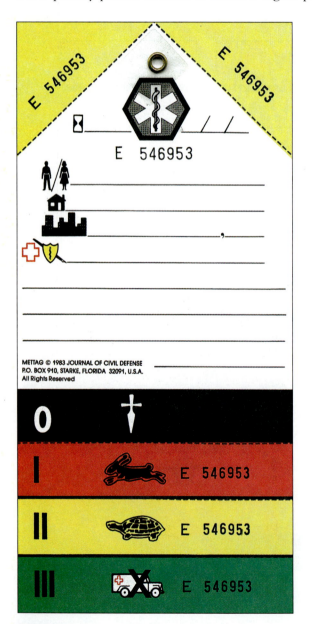

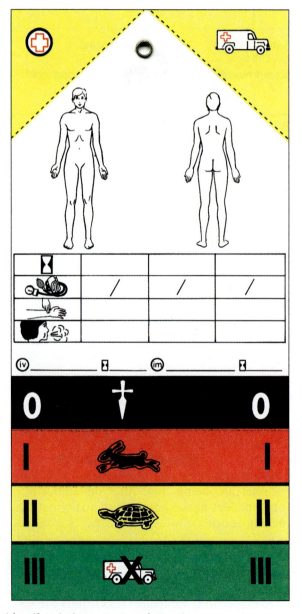

Figure 28-8 METTAG® triage tag (front and back) used to identify Priority 1, 2, 3, and 0 patients.

Figure 28-9 EMS disaster tag (front and back).

events, it is equally important that different services in the same region use the same coding system. If each agency were to use a different system, it would be impossible to correctly coordinate the order in which patients are to receive care.

Patients are usually divided into the following four categories:

- **Priority One (P-1).** The red color designation indicates that the patient has life-threatening critical injuries or illnesses such as airway and breathing difficulties, uncontrolled or severe bleeding, decreased mental status, severe medical problems, shock (hypoperfusion), or severe burns. Whenever possible, these patients should be transported to the hospital first.

- **Priority Two (P-2).** The yellow color designation identifies patients with unstable or potentially unstable injuries such as burns without airway problems, major or multiple bone or joint injuries, or back injuries with or without spinal cord damage. Whenever possible, these patients should be transported as soon as the P-1 patients have been removed from the scene.

- **Priority Three (P-3).** The green color designation identifies the "walking wounded," such as patients with minor painful, swollen, deformed extremities; minor soft-tissue injuries; and psychological trauma. Whenever possible, isolate these patients from the P-1 and P-2 patients to limit their psychological trauma as well as to unclutter the scene. Many services routinely dispatch a school bus to transport the P-3 patients to a distant hospital for further evaluation and treatment. While this is helpful, ensure that these patients are reevaluated prior to allowing them to ride the bus and that medical personnel are placed on the bus in case a patient's condition changes.

- **Priority Zero (P-0).** The color black identifies the dead and includes victims with exposed brain matter, cardiac arrest for over 20 minutes except with cold-water drowning or severe hypothermia, decapitation, severed trunk, and incineration. In a situation where there is a limited number of responders compared to the large number of patients, a patient with a critical injury may initially be prioritized as a P-3 and then, when ample help is available, either worked as a P-1 or left as a P-0. The basic principle of triage is to help as many of the seriously injured as possible. Dedicating an EMT-B crew to a cardiac-arrest patient when there are many, many serious patients who need their help would violate the basic principle of triage.

The Treatment Sector

The **Treatment Sector Officer** is responsible for setting up treatment areas as requested and warranted by the site and transportation considerations. This officer supervises the area established to hold patients prior to transportation from the scene, as well as coordinates activities of all EMS personnel assigned to the sector.

The treatment officer and assistants triage the patients in that sector to determine the order in which they will receive treatment. During secondary triage, it may be necessary to recategorize to a higher or lower priority a patient whose condition has deteriorated or improved or who was incorrectly diagnosed. This necessitates moving the patient to the proper treatment sector as resources permit. During secondary triage, some services use a different tag on which more detailed information about the patient can be recorded. Other services set up their treatment sector by using red, yellow, green, and black tarps to separate the patients while they wait for transportation. The treatment officer appoints treatment personnel, directly oversees the patient care provided, determines the need for additional personnel and equipment, and coordinates movement of patients to ambulances with the transport sector.

The Transport Sector

The **Transport Sector Officer** establishes and maintains ambulance loading areas. This officer is responsible for supervising patient movement in conjunction with the treatment sector officer, monitoring local hospital capabilities, and determining patient destinations. The transport sector officer also coordinates helicopter evacuations if they are used at the incident. No ambulance should proceed to a treatment sector without having been requested by the transport officer and directed by the staging officer. It is also vital that no ambulance transport any patient without the approval of the transport officer, since the transport officer maintains documentation of all patient destinations through a patient log or copies of the triage tags.

The transport officer also supervises the hospital communications network, which may involve appointing a hospital communicator to operate the hospital communications network, maintaining hospital status and capability, and providing patient information to hospitals via radio or cellular phone. During a major incident, individual ambulances should not communicate directly with the hospital. This will be done directly by the hospital communicator in an abbreviated manner. The hospital may be told only that they are receiving a Priority-1 patient with respiratory problems. The transport officer also appoints vehicle loaders to facilitate patient loading and ambulance movement from the scene.

> ### PRECEPTOR PEARL
>
> Encourage new EMT-Bs to practice declaring EMS Command, establishing a triage sector, donning sector vests, giving an arrival report to dispatch, and applying triage tags at all incidents involving three or more ambulances. In this way, the procedures will be second nature to them at larger incidents.

Freelancing

Individuals at the scene will be assigned to particular roles in one of the sectors. Upon arrival, you should report to the sector officer for specific duties. Once assigned a specific task, you should complete the task and report back to the sector officer. At an MCI, never go off and do just anything you want. This is called "freelancing" and leads to confusion, lack of coordination of resources, and the potential for injury to the EMT-B.

Psychological Aspects of MCIs

During MCIs, you often encounter psychologically stressed patients. While these patients may outwardly exhibit few signs of injury, they undoubtedly have been subjected to devastating circumstances. Proper early management of the psychologically stressed patient supports later treatment and helps ensure a faster recovery. Some services will automatically dispatch a clergy member or a psychologist who has been oriented to emergency services work to assist these patients at the scene.

Adequately managing a patient during an MCI may require you to administer "psychological first aid." This may take the form of talking with a terrified parent, child, or witness. A compassionate, honest demeanor can reassure the patient, as will listening to the patient and acknowledging his or her fears. Often this is all the patient needs.

LIFESPAN DEVELOPMENT

At MCIs involving children, it is a good idea to move the children who have been evaluated as having no problem or the lowest priority away from the higher priority patients as soon as possible. Doing this can help limit emotional injuries to these children and the need to transport larger numbers of patients to the hospital.

Patients are not the only ones to sustain emotional scars during an MCI. Emergency responders do, too. Large-scale or horrific MCIs may affect rescuers as much as, if not more than, non-rescuers. No one gets used to walking through body parts at the scene of a plane crash. It is not a sign of weakness to talk about your feelings after a major incident.

Treat co-workers who become emotionally incapacitated as patients and remove them to an area where they can rest without viewing the scene. Ensure that these patients are monitored by an EMS provider until a clinically competent provider can take over. Do not allow these EMT-Bs to return to duty without first being evaluated by a psychologist. Critical incident stress debriefing (CISD) teams are a resource that can provide the emotional and psychological support needed by these patients. Intervention by a CISD team may help to prevent post-traumatic stress disorder and help put the individual back in service more quickly.

HAZMAT AWARENESS

What Is a Hazardous Material?

The definition of hazardous materials varies, depending on the regulations or standards of the defining agency. The U.S. Department of Transportation (DOT) defines a **hazardous material** as "any substance or material in a quantity or form which poses an unreasonable risk to health, safety, and property when transported in commerce." This definition is appropriate for DOT because it regulates commercial means of transportation. However, the Environmental Protection Agency (EPA), because it regulates the environment, defines a **hazardous substance** as "any substance designated under the Clean Water Act and Comprehensive Environmental Response Compensation and Liability Act as posing a threat to waterways and the environment when released." The EPA goes on to define **hazardous waste** as "any waste or combination of wastes which pose a substantial present or potential hazard to human health or living organisms because such wastes are non-degradable or persistent in nature, or because they can biologically magnify, or because they may otherwise cause or tend to cause detrimental cumulative effects."

Perhaps the most encompassing definition of a hazardous material is the National Fire Protection Association's (NFPA) in Standard #472. It defines it as "any substance that causes or may cause adverse effects on the health or safety of employees, the general public, or the environment; any biological agent and other disease-causing agent, or a waste or combination of wastes." Examples of hazardous materials appear in Table 28-1.

Recognizing the Risks of Hazardous Materials

Preparing to respond to a call that involves a hazardous material is more than having the money to buy protective encapsulated ("Gumby") suits. Hazmat training—as well as analyzing the hazmat risks in your community—is required by the Occupational Safety and Health Administration (OSHA). Hazardous materials are all around us, and the number of chemicals is constantly growing. Consider the case of a brewery in Golden, Colorado, where, in July of 1991, two anhydrous ammonia leaks occurred within a month, producing over 32 inhalation injuries. Could this happen in your area? Although there may not be a brewery in your district, what other manufacturers use anhydrous ammonia in the manufacture of their products?

Have you ever observed the trucks passing through your district? Consider the case of the tanker truck which, when one of its three cells split open on the New Jersey Turnpike during rush-hour traffic, spilled 4,000 gallons of hydrochloric acid on the highway. In addition to the closing of 15 miles of packed highway, five police officers, seven firefighters, and more than a dozen motorists were hospitalized for severe respiratory burns.

Table 28-1   **Examples of Hazardous Materials**

Material	Possible Hazard
Benzene (benzol)	Toxic vapors can be absorbed through the skin; destroys bone marrow
Benzoyl peroxide	Fire and explosion
Carbon tetrachloride	Damages internal organs
Cychohexane	Explosive; eye and throat irritant
Diethyl ether	Flammable and can be explosive; irritant to eyes and respiratory tract; can cause drowsiness or unconsciousness
Ethyl acetate	Irritates eyes and respiratory tract
Ethylene chloride	Damages eyes
Ethylene dichloride	Strong irritant
Heptane	Respiratory irritant
Hydrochloric acid	Respiratory irritant; explosive to high concentration of vapors can produce pulmonary edema; can damage skin and eyes
Hydrogen cyanide	Highly flammable; toxic through inhalation or absorption
Methyl isobutyl ketone	Irritates eyes and mucous membranes
Nitric acid	Produces a toxic gas (nitrogen dioxide); skin irritant; can cause self-ignition of cellulose products (e.g., sawdust)
Organochloride (Chlordane, DDT, Dieldrin, Lindane, Methoxyclor)	Irritates eyes and skin; fumes and smoke toxic
Perchloroethylene	Toxic if inhaled or swallowed
Silicon tetrachloride	Water-reactive to form toxic hydrogen chloride fumes
Tetrahydrofuran (THF)	Damages eyes and mucous membranes
Toluol (toluene)	Toxic vapors; can cause organ damage
Vinyl chloride	Flammable and explosive; listed as carcinogen

Maybe your town is divided by a railroad and each year your service practices for a train multiple-casualty incident (MCI). Watch as the trains go by and pay attention to the markings on the cars. To emphasize the importance of observing passing trains, consider an incident that took place in Murdock, Illinois. After a freight train carrying sulfuric acid, alcohol, and propane derailed, a fireball resulted that was visible for 20 miles. The explosion was so powerful that it threw a large portion of a tank car almost half a mile, and it required the evacuation of a four-mile area. Eight emergency workers required treatment for chemical exposure.

Take time to review what chemicals are manufactured and stored in or transported through your community. Do you have major interstate routes through your district? Does it have railroads, chemical plants, fertilizer storage facilities, waterways, airports, hospitals, water-treatment plants, refineries, nuclear plants, a nursery, or corner gas stations? What, exactly, is stored in those warehouses on the edge of town?

However, do not mistakenly think that dangerous goods are carried only in 55-gallon drums, in tankers, or in rail cars. Some chemicals can be very hazardous in small quantities. Keep in mind that some small-package shippers in the United States, aware of the rules and regulations for shipping hazardous materials, very carefully and properly load their vehicles with less than the amount of chemical that would require a hazmat placard on the outside of their trucks. Even the local high school chemistry class easily illustrates the volatility of small quantities of chemicals if they are improperly mixed (Figure 28-10). The local school lab can be very hazardous if not properly supervised. So be aware of the range of potential hazmat incident sites in your community.

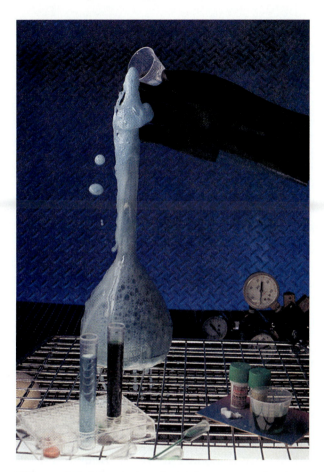

Figure 28-10 A chemistry laboratory can be the site of a hazmat incident.

LIFESPAN DEVELOPMENT

Not all MCIs are as initially evident as major vehicle collisions, downed planes, or building explosions. EMT-Bs frequently respond to traumatic calls which have multiple patients. It is unusual, however, to have multiple patients with similar medical complaints, such as headaches, vomiting, chest pain or difficulty breathing, at the same call. Whenever you arrive on the scene and there are multiple patients with medical complaints, think "POISON" right away. Your first priority should be self protection. Determine if the problem may be in the air and a hazard to you and your crew. In some cases where family members present with headaches, nausea, or vomiting, there may be poison in the air such as carbon monoxide from an improperly vented heating system.

Hazmat Rules and Standards

Because of a few "high profile" incidents in the United States, the storage, transportation, and response to emergencies involving chemicals have come under the regulation of many government agencies.

SARA Title III: Planning Regulations

The Superfund Amendments and Reauthorization Act of 1986 (SARA) is a federal law. Title III of this law—the Emergency Planning and Community Right-to-Know Act—established hazardous chemical requirements for local, state, and federal governments, as well as industry, in the areas of emergency planning, emergency notification, community right-to-know reporting requirements, and toxic-chemical release reporting emissions inventory. The emergency planning section of SARA was designed to develop state and local preparedness and response capabilities through better coordination and planning. The governor of each state appointed a State Emergency Response Commission which, in turn, designated **local emergency planning committees (LEPCs).** Your ambulance service may have some involvement in LEPCs, which are responsible for:

■ Identifying facilities, transportation routes, and secondary facilities

■ Establishing facility and community response procedures

■ Designating facility and community emergency coordinators

■ Developing facility and public notification procedures

■ Developing methods for determining release and impact areas

■ Describing emergency equipment and personnel at facilities and in the community

■ Developing evacuation plans

■ Developing training programs and schedules

■ Designing methods and schedules for exercising plans

OSHA Regulations

In 1989, OSHA put in place 29 CFR Part 1910.120, which deals with the Emergency Response to Hazardous Substance Releases. These regulations:

■ Spell out training requirements for five levels of responders to hazmat incidents

■ Specify who can teach the training programs

■ Set out refresher training requirements

■ Specify medical surveillance and consultation requirements

■ Specify chemical protective clothing and post-emergency response operations

These regulations were designed for the first response agencies to a hazardous materials incident, such as police departments, fire departments, and ambulance services. The regulations frequently use the terms "employer" and "employee." In some states, the courts have determined that volunteer agencies are employers and their members are employees, even if they do not receive remuneration for their services.

The training is broken into the following five levels:

- **First Responder Awareness.** Four to six hours of training for rescuers who are likely to witness or discover a hazardous substance release. They are trained only to recognize the problem and initiate a response from the proper organizations.

- **First Responder Operations.** Eight hours of training for those who initially respond to releases or potential releases of hazardous materials, in order to protect people, property, and the environment. These responders stay at a safe distance, keep the incident from spreading, and protect people from any exposures.

- **Hazardous Materials Technician.** Twenty-four hours of training for those who actually plug, patch, or stop the release of a hazardous material.

- **Hazardous Materials Specialist.** Twenty-four hours of training for those expected to respond with and provide support to hazardous material technicians. Their duties parallel those of the technician. However, specialists require a more directed or specific knowledge of the various substances they may be called upon to contain. They also act as the site liaison with federal, state, and local government authorities in regard to site activities.

- **On-Scene Incident Commander.** This training level is for the rescuer who will assume control of the incident. Training includes the first responder operations level in addition to competency in the following:

  - Know and be able to implement the employer's incident command system

  - Know how to implement the employer's emergency response plan

  - Know and understand the hazards and risks associated with employees working in chemical-protective clothing

  - Know how to implement the local emergency response plan

  - Know the state emergency response plan and the plan of the Federal Regional Response Team

  - Know and understand the importance of decontamination procedures

Employees are expected to be adequately trained at the level in which they will participate prior to being involved in an incident. Each EMS agency is responsible for training its EMT-Bs in at least the awareness level, if your original EMT-B training did not also include hazmat training. Some services show a video, run a drill, and review the hazmat plan. Then each employee is given a written test on the objectives they must pass, which is then inserted in the employee's file. In addition, OSHA requires that trainees at each level demonstrate their competencies annually.

National Fire Protection Association's Standards

The National Fire Protection Association (NFPA) sets voluntary standards for the fire service that are often adopted by local municipalities. Why is the NFPA writing safety standards for EMS? Because in the United States, more than 50% of prehospital EMS is provided by the fire service. The NFPA standards most relevant to EMS are Standards 472, 473, and 704.

Standard 472: Professional Competence of Responders to Hazardous Materials Incidents preceded and set the stage for OSHA 1910.120. Standard 473: Competencies for EMS Personnel Responding to Hazardous Materials Incidents established two levels of EMS hazmat responder above the awareness level and was the first standard to specifically address the role of EMS personnel. This standard is also the best predictor of the next OSHA regulations for EMS personnel. Standard 704: This defines a method of classifying hazards discussed later in this module.

EMT-B's First Responder Role

Establish Command and Control Zones

When you arrive on the scene of a hazmat emergency, take a defensive position in a safe place far enough from the site to ensure your safety. Try to position your vehicle upwind and at a higher level than the incident to avoid providing an ignition source for gases that stay near the ground and to prevent your inhaling potentially toxic fumes escaping from the area. Secure the scene without entering the area of contamination, commonly called the **hot zone.** Do what you can to isolate the area, establish a perimeter, evacuate people if necessary, assure the safety of your crew, and direct bystanders to a safe area. Call for the hazmat team capable of entering the hot zone to rescue the injured and control the incident.

While help is on the way, implement your agency's incident management system and establish an EMS commander and a unified command post. Establish control zones, isolating a hot zone as well as a decontamination corridor, or **warm zone.** This warm zone provides the only way into and out of the hot zone. It is in this zone that the hazmat team and all patients who have been removed from the hot zone may need to be decontaminated, depending on the specific chemicals to which they were exposed. Properly dressed personnel in the decontamination corridor systematically remove the patients' clothing and bathe them with the appropriate agents for the chemical to which they were exposed. A sample of the stages in the decon corridor is illustrated in Figure 28-11.

Equipment, other emergency rescuers, and the command post should be staged in the next adjacent area, called the **cold zone.**

Identify the Substance Involved

An attempt must be made to identify the hazardous material and assess the severity of the situation. Until that is done, it will be difficult to determine the risk to the public, rescuers, patients, and the environment. You must try to find out what the substance is and its properties and dangers; whether or not there is imminent danger of the contamination spreading; what you hear, see, and smell; how many victims are involved; and if there is any danger of secondary contamination from the victims. Secondary contamination occurs when a contaminated person makes contact with someone who previously was "clean."

An important piece of scene assessment equipment is a simple pair of binoculars (Figure 28-12). They may allow a visual inspection of the hot zone

from a safe distance so you can spot identifying labels, tank styles, and placards.

If you are approached by victims leaving the hot zone, listen very carefully to them; they are a good source of information. Often these people have been ignored, only for rescuers to discover later in the incident that one of the first people to exit the scene identified the hazardous material. Perhaps it was a chemist who knew exactly which chemicals were mixed or a factory worker who knew exactly the amount and type of bulk chemicals stored in a particular corner of the factory.

Be especially careful when something about the scene just does not add up or you get a funny feeling in your gut that something is wrong. As an EMT-B, you respond to many trauma scenes with multiple patients, yet it is unusual to respond to a medical call with multiple patients. Any time you arrive on the scene to find multiple patients with chest pain, breathing difficulty, or stomach cramps, stop and consider that they may have been poisoned in some manner. For example, it could be the air you are about to inhale that poisoned them. Thinking ahead will prevent you from becoming the next victim. The smart rescuer will size up the situation and call for and wear self-contained breathing apparatus (SCBA) *before* removing the patients to a safe spot for treatment.

Establish a Rehab Sector in the Cold Zone

In order to enter the hot zone safely, the hazmat team will need to determine the most appropriate level of chemical-protective clothing. Specialized hazmat clothing is very hot inside, causing its wearer to sweat excessively, which can lead to dehydration. The OSHA regulations require that medical surveillance and consultation be provided for the members of the hazmat team, as well as emergency response employees, who exhibit signs or symptoms that may have resulted from an exposure to a chemical. This surveillance and consultation takes place in the rehab sector located in the cold zone.

The **rehab sector** should be protected from inclement weather conditions and be easily accessible to ambulances. The area should be upwind of the incident and free from exhaust fumes. Make sure the rehab sector has plenty of room in case it must be transformed into a treatment sector for a large number of injured or exhausted responders.

While treating decontaminated patients and hazmat team members in the cold zone, you may be asked to assist in medical monitoring. Medical monitoring involves a pre- and post-suiting up medical exam of the rescuers including: respiration, pulse, BP, mental status, ECG by ALS personnel, motor skills, hydration status, and weight (using a portable scale carried by the hazmat team). If a rescuer's heart rate exceeds 110 beats per minute, an oral temperature

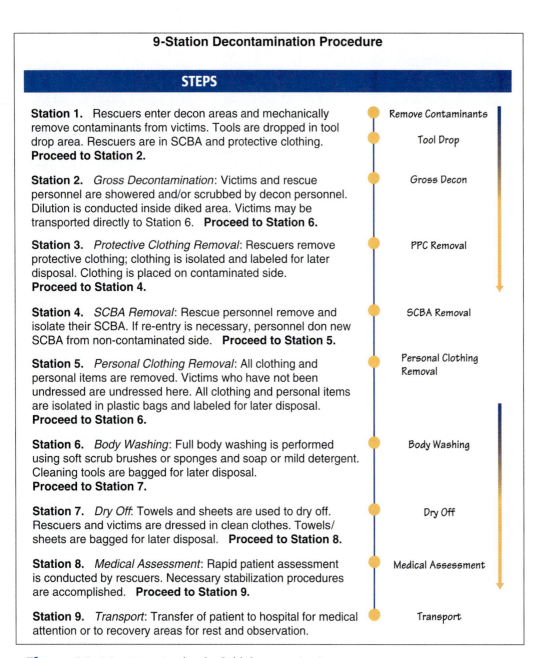

9-Station Decontamination Procedure

STEPS

Station 1. Rescuers enter decon areas and mechanically remove contaminants from victims. Tools are dropped in tool drop area. Rescuers are in SCBA and protective clothing. **Proceed to Station 2.**

Remove Contaminants

Tool Drop

Station 2. *Gross Decontamination*: Victims and rescue personnel are showered and/or scrubbed by decon personnel. Dilution is conducted inside diked area. Victims may be transported directly to Station 6. **Proceed to Station 6.**

Gross Decon

Station 3. *Protective Clothing Removal*: Rescuers remove protective clothing; clothing is isolated and labeled for later disposal. Clothing is placed on contaminated side. **Proceed to Station 4.**

PPC Removal

Station 4. *SCBA Removal*: Rescue personnel remove and isolate their SCBA. If re-entry is necessary, personnel don new SCBA from non-contaminated side. **Proceed to Station 5.**

SCBA Removal

Station 5. *Personal Clothing Removal*: All clothing and personal items are removed. Victims who have not been undressed are undressed here. All clothing and personal items are isolated in plastic bags and labeled for later disposal. **Proceed to Station 6.**

Personal Clothing Removal

Station 6. *Body Washing*: Full body washing is performed using soft scrub brushes or sponges and soap or mild detergent. Cleaning tools are bagged for later disposal. **Proceed to Station 7.**

Body Washing

Station 7. *Dry Off*: Towels and sheets are used to dry off. Rescuers and victims are dressed in clean clothes. Towels/sheets are bagged for later disposal. **Proceed to Station 8.**

Dry Off

Station 8. *Medical Assessment*: Rapid patient assessment is conducted by rescuers. Necessary stabilization procedures are accomplished. **Proceed to Station 9.**

Medical Assessment

Station 9. *Transport*: Transfer of patient to hospital for medical attention or to recovery areas for rest and observation.

Transport

Figure 28-11 An example of a field decontamination process.

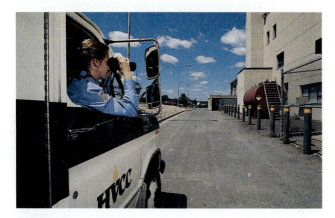

Figure 28-12 Binoculars may allow a visual inspection of the hot zone from a safe distance.

should be taken. If the rescuer's temperature exceeds 100.6°F or pulse exceeds 120, he or she must stay in the rehab sector until temperature and pulse stabilize.

Advise the hazmat team of the specific dangers and early signs and symptoms of exposure. Make sure the team members are well informed about dehydration and heat exhaustion. Hazmat experts suggest encouraging team members to drink plenty of water prior to suiting up to help prevent dehydration. During periods of high heat stress and physical exertion, at least one quart of water per hour should be consumed. Electrolyte sport drinks are helpful but not essential; if used, they should be diluted to half strength. Do not allow team members to drink caffeinated beverages, since these promote dehydration.

If the incident lasts for an extended period of time, rescuers should consider eating fruits and foods that are low in salt and saturated fats. In cold environments, soups and stews are more easily eaten and digested than sandwiches, greasy hamburgers, or hot dogs.

If team members think they may have been exposed to a chemical, advise them to seek follow-up medical examinations per your local protocol. Carefully document all examinations you conduct on a prehospital care report (PCR). Your PCR may prove to be the only documentation of an exposure when, years later, rescuers or patients suffer from medical problems that appear to have resulted from the particular incident. For example, this documentation may be needed in order for the rescuers to obtain workers' compensation.

EMS personnel should assist the incident commander or safety officer with the monitoring of team members via binoculars and radio. Look for central nervous system symptoms of exposure to the chemicals involved. Watch for, and listen for on the radio, signs such as clumsiness, disorientation, slurred speech, dizziness, or fatigue from heat exhaustion. Should any team member appear disoriented, both the team member and partner should exit the incident and report to the decontamination corridor immediately. The suggested maximum period of work time before team members should report back to the rehab sector for rest is 45 minutes.

Sources for Identifying Hazardous Materials

There are at least five types of clues to help you detect and identify the presence of hazardous materials. They are container shapes, occupancy or location type, placards and labels, markings and colors, and shipping papers and documents.

Container Shapes

Knowledge of the typical shapes of tankers and rail cars can be a clue to how dangerous the substance inside or leaking out is. Study Figure 28-13, which shows the typical shapes of tankers and their contents. Learning to recognize these types of tankers will give you a clue about the type of chemicals inside the containers:

- **MC-306 Atmospheric Pressure Cargo Tank.** The oval cross section of this tank indicates a non-pressurized tank of single-shell aluminum construction holding up to 9,000 gallons of petroleum products or class B poisons.
- **MC-307 Low-Pressure Chemical Cargo Tank.** This low-pressure tank has a circular cross section and typically a double-shell construction with an

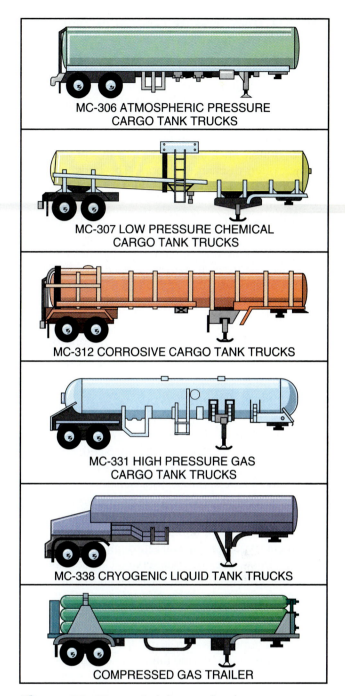

Figure 28-13 Typical shapes of tankers.

insulation layer and one or two sections. A cargo tank holds a maximum of 7,000 gallons of flammable or combustible liquids, mild corrosives, and most chemicals.

- **MC-312 Corrosive Cargo Tank.** The corrosive cargo tank has a smaller-diameter circular cross section, with external ribs that are often visible. When insulated, the tank may not appear circular. The design includes overturn and splash protection at the dome cover valve locations. The tank carries up to a maximum of 6,000 gallons of strong corrosives.

- **MC-331 High-Pressure Gas Cargo Tank.** The high-pressure tank has a circular cross section with rounded ends made of a single non-insulated shell. The upper two-thirds is usually painted white or a highly reflective color. The tank has an 11,500 gallon capacity of either LP gases or anhydrous ammonia.
- **MC-338 Cryogenic Liquid Tank.** This well-insulated, double-shell tank has relief valve protection, which often discharges vapors. The ends are flat. Such tanks usually transport liquid carbon dioxide, nitrogen, or argon.
- **Compressed Gas Trailer.** This truck carries cylinders that are stacked and held together by a manifold on the rear of the trailer. It is not uncommon for the gases to be pressurized to 5,000 psi. These trailers usually carry oxygen, hydrogen, or nitrogen and are often found at construction or industrial sites.

Rail cars also come in pressurized, nonpressurized, and cryogenic tank cars carrying similar materials in larger quantities.

Occupancy or Location Type

By law, the facilities that store chemicals are required to inform the local fire department of the types of chemicals they use, the volume involved, and the specific location in their facility. Chemical plants, gardening supply stores, public pools, chemical labs, factories, and other industrial sites occur throughout our communities. So when planning for EMS at potential hazmat sites in your community, work with your fire department. Arrange for walk-through drills so you and other employees of your service can become familiar with potential hazmat sites that are local.

Suppose there is a warehouse store that sells pool supplies in your district. A can of chlorine is spilled and the store employees wet-mop the powder in an attempt to clean it up. Your ambulance is called because the chlorine fumes are throughout the building and both the employees and the customers are getting sick from inhaling them. Think about how this hazmat might be handled in your community.

Placards and Labels

There are several types of placards and labels generally used—the nine United Nations (U.N.) classes of hazardous materials, which are used in the transportation of chemicals, the U.S. Department of Transportation's placard system, and the NFPA 704 system, which is generally reserved for fixed facilities or labels.

The U.N. placards are diamond shaped and 10-3/4″ in size. A placard provides easy recognition through a combination of a colored background, a symbol on the top of the placard, and a U.N. class number on the bottom of the placard. There are also labels required by federal laws that are found on the containers of chemicals. The colors and symbols that appear each have a significance. The nine classes of hazardous materials found on both labels and placards are shown in Table 28-2.

The NFPA 704 Hazard Classification System was originally developed for voluntary use but has since been adopted by many municipalities as the standard for classifying fixed facilities that contain hazardous materials. The system incorporates a diamond-shaped diagram (Figure 28-14) divided into four quadrants to identify the health or toxicity, flammability, reactivity, and any special warnings about chemicals. Although this system does not identify chemicals, it does provide valuable information through the use of the numbers 0 to 4 placed in each

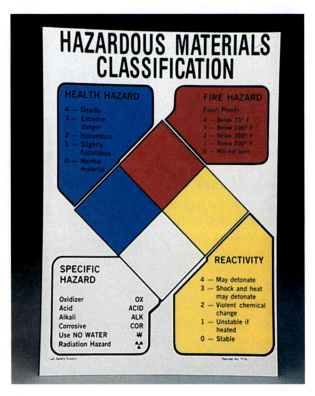

Figure 28-14 Key to the National Fire Protection Association (NFPA) 704 System of numeric and color codes.

Table 28-2 Hazard Classification System

Class 1—Explosives

Division 1.1	Explosives with a mass explosion hazard
Division 1.2	Explosives with a projection hazard
Division 1.3	Explosives with predominantly a fire hazard
Division 1.4	Explosives with no significant blast hazard
Division 1.5	Very insensitive explosives; blasting agents
Division 1.6	Extremely insensitive detonating articles

Class 2—Gases

Division 2.1	Flammable gases
Division 2.2	Non-flammable, non-toxic compressed gases
Division 2.3	Gases toxic by inhalation
Division 2.4	Corrosive gases

Class 3—Flammable Liquids and Combustible Liquids
Class 4—Flammable Solids; Spontaneously Combustible Materials; Dangerous-When-Wet Materials

Division 4.1	Flammable solids
Division 4.2	Spontaneously combustible materials
Division 4.3	Dangerous-when-wet materials

Class 5—Oxidizers and Organic Peroxides

Division 5.1	Oxidizers
Division 5.2	Organic peroxides

Class 6—Toxic Materials and Infectious Substances

Division 6.1	Toxic materials
Division 6.2	Infectious substances

Class 7—Radioactive Materials
Class 8—Corrosive Materials
Class 9—Miscellaneous Dangerous Goods

Division 9.1	Miscellaneous dangerous goods
Division 9.2	Environmentally hazardous substances
Division 9.3	Dangerous wastes

section of the placard or label. Study the placard as you read about each category below:

- **Health "Blue Quadrant."** The assignment of numbers from 0 to 4 in this category illustrates the effect of a single exposure on a person's health when firefighting over the time frame of a few seconds to an hour. The physical exertion demanded in firefighting or other emergency conditions may be expected to intensify the effects of any exposure. Only hazards arising out of an inherent property of the material are considered. For example, if there was a "2" in this section of the placard, it would indicate: "Materials hazardous to health, but areas may be entered freely, with full-faced mask, self-contained breathing apparatus which provides eye protection."

- **Flammability "Red Quadrant."** Assignment of numbers from 0 to 4 in this category rates the susceptibility to burning. The method of attacking a fire is influenced by this susceptibility factor. For example, if there was a "4" in this section of the placard, it would indicate: "Very flammable gases or very volatile flammable liquids. Shut off flow and keep cooling water streams on exposed tanks or containers."

- **Reactivity/Stability "Yellow Quadrant."** Assignment of numbers from 0 to 4 in this category illustrates the susceptibility of materials to release energy either by themselves or in combination with water. For example, if there was a "4" in this section of the placard, it would indicate: "Materials that by themselves are readily capable of detonation or of explosive decomposition or explosive reaction at normal temperatures and pressures. Includes materials which are sensitive to mechanical or localized thermal shock." If a chemical with this hazard rating is in an advanced or massive fire, the area should be evacuated.

■ **Specific Hazards "White Quadrant."** Specific hazards, such as "OX" (the chemical is an oxidizer), or a "W" with a line through it (do not add water to this chemical), or a radioactive symbol.

Markings and Colors

The U.S. DOT requires that packages, storage containers, and vehicles containing hazardous materials bear labels or placards with markings that identify the nature of the contents (Figure 28-15). Diamond-shaped placards not only show the hazard class, such as "explosives," "flamable gas," "poison" or other, but also bear identification numbers.

Since 1981, the United Nations (U.N.) system for identifying hazardous materials has been required on all portable tanks, cargo tanks, and tank cars carrying hazardous materials. There are three methods of displaying the four-digit U.N. numbers:

■ Orange panel adjacent to the placards. Panel is 5-7/8″ × 15-3/4″ with four-inch-high letters.

■ Center of appropriate placard. Placards on combustible materials that display a number will have a white area under the number to differentiate them from the flammable liquids.

■ Center of a placard-sized white panel for hazardous substances and wastes not requiring a placard.

The color of portable gas tanks is also standardized. As an EMT-B, you are already familiar with the green steel tanks used for oxygen. Other pressurized gases are contained in tanks of specific colors also.

Shipping Papers and Documents

Shipping papers can be helpful in identifying the materials at a hazmat incident. A typical shipping paper must contain the following information:

■ Proper shipping number

■ Hazard classification

■ U.N. identification number

■ Number of packages

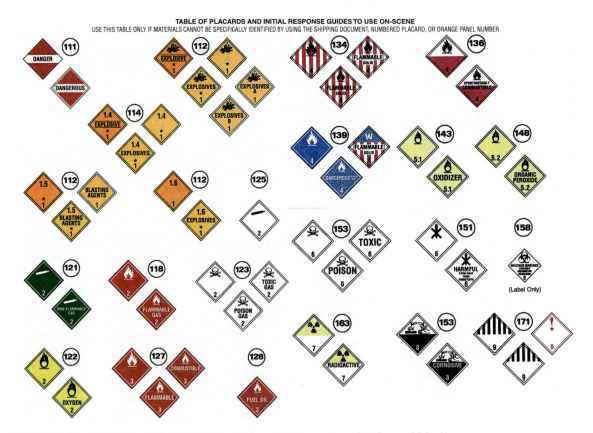

Figure 28-15 The U.S. Department of Transportation (DOT) requires that hazard labels or placards be displayed on packages, storage containers, and vehicles containing hazardous materials.

- Type of packages
- Correct weight
- Emergency response telephone number

The following emergency response information must be attached to the shipping papers:

- Description of the material
- Risks of fire or explosion
- Immediate hazards to health
- Immediate methods for handling small or large fires
- Immediate precautions to be taken in the event of an accident
- Initial methods for handling spills or leaks in the absence of a fire
- Preliminary first-aid measures

To find the shipping papers on a train, look for the waybill in the engine car. In a ship, check the mailbox, which is located on the bridge of the vessel. On an aircraft, the pilot is responsible for the shipping papers. The bill of lading can be found in the cab of a truck. If the shipping papers are not easily accessible, never put yourself or your crew members in danger trying to locate them.

Emergency Response Guidebook

All emergency vehicles should carry a copy of the *Emergency Response Guidebook* (Figure 28-16). You may already be familiar with this book since it is often your first method of identifying a hazardous material. Over 2,500 chemicals are listed both alphabetically (blue section) and in numerical order by the U.N. identification number (yellow section). Once you locate a chemical in the book, it will refer you to a guide in the book's orange section. That section provides general information about what to do in the first few minutes of a hazmat incident that involves the chemical. If a chemical listing is highlighted, you must immediately refer to the back of the book (green section) to obtain information about evacuation distance needed to protect people from being harmed by the chemical.

CHEMTREC

When shipping papers are not accessible or an emergency response number has not been listed on the papers, the incident commander should assign someone to contact the Chemical Transportation Emergency Center (CHEMTREC), which is a chemical industry service. CHEMTREC will give you immediate initial advice and contact the shipper of the materials involved for further advice. It is also able to provide state or federal resources for radiological incidents. When calling CHEMTREC, a 24-hour, 7-day-a-week toll-free number (1-800-424-9300), be prepared to provide the following information to the operator:

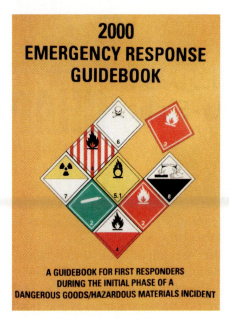

Figure 28-16 Keep the latest edition of the *Emergency Response Guidebook* in your vehicle at all time.

- Your name and call-back telephone number
- Location and nature of problem
- Name of material(s) involved
- Shipper or manufacturer
- Container type
- Rail car or truck number
- Carrier name
- Consignee
- Local conditions

Material Safety Data Sheets (MSDS)

Another section of OSHA regulations is the Hazard Communication standard, or CFR 1910.1200, which requires that employers must make available to employees information on the chemicals that are used in their workplaces. There also are annual training requirements in this regulation. Employers are required to post **material safety data sheets (MSDS)** that provide information about the chemicals. These sheets can be helpful when you respond to a hazmat incident at a factory. So always request them. Unfortunately, there is no standardized format for the MSDS, although the manufacturer of the chemical is required to provide the name of the substance, its physical properties, fire and explosion hazard information, and emergency first-aid treatment.

Regional Poison Control Center

Another available resource is the regional poison control center. If contacted from the scene, it can help you determine the most appropriate course of treatment for patients exposed to specific chemicals.

SUMMARY

- Understand your role in your agency's MCI or disaster plan.
- Realize the importance of practicing implementation of your agency's MCI plan.
- You should become keenly aware of the role of each of the sector officers and how to use triage tags.
- Recognize a hazmat incident early, and call for the appropriate back-up assistance in your community.

- Understand the importance of establishing command and control zones, identifying the substance involved, and establishing a rehab sector in the cold zone of a hazardous materials incident.

REVIEW QUESTIONS

1. Which one of the following divisions at an MCI includes staging, treatment, transport, and extrication?
   a. operations
   b. EMS command
   c. staging
   d. triage

2. At the scene of an MCI, a patient with airway and breathing difficulties may be classified as a priority:
   a. one.
   b. two.
   c. three.
   d. zero.

3. The EMS _____ sector officer directly oversees patient care and coordinates movement of patients to ambulances:
   a. staging
   b. triage
   c. safety
   d. treatment

4. The rehab sector should be established in the _____ zone.

  a. hot

  b. cold

  c. warm

  d. temperate

5. The oval cross section of a(n) _____ indicates a nonpressurized tank of single-shell aluminum construction holding up to 9,000 gallons of petroleum products or class B poisons.

  a. compressed gas trailer

  b. MC-338 cryogenic liquid tank

  c. MC-331 high-pressure gas cargo tank

  d. MC-306 atmospheric pressure cargo tank

WEB MEDIC

Visit Brady's *Essentials of Emergency Care* web site for direct web links. At **www.prenhall.com/limmer,** you will find information related to the following Chapter 28 topics:

- The Incident Command System
- Medical priority systems
- Critical incident stress management
- OSHA hazmat regulations
- Exposure to environmental chemicals

Chapter Twenty-Nine

ADVANCED AIRWAY MANAGEMENT

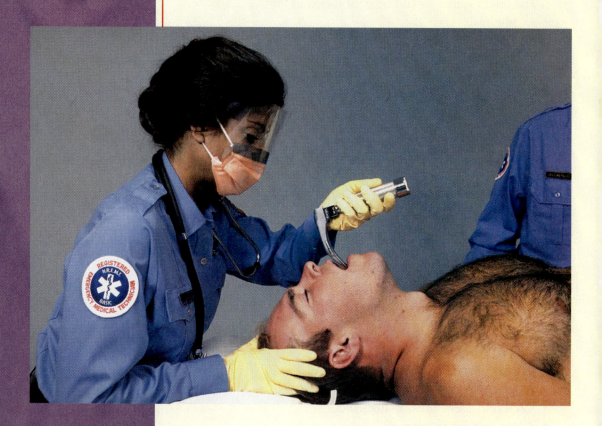

ESSENTIAL ELECTRONIC EXTRAS

CD ESSENTIALS

For preview and review of chapter material, see the student CD-ROM for

- Pretest
- Chapter quizzes
- Posttest

WEB ESSENTIALS

For additional review and enrichment, visit www.prenhall.com/limmer for

- Interactive student quizzes
- Links to online EMS resources
- Online case studies
- Audio glossary

Airway control is the highest priority in managing any critically ill or injured patient, because without an adequate airway the patient will die—no matter what other care you provide.

ANATOMY AND PHYSIOLOGY

There are specific aspects of both airway anatomy and physiology that the EMT-B who performs advanced airway skills must understand in greater depth in order to perform these skills effectively and successfully.

Anatomy

Air that enters through the nose passes through the **nasopharynx** and enters the respiratory tract; air that enters through the mouth passes through the **oropharynx** and also travels on to the respiratory tract. The **hypopharynx** is the area directly above the openings of both the trachea and the esophagus. The leaf-shaped epiglottis protects the airway by covering the entrance to the trachea when swallowing occurs. Anterior to the epiglottis is a groove-like structure called the **vallecula.**

The epiglottis allows air to pass into the opening of the trachea and through the larynx, or voice box. The larynx contains the two vocal cords.

Giving support to the larynx and trachea are several rigid pieces of cartilage. The thyroid cartilage is a shield-shaped structure at the anterior of the larynx. Multiple horseshoe-shaped cartilages give support to the trachea. **The cricoid cartilage** is a cartilage at the lower portion of the larynx. It is unique in that it is the only cartilage that completely surrounds the trachea.

Once air has passed through the larynx, it proceeds through the trachea until the trachea bifurcates, or splits, into the two **mainstem bronchi** at the level of the **carina.** The right mainstem bronchus splits off the carina at less of an angle than the left mainstem bronchus. Because of the angle of the right mainstem bronchus, objects that pass all the way down the trachea (such as aspirated food) tend to lodge in the right rather than the left mainstem bronchus. The mainstem bronchi subsequently divide into smaller air passages until reaching the level of the alveoli, where the exchange of oxygen and carbon dioxide takes place.

When learning the anatomy of the airway, remember that the majority of the time you are managing a critical airway problem the patient will be supine, or lying flat. For this reason it is important to visualize the anatomy in both the traditional upright "anatomical position" (Figure 29-1) and in the supine position (Figure 29-2).

Physiology

The most important aspect of respiratory physiology for the EMT-B who uses advanced airway skills is an understanding of what can cause the respiratory system to fail so severely that an advanced airway is necessary.

When the respiratory system functions properly, adequate breathing is the result of many factors including the following:

- A functioning brain stem, where the brain's centers of respiratory control are located
- An open airway
- An intact chest wall
- The ability of gas exchange to take place at the alveoli

Injuries or illnesses that affect any of these components can result in inadequate breathing and respiratory failure. For example, a massive head injury could result in both brain-stem injury and an airway

CORE CONCEPTS

In this chapter, you will learn about the following topics:

- The purpose and procedure for nasogastric tubes
- The purpose and procedure for orotracheal intubation
- How to perform Sellick's maneuver
- How to use the Combitube® airway
- The usefulness of an automatic transport ventilator
- How to use the laryngeal mask airway

DOT OBJECTIVES

There are no DOT refresher objectives for this chapter.

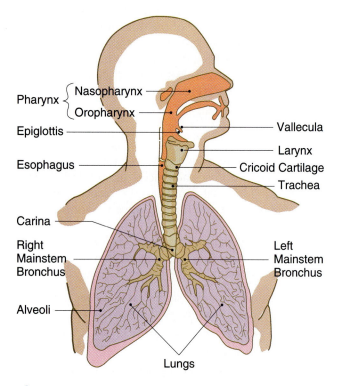

Pharynx
Nasopharynx
Oropharynx
Epiglottis
Vallecula
Larynx
Esophagus
Cricoid Cartilage
Trachea
Carina
Right Mainstem Bronchus
Left Mainstem Bronchus
Alveoli
Lungs

Figure 29-1 The airway, anatomical position.

Cricoid cartilage
Larynx
Trachea
Vallecula
Mainstem bronchi
Pharynx
Nasopharynx
Oropharynx
Hypopharynx
Epiglottis
Esophagus
Carina
Lungs

Figure 29-2 The airway, supine position.

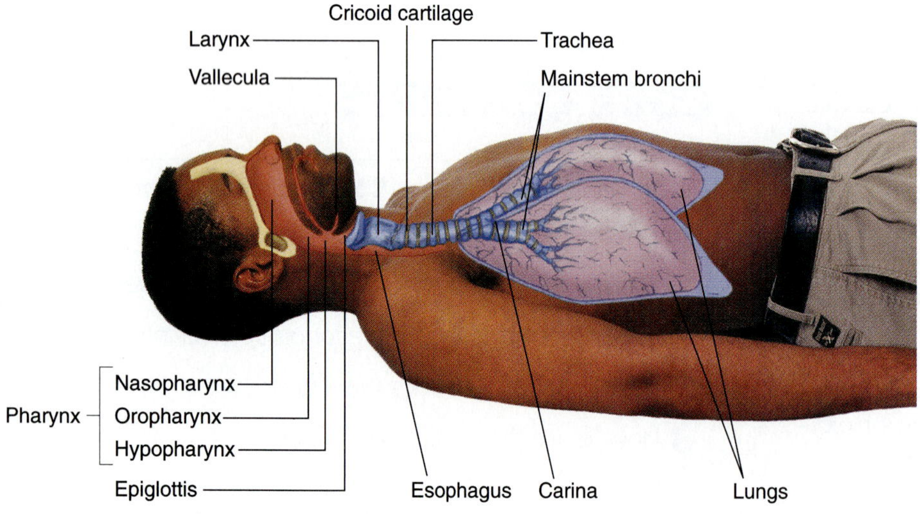

obstructed by blood and broken teeth. Similarly, a patient with massive pulmonary edema from congestive heart failure can go into respiratory failure because edema prevents adequate gas exchange at the level of the alveoli.

Assessing the adequacy of a patient's breathing is an essential skill when making decisions about what basic and advanced airway management is indicated. A patient's respiratory status can range anywhere from normal, unlabored breathing to respiratory arrest. Recognition of adequate breathing and respiratory arrest is rarely a challenge for the EMT-B. It is recognizing the more subtle signs and symptoms of inadequate breathing that is an essential skill for the EMT-B.

In general, when assessing the adequacy of breathing you should carefully observe the rate, rhythm, quality, and depth of the patient's respirations. The normal rate of breathing is dependent on the age of the patient (Table 29-1). An adequately breathing patient will normally be breathing in a regular rather than an irregular rhythm. The quality of a patient's breathing should be assessed by listening for breath sounds and observing chest expansion and effort of breathing. The adequately breathing patient will have breath sounds that are equal and present bilaterally. In addition, when observing the patient's chest during normal breathing you will note equal and full expansion of the chest and a lack of any accessory muscle use in the chest or neck during inspiration. Finally, the depth of breathing (tidal volume) will normally be sufficient not only to expand the lungs, but also to assure adequate delivery of oxygen and removal of carbon dioxide at the level of the alveoli.

When a patient is in respiratory distress because of inadequate breathing, the following variations in rate, rhythm, quality, and depth of breathing will be noted:

Table 29-1 Normal Rates of Breathing

Adult—12–20 breaths per minute
Child—15–30 breaths per minute
Infant—25–50 breaths per minute

- **Rate** Outside the normal range: either too fast or too slow
- **Rhythm** Irregular pattern of breathing
- **Quality**
  - Breath sounds: diminished, unequal, or absent
  - Chest expansion: unequal or inadequate
  - Effort of breathing: increased effort evidenced by use of accessory muscles and inability to speak in full sentences
- **Depth** Shallow

You may also note the following signs and symptoms in the patient with inadequate breathing:

- Cyanosis in the lips, nail beds, and finger tips
- Cool and clammy skin
- Agonal breathing (gasping breaths which occur just prior to respiratory arrest)

Pediatric Anatomy and Physiology

As you reviewed in Chapter 25, the anatomy and physiology of the pediatric respiratory system differs from those of adults (Figure 29-3). Younger patients may also have different signs and symptoms of respiratory failure than adults. Unique features of the pediatric versus the adult airway include the following:

- All structures in the mouth and nose are smaller in the child and can be more easily obstructed.
- The tongue is proportionately larger, occupying more of the mouth and pharynx.
- The trachea is softer and more flexible, allowing the airway to be closed off if the neck is extended too far when opening the airway.
- The trachea is narrower, allowing the airway to become more easily obstructed if swelling occurs.
- The narrowest area in the airway is at the level of the cricoid cartilage.
- Because the chest wall is softer, the diaphragm is relied on heavily for the work of breathing.

Although infants and children may manifest inadequate breathing with the signs and symptoms mentioned above, they also frequently show respiratory distress in other ways, including:

- A slower than normal heart rate
- Weak or absent peripheral pulses
- Retractions between and below the ribs, above the clavicles and sternal notch
- Nasal flaring, in which the nostrils "flare" open with exhalation and clamp almost shut with inhalation
- So-called "seesaw" breathing, in which the chest and abdomen move in opposite directions during breathing

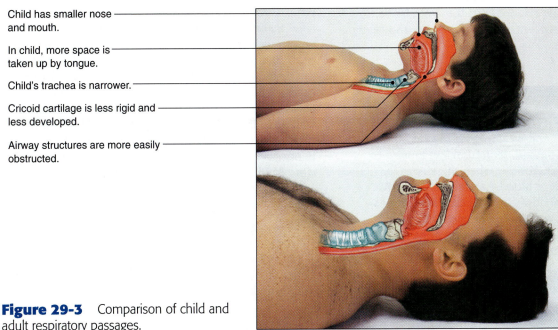

Child has smaller nose and mouth.

In child, more space is taken up by tongue.

Child's trachea is narrower.

Cricoid cartilage is less rigid and less developed.

Airway structures are more easily obstructed.

Figure 29-3 Comparison of child and adult respiratory passages.

MANAGEMENT OF THE AIRWAY

Although this chapter is about advanced airway management, it cannot be overemphasized that the primary management of any airway is done with basic techniques such as opening and suctioning the airway, administering oxygen, and using oro- and nasopharyngeal airways.

Oropharyngeal Suctioning

The goal of airway management is keeping the airway open and free of obstructions. If the airway is obstructed with secretions, blood, or foreign materials, it will have to be suctioned. Suction equipment should always be within easy reach when managing any critical patient. If the patient is outside the ambulance, a suctioning device should be brought to the patient's side. If the patient is in the ambulance, the on-board suction system should be set up and ready for immediate use.

Orotracheal Intubation

An **endotracheal tube,** or ET tube, is a tube designed to be inserted into the trachea (*endo* means "into"). Oxygen, medication, or a suction catheter can be directed into the trachea through the endotracheal tube. **Intubation** means the insertion of a tube. **Orotracheal intubation** is the placement of an endotracheal tube orally; that is, placement by way of the mouth (*oro* means "mouth"), then through the vocal cords and into the trachea.

Orotracheal intubation allows direct ventilation of the lungs through the endotracheal tube, bypassing the entire upper airway. The endotracheal tube is placed through the vocal cords with direct visualization of the process. A laryngoscope is an illuminating instrument that is inserted into the pharynx and allows you to visualize the pharynx and larynx.

The advantages of orotracheal intubation of the apneic patient include:

- Allows complete control of the airway by inserting the tube directly into the trachea, which prevents the tongue, blood, or debris that may be present in the upper airway from interfering with the passage of air into the trachea and lungs
- Minimizes the risk of aspiration by blocking vomitus or foreign matter from being aspirated
- Allows for direct oxygen delivery to the lungs
- Allows for deep suctioning of the airway by passing a flexible suction catheter through the endotracheal tube to suction the trachea to the level of the carina

Complications

Although orotracheal intubation is frequently a lifesaving procedure, it has many potential complications. Orotracheal intubation is considered an "invasive technique" because it requires placement of equipment inside the body cavity. Whenever you perform an invasive procedure you must be aware of the potential complications and be prepared to recognize and treat them should they arise. These concerns about invasive procedures are never more critical than in orotracheal intubation, since improper placement of the endotracheal tube in the apneic patient, if it is not immediately detected and corrected, can rapidly result in the patient's death.

Specific complications of orotracheal intubation include:

- **Slowing of the heart rate.** Stimulation of the airway with the laryngoscope and the endotracheal (ET) tube can lead to a slowing of the heart. The patient's heart rate should be monitored throughout the intubation.

- **Soft-tissue trauma to the teeth, lips, tongue, gums, and airway structures**
- **Hypoxia.** Prolonged attempts at intubation may lead to inadequate oxygenation, or oxygen starvation, known as **hypoxia.** To prevent this, you should hyperventilate the patient with high-concentration oxygen (ventilations provided at about double the normal rate, or 24 ventilations per minute) prior to intubation, and intubation attempts should be limited to 30 seconds from the time ventilations cease until the patient is ventilated through the endotracheal (ET) tube.
- **Vomiting.** Stimulation of the airway may cause the patient to gag and vomit.
- **Right mainstem intubation.** The endotracheal (ET) tube has to remain superior to the carina (before the point where the right and left mainstem bronchi branch off) in order to send air into both lungs. If the ET tube is advanced too far, the tube is likely to go down the steep right mainstem bronchus. Mainstem intubation results in only one lung being ventilated and the development of hypoxia (oxygen starvation).
- **Esophageal intubation.** This is the most serious complication, since the unrecognized placement of the ET tube in the esophagus rather than the trachea will rapidly result in death.
- **Accidental extubation.** Even if the ET tube is properly placed initially, it can become dislodged while moving the patient or by the patient if consciousness is regained. Be sure to reassess chest wall movement and breath sounds of the intubated patient after every major move, such as down the stairs or from the floor to the stretcher.

Mask and Eye Protection

Due to the high risk of splattering of sputum or blood during intubation, it is essential that BSI precautions be taken. This means that a mask and goggles or other protective eyewear be worn in addition to gloves (Figure 29-4). This is mandatory, since your face will be in direct line with the path of secretions, blood, and vomit coming from the patient's mouth while you attempt to visualize the airway.

Laryngoscope

A **laryngoscope** is made up of two components: the handle that contains the batteries and the blade that is inserted in and illuminates the airway. In most laryngoscopes the handle and the blades are two separate pieces that need to be assembled with each use. In these devices the blade is placed parallel to the handle; the notch at the base of the blade is attached to the bar on the handle. The blade is then lifted to a 90° angle

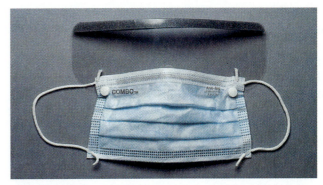

Figure 29-4 BSI precautions must include gloves, mask, and protective eyewear when managing a patient's airway.

with the handle (Figure 29-5) and, as the blade locks into place, the light at the tip of the blade illuminates. Always check the light at the end of the blade to assure that it illuminates with a bright white color and that the bulb is tightly secured to the blade.

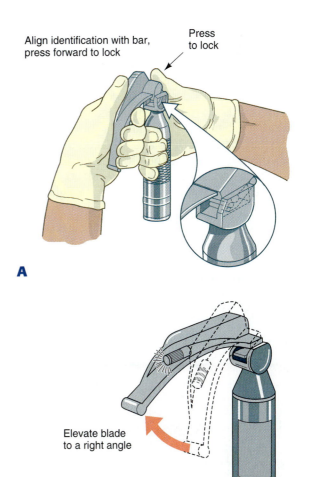

Align identification with bar, press forward to lock

Press to lock

A

Elevate blade to a right angle

B

Figure 29-5 (A) First, affix the laryngoscope blade. (B) Then, elevate the laryngoscope blade.

Some disposable laryngoscopes are pre-assembled with the handle and blade as a single fixed unit. No matter what type of laryngoscope you use, it is essential that you conduct a daily check of the device to assure that it is working properly. Spare batteries and bulbs should always be stored with the laryngoscope.

Laryngoscope blades are specifically designed to fit into the anatomy of the airway and provide optimal illumination of the vocal cords to enable you to pass the ET tube between them. Most commercially available blades are designed with the light on the right side of the blade. This requires that the handle of the scope be held in the left hand to provide optimal illumination of the airway.

There are two general types of blades: straight and curved. Both types of blades come in assorted sizes ranging from the smallest size (0) to the largest (4). The size of the blade used depends on the size of the patient. Most adult patients can be intubated using a size 2 or 3 straight blade or a size 3 curved blade (pediatric blade sizes will be discussed later in this chapter). The decision as to whether to use a straight or curved blade depends on individual preference; however, straight blades are preferred for pediatric orotracheal intubation and trauma intubations.

Each blade type is designed to enable you to visualize the cords by taking advantage of different anatomical mechanisms. The straight blade is designed so that the tip of the blade is placed under the epiglottis to lift it and bring the **glottic opening** (the entrance to the trachea) and the vocal cords into view (Figure 29-6). The curved blade is designed so

that the tip of the blade is inserted into the vallecula and the lifting of the laryngoscope handle in an upward fashion brings the glottic opening and the vocal cords into view (Figure 29-7).

Endotracheal Tube

The endotracheal (ET) tube (Figure 29-8) is comprised of a single lumen (tube) through which air and supplemental oxygen are delivered. At the proximal end of the tube (the end that will remain outside the patient, nearest to you) is a standard 15 millimeter adapter for connection to the bag valve.

At the distal end of the tube (the end farthest from you that will go into the patient) is a cuff. The cuff is designed to be inflated after the tube is placed to prevent leakage of air and fluid around the tip of the tube. The cuff holds approximately 10 cc of air and should be inflated only enough to prevent air from leaking around the tube. The cuff of the tube is filled with a 10 cc syringe at the inflation valve. Just below the inflation valve is the pilot balloon, which fills with air when the cuff is inflated. Since the cuff is inside the patient's trachea, you will not be able to see if it is inflated, but the inflation of the pilot balloon will verify that there is air in the cuff. If the pilot balloon does not hold air, then you must assume that the cuff at the end of the tube has also failed.

ET tubes used on infants and children less than 8 years old do not have a cuff. Many ET tubes have a small hole on the left side of the tube on the opposite side of the bevel, known as a **Murphy eye.** This feature is designed to lessen the chances of tube obstruction.

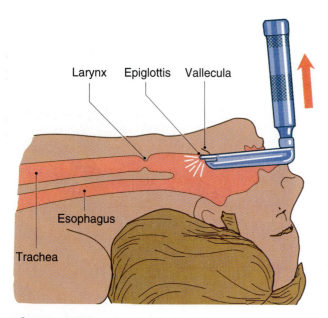

Figure 29-6 The straight blade brings the glottic opening and vocal cords into view by lifting the epiglottis.

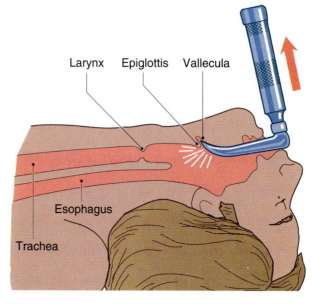

Figure 29-7 The curved blade brings the glottic opening and vocal cords into view by lifting the vallecula.

Figure 29-8 The endotracheal [ET] tube.

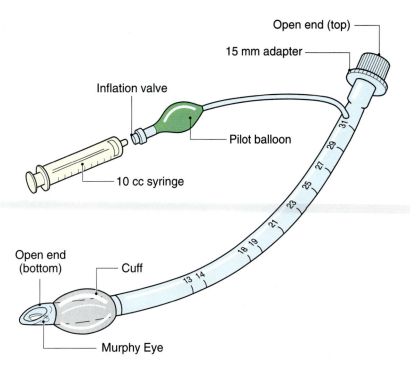

Endotracheal tubes come in various diameters, from 2.0 millimeters (used on premature infants) to 10.0 millimeters (used on large adults). The diameter measured is the distance from one internal wall of the tube to the other: called the **internal diameter,** or "i.d." No matter what the internal diameter of the tube, the standard 15 millimeter adapter is affixed to the end of the tube. When determining the proper size of the ET tube in the adult patient, the rule of thumb is: in an emergency use a 7.5 mm tube. For more precise sizing of the ET tube, it is generally accepted that the adult male should receive either an 8.0 or an 8.5 mm tube and the adult female should receive from a 7.0 to an 8.0 mm tube. The sizing of pediatric ET tubes will be discussed later in this chapter.

The adult endotracheal tube is a standard length of 33 centimeters. The side of the tube is marked in centimeters starting from the tip of the tube. The most important measurement to remember is that, as a general rule, a properly placed ET tube will have the 22 centimeter mark at the teeth. This position assures that the tip of the tube is in the trachea above the carina. (As you will learn, assuring proper placement of the tube is a critical skill, and checking the length marking is only a small part of this procedure.) It may be helpful to envision the depth of tube placement by reviewing the following distances in the average adult.

- 15 centimeters from the teeth to the vocal cords
- 20 centimeters from the teeth to the sternal notch
- 25 centimeters from the teeth to the carina

As you can see, there is very little room for error when placing the ET tube, since only a few centimeters can mean the difference between the proper placement and the tube being placed past the carina into the mainstem bronchus.

Accessories to the Endotracheal Tube

There are several accessories to the endotracheal tube with which you need to be familiar. These include the stylet, lubricant, a 10 cc syringe, devices for assuring proper placement of the tube, devices for securing the tube once it is placed, and a suction device.

Because the ET tube is made of relatively flexible plastic, it is generally recommended that a **stylet**—which is a long, thin, bendable metal probe (Figure 29-9)—be inserted into the tube prior to intubation to help stiffen it and provide it with a shape that will ease its insertion through the vocal cords. It is recommended that the stylet be lubricated with water-soluble lubricant, such as K-Y® jelly, Lubifax®, or Surgilube®, prior to insertion into the tube to allow for a smooth withdrawal of the stylet once the tube is successfully placed. A silicone-based lubricant or a petroleum-based lubricant such as Vaseline® must not be used because it will cause aspiration pneumonia.

Once the lubricated stylet is inserted, the ET tube should be shaped into a "hockey stick" configuration. To avoid trauma to the airway, the stylet should not be inserted past the tip of the tube. Since all stylets are longer than the ET tube, it is easy to inadvertently allow the tip to extend beyond the end of the tube.

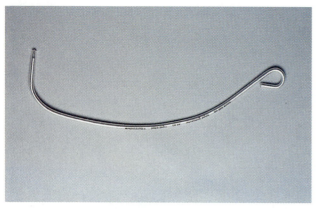

A

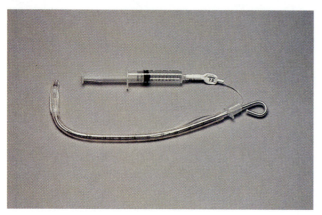

B

Figure 29-9   (A) The stylet. (B) The stylet in place.

Such an error, however, could cause a puncture of the trachea. To avoid this complication, the tip of the stylet should not be inserted beyond the proximal end of the Murphy eye and the excess length bent over the 15 mm adapter.

When performing orotracheal intubation, excessive oral secretions often obstruct an adequate view of the vocal cords. Paradoxically, airways are sometimes very dry, thus making insertion of the ET tube difficult because of friction between the end of the tube and the patient's pharynx and glottis. For these reasons, it is important both that a wide-bore suction device be operational and within easy reach during intubation attempts, and that a water-soluble lubricant be applied to the outside of the distal portion of the tube. The suction device should be turned on and placed by your right hand. In general, you can use half a packet of lubricant on the stylet and the other half of the packet on the outside of the ET tube.

Another piece of essential equipment for use with the ET tube is a 10 cc syringe. As mentioned above, the syringe is used to inflate the cuff through the inflation valve. The syringe should also be used to test that the cuff is intact and holds air prior to inserting the tube. Once the integrity of the cuff has been assured, the air should be withdrawn, but the syringe should remain attached to the tube so that it is easily found when it is time to reinflate the cuff after the patient is intubated. It should be noted that, following final inflation of the cuff, the 10 cc syringe should be detached from the inflation valve to prevent any subsequent leakage of air out of the cuff and back into the syringe.

One of the final steps in orotracheal intubation is securing the tube to the patient so that it does not move or become dislodged. This is especially important in the prehospital setting where the tube can easily be dislodged during patient movement. Prior to securing the ET tube, an oral airway or similar device should be inserted as a *bite block* in case the patient becomes responsive and gnaws at the tube. There are a number of methods for securing ET tubes. These range from cloth tape to commercially available devices. The manner in which ET tubes are secured is usually dictated by the medical direction authorities of the EMS system you work in. Whatever system you use, make sure the tube is firmly secured in place and able to withstand the tugs and pulls that are routine during moves of critically ill patients.

Indications

When properly performed, orotracheal intubation is clearly a life-saving technique. It is essential, however, that you know under what conditions a patient needs to be intubated. Indications for orotracheal intubation include:

- Inability to ventilate the apneic patient
- To protect the airway of a patient without a gag reflex or cough
- To protect the airway of a patient unresponsive to any painful stimuli
- Cardiac-arrest patient

Technique of Insertion—The Adult Patient

Orotracheal intubation is the most complicated and difficult procedure the EMT-B is expected to perform. Properly performed, it is truly a life-saving procedure. Incorrectly performed, the EMT-B's actions can easily result in the patient's death. Because many EMT-Bs will only rarely perform orotracheal intubation, it is essential that you not only learn and practice the technique extensively during your training but also practice the technique on a regular basis. If you do not intubate actual patients frequently, the skill should be refreshed often on a mannequin and under the supervision of a qualified instructor.

The following is a step-by-step guide to orotracheal intubation of the adult patient (Skill Summary 29-1):

Preparation

1. Take BSI precautions. This should include gloves, goggles or other protective eyewear, and a mask.

2. Assure that adequate ventilation with a BVM and high-concentration oxygen is being performed.

3. Hyperventilate the patient at a rate of 24 breaths per minute prior to any intubation attempts.

4. Assemble, prepare, and test all equipment including:
   - A suction unit with a large-bore rigid tip, which should be functional and positioned so that it is within easy reach of your right hand if needed
   - The cuff on the ET tube, which should be tested and then deflated, with the 10 cc syringe left attached to the inflation valve
   - The assembled laryngoscope with a bright and constant light
   - The device that will be used to secure the tube after successful intubation

5. Position yourself at the patient's head so that, during intubation, left and right are your left and right as well as the patient's left and right.

Visualizing the Glottic Opening and Vocal Cords

6. Preposition the patient's head to assure good visualization of the vocal cords.
   - If trauma is not suspected, tilt the head, lift the chin, and attempt visualization of the cords. If the cords cannot be seen, raise the patient's shoulders approximately 1 inch by placing a towel beneath them and attempt visualization again.
   - If trauma is suspected, the patient will have to be intubated with the head and neck in a neutral position with a second rescuer maintaining in-line stabilization of the neck and head.

7. Hold the laryngoscope in your left hand and insert the laryngoscope into the right corner of the patient's mouth.

8. Use a sweeping motion to lift the tongue upward and to the left, out of the way, to enable visualization of the glottis.

9. Insert the blade into the proper anatomical location:
   - Curved blade into the vallecula
   - Straight blade lifts the epiglottis

10. Lift the scope up and away from the patient.

11. Avoid using the teeth as a fulcrum.

12. Application of the cricoid pressure, or **Sellick's maneuver,** during intubation attempts may be beneficial. Sellick's maneuver is performed by a second rescuer who uses an index finger and thumb to exert direct pressure on the patient's cricoid cartilage (Figure 29-10). Since the cricoid cartilage is the only cartilage in the neck that

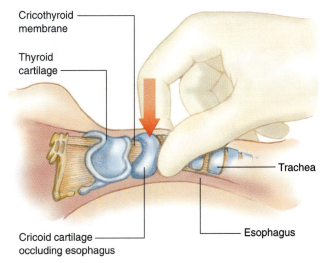

Cricothyroid membrane

Thyroid cartilage

Trachea

Cricoid cartilage occluding esophagus

Esophagus

A

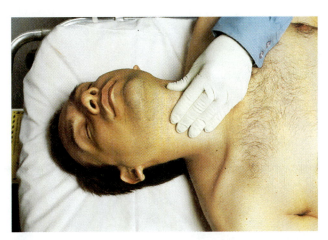

B

Figure 29-10   (A) The cricoid cartilage rings the trachea at the lower end of the larynx. (B) Sellick's maneuver is placing pressure on the cricoid cartilage to help suppress vomiting and to help bring the glottic opening into view.

Orotracheal Intubation—Adult Patient

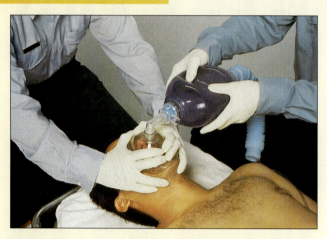

▲ **1.** Hyperventilate the patient.

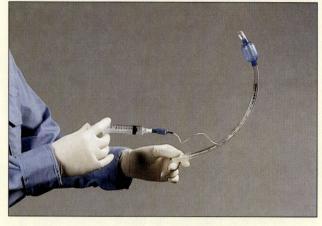

▲ **2.** Assemble, prepare, and test all equipment.

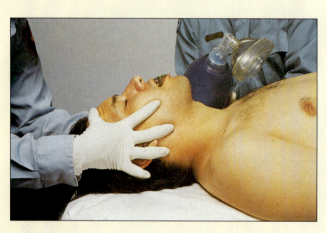

▲ **3.** Position the patient's head.

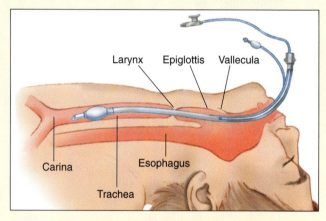

Larynx Epiglottis Vallecula

Carina Esophagus

Trachea

▲ **4.** Make sure the airway is aligned. (If trauma is suspected, keep patient's head and neck in a neutral position with manual stabilization.)

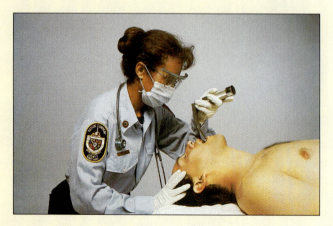

▲ **5.** Insert the laryngoscope blade.

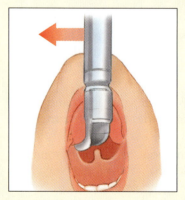

▲ **6.** Lift the tongue out of the way.

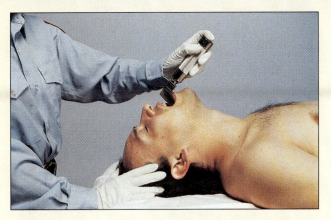

▲ **7.** Insert the blade (curved blade into vallecula, straight blade under epiglottis) and lift to bring glottic opening into view.

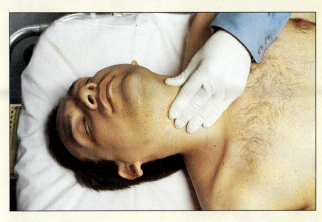

▲ **8.** A second rescuer may perform Sellick's maneuver (cricoid pressure) during intubation to suppress vomiting and aid visualization.

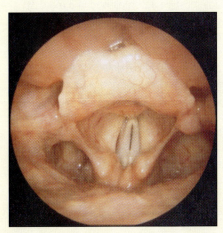

▲ **9.** Visualize the glottic opening.

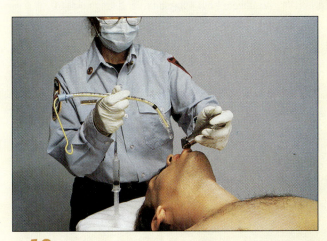

▲ **10.** Insert the endotracheal (ET) tube with stylet.

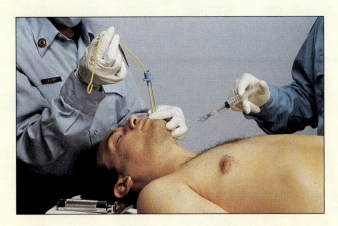

▲ **11.** Remove the laryngoscope and stylet. Inflate the cuff with 5-10 cc of air. NOTE: If an esophageal intubation detector device is employed, use it prior to inflating the cuff.

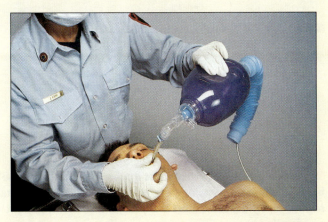

▲ **12.** Attach the bag-valve unit or other ventilation device to tube.

(continued)

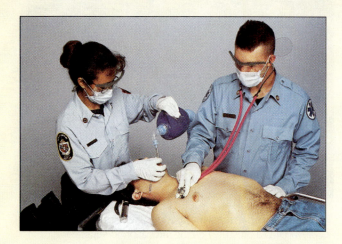

▲ **13.** Auscultate both epigastrium and lung fields to confirm correct placement.

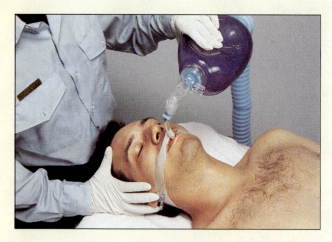

▲ **14.** If correct placement is confirmed, secure tube in place. A commercial tube restraint is the preferred method of securing the tube.

CONFIRM CORRECT PLACEMENT OF TUBE

- Observe rise and fall of chest.
- Auscultate epigastrium for absence of breath sounds.
- Auscultate over both lungs for breath sounds. The sounds should be equal when comparing the left and right sides.
- Observe patient for signs of deterioration, such as cyanosis.
- Use measures such as an end tidal carbon dioxide detector (Figure 29-11), a Tube Check® device (Figure 29-12), or pulse oximetry per local protocols. If a Tube Check® (esophageal intubation detector device) is used, it should be applied and the suction aspirated prior to the first ventilation with the BVM. This adds time to the intubation attempt which already must be accomplished in a mere 30 seconds, from stopping the hyperventilation of the patient to beginning to ventilate the now tubed patient. Be sure to practice applying the Tube Check® device, withdrawing it to see if there is condensation in the device. It also should be easy to withdraw, which would indicate a tracheal intubation. Difficulty in withdrawal is due to the flat esophagus collapsing and fluid from stomach contents collecting in the device, which would indicate a misplaced tube in the esophagus. If a tube is found to be misplaced in the esophagus, immediately remove it and reventilate the patient.

CORRECT ANY INCORRECT PLACEMENT OF TUBE

- Breath sounds present on right, diminished or absent on left means the right mainstem bronchus is probably intubated. Deflate cuff, gently withdraw tube (continue ventilation) until breath sounds are equal right and left.
- Breath sounds in epigastrium means the esophagus is intubated. Withdraw tube. Hyperventilate 2–5 minutes.

NOTE: Make only two attempts at intubation. If both attempts fail, insert an oral airway and continue to ventilate with bag-valve-mask device. Aggressively suction the airway. If tube has been correctly placed and secured, reassess breath sounds and placement after every major move with patient. Offer reassurance and emotional support to the patient and family.

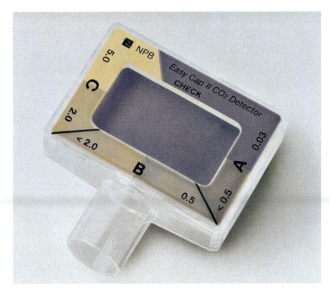

Figure 29-11 An Easy Cap® CO_2 Detector, an end-tidal CO_2 detector device. (Photo reprinted by permission of Nellcor Puritan Bennett, Pleasanton, California.)

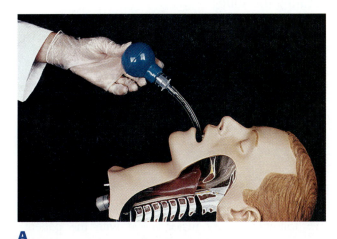

A

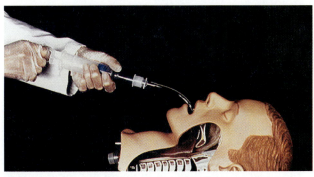

B

Figure 29-12 (A) A Tube Check®, a bulb syringe-type device. (B) A Tube Check®, syringe-type device.

completely encircles the trachea, direct pressure helps to compress the esophagus, which is anterior to (behind) the trachea, lowering the risk of vomiting. In addition, the pressure often brings the vocal cords into better view. Cricoid pressure should be maintained until the patient is intubated.

13. Visualize the glottic opening and vocal cords. Once the cords come into view, do not lose sight of them!

Inserting the Endotracheal Tube

14. With the right hand, carefully insert the ET tube through the vocal cords. The tube should be inserted just deep enough so that the cuff material is past the cords. Verify that the ET tube is at about 22 cm at the gums and teeth.

15. Remove the laryngoscope and extinguish the lamp.

16. Remove the stylet, if used. Then assure placement with a Tube Check® device or capnography.

17. Inflate the cuff with 5 cc to 10 cc of air, and remove the syringe.

18. Continue to hold onto the ET tube. Never let go of the tube until it is secured in place with a commercial tube restraint device.

19. Have a partner attach the bag valve to the ET tube and deliver artificial ventilations.

Assuring Correct Tube Placement

20. The single most accurate way of assuring proper tube placement is visualizing the ET tube passing through the vocal cords. All the following methods are for verification of tube placement:

- Observe the patient's chest rise and fall with each ventilation.
- Auscultate for the presence of breath sounds as follows: Begin over the epigastrium; no breath sounds should be heard here during ventilations. Listen over the left apex (top of the left lung area) and compare the breath sounds with those at the right apex; breath sounds should be heard equally on both sides. Listen over the left base (bottom of the lung area) and compare the breath sounds with those at the right base; breath sounds should be heard equally on both sides.
- Observe the patient for signs of deterioration after tube placement, such as becoming combative or developing cyanosis. Both are signs of hypoxia (oxygen starvation) and probable incorrect tube placement.

Misplacing an ET tube into the esophagus occasionally occurs. This problem can be quickly detected and the tube removed so that it can be properly placed after a minute or two of BVM ventilations to oxygenate the patient. If the ET tube is placed in the esophagus and the problem is not recognized, the patient will die! This is one of the few fatal errors an EMT-B could potentially make if not following the proper procedures of intubation. When this error occurs, so generally does a lawsuit. Some of these errors have been very high profile and explored by the media. Most medical legal experts would agree that the standard for assuring tube placement is rapidly changing to involve more methods than just watching the tube go through the vocal cords and hearing lung sounds on both sides! The authors of this text strongly recommend that tube placement be assured by:

- **Visualization.**
- **Auscultation over the lung fields and epigastrium.**
- **Use of either a colormetric end-tidal CO_2 monitoring device, such as an Easy Cap® CO_2 Detector (Figure 29-11), a Tube Check® device (Figure 29-12), or a capnography device (Figure 29-13).**
- **Never letting go of the tube until it is properly secured in place.**
- **Frequent re-auscultation during the management of the patient.**
- **Utilization of a pulse oximeter whenever available.**
- **Always ensuring removal of the BVM from the ET tube prior to defibrillation attempts.**
- **PCR documentation of efforts to assure that the tube was properly placed throughout the prehospital care of the patient.**

Your local medical direction should address this subject proactively rather than reactively!

Detecting and Correcting Incorrect Tube Placements

21. If breath sounds are diminished or absent on the left but present on the right, it is likely the tube has advanced beyond the carina and intubated the right mainstem bronchus. If this occurs

- Deflate the cuff and gently withdraw the tube while artificially ventilating and auscultating over the left apex of the chest.
- Take care not to completely remove the endotracheal tube.
- When the breath sounds become equal at both the left and right apex, reinflate the cuff and follow the above directions for securing the tube.

22. If breath sounds are present only in the epigastrium, the esophagus has been intubated and air is being sent into the stomach instead of the lungs. Since esophageal intubation is a fatal occurrence, immediately deflate the cuff and withdraw the tube. The patient should then be hyperventilated for at least 2 to 5 minutes prior to your second attempt to intubate.

23. The EMT-B should make only two attempts at orotracheal intubation. If both attempts fail, insert an oral airway, continue to ventilate the patient with high-concentration oxygen via BVM, and aggressively suction the airway.

Securing the Tube

24. If breath sounds are heard bilaterally and no sounds are heard over the epigastrium, the ET tube should be secured in place using a commercial tube restraint device. An oral airway may be inserted as a bite block to protect the tube. Note the depth of the tube at the teeth, both before and after securing it, to assure the tube has not been dislodged during the procedure.

Ongoing Assessment

25. Be sure to assess and reassess the breath sounds following every major move with the patient. A capnograph can be helpful in monitoring tube position (Figure 29-13).

It cannot be overemphasized that inadvertent esophageal intubation will likely result in the patient's death. Because of the magnitude of this complication, tell new EMT-Bs that if at any time—despite the best efforts to properly assess tube placement—they are in doubt of proper tube placement, immediately withdraw the tube and manage the airway with basic airway adjuncts.

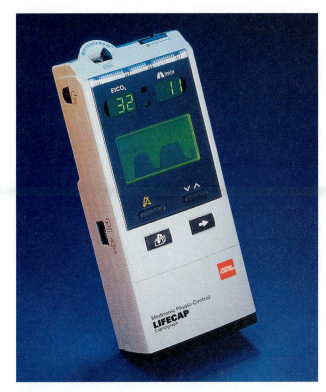

Figure 29-13 A capnograph is used to measure end-tidal CO_2.

Orotracheal Intubation of an Infant or Child

Although the goal of orotracheal intubation is identical in both adult and pediatric patients, intubation of the infant and child requires special training because of various considerations of anatomy, physiology, and size.

The specific anatomy and physiology of the pediatric airway has been discussed earlier in this chapter. The importance of these factors as they relate to orotracheal intubation is as follows:

- It is often difficult to create a single clear visual plane from the mouth through the pharynx and into the glottis for orotracheal intubation because of such factors as the relatively large size of the tongue of the infant and child.

- Because of size differences among infants and children as well as the fact that the narrowest portion of the airway is at the level of the cricoid ring, the proper sizing of the ET tube is crucial.

- Because infants and children tend to develop hypoxia (oxygen starvation) and bradycardia (slowed heartbeat) easily during intubation attempts, pediatric intubations require careful monitoring coupled with swift and accurate technique.

The indications for orotracheal intubation of the infant and child are similar to those for the adult patient:

- When prolonged artificial ventilation is required
- When adequate artificial ventilation cannot be achieved by other means
- To ventilate the clearly apneic patient
- To ventilate the cardiac-arrest patient
- To control the airway of unresponsive patients who have no cough or gag reflex

The laryngoscope blades and the ET tubes necessary for the orotracheal intubation of infants and children must be carefully sized to the patient. In general the straight blade, usually a size 1, is preferred in infants and small children because it provides for greater displacement of the tongue and better visualization of the glottis. As in adults, the blade lifts the epiglottis, bringing the vocal cords into view. In older children the curved blade is often preferred because the blade's broad base displaces the tongue better, allowing improved visualization of the vocal cords once the blade is placed into the vallecula and lifted.

Assorted sizes of ET tubes should always be stocked in the pediatric airway kit. As previously mentioned, the proper sizing of the tube is essential in children.

A formula—(patient's age + 16)/4 = tube size—can be used to estimate the proper size. Also, using the diameter of the patient's little finger or the diameter of the nasal opening are alternative techniques for estimating correct tube size.

Because infants are often the pediatric patients who require orotracheal intubation, it is helpful to simply memorize that newborns and small infants generally require a 3.0 to a 3.5 tube, and a 4.0 tube can be used for older infants up to the age of one year. No matter what system you use in determining tube size, it is always prudent to have one half-size larger tube and one half-size smaller tube on standby, since the size of the glottic structures does vary in infants and children.

ET tubes come in both cuffed and uncuffed versions. Cuffed tubes are always used in adult patients.

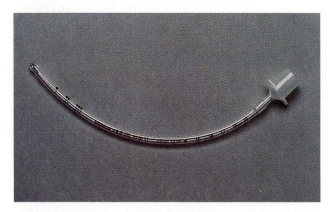

Figure 29-14 An uncuffed endotracheal (ET) tube is used for patients under 8 years of age.

In the pediatric population, cuffed tubes are reserved for children 8 years of age and older. For younger children and infants, uncuffed tubes are used since the narrowing of the airway at the level of the cricoid cartilage serves as a functional cuff, snugging the tube in the airway. Uncuffed tubes (Figure 29-14) should display a vocal cord marker to assure proper placement. This marker is designed so that the vocal cords are at the level of the translucent marker-break in the tube. If the patient is old enough to get a cuffed tube, it should be inserted, like the adult tube, just deep enough so that the cuff material is distal to the cords.

The depth of proper tube placement at the teeth to assure that the ET tube is at the level of the mid-trachea can also be approximated by age (Table 29-2). However, direct visualization of the tube being placed properly is the best measure of tube depth.

Table 29-2 **Length of Endotracheal Tubes in Pediatrics**

Measurement of Endotracheal Tube at the Teeth

6 months–1 year: 12 cm teeth to midtrachea

2 years: 14 cm teeth to mid-trachea

4–6 years: 16 cm teeth to mid-trachea

6–10 years: 18 cm teeth to mid-trachea

10–12 years: 20 cm teeth to mid-trachea

The step-by-step procedure for orotracheal intubation of infants and children is very similar to the procedure outlined for adults. There are, however, some important differences that you must keep in mind when performing a pediatric intubation:

- The rate of hyperventilation both before and after intubation must be adjusted to the patient's age.

- The patient's heart rate must be continuously monitored during intubation attempts since mechanical stimulation of the airway and hypoxia can both slow the heart rate. If the heart rate slows, the blade should immediately be withdrawn and the infant or child reventilated with high-concentration oxygen.

- The optimal positioning of the patient's head is to gently tilt the head forward and lift the chin into the "sniffing" position (Figure 29-15).

- Very little force is needed to intubate the infant or child. Gentle finesse is the rule, not the exception.

- Sellick's maneuver is also often beneficial, but the landmarks may be difficult to locate in the infant and child. In addition, excessive pressure on the relatively soft cartilage may cause tracheal obstruction.

- When using a straight blade, remember that the epiglottis in infants and children is not as stiff as in adults and may partially obscure a clear view of the vocal cords.

- Since distances in the infant and child are small, be certain to hold onto the tube until you are assured it is well secured. This is especially true in pediatric patients who often have lots of secretions, which make the tube very slippery. As with adults, reassess tube placement every time you move the patient.

- In infants and children, the best indicator of tube placement is symmetrical rise and fall of the chest during ventilation.

- Breath sounds in infants and children can often be misleading, since the chest is small and sounds are easily transmitted from one area to another.

- Observe the patient for increased heart rate and improving color after intubation. An infant or child who becomes dusky in color and whose heart rate

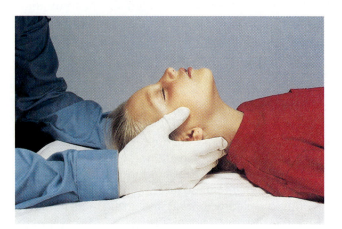

Figure 29-15 Place the pediatric (non-trauma) patient's head in the "sniffing" position for intubation.

slows after intubation is likely not to be properly intubated.

- Once tube placement is confirmed, the patient should be secured to an appropriate device to prevent any head movement from dislodging the tube.
- If the tube is properly placed but there is inadequate chest expansion, seek out one of the following causes:
  - The tube is too small and there is an air leak around the tube at the glottic opening. This is detected by auscultating over the neck. The tube should be replaced by a larger tube.
  - The pop-off valve on the bag-valve device has not been deactivated.
  - There is a leak in the bag-valve device.
  - The ventilator is delivering an inadequate volume of air/oxygen.
  - The tube is blocked with secretions. This can be treated initially with endotracheal suctioning. If suctioning fails, the tube should be removed.
- Infants and children are at risk for the same complications of orotracheal intubation as adult patients. Inadvertent esophageal intubation is perhaps even more rapidly fatal in infants and children than adults. In addition, barotrauma from over-inflation of the lungs can result in collapse of the lung, which can further compromise your ability to ventilate the patient.

Nasogastric Tube Placement in the Pediatric Patient

An additional procedure you will have to master in conjunction with orotracheal intubation of an infant or child is the placement of a **nasogastric tube,** or NG tube. A nasogastric (NG) tube is inserted through the nose into the infant's or child's stomach. The most common use of the NG tube in advanced airway management is to decompress the stomach and proximal bowel of air. In infants and children, air frequently fills the stomach and bowel after overly aggressive artificial ventilation or as a result of air swallowing. The NG tube provides an escape route for excess air. The NG tube also can be used to drain the stomach of blood or other substances. In the hospital setting, NG tubes can be used to give medication and provide a route for nutrition as well.

The indications for insertion of the NG tube in pediatric patients are as follows:

- Inability to adequately ventilate the patient because of distention of the stomach
- An unresponsive patient with gastric distention

Many experts believe that the NG tube should be inserted only after the trachea has been secured with

Table 29-3 Equipment for Nasogastric Intubation
Equipment for Nasogastric Tube Placement
Nasogastric tubes of various sizes:
Newborn/infant: 8.0 French
Toddler/preschool: 10.0 French
School age: 12 French
Adolescent: 14-16 French
20 cc syringe
Water-soluble lubricant
Emesis basin
Tape
Stethoscope
Suction unit with connecting tubing

an endotracheal tube in order to prevent incorrect placement of the NG tube into the trachea instead of the esophagus. Other possible complications of NG intubation include trauma to the nose, triggering vomiting and, in very rare cases, passing the tube into the cranium through a basilar skull fracture. Because of the risk of cranial intubation with the NG tube, the presence of major facial trauma or head trauma is considered a contraindication to the NG tube. In such cases, should the infant or child require gastric decompression, the insertion of the tube through the mouth (orogastric technique) is preferred if allowed by local protocol.

The equipment required for NG tube insertion is listed in Table 29-3.

The procedure for insertion of the NG tube is as follows (Skill Summary 29-2):

1. Prepare and assemble all equipment.

2. Assure that the patient is well oxygenated prior to the procedure.

3. Measure the tube from the tip of the nose and around the ear to below the xiphoid process. (If the tube will be inserted by way of the orogastric technique, measure from the lips.) This length will determine the depth the tube will be inserted.

4. Lubricate the end of the tube.

5. Pass the tube gently downward along the nasal floor.

6. Confirm that the tube is in the stomach by:
  - Aspirating stomach contents
  - Auscultating a rush of air over the epigastrium while injecting 10 cc to 20 cc of air into the tube

Nasogastric Intubation of the Pediatric Patient

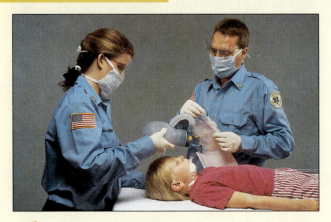

▲ **1.** Oxygenate the patient.

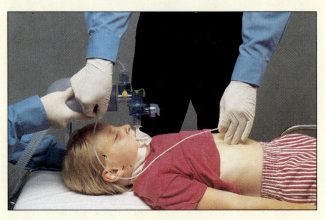

▲ **2.** Measure NG tube from tip of patient's nose, over ear, to below xiphoid process.

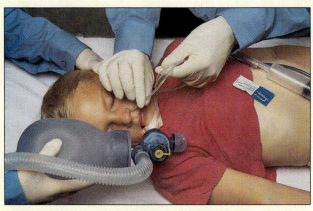

▲ **3.** Pass lubricated tube gently downward along nasal floor into stomach.

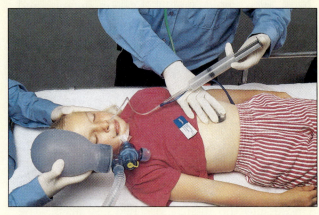

▲ **4.** To confirm correct placement, auscultate over epigastrium. Listen for bubbling while injecting 10–20 cc air into tube.

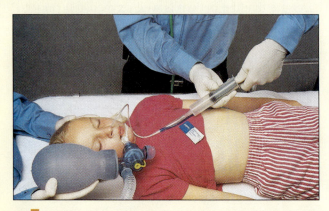

▲ **5.** Use suction to aspirate stomach contents.

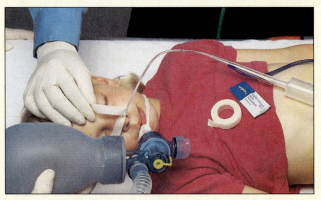

▲ **6.** Secure tube in place.

7. Aspirate gastric contents by attaching the tube to suction.

8. Secure the tube in place with tape.

Orotracheal Suctioning

In conjunction with your training in advanced airway management, you may also be trained in the techniques of **orotracheal suctioning.** For this procedure, a flexible soft suction catheter is used to suction the trachea, usually down to the level of the carina in the artificially ventilated patient. This procedure is sometimes referred to as **deep suctioning** to set it apart from the basic airway management procedure—suctioning of the oropharynx (mouth and pharynx), in which suctioning does not advance as far as the trachea.

The indications for orotracheal suctioning are as follows:

- **Obvious secretions in the airway.** This may be detected by either moist bubbling sounds during ventilation with the bag-valve-mask device or by visible secretions inside the ET tube after the patient has been intubated.
- **Poor compliance with bag-valve-mask ventilation.** Resistance to ventilation may be caused by secretions below the level of the larynx in the trachea.

The technique for orotracheal suctioning is as follows (Skill Summary 29-3):

1. Take BSI precautions. Be especially mindful to have eye protection, as splattering during deep suctioning is common.

2. Pre-oxygenate the patient with high-concentration oxygen prior to attempting suction.

3. Hyperventilate the patient prior to suctioning.

4. Check that all equipment is operating correctly.

5. Use a sterile technique.

6. Approximate the desired length of the catheter to be inserted by measuring from the lips to the ear to the nipple line. This will approximate the level of the carina.

7. Advance the catheter to the desired location.

8. Apply suction and withdraw the catheter in a twisting motion.

9. Resume ventilations.

10. To prevent hypoxia, attempts at deep suctioning should not exceed 15 seconds.

Deep suctioning techniques are not without potential complications. Most of the serious complications relate to the fact that the ventilated patient is deprived of oxygen during suctioning. Hyperventilation prior to suctioning, careful technique, and limiting suctioning to 15 seconds can help prevent the following complications of deep suctioning:

- Cardiac dysrrhythmias
- Hypoxia
- Coughing
- Damage to the lining (mucosa) of the airway
- Spasm of the bronchioles (bronchospasm) if the catheter extends past the carina
- Spasm of the vocal cords (laryngospasm) during orotracheal suctioning

Automatic Transport Ventilators

Automatic transport ventilators, or ATVs (Figure 29-16) have been used extensively in Europe for a number of years. The devices are rapidly gaining popularity in the United States, as recent studies have demonstrated them to be superior in some respects to manual ventilation with the BVM.

ATVs are compact devices with controls that set both the rate of ventilation and the tidal volume. Tidal volumes are determined by the patient's weight. A number of different ATV models are commercially available. The American Heart Association recommends that ATVs should meet certain minimal standards. They should:

- Have the ability to deliver 100% oxygen
- Be able to provide at least two rates of ventilation—10 breaths per minute for adults and 20 breaths per minute for children
- Be lightweight (≤4 kg), rugged, and compact
- Be capable of generating under extremes of temperature
- Have a default inspiratory time of 2 seconds in adults and 1 second in children
- Be equipped with an audible alarm to alert the user to problems in ventilation
- Have a standard 15 mm/22 mm coupling to connect with a mask or ET tube

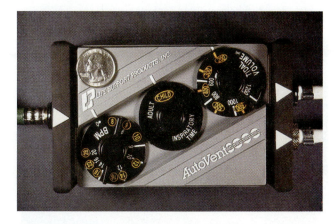

Figure 29-16 The automatic transport ventilator (ATV). (NOTE: The quarter in the photo is meant to give you an idea of the actual size of the device.)

Orotracheal Suctioning

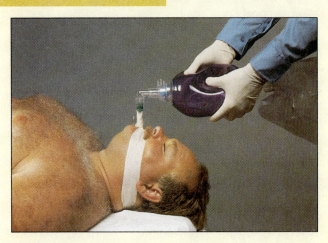

▲ **1.** Hyperventilate the patient.

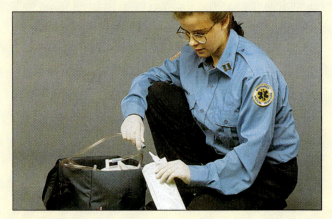

▲ **2.** Carefully check equipment.

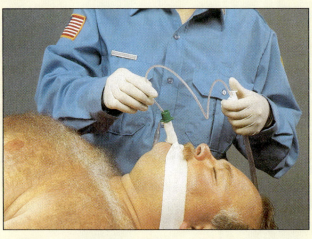

▲ **3.** Insert catheter without applying suction.

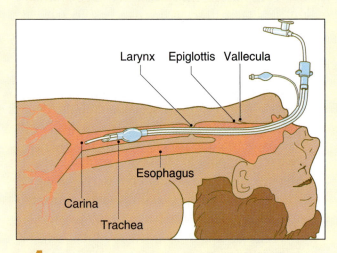

Larynx   Epiglottis   Vallecula

Esophagus

Carina

Trachea

▲ **4.** Catheter may be advanced as far as carina level.

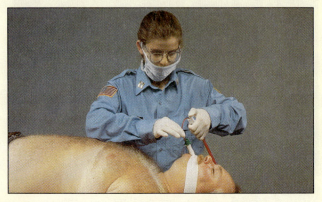

▲ **5.** Advance catheter to desired level, apply suction, and withdraw catheter with a twisting motion.

▲ **6.** Resume ventilation. Suctioning procedure should interrupt ventilation for no more than 15 seconds.

Although some units are marketed for pediatric use with controls for lower tidal volumes, the device is not suitable for children less than 5 years of age.

Because ATVs require some additional training for safe use, the decision to use ATVs in an EMS system and the establishment of ATV protocols should be made by the medical director.

Other Types of Advanced Airways

In some EMS systems, medical direction may elect to allow the EMT-B to use another type of advanced airway such as the esophageal-tracheal Combitube® (ETC) or the laryngeal mask airway (LMA). Other devices, which are not shown in this text since they are seldom used, include the esophageal obturator airway (EOA), the esophageal gastric tube airway (EGTA), and pharyngotracheal lumen airway (PTL). The EOA and EGTA have been problematic because of their reliance on a mask seal. Although these other types of advanced airways do not provide the definitive airway control of the ET tube, when properly used they provide superior ventilation of the apneic patient as compared with a simple oral airway (OPA).

The Esophageal Tracheal "Combitube®" (ETC)

The **esophageal tracheal Combitube®** or, more commonly, the "Combitube®" (see Figure 29-17) has a double lumen airway where the two lumens are separated by a partition wall.

In one lumen of the Combitube®, the distal end is sealed and there are perforations in the area that would be in the pharynx. When the tube is in the esophagus, ventilations are delivered through it. The sealed end prevents ventilations from entering the esophagus and stomach and diverts them through the perforations into the pharynx, from which they flow into the trachea and the lungs.

In the other lumen of the Combitube®, the distal end is open. When the tube is in the trachea, ventilations are delivered through this tube.

The Combitube® has a distal cuff that inflates to seal the esophagus or trachea, depending on which passageway it is in. When the trachea is sealed, the cuff prevents stomach contents from being aspirated, but it does not prevent ventilations from entering the trachea via the tube that passes through the cuff.

The Combitube® should not be used on a patient who:

■ Is alert, verbally responsive, or who responds to painful stimuli and also still has a gag reflex. Vomiting and aspiration are likely.

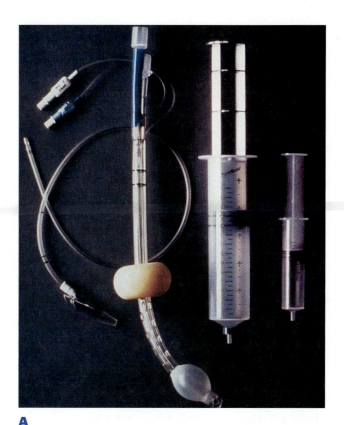

A

B

Figure 29-17 (A) The esophageal tracheal Combitube®. (B) The Combitube® ETC in place.

- Is less than 4 feet. There are 2 sizes of the device: 37 French (patients from 4–6 feet) and 41 French (for over 6 feet).
- Has ingested a corrosive substance. A corrosive could perforate the tip of the device, or may weaken the esophagus so that the device could perforate the esophagus wall.
- Has a known esophageal disease or cancer of the esophagus.
- Has esophageal varices, which weaken the wall of the esophagus and increase the chance for a ruptured esophagus.
- Has significant upper airway bleeding. Blood flowing from the nose or mouth will pass directly into the lungs once the inflated cuff has closed off the esophagus.
- Has airway trauma.

Follow these steps to insert the Combitube®:

1. Insert it blindly, watching for the two black rings on the Combitube® that are used for measuring the depth of insertion. These rings should be positioned between the teeth and the bony cavities where the teeth have their roots.
2. Use the large syringe to inflate the pharyngeal cuff with 100 cc of air. On inflation, the device will seat itself in the posterior pharynx behind the hard palate.
3. Use the smaller syringe to fill the distal cuff with 10 cc to 15 cc of air.
4. Usually the tube will have been placed in the esophagus. On this assumption, ventilate through the esophageal connector. It is the external tube that is the longer of the two and is marked "#1." You must listen for the presence of breath sounds in the lungs and the absence of sounds from the epigastrium in order to be sure that the tube is, in fact, placed in the esophagus.
5. If there is an absence of lung sounds and presence of sounds in the epigastrium, the tube has been placed in the trachea. In this case, change the ventilator to the shorter tracheal connector, which is marked "#2." Listen again to be sure of proper placement of the tube.

An advantage of the Combitube® is that no stylet must be withdrawn from the open-ended esophageal lumen before suctioning of the stomach can take place, making this process quicker. Another advantage is the automatic seating of the pharyngeal cuff. The biggest advantage is that rapid intubation is possible independent of the position of the patient, which is helpful for trauma patients requiring limited cervical-spine movement.

If the patient becomes conscious, you must remove the Combitube®. Remember that extubation is likely to cause vomiting. Have suction equipment ready. Follow the same guidelines as for removal of the other airway devices.

The Laryngeal Mask Airway (LMA)

The laryngeal mask airway (LMA) is composed of a tube with a cuffed mask-like projection on the distal end. It is designed to provide a more secure and reliable means of ventilation than the face mask. Although the LMA does not ensure the airway is protected from aspiration, it has been studied and shown to be helpful in limiting regurgitation and subsequent aspiration during ventilation. Used in the operating room setting for many years, this device is new to the prehospital arena since its introduction in the American Heart Association's Guidelines 2000.

Each service's medical direction will need to evaluate the LMA and decide if this is an appropriate device to train their EMT-Bs to use. The device is easy to use and the "LMA-Unique™" model has been designed for field use. LMAs come in many sizes so they can be used in both pediatric patients as well as adults. The procedure for insertion of the device is shown in Skill Summary 29-4. Additional training manuals and a video are also available from the manufacturer of the device.

PRECEPTOR PEARL

Remind new EMT-Bs that whenever a Combitube® or LMA is inserted or extubated, gloves, mask, and goggles should be worn to protect the EMT-B from the potential spraying of body fluids.

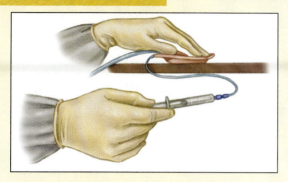

▲ **1.** Tightly deflate the cuff so that it forms a smooth "spoon-shape." Lubricate the posterior surface of the mask with water-soluble lubricant.

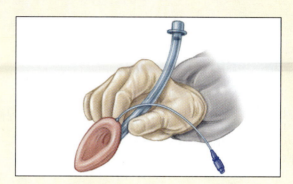

▲ **2.** Hold the LMA like a pen, with the index finger at the junction of the cuff and the tube.

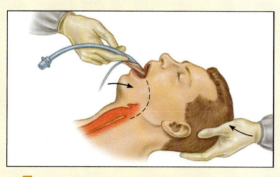

▲ **3.** With the patient's head extended and the neck flexed, carefully flatten the LMA tip against the hard palate.

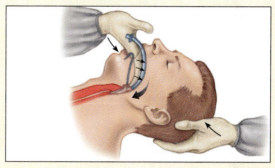

▲ **4.** Use the index finger to push cranially, maintaining pressure on the tube with the finger. Advance the mask until definite resistance is felt at the base of the hypopharynx.

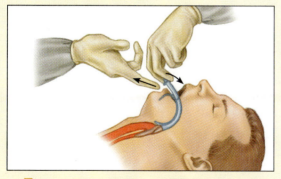

▲ **5.** Gently maintain cranial pressure with the one hand while removing the index finger.

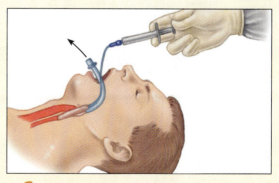

▲ **6.** Without holding the tube, inflate the cuff with just enough air to obtain a seal (to a pressure of approximately 60 cm H_2O).

Maximum LMA Cuff Inflation Volumes

LMA Size	Cuff Volume(air)	LMA Size	Cuff Volume(air)
1	up to 4 ml	3	up to 20 ml
1½	up to 7 ml	4	up to 30 ml
2	up to 10 ml	5	up to 40 ml
2½	up to 14 ml	6	up to 50 ml

Souce: LMA Instuction Manual, Table 5, p. 28

SUMMARY

- The placement of an endotracheal (ET) tube permits complete control of the airway, minimizes the risk of aspiration, allows for better oxygen delivery, and allows for deep suctioning of the trachea.

- The procedure for endotracheal intubation of pediatric patients is similar to the procedure for adults, but you should keep these differences in the airways of infants and children in mind: all structures in the mouth an nose are smaller; the tongue is proportionately larger; the trachea is softer, more flexible, and narrower; the airway is especially narrow at the cricoid cartilage, and the chest wall is softer.

- The differences in the pediatric airways result in the airways being more easily obstructed,

in the use of uncuffed ET tubes in patients under the age of 8, and in distinctive breathing patterns.

- Pediatric patients are more susceptible to damage from incorrect placement of a tube and to interruptions of the supply of oxygen; they, therefore, must be monitored especially carefully during intubation and suctioning procedures.

- Alternatives to the ET tube, which EMTs may be taught to use, include the Combitube® airway and the laryngeal mask airway (LMA).

- Whenever a patient is intubated, it is essential to verify and monitor the position of the tube because it may easily be dislodged and the consequences may be fatal if unrecognized.

REVIEW QUESTIONS

1. An advantage of orotracheal intubation of the apneic patient includes:
   a. allowing for deep suctioning.
   b. maximizing the risk of aspiration.
   c. preventing oxygen delivery to the lungs.
   d. all of the above.

2. Complications of orotracheal intubation may include any of the following EXCEPT:
   a. gagging and vomiting.
   b. slowing of the heart rate.
   c. soft-tissue trauma to the nose.
   d. inadequate oxygenation, or oxygen starvation.

3. Why is it important to frequently reassess lung sounds after placing an ET tube?
   a. Sometimes they will disappear.
   b. The tube may become accidentally dislodged.
   c. The tube frequently moves into the left mainstem bronchus.
   d. All of the above.

4. The standard length of an adult ET tube is _____ centimeters.
   a. 20
   b. 25
   c. 33
   d. 38

5. A properly placed ET tube in an adult will have the _____ centimeter mark at the teeth.
   a. 18
   b. 22
   c. 31
   d. 35

6. The indications for orotracheal intubation include:
   a. a gag reflex in your patient.
   b. a patient in cardiac arrest.
   c. a patient responsive to painful stimuli.
   d. adequate ventilations in an apneic patient.

7. If breath sounds are heard only in the epigastrium area during ventilation, the ET tube:

a. has probably found a pneumothorax.

b. is properly placed and should be left alone.

c. is probably in the esophagus and should be removed.

d. is probably in the trachea but should be removed.

8. When intubating infants, usually the _____ blade in size _____ is preferred.

a. straight, 1

b. straight, 2

c. curved, 1

d. curved, 2

9. Stimulation of the airway can lead to:

a. vomiting.

b. gagging.

c. slowing of the heart rate.

d. any of the above.

10. An NG tube should be measured from the:

a. tip of the nose and around the ear to below the xiphoid process.

b. tip of the nose down the midline of the body to the umbilicus.

c. bridge of the nose to the angle of the jaw to the mouth.

d. corner of the mouth to the xiphoid process.

WEB MEDIC

Visit Brady's *Essentials of Emergency Care* web site for direct web links. At **www.prenhall.com/limmer,** you will find information related to the following Chapter 29 topics:

• Capnography

• End-tidal CO_2 monitoring devices

• The Combitube®

• The LMA™

RESEARCH IN EMS

Anti-shock trousers are good. Anti-shock trousers are bad. Intravenous fluids are good. Intravenous fluids are bad. EMS providers hear these and other similar statements all the time. Newspapers and the television news pick up stories about articles in medical journals and report them to the public. How much of these reports can an EMT-B believe? Do they apply to all EMS systems? Should they be the basis for changes in prehospital practice?

Research is an increasingly more important part of EMS. Many of our ideas about patient care are the result of tradition and have never been evaluated. This is true not just of EMS, but also of medicine in general and emergency medicine in particular. Only in the last few years has anyone paid significant attention to laying the foundation for research-proven quality care in EMS. This appendix will describe three aspects of research as it applies to EMS. First, it will introduce you to the subject of interpreting research. This will help you understand what to look for in a piece of published research, such as whether to believe the conclusions of the paper and how to apply the research to your EMS system. Second, it will describe what you need to know if you participate in a research project. More and more EMS systems are participating in the research needed to determine how best to care for our patients and to justify what we do. Third, it will list a number of resources where you can learn more about research and how it is interpreted.

INTERPRETING RESEARCH

How a Field Advances

Every area of medicine is changing today, and EMS is no exception. One of the ways in which a field advances is by common sense. No one has to do a study to realize that placing heavy sand bags on the sides of an immobilized patient's head can lead to harm if the patient and backboard must be turned on their side. In this case, using something sturdy and lightweight makes a great deal more sense. Similarly, it is obvious that glass IV bottles are much more likely to break in a moving ambulance than plastic IV bags.

However, common sense has limits. It was common sense only 20 years ago to believe that raising the blood pressure of a patient in shock by inflating anti-shock trousers was going to improve survival. Unfortunately, no one has been able to show improved survival in this group of patients and experts are divided about how best to treat shock. It was also common sense then to put a soft cervical collar around the neck of a patient with a suspected cervical-spine injury. That belief is no longer considered valid. Today's common sense tells us that using a collar that restricts motion of the head and neck prevents spine injuries from becoming spinal-cord injuries. It remains to be seen whether this belief will be verified by evidence or if someone will find a better approach.

Sometimes we have to rely on something a little more substantive than common sense, even when we don't have the hard data to make a definitive statement. In this case, we may try to get a consensus of experts in the field. The U.S. DOT's 1994 "EMT-Basic: National Standard Curriculum" was developed using this method. Two panels of experts, one consisting of physicians and the other of curriculum developers, discussed and agreed on what should and should not be included in this curriculum. This approach is used often in medicine when there is conflicting and missing information or when there have been many changes in a short time. The American Heart Association, for example, also uses this approach in updating its guidelines for basic and advanced cardiac life support every few years.

Scientific studies are another way of improving the care our patients receive. To many people, this is the best way to advance a field because it allows practitioners to see exactly how an idea was tested. When done well, a piece of research can have a significant impact on many people's lives. EMS has only recently begun to lay this foundation and establish credibility for itself. In recent years, some of the areas that have received attention from EMS researchers include defibrillation, anti-shock trousers, spine immobilization, aeromedical transport (helicopters), triaging of patients to trauma centers, and intravenous fluids.

Types of Studies

There are four types of studies you are likely to encounter: descriptive, case-control, cohort, and intervention studies. Each type of study has its strengths and weaknesses.

Descriptive Studies

In a **descriptive study,** researchers do not attempt to change anything or discover the effects of any intervention. Instead, they carefully evaluate a particular subject according to carefully spelled out criteria. This yields a report that describes the current state of affairs in a particular area. For example, an EMS agency may wish to learn how many defibrillators to purchase and where to place them. To accomplish this, they review their run reports for the last three years to determine how many cardiac arrests the service had and where those arrests occurred. The results give the organization the information it needs in order to station enough defibrillators in the right places. This will increase the likelihood that a defibrillator will be nearby when a patient goes into cardiac arrest.

Descriptive studies are relatively inexpensive and simple to conduct because they usually involve reviewing a data base or conducting a survey. They are limited, though, in their scope and applicability because they typically look only at a single system, which may be very different from other systems, and because like a snapshot it shows conditions at only one particular point in time. Because they are very weak in their ability to draw conclusions about cause and effect, descriptive studies are not very useful for investigating hypotheses. Instead, they are better suited for laying the foundation for research in a particular area and for suggesting research questions for the future.

Case-Control Studies

A **case-control study** is an example of retrospective research, which looks backward in time. By finding patients who have a particular disease or condition and comparing them to people who do not have the disease or condition, a case-control study can allow investigators to determine which factors place someone at risk for developing the disease. An example of this was a landmark study on the effects of cigarette smoking published in 1950. The investigators looked at the health history, including smoking history, of more than 700 patients hospitalized for lung cancer and compared this to the same information obtained from a large number of patients hospitalized for other conditions. They found that patients with lung cancer were significantly more likely to have smoked than those without lung cancer.[1]

One of the criticisms of case-control studies is a phenomenon called **recall bias.** If you ask someone with lung cancer how long and how much he has smoked, he may, either consciously or unconsciously, give inaccurate answers, depending on whether he believes smoking caused his condition and which answers he believes the investigator wants. He may also not want to admit he was unable to quit smoking and so may be less than completely truthful. Alternatively, he may wish to exaggerate the role smoking played in causing his condition so that others will not imitate him. The person without lung cancer is presumably less likely to be subject to these feelings, but may still be subject to recall bias. Even the most carefully conducted study can fall victim to this kind of distortion, so it is important that researchers take it into consideration and do everything they can to minimize it.

---

[1] Doll, R., and A.B. Hill. Smoking and carcinoma of the lung: Preliminary report. *Br Med J.* 2:739, 1950.

Cohort Studies

Like case-control studies, **cohort studies** look at certain characteristics of study subjects (potential risk factors) and development of disease. In this case, though, we don't know yet whether the study subjects have the disease we are studying. Instead, we record which potential risk factors patients have or were exposed to and follow them to see which ones develop the disease being studied.

This can be quite time consuming since many conditions take years to develop. Over a long period of time, study subjects may also move away from the investigators or in other ways be lost to follow-up. This can make such a study quite expensive. Probably one of the best known examples of this type of study is the Framingham Heart Study.[2]

In the early 1950s investigators began studying more than 5,000 middle-aged adults without cardiovascular disease in the Framingham, Massachusetts, area. These people have been followed and periodically examined for heart disease. Since the researchers did not (and could not) know at the beginning of the study which patients with which risk factors would develop heart disease, this study has given scientists very strong evidence about the roles of cigarette smoking, cholesterol, and high blood pressure in the development of heart disease.

Intervention Studies

In case-control studies, investigators look at patients who have a disease and look back in time to determine risk factors for development of the disease. In cohort studies, patients are selected on the basis of whether or not they have been exposed to risk factors and followed forward in time for the development of disease. In **intervention studies,** the situation is quite different. In these studies, the investigators determine whether or not a subject is exposed (or treated) instead of depending on nature to decide this. This kind of study, when designed and conducted properly, yields extremely strong evidence about the effects of certain interventions. For this reason, it is often considered the gold standard in research methodology.

The investigators begin, just as they do with case-control and cohort studies, by deciding on a study hypothesis. This consists of an idea that they can test in an objective manner. For instance, a number of years ago, clinicians in King County, Washington,

wished to test the hypothesis that EMTs with automated external defibrillators (AEDs) could increase survival from cardiac arrest just as well as EMTs with manual defibrillators.[3] They trained EMTs to use both machines, set up protocols for their use, decided exactly what data they were going to record, and planned how they were going to be able to tell if their hypothesis was correct (through selection of the proper statistical tests). They did this very carefully and planned how to conduct the study so that irrelevant factors were eliminated or minimized.

Since the researchers wanted to find out whether EMTs could operate AEDs, they used just one brand of AED. This eliminated one potential source of confounding. A variable that is not being studied but which may have an effect on the result is called a **confounding variable.** In this case, the researchers made sure that no one could say increased (or decreased) survival could be attributed to one brand of AED over another since only one AED was being used.

Whenever possible, researchers performing clinical trials attempt to randomize the intervention so that there is less chance of interference from a confounding variable. For example, a number of EMTs in King County had been using manual defibrillators for several years and preferred using them. If they had a choice as to which defibrillator they could use, they might select the manual defibrillator for patients with short down times and the automated defibrillator for long or unknown down times. The researchers took this into account by telling the EMTs to use one of the machines for 75 days and then the other for the next 75 days. Although this is not true randomization in the strictest sense of the word, this alternation design is an acceptable means of preventing this type of confounding.

All clinical trials compare one group which receives an intervention (the **study group**) against at least one other group that does not receive the intervention being studied (the **control group**). In many studies, the control group receives a **placebo,** something that resembles the intervention but has no physical effect on the study subject. In drug trials, for instance, a placebo is sometimes a sugar pill. In the case of an AED study, it would have been unethical to deny defibrillation to cardiac-arrest patients in the control group since there was clear evidence that manual defibrillation was saving some lives. So the researchers used manual defibrillation as their control.

[2] Dawber, T.R. *The Framingham Study: The Epidemiology of Atherosclerotic Disease*. Cambridge, MA: Harvard University Press, 1980.

[3] Cummins, R.O., M.S. Eisenberg, P.E. Litwin, *et al*. Automatic external defibrillators used by emergency medical technicians. *JAMA* 1987; 257: 1605-1610.

Something else researchers attempt to incorporate into their study designs whenever possible is **blinding.** This refers to whether or not someone knows which is being used, a placebo or an active agent. **Single blinding** occurs when the patient does not know what he is receiving, but the researcher does. **Double blinding** means that neither the patient nor the researcher knows what the patient is receiving. In the case of a drug study, it can be very important to blind the study subjects and the investigators because of the possibility of **observation bias.** This occurs when, either consciously or unconsciously, someone (either the subject or the investigator) reports an effect because they believe there should be one. This is called the **placebo effect.** Study subjects who receive placebos often report feeling better, even though they did not receive any medication. This effect can occur in as many as a quarter of study subjects and may persist for years afterward.

In a study where the outcome being studied is as objective as death or survival, there is little or no need for blinding. If, however, a subjective outcome like quality of life after cardiac arrest was being studied, there would be a lot more potential for observation bias. In this case, it would be important to make sure the investigators determining the quality of life do not know which intervention a patient receives, if at all possible.

Another way in which the King County researchers demonstrated good study design was the way they planned their data collection and statistical analysis. Even with randomization, study subjects may differ from the control subjects in important ways. It thus becomes important for researchers to evaluate the two groups for differences that may confound the results. In this case, they looked at a number of variables, including age, sex, whether or not the arrest was witnessed, initial EKG rhythm, and response times. They found that the two groups were significantly different in a few ways, but they were able to use some sophisticated statistical methods to determine that in this case those differences did not affect patient outcome.

One of the other things they did was to calculate the sample size they would need to detect a difference in survival rates. They calculated that in order to have an 80% chance of detecting a difference in survival of more than 15% (if a difference truly existed), they would need to have at least 150 patients in each group. This allowed them to plan approximately how long the study would take. The figure of 80% is sometimes referred to as the "power of the study" and is directly related to how willing the investigators are to avoid making an error in their conclusions.

There are two types of **statistical error** that researchers can make. A Type I, or alpha, error is rejecting the hypothesis when it is true. A Type II, or beta, error is accepting the hypothesis when it is false. The Type I error rate, called "alpha," is set at 0.05 or 5% in most research. A commonly accepted Type II error rate, called "beta," is 20% or 0.2. The power of a study is equal to 1 − beta. Since many studies set beta at 0.2, the power is 1 − 0.2 = 0.8 or 80% to detect a difference at the magnitude specified by the investigators if a difference truly exists. The Type I and Type II error rates have an inverse relationship; that is, the lower the Type I error rate the investigator wishes to have, the higher the Type II error rate the investigator will have to tolerate, all other factors being equal. The reverse is also true.

The Type I error rate, or alpha, receives a great deal of attention in published research. Most investigators set alpha at 0.05. This means the researchers will say there is a difference and consider the study to have statistically significant results only if there is a 5% chance or less of getting the results they obtained. Another way of looking at a Type I error rate, or alpha, of 0.05 is that there is only a 5% chance of rejecting the study hypothesis when it is false, assuming the hypothesis is true.

Many studies report not just the acceptable alpha of 0.05, but also the actual probability of getting the results obtained in the study. You may see this written as "$P < .01$." This means the probability of finding such a difference in the study groups is less than 1% assuming the hypothesis is true. Some people have misinterpreted P values in two ways.

First, they conclude that because the P value is so small the hypothesis is absolutely proven beyond a shadow of a doubt. This is not true. No study can definitively prove its hypothesis. All a study can do is assign certain probabilities to the conclusions. All studies also make certain assumptions, such as the type of data to be collected, accuracy of the data, and whether or not samples were selected randomly and independently. If these assumptions are violated, the study's conclusions are suspect.

Second, some people conclude that because there is *statistical* significance (because the P value is so small) there must be *clinical* significance. This is not the case. The researcher determines whether or not there is statistical significance by deciding how much Type I error is acceptable. The researcher and the reader must then determine if there is clinical significance by evaluating the effect of this difference on patient care.

For example, suppose a new drug for hypertension is studied. The investigators find statistically significant differences between the blood pressures in the treated and untreated subjects with $P \ll .01$ (P much less than 1%). In other words, if there was no difference between the drug and the control, these results would occur much less than 1% of the time. On looking at the data, the reader finds that the experimental drug lowers diastolic blood pressure 0.1 mmHg. Is this a clinically significant difference? Not likely. To see a change that is significant enough to affect patient outcome, the difference would have to be greater.

The Type II error rate, or beta, receives much less attention in most published research. This oversight is unfortunate because in some cases investigators fail to get a large enough sample size and so are unable to find a difference even though it exists. A good way to reduce both error rates is to increase the sample size. This solution can lead to some other problems, though.

With greater sample size come the difficulties of more data collection, longer times required to conduct the study, and increased expense. Additionally, it may become easier to find differences that are irrelevant. This occurs because a larger sample allows smaller differences to be detected.

Another problem that can arise in clinical trials is violation of protocol. Despite the planning and precautions of the investigators in the King County study, there were some instances in which EMTs used the manual defibrillator when they were supposed to use the AED. In their analysis of the data, they evaluated these cases as a separate group and also with the AED group to which they should have belonged. This is called **intention to treat** analysis and is an appropriate way to manage protocol violations. This approach does increase the difficulty of finding a difference, but this is usually safer than the opposite approach of including these cases in the other treatment group. In this case, when the investigators analyzed the data, they found that the violations did not have an effect on the overall outcome.

In the end, the King County study found that there was no significant difference in survival between the group treated with the manual defibrillator and the group treated with the AED. Since AEDs are less expensive, require less training to operate, are extremely consistent in performance, and can be used in areas where there are fewer cardiac arrests, the investigators concluded that AEDs can make early defibrillation possible for more patients and should be encouraged. This is an example of a study that, because it showed there was no statistically significant difference between two treatments, had great clinical significance.

Table A-1 summarizes the advantages and disadvantages of different types of studies.

Table A-1 Advantages and Disadvantages of Different Types of Studies

Study Type	Advantages	Disadvantages
Descriptive	Inexpensive. Relatively easy to conduct. Can be done in relatively short time.	Not good for testing hypotheses. Very system-specific.
Case-control	Good for testing hypothesis regarding uncommon or rare conditions. Lays groundwork for cohort and intervention studies.	Subject to recall bias.
Cohort	Can provide very strong evidence for effects of risk factors.	Not good for uncommon or rare conditions. Can be very time-consuming. Expensive.
Intervention	Provides strongest kind of evidence research can produce. Can minimize bias through randomization and blinding.	Expensive. Need to protect study subjects may prolong time needed to conduct study. Study conditions may not be similar to real-life conditions.

Common Statistical Tests

A number of computer programs are available to calculate statistical tests for researchers and others. This section will briefly describe in layperson's terms a few of the more common tests you will find in reading research papers. The most common one you will encounter is the **mean,** or average. It is computed by adding the values and dividing by the number of values involved. This gives a look at the average or typical value of a group of numbers in many cases. The mean is especially well suited when the data are what statisticians call "normally distributed." This means that if you graphed the data, they would form a shape similar to a bell curve. Height of individuals is an example of a normally distributed variable. Most people have a height close to the average, with a few very short and a few very tall people at each end of the graph.

When the data are not normally distributed, the **median** is a better way of finding a typical value. To compute the median, put the values into numerical order and find the middle value. This is the median, also known as the "fiftieth percentile." For example, if you have seven exam scores, to find the median, you put the scores in order and find the fourth highest (or fourth lowest, since it is the same).

Here is an example of how the median can be more useful than the mean in some situations: In many states the number of emergency calls received by EMS agencies is not normally distributed. There are frequently a few very busy services in urban areas, a good number of moderately busy services, and a larger number of services in rural areas that receive a much smaller number of calls. If you were to compute the mean, or average, it would be skewed by the very busy services, even though there are only a few of them. However, if you computed the median, you would get a smaller number that would better reflect the number of calls received by a typical service.

The mean and the median tell only one part of the story. They are called **measures of central tendency** because they indicate the center of the group in one way or another. A different but very important quality to know about a group is how spread out it is, or how dispersed the data are. There are two closely related measures of this that you are likely to see. The first is called the **variance.** To get it, we take each value and subtract the mean from it. We can't take the average of these numbers and get anything useful because the negative numbers will cancel out the positive numbers and we will get zero. To overcome this, we multiply each number by itself (square it) and add up the squared numbers. We then divide this sum by the number of values we started with (for

reasons statisticians can describe, when we are working with samples, we usually divide by one less than the number of values). This is the variance. To get the **standard deviation** (SD), the other common measure of dispersion, we take the square root of the variance. See Figure A-1 on page 516 for two examples of variance and standard deviation.

The standard deviation gives us valuable information about the data. If two groups of data have the same mean but the second has a standard deviation much larger than the first, the data in the second group are much more spread out than the data in the first group. The SD is also used in many statistical formulas.

When researchers find that something occurs with a certain frequency, they usually report this proportion as a percentage. For example, survival from cardiac arrest caused by ventricular fibrillation (VF) may be 20% in a particular study. But since the study looked at a sample of patients in VF, this proportion is only an estimate and may in reality be higher or lower. Investigators can calculate how much variability exists in this percentage based on the number of observations, the actual data, and how reliable they wish the estimate to be. This variability (not the same as the variance) can then be added and subtracted to the original proportion to give what is called a **confidence interval.** For example, suppose the investigators calculated the variability in the example above with 95% confidence and found it was 6%. Then we would have a 95% confidence interval of 20% plus or minus 6%. This means that, assuming the hypothesis is true, we can be 95% confident that the actual rate of survival under the conditions studied was between 14% and 26%.

Confidence intervals are very important in interpreting the value of the research results. If the confidence interval for a proportion like the one above included zero, then there would be a real possibility that there is no actual difference between the study group outcome and the control group outcome. We would conclude that the results are not statistically significant and that there is insufficient reason to believe there is a difference between the two groups.

There are many tests for finding differences between groups, including the **t test** and the **chi square test.** Which test is used depends to a great extent on the kind of data involved and the kinds of differences the investigators are looking for. We will not describe these tests here, but the interested reader can consult some of the sources listed at the end of this appendix.

Another test you may see is the **odds ratio.** This is used in case-control studies and consists of the odds of having a risk factor if the condition is present divided by the odds of having the risk factor if the condition is not present. Simply put, the odds ratio describes how strong the association is between a risk factor and the condition it is associated with. The larger the risk factor, the stronger the association. When you see an odds ratio, look for the confidence interval. Since an odds ratio of 1 indicates that there is no risk associated with the risk factor, if the confidence interval includes 1, there is no statistically significant risk.

For example, suppose investigators surveyed EMT-B students regarding how much education they had received before enrolling in their course. They wished to test the hypothesis that having at least a high school diploma is associated with passing the EMT-B certification exam. After the course is over, they perform the proper calculations and determine that the odds ratio is 1.6. This means a student who passes is 1.6 times as likely to have at least a high school diploma compared to someone who doesn't pass the exam. The 95% confidence interval, though, is 0.8 to 2.4. This means we are 95% confident the true odds ratio lies between 0.8 and 2.4. Since the interval includes 1 (keep in mind an odds ratio of 1 means there is no association), we cannot be 95% confident that there really is an association, and so we conclude there is no statistically significant relationship between having at least a high school diploma and passing the EMT-B exam in this group. On the other hand, if the 95% confidence interval had been 1.2 to 2.0, an interval that does not include 1, we would have concluded with 95% confidence that there is a statistically significant relationship and that a person who passes the EMT-B exam is between 1.2 and 2.0 times as likely to have at least a high school diploma.

Many other statistical tests are used for different kinds of studies and different kinds of data. The references section at the end of this appendix lists several sources where you can learn more about them.

Format of Research Papers

When authors submit their findings to a journal, they structure their results in a standardized fashion that allows others to quickly understand what the researchers did and what they found (Table A-2). The first thing to appear after the title and names of the authors is the **abstract.** This is a brief paragraph that summarizes the need for the study, the research methods used, and the results encountered. Many people use the abstract to determine whether or not the paper is one of interest to them and therefore worth reading.

The **introduction** is the first section of the paper itself. This is a brief description of pertinent previously published papers on the subject of the

investigation. It should describe why the study was undertaken and what the purpose of the study was and what hypothesis the authors wanted to test.

Next comes the **methods** section. This describes exactly how the authors conducted the study, including how patients were selected (and excluded) and what intervention was performed, if any. There should be enough information for interested readers to repeat the experiment. The authors should also describe how they determined the sample size, how much statistical power there was to detect a difference, which statistical tests they used to analyze the data, and what level of significance they chose for their statistical tests.

The **results** come next. Here the researchers provide their data (or a summary of the data), frequently with tables, charts, and graphs to help make sense of the information they gathered. This section presents the data, but does not elaborate on it.

Table A-2 Outline of Research Paper Format

Abstract
Introduction
Methods
Results
Discussion
Summary

The **discussion** section is where the authors interpret their findings and describe the significance of them. There is usually a description of how this new information fits into the field of study and whether it supports or refutes previous research. There should also be a discussion of the limitations of the study, frequently followed by a call for further research to answer the questions raised by the study.

The **summary,** or conclusion, is a very brief (no more than a few sentences) recap of the main findings of the study.

How a Research Paper Is Published

Once the authors of a study have drafted their paper, they submit it to a scientific journal for publication. Each journal has its own particular rules, but all peer-reviewed journals follow the same general procedure. After receiving the paper, the editor sends it to one or more members of a review board, people who have significant expertise either in the field covered by the journal or a related area, such as statistics

Examples of Variance and Standard Deviation

To see how the variance and standard deviation can give valuable information about data, consider this example: Two different EMT-B classes take the same mid-term exam. The classes are the same size (seven students each) and have the same mean (or average) score, 85%. If we didn't look any further, we might think the two classes performed the same on the exam. By looking at the variance and standard deviation, though, we can see that they are actually quite different.

CLASS 1			
Score	Mean	Score−mean	(Score−mean)^2
78	85	−7	49
81	85	−4	16
82	85	−3	9
84	85	−1	1
87	85	2	4
89	85	4	16
94	85	9	81
Sum 595		0	176

Recall that to get the variance we must find the mean, then find the differences between the scores and the mean, square these differences, add them up, and divide by one less than the number of scores. The mean is included in the second column to make it easier to calculate the difference between each score and the mean. The variance is then 176/6 = 29.3. The standard deviation is the square root of 29.3, which is 5.4.

Figure A-1

CLASS 2			
Score	Mean	Score−mean	(Score−mean)^2
82	85	−3	9
83	85	−2	4
84	85	−1	1
85	85	0	0
86	85	1	1
87	85	2	4
88	85	3	9
Sum 595		0	28

Again, to get the variance, we sum the squared differences in the last column and divide by one less than the number of scores: 28/6 = 4.7. The standard deviation is the square root of 4.7, or 2.2, less than half the standard deviation of the first class.

This implies that the scores in the first class are much more spread out than the scores in the second class. When we graph the scores, we can see that this is true:

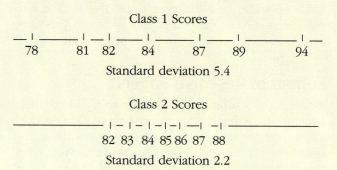

Class 1 Scores

78 81 82 84 87 89 94

Standard deviation 5.4

Class 2 Scores

82 83 84 85 86 87 88

Standard deviation 2.2

or research methodology. The reviewers read the paper and evaluate it for its adherence to standards of research methods, its pertinence to the field, and the potential value it has for practitioners. The reviewers send their comments to the editor, who then decides whether to publish it, send it back for revisions, or reject it. A copy editor may go over it for grammar, spelling, and syntax at some point in the process. Many papers submitted by researchers are not published and some journals have reputations for being very selective.

The peer review process has recently begun to receive greater attention than it has in the past. This has been the result, ironically enough, of several studies looking at the quality of published papers. A surprisingly large number of papers, when evaluated objectively for adherence to principles of research methodology, have been shown to be deficient. This has led at least one journal, *Annals of Emergency Medicine,* to review and revamp its review procedures.[4] Reviewers now get training in what to look for and how to evaluate papers, and closer attention will be paid to how statistics are used. This may be the beginning of a trend that should improve the quality of the research that is conducted and published.

What to Look for When Reviewing a Study

Questions to ask when reviewing a study include the following (Table A-3):

- *Was there a clear hypothesis or study purpose?* The paper should have a clear description of exactly what the investigators were evaluating and what their study hypothesis was. When a hypothesis is not clearly spelled out, it is very easy for the investigators to draw unjustified conclusions.

- *Was the study type appropriate?* Not every investigation lends itself to the format of the randomized controlled clinical trial. It may be necessary, for ethical or financial reasons, to use another format. Evaluate whether the questions the investigators asked were well suited to the type of study they conducted.

- *Were patients assigned to control and study groups properly?* The effects of bias and confounding must be taken into account for the study to yield worthwhile results. In particular, ask yourself:

---

[4] Waeckerle, J.F. and M.L. Callaham. Medical journals and the science of peer reviewing: Raising the standard. Ann Emerg Med July 1996; 28: 75-77.

Table A-3 Questions to Ask When Reviewing a Study
■ Was there a clear hypothesis or study purpose?
■ Was the study type appropriate?
■ Were patients assigned to control and study groups properly?
• For case-control and cohort studies, were selection bias and recall bias taken into account?
• For randomized controlled studies, were randomization and blind assignment maintained?
■ Were the control and study groups the proper size?
■ Were the effects of confounding variables taken into account?
■ Were data analyzed with the proper statistical test?
■ Were the results reported properly (e.g., 95% confidence interval)?
■ How likely is it that the study results would occur by chance alone?

- For case-control and cohort studies, were selection bias and recall bias taken into account?
- For randomized controlled studies, were randomization and blind assignment maintained?

- *Were the control and study groups the proper size?* Did the investigators describe the sample size necessary to produce sufficient power to avoid a Type II error? What was the power of the study?

- *Were the effects of confounding variables taken into account?* Did the investigators describe potential confounders and how they prevented them from interfering with the study?

- *Were the data analyzed with the proper statistical test?* There are many tests available and more than one may be appropriate for the conditions at hand. You may need to consult a statistician or researcher to determine whether or not the investigators used the right tests on the data. Did the investigators clearly determine before data collection took place which tests they were going to use? When the data fail to provide statistically significant results, it is very tempting to perform more tests until one shows significant results. This kind of retrospective testing is called **data snooping** or **data dredging.** If one continues to perform statistical tests, eventually one will be significant just by chance alone. This inappropriate use of statistics is to be avoided.

- *Were the results reported properly?* When a paper includes a proportion or an odds ratio, is there also a 95% confidence interval?

- *How likely is it that the study results would occur by chance alone?* Remember that a *P* value reflects only the chance of seeing the results of a particular piece of research if the study hypothesis is true. A small *P* value may be very impressive, but it does not prove the study hypothesis. Keep in mind also the difference between association and causation. For example, it would be easy to show that the number of drownings increases with sales of ice cream. An inattentive reader might conclude that the sale of more ice cream causes more drownings to occur. In reality, this is an example of association, not causation. Ice cream sales go up when the weather gets warmer, which is also when more people go swimming and drown. This is also an example of confounding.

Applying Study Results to Your Practice

Once you have evaluated a study, you are in a better position to determine whether or not it should change your practice. Before you do so, though, you need to consider several factors. Rarely do clinicians make significant changes on the basis of just one study. Since no study can definitively prove a hypothesis, the reader must look at other studies and his own experience in order to construct an informed opinion. If every other study published on a particular topic comes to very different conclusions than the study at hand, the reader has to wonder whether the study was poorly designed, subject to bias of some sort, affected by unknown confounding variables, or just the result of chance. One must evaluate the field and its knowledge base in order to make an informed decision about how to interpret a piece of research.

The clinical significance is another important piece of the puzzle to consider. A *P* value with lots of zeroes (e.g., *P* < 0.0001) may be very impressive, but not very pertinent. Distinguish between the statistical significance and the clinical significance of the study. Was the difference found in the study large enough to make a real difference to patients?

When investigators conduct their experiments, they have the luxury of selecting patients who meet their criteria and excluding patients who don't. In the real world, things aren't quite so tidy. Before we can apply the results of a piece of research to a particular patient, we must be sure the patient is similar enough to the study group to benefit from the intervention.

Finally, EMS providers do not function in a vacuum. Before implementing any significant changes in your practice, speak to the management of your organization and especially to your medical director. You are responsible not only to your patients, but also to your bosses and your medical director. Including them in decision making of this nature is essential and will pay off in better patient care overall.

PARTICIPATING IN RESEARCH

Many EMS systems are not content to watch other people advance their field. They have decided to conduct research themselves. They have found that by executing well-designed studies, they can not only improve care in their coverage areas, but also improve prehospital care throughout the nation, sharpen the skills of their providers, and rekindle their providers' interest by doing something new and potentially groundbreaking.

Before you participate in such a study, there are certain things you should find out (Table A-4). Clearly, the goal or hypothesis of the study is important to know so that you can understand what the researchers are evaluating. You also need to know the name of the principal investigator and how to contact him or her. This is usually, though not always, a physician. Many EMS physicians who conduct field research will recruit a field provider to researchers are evaluating. You also need to know   researchers are evaluating. You also need to know researchers

---

Table A-4   Things to Know about a Study Before You Participate in It

- Goals
- Name of principal investigator(s) and how to contact
- Anticipated length of time for completion
- Type of study
- Data collection
- Patient assignment methods
- Interventions (including placebos)
- Approval of appropriate agencies: medical director, institutional review board(s), head of service
- Inclusion and exclusion criteria
- Effect on patient care in general
- Risks and potential benefits to patients in study

researchers are evaluating. You also need to know the name of the principal investigator and how to contact him or her. This is usually, though not always, a physician. Many EMS physicians who conduct field research will recruit a field provider to coordinate and assist with data collection. A good **principal investigator** (PI) will meet with the EMS providers who are administering the study intervention and collecting the data. The PI should make sure you know how long the study is expected to last. This allows you to make plans and perhaps re-schedule certain activities you had anticipated in the future. The PI should also inform you about the type of study (e.g., case-control or randomized controlled trial), how data collection will take place (will you have to fill out any more forms?), how patients will be assigned to the study and control groups, and which intervention you will be administering (including placebos). The PI should be able to tell you that the study has the approval of the appropriate agencies, including the medical director, the head of the service, and an **institutional review board** (IRB). An IRB is a group of people, usually at a hospital or university, who review study proposals to insure that patients are protected when they participate in research as study subjects. Other things to find out include the inclusion and exclusion criteria for enrolling patients in the study, the effect of the study on patient care in general, and the risks and potential benefits to patients in the study. Once you understand these factors, you will be prepared to participate in the study.

LEARNING MORE ABOUT RESEARCH

There are many ways you can learn more about interpreting and conducting research. Two methods in particular are aimed at prehospital providers. Ferno-Washington of Wilmington, Ohio, published a manual in 1994 by James Menegazzi called *Research: The Who, What, Why, When, and How . . .* It is an excellent introduction to this topic and includes the proceedings of the 1992 Winter Assembly of the National Association of EMS Physicians on Research in Prehospital Care Systems. Another excellent source of information for EMS providers is the *EMS Journal Club*. This is a monthly publication which collects articles of EMS interest from many different journals and summarizes them. It comes with an audio tape of a paramedic and an EMS physician discussing the articles. They describe the good points and the shortcomings of the articles and suggest ways to interpret their results.

A number of peer-reviewed medical journals publish articles regarding prehospital care. Two that publish many such articles are *Prehospital Emergency Care* and *Annals of Emergency Medicine*.

Sometimes the *New England Journal of Medicine* and the *Journal of the American Medical Association* also publish articles of an EMS nature. All of these journals should be available at the library of your local hospital or medical school.

For the advanced reader who is not afraid of a challenge, there is *Emergency Medical Abstracts*. This is a monthly collection of forty abstracts of articles pertaining to emergency medicine. Only a few of the articles are directly related to EMS, but for the interested reader the real prize is the audio tape that comes with the abstracts. On the tape, two emergency physicians discuss the abstracts for that month in an educational and frequently humorous fashion. The frequent criticisms of the methodologies used in the articles can enlighten even the most experienced clinician.

An excellent book for those interested in learning about research methodology is *Studying a Study and Testing a Test: How to Read the Medical Literature* by Richard Riegelman and Robert Hirsch. It includes a great deal more information about many of the topics discussed above.

Probably the most humorous book you will ever see about statistics is *PDQ Statistics* by Geoffrey Norman and David Streiner. This book does not go into detail about how to calculate statistics, but instead concentrates on describing these tests in lay terms so that the reader can gain a fuller understanding of what statisticians do.

Finally, talk to others who have an interest in research. Emergency physicians are an especially good source of information about what is new and how to interpret it. EMS is performed by teams and learning how to do it better is often best done in teams, too.

More information on the sources mentioned above:

Emergency Medical Abstracts. Center for Medical Education, P.O. Box 600, Creamery, PA 19430. Phone 1-800-458-4779.

EMS Journal Club. Department of Emergency Medicine, SUNY Health Science Center, 750 East Adams Street, Syracuse, NY 13210. Phone 1-800-755-3675.

Menegazzi, J. Research: *The Who, What, Why, When, and How*. Ferno-Washington, Wilmington, Ohio, 1994.

Norman, G.R., and D.L. Streiner. *PDQ Statistics*. B. C. Decker Inc., 1986.

Riegelman, R.K., and R.P. Hirsch. *Studying a Study and Testing a Test: How to Read the Medical Literature,* Third Edition. Little, Brown and Company, 1996.

APPENDIX B

NATIONAL REGISTRY PRACTICAL EXAMINATION

The National Registry of Emergency Medical Technicians is an organization founded in 1970, one of whose goals is to establish nationwide professional standards for EMTs. Many state EMS systems use examinations developed by the National Registry to establish certification of EMTs.

The National Registry has prepared a certification examination correlated to the 1994 Department of Transportation Emergency Medical Technician-Basic: National Standard Curriculum. The examination includes both a written portion and a practical portion that consists of a series of performance-based skill stations.

To assist students in preparing for the skill stations that are part of the EMT-Basic examination, as well as to establish guidelines and parameters for those who will evaluate students' performance at the skill stations, the National Registry has developed a series of skill sheets. Each skill sheet contains a set of directions, the skill criteria, and the critical criteria that if not met by the student result in immediate failure of the station.

In studying for the National Registry examination, you should use these skills sheets in conjunction with the material presented in the textbook and not as the sole means of learning the individual skills. The skill sheets will aid you in organizing the steps necessary to perform each skill and in identifying the criteria that will be used to evaluate your performance. You can use these sheets to evaluate your own performance when practicing these skills and preparing for your practical skills evaluation.

Note: Three skill sheets regarding advanced airway management are included. The use of these skills will vary based on your medical director, training program, and local protocol.

ORGANIZATION OF THE NATIONAL REGISTRY EXAMINATION

The practical examination consists of six stations, five mandatory stations and one random basic skill station consisting of both skill-based and scenario-based testing. The random skill station is conducted so the candidate is totally unaware of the skill to be tested until he or she arrives at the test site.

The candidate will be tested individually in each station and will be expected to direct the actions of any assistant EMTs who may be present in the station. The candidate should pass or fail the examination based solely on his or her actions and decisions.

On page 522 is a list of the stations and their established time limits. The maximum time is determined by the number and difficulty of tasks to be completed.

INSTRUCTIONS TO THE CANDIDATE
PATIENT ASSESSMENT/MANAGEMENT–TRAUMA

This station is designed to test your ability to perform a patient assessment of a victim of multi-system trauma and voice-treat all conditions and injuries discovered. You must conduct your assessment as you would in the field, including communicating with your patient. You may remove the patient's clothing down to shorts or swimsuit if you feel it is necessary. As you conduct your assessment, you should state everything you are assessing. Clinical information not obtainable by visual or physical inspection, for example, blood pressure, will be given to you after you demonstrate how you would normally gain that information. You may assume that you have two EMTs working with you and that they are correctly carrying out the verbal treatments you indicate. You have (10) ten minutes to complete this skill station. Do you have any questions?

PATIENT ASSESSMENT/MANAGEMENT– MEDICAL

This station is designed to test your ability to perform a patient assessment of a victim with a chief complaint of a medical nature and voice-treat all conditions and injuries discovered. You must conduct your assessment as you would in the field including communicating with your patient. As you conduct your assessment, you should state everything you are assessing. Clinical information not obtainable by visual or physical inspection, for example, blood pressure, will be given to you after you demonstrate how you would normally gain that information. You may assume that you have two EMTs working with you and that they are correctly carrying out the verbal treatments you indicate. You have (10) ten minutes to complete this skill station. Do you have any questions?

CARDIAC ARREST MANAGEMENT/AED

This station is designed to test your ability to manage a pre-hospital cardiac arrest by integrating CPR skills, defibrillation, airway adjuncts, and patient/scene management skills. There will be an EMT assistant in this station. The EMT assistant will only do as you instruct him. As you arrive on the scene you will encounter a patient in cardiac arrest. A first responder will be present performing single rescuer CPR. You must immediately establish control of the scene and begin resuscitation of the patient with an automated external defibrillator. At the appropriate time, you must control the airway and ventilate the patient using adjunctive equipment. You may not delegate this action to the EMT assistant. You may use any of the supplies available in this room. You have (15) fifteen minutes to complete this skill station. Do you have any questions?

AIRWAY, OXYGEN, VENTILATION SKILLS BAG-VALVE-MASK APNEIC PATIENT WITH PULSE

This station is designed to test your ability to ventilate a patient using a bag-valve-mask. As you enter the station you will find an apneic patient with a palpable central pulse. There are no bystanders and artificial ventilation has not been initiated. The only patient intervention required is airway management and ventilatory support using a bag-valve-mask. You must initially ventilate the patient for a minimum of 30 seconds. You will be evaluated on the appropriateness of ventilator volumes. I will inform you that a second rescuer has arrived and will instruct you that you must control the airway and the mask seal while the second rescuer provides ventilation. You may use only the equipment available in this room. You have (5) five minutes to complete this procedure. Do you have any questions?

SPINAL IMMOBILIZATION–SUPINE PATIENT

This station is designed to test your ability to provide spinal immobilization on a patient using a long spine immobilization device. You arrive on the scene with an EMT assistant. The assistant EMT has completed the scene size-up as well as the initial and focused assessments. As you begin the station there are no airway, breathing, or circulatory problems. You are required to treat the specific, isolated problem of an unstable spine using a long spine immobilization device. When moving the patient to the device, you should use the help of the assistant EMT and the evaluator. The assistant EMT should control the head and cervical spine of the patient while you and the evaluator move the patient to the immobilization device. You are responsible for the direction and subsequent action of the EMT assistant. You may use any equipment available in this room. You have (10) ten minutes to complete this procedure. Do you have any questions?

SPINAL IMMOBILIZATION–SEATED PATIENT

This station is designed to test your ability to provide spinal immobilization on a patient using a half spine immobilization device. You arrive on the scene with an EMT assistant. The assistant EMT has completed the scene size-up, initial and focused assessments. As you begin the station, there are no airway, breathing, or circulatory problems. You are required to treat the specific, isolated problem of an unstable spine using a half spine immobilization device. Continued assessment of airway, breathing, and central circulation is not necessary. You are responsible for the direction and subsequent actions of the EMT assistant.

Transferring the patient to the long spine board should be accomplished verbally. You may use any equipment available in this room. You have (10) ten minutes to complete this procedure. Do you have any questions?

Station 1:	Patient Assessment/Management—Trauma	10 min
Station 2:	Patient Assessment/Management—Medical	10 min
Station 3:	Cardiac Arrest Management/AED	15 min
Station 4:	Bag-Valve-Mask Apneic Patient	10 min
Station 5:	Spinal Immobilization Station	
	Spinal Immobilization—Supine Patient	10 min
	Spinal Immobilization—Seated Patient	10 min
Station 6:	Random Basic Skill Verification	
	Long Bone Injury	5 min
	Joint Injury	5 min
	Traction Splint	10 min
	Bleeding Control/Shock Management	10 min
	Upper Airway Adjuncts and Suction	5 min
	Mouth-to-Mask with Supplemental Oxygen	5 min
	Supplemental Oxygen Administration	5 min

IMMOBILIZATION—LONG BONE INJURY

This station is designed to test your ability to properly immobilize a closed, non-angulated long bone injury. You are required to treat only the specific, isolated injury. The scene size-up and initial assessment have been completed and during the focused assessment a closed, non-angulated injury of the _____ (radius, ulna, tibia, fibula) was detected. Ongoing assessment of the patient's airway, breathing, and central circulation is not necessary. You may use any equipment available in this room. You have (5) five minutes to complete this procedure. Do you have any questions?

IMMOBILIZATION—JOINT INJURY

This station is designed to test your ability to properly immobilize a non-complicated shoulder injury. You are required to treat only the specific, isolated injury. The scene size-up and initial assessment have been accomplished on the patient and during the focused assessment a shoulder injury was detected. Ongoing assessment of the patient's airway, breathing, and central circulation is not necessary. You may use any equipment available in this room. You have (5) five minutes to complete this procedure. Do you have any questions?

IMMOBILIZATION—0TRACTION SPLINTING

This station is designed to test your ability to properly immobilize a mid-shaft femur injury with a traction splint. You will have an EMT assistant to help you in the application of the device by applying manual traction when directed to do so. You are required to treat only the specific, isolated injury. The scene size-up and initial assessment have been accomplished on the patient, and during the focused assessment a mid-shaft femur deformity was detected. Ongoing assessment of the patient's airway, breathing, and central circulation is not necessary. You may use any equipment available in this room. You have (10) ten minutes to complete this procedure. Do you have any questions?

BLEEDING CONTROL/SHOCK MANAGEMENT

This station is designed to test your ability to control hemorrhage. This is a scenario-based testing station. As you progress through the scenario, you will be offered various signs and symptoms appropriate for the patient's condition. You will be required to manage the patient based on these signs and symptoms. A scenario will be read aloud to you, and you will be given an opportunity to ask clarifying questions about the scenario; however, you will not receive answers to any questions about the actual steps of the procedures to be performed. You may use any of the supplies and equipment available in this room. You have (10) ten minutes to complete this skill station. Do you have any questions?

AIRWAY, OXYGEN, VENTILATION SKILLS
UPPER AIRWAY ADJUNCTS AND SUCTION

This station is designed to test your ability to properly measure, insert, and remove an oropharyngeal and a nasopharyngeal airway as well as suction a patient's upper airway. This is an isolated skills test comprised of three separate skills. You may use any equipment available in this room. You have (5) five minutes to complete this skill station. Do you have any questions?

AIRWAY, OXYGEN, VENTILATION SKILLS MOUTH-TO-MASK WITH SUPPLEMENTAL OXYGEN

This station is designed to test your ability to ventilate a patient with supplemental oxygen using a mouth-to-mask technique. This is an isolated skills test. You may assume that mouth-to-mouth ventilation is in progress and that the patient has a central pulse. The only patient management required is ventilatory support using a mouth-to-mask technique with supplemental oxygen. You must ventilate the patient for at least 30 seconds. You will be evaluated on the appropriateness of ventilatory volumes. You may use any equipment available in this room. You have (5) five minutes to complete this skill station. Do you have any questions?

AIRWAY, OXYGEN, VENTILATION SKILLS SUPPLEMENTAL OXYGEN ADMINISTRATION

This station is designed to test your ability to correctly assemble the equipment needed to administer supplemental oxygen in the pre-hospital setting. This is an isolated skills test. You will be required to assemble an oxygen tank and regulator and administer oxygen to a patient using a nonrebreather mask. At this point you will be instructed to discontinue oxygen administration by the nonrebreather mask because the patient cannot tolerate the mask and start oxygen administration using a nasal cannula. Once you have initiated oxygen administration using a nasal cannula, you will be instructed to discontinue oxygen administration completely. You may use only the equipment available in this room. You have (5) five minutes to complete this skill station. Do you have any questions?

PATIENT ASSESSMENT/MANAGEMENT—TRAUMA

Start Time: _____
Stop Time: _____ Date: _____
Candidate's Name: _____
Evaluator's Name: _____

	Points Possible	Points Awarded
Takes, or verbalizes, body substance isolation precautions	1	
SCENE SIZE-UP		
Determines the scene is safe	1	
Determines the mechanism of injury	1	
Determines the number of patients	1	
Requests additional help if necessary	1	
Considers stabilization of spine	1	
INITIAL ASSESSMENT		
Verbalizes general impression of patient	1	
Determines responsiveness/level of consciousness	1	
Determines chief complaint/apparent life threats	1	
Assesses airway and breathing — Assessment	1	
Assesses airway and breathing — Initiates appropriate oxygen therapy	1	
Assesses airway and breathing — Assures adequate ventilation	1	
Assesses airway and breathing — Injury management	1	
Assesses circulation — Assesses/controls major bleeding	1	
Assesses circulation — Assesses pulse	1	
Assesses circulation — Assesses skin (color, temperature, and condition)	1	
Identifies priority patients/makes transport decision	1	
FOCUSED HISTORY AND PHYSICAL EXAM/RAPID TRAUMA ASSESSMENT		
Selects appropriate assessment (*focused or rapid assessment*)	1	
Obtains or directs assistant to obtain baseline vital signs	1	
Obtains S.A.M.P.L.E. history	1	
DETAILED PHYSICAL EXAMINATION		
Assesses the head — Inspects and palpates the scalp and ears	1	
Assesses the head — Assesses the eyes	1	
Assesses the head — Assesses the facial areas including oral and nasal areas	1	
Assesses the neck — Inspects and palpates the neck	1	
Assesses the neck — Assesses for JVD	1	
Assesses the neck — Assesses for tracheal deviation	1	
Assesses the chest — Inspects	1	
Assesses the chest — Palpates	1	
Assesses the chest — Auscultates	1	
Assesses the abdomen/pelvis — Assesses the abdomen	1	
Assesses the abdomen/pelvis — Assesses the pelvis	1	
Assesses the abdomen/pelvis — Verbalizes assessment of genitalia/perineum as needed	1	
Assesses the extremities — 1 point for each extremity	4	
includes inspection, palpation, and assessment of motor, sensory and circulatory function		
Assesses the posterior — Assesses thorax	1	
Assesses the posterior — Assesses lumbar	1	
Manages secondary injuries and wounds appropriately		
1 point for **appropriate management** of secondary injury/wound	1	
Verbalizes re-assessment of the vital signs	1	
	Total: 40	

Critical Criteria

____ Did not take, or verbalize, body substance isolation precautions
____ Did not determine scene safety
____ Did not assess for spinal protection
____ Did not provide for spinal protection when indicated
____ Did not provide high concentration of oxygen
____ Did not find, or manage, problems associated with airway, breathing, hemorrhage or shock (hypoperfusion)
____ Did not differentiate patient's need for transportation versus continued assessment at the scene
____ Did other detailed physical examination before assessing airway, breathing, and circulation
____ Did not transport patient within (10) minute time limit

PATIENT ASSESSMENT/MANAGEMENT—MEDICAL

Start Time: _____
Stop Time: _____ Date: _____
Candidate's Name: _____
Evaluator's Name: _____

	Points Possible	Points Awarded
Takes, or verbalizes, body substance isolation precautions	1	
SCENE SIZE-UP		
Determines the scene is safe	1	
Determines the mechanism of injury/nature of illness	1	
Determines the number of patients	1	
Requests additional help if necessary	1	
Considers stabilization of spine	1	
INITIAL ASSESSMENT		
Verbalizes general impression of patient	1	
Determines responsiveness/level of consciousness	1	
Determines chief complaint/apparent life threats	1	
Assesses airway and breathing — Assessment	1	
Assesses airway and breathing — Initiates appropriate oxygen therapy	1	
Assesses airway and breathing — Assures adequate ventilation	1	
Assesses circulation — Assesses/controls major bleeding	1	
Assesses circulation — Assesses pulse	1	
Assesses circulation — Assesses skin (color, temperature, and condition)	1	
Identifies priority patients/makes transport decision	1	

FOCUSED HISTORY AND PHYSICAL EXAM/RAPID ASSESSMENT

Signs and symptoms (*Assesses history of present illness*)

Respiratory	Cardiac	Altered Mental Status	Allergic Reaction	Poisoning/ Overdose	Environmental Emergency	Obstetrics	Behavioral
•Onset?	•Onset?	•Description of the episode	•History of allergies?	•Substance?	•Source?	•Are you pregnant?	•How do you feel?
•Provokes?	•Provokes?	•Onset?	•What were you exposed to?	•When did you ingest/become exposed?	•Environment?	•How long have you been pregnant?	•Determine suicidal tendencies
•Quality?	•Quality?	•Duration?	•How were you exposed?	•How much did you ingest?	•Duration?	•Pain or contractions?	•Is the patient a threat to self or others?
•Radiates?	•Radiates?	•Associated symptoms?	•Effects?	•Over what time period?	•Loss of consciousness?	•Bleeding or discharge?	•Is there a medical problem?
•Severity?	•Severity?	•Evidence of trauma?	•Progression?	•Interventions?	•Effects— General or local?	•Do you feel the need to push?	•Interventions?
•Time?	•Time?	•Interventions?	•Interventions?	•Estimated weight?		•Last menstrual period?	
•Interventions?	•Interventions?	•Seizures?					
		•Fever?					

	Points Possible	Points Awarded
Signs and symptoms row	1	
Allergies	1	
Medications	1	
Past pertinent history	1	
Last oral intake	1	
Events leading to present illness (rule out trauma)	1	
Performs focused physical examination	1	
(assesses *affected body part/system* or, if indicated, completes *rapid assessment*)		
Vitals (obtains baseline vital signs)	1	
Interventions (obtains medical direction or verbalizes standing orders for medication interventions and verbalizes proper additional intervention/treatment)	1	
Transport (re-evaluates transport decision)	1	
Verbalizes the consideration for completing a detailed physical examination	1	
ONGOING ASSESSMENT (verbalized)		
Repeats initial assessment	1	
Repeats vital signs	1	
Repeats focused assessment regarding patient complaint or injuries	1	
	Total: 30	

Critical Criteria

____ Did not take, or verbalize, body substance isolation precautions when necessary
____ Did not determine scene safety
____ Did not obtain medical direction or verbalize standing orders for medication interventions
____ Did not provide high concentration of oxygen
____ Did not find or manage problems associated with airway, breathing, hemorrhage or shock (hypoperfusion)
____ Did not differentiate patient's need for transportation versus continued assessment at the scene
____ Did detailed or focused history/physical examination before assessing airway, breathing and circulation
____ Did not ask questions about the present illness
____ Administered a dangerous or inappropriate intervention

CARDIAC ARREST MANAGEMENT/AED

Start Time: _____
Stop Time: _____
Candidate's Name: _____ Date: _____
Evaluator's Name: _____

	Points Possible	Points Awarded
ASSESSMENT		
Takes, or verbalizes, body substance isolation precautions	1	
Briefly questions the rescuer about arrest events	1	
Directs rescuer to stop CPR	1	
Verifies absence of spontaneous pulse **(skill station examiner states "no pulse")**	1	
Directs resumption of CPR	1	
Turns on defibrillator power	1	
Attaches automated defibrillator to the patient	1	
Directs rescuer to stop CPR and ensures all individuals are clear of the patient	1	
Initiates analysis of the rhythm	1	
Delivers shock (up to three successive shocks)	1	
Verifies absence of spontaneous pulse **(skill station examiner states "no pulse")**	1	
TRANSITION		
Directs resumption of CPR	1	
Gathers additional information about arrest event	1	
Confirms effectiveness of CPR (ventilation and compressions)	1	
INTEGRATION		
Verbalizes or directs insertion of a simple airway adjunct (oral/nasal airway)	1	
Ventilates, or directs ventilation of, the patient	1	
Assures high concentration of oxygen is delivered to the patient	1	
Assures CPR continues without unnecessary/prolonged interruption	1	
Re-evaluates patient/CPR in approximately one minute	1	
Repeats defibrillator sequence		
TRANSPORTATION		
Verbalizes transportation of patient	1	
Total:	21	

Critical Criteria

_____ Did not take, or verbalize, body substance isolation precautions
_____ Did not evaluate the need for immediate use of the AED
_____ Did not direct initiation/resumption of ventilation/compressions at appropriate times
_____ Did not assure all individuals were clear of patient before delivering each shock
_____ Did not operate the AED properly (inability to deliver shock)
_____ Prevented the defibrillator from delivering indicated stacked shocks

---

BAG-VALVE-MASK
APNEIC PATIENT

Start Time: _____
Stop Time: _____
Candidate's Name: _____
Evaluator's Name: _____ Date: _____

	Points Possible	Points Awarded
Takes, or verbalizes, body substance isolation precautions	1	
Voices opening the airway	1	
Voices inserting an airway adjunct	1	
Selects appropriately sized mask	1	
Creates a proper mask-to-face seal	1	
Ventilates patient at no less than 800 ml volume *(The examiner must witness for at least 30 seconds)*	1	
Connects reservoir and oxygen	1	
Adjusts liter flow to 15 liters/minute or greater	1	
The examiner indicates the arrival of second EMT. The second EMT is instructed to ventilate the patient while the candidate controls the mask and the airway.		
Voices re-opening the airway	1	
Creates a proper mask-to-face seal	1	
Instructs assistant to resume ventilation at proper volume per breath *(The examiner must witness for at least 30 seconds)*	1	
Total:	11	

Critical Criteria

_____ Did not take, or verbalize, body substance isolation precautions
_____ Did not immediately ventilate the patient
_____ Interrupted ventilations for more than 20 seconds
_____ Did not provide high concentration of oxygen
_____ Did not provide, or direct assistant to provide, proper volume/breath *(more than two(2) ventilations per minute are below 800 ml)*
_____ Did not allow adequate exhalation

SPINAL IMMOBILIZATION
SUPINE PATIENT

Start Time: _____ Date: _____
Stop Time: _____
Candidate's Name: _____
Evaluator's Name: _____

	Points Possible	Points Awarded
Takes, or verbalizes, body substance isolation precautions	1	
Directs assistant to place/maintain head in neutral in-line position	1	
Directs assistant to maintain manual immobilization of the head	1	
Re-assesses motor, sensory and circulatory function in each extremity	1	
Applies appropriately sized extrication collar	1	
Positions the immobilization device appropriately	1	
Directs movement of the patient onto the device without compromising the integrity of the spine	1	
Applies padding to voids between the torso and the board as necessary	1	
Immobilizes the patient's torso to the device	1	
Evaluates the pads behind the patient's head as necessary	1	
Immobilizes the patient's head to the device	1	
Secures the patient's legs to the device	1	
Secures the patient's arms to the device	1	
Reassesses motor, sensory and circulatory function in each extremity	1	
Total:	14	

Critical Criteria

____ Did not immediately direct, or take, manual immobilization of the head
____ Released, or ordered release of, manual immobilization before it was maintained mechanically
____ Patient manipulated, or moved excessively, causing potential spinal compromise
____ Patient moves excessively up, down, left or right on the patient's torso
____ Head immobilization allows for excessive movement
____ Upon completion of immobilization, head is not in the neutral position
____ Did not reassess motor, sensory, and circulatory function in each extremity after immobilization to the device
____ Immobilized head to the board before securing the torso

SPINAL IMMOBILIZATION
SEATED PATIENT

Start Time: _____ Date: _____
Stop Time: _____
Candidate's Name: _____
Evaluator's Name: _____

	Points Possible	Points Awarded
Takes, or verbalizes, body substance isolation precautions	1	
Directs assistant to place/maintain head in neutral in-line position	1	
Directs assistant to maintain manual immobilization of the head	1	
Reassesses motor, sensory and circulatory function in each extremity	1	
Applies appropriately sized extrication collar	1	
Positions the immobilization device behind the patient	1	
Secures the device to the patient's torso	1	
Evaluates torso fixation and adjusts as necessary	1	
Evaluates and pads behind the patient's head as necessary	1	
Secures the patient's head to the device	1	
Verbalizes moving the patient to a long board	1	
Reassesses motor, sensory and circulatory function in each extremity	1	
Total:	12	

Critical Criteria

____ Did not immediately direct, or take, manual immobilization of the head
____ Released, or ordered release of, manual immobilization before it was maintained mechanically
____ Patient manipulated, or moved excessively, causing potential spinal compromise
____ Device moved excessively up, down, left or right on patient's torso
____ Head immobilization allows for excessive movement
____ Torso fixation inhibits chest rise, resulting in respiratory compromise
____ Upon completion of immobilization, head is not in the neutral position
____ Did not reassess motor, sensory and circulatory function in each extremity after voicing immobilization to the long board
____ Immobilized head to the board before securing the torso

IMMOBILIZATION SKILLS
LONG BONE INJURY

Start Time: _____
Stop Time: _____
Candidate's Name: _____ Date: _____
Evaluator's Name: _____

	Points Possible	Points Awarded
Takes, or verbalizes, body substance isolation precautions	1	
Directs application of manual stabilization of the injury	1	
Assesses motor, sensory and circulatory function in the injured extremity	1	
Note: The examiner acknowledges "motor, sensory and circulatory function are present and normal."		
Measures the splint	1	
Applies the splint	1	
Immobilizes the joint above the injury site	1	
Immobilizes the joint below the injury site	1	
Secures the entire injured extremity	1	
Immobilizes the hand/foot in the position of function	1	
Reassesses motor, sensory and circulatory function in the injured extremity	1	
Note: The examiner acknowledges "motor, sensory and circulatory function are present and normal."		
Total:	10	

Critical Criteria

____ Grossly moves the injured extremity
____ Did not immobilize the joint above and the joint below the injury site
____ Did not reassess motor, sensory and circulatory function in the injured extremity before and after splinting

---

IMMOBILIZATION SKILLS
JOINT INJURY

Start Time: _____
Stop Time: _____
Candidate's Name: _____ Date: _____
Evaluator's Name: _____

	Points Possible	Points Awarded
Takes, or verbalizes, body substance isolation precautions	1	
Directs application of manual stabilization of the shoulder injury	1	
Assesses motor, sensory and circulatory function in the injured extremity	1	
Note: The examiner acknowledges "motor, sensory and circulatory function are present and normal."		
Selects the proper splinting material	1	
Immobilizes the site of the injury	1	
Immobilizes the bone above the injured joint	1	
Immobilizes the bone below the injured joint	1	
Reassesses motor, sensory and circulatory function in the injured extremity	1	
Note: The examiner acknowledges "motor, sensory and circulatory function are present and normal."		
Total:	8	

Critical Criteria

____ Did not support the joint so that the joint did not bear distal weight
____ Did not immobilize the bone above and below the injured site
____ Did not reassess motor, sensory and circulatory function in the injured extremity before and after splinting

IMMOBILIZATION SKILLS
TRACTION SPLINTING

Start Time: _____

Stop Time: _____ Date: _____

Candidate's Name: _____

Evaluator's Name: _____

	Points Possible	Points Awarded
Takes, or verbalizes, body substance isolation precautions	1	
Directs application of manual stabilization of the injured leg	1	
Directs the application of manual traction	1	
Assesses motor, sensory and circulatory function in the injured extremity	1	
Note: The examiner acknowledges "motor, sensory and circulatory function are present and normal"		
Prepares/adjusts splint to the proper length	1	
Positions the splint next to the injured leg	1	
Applies the proximal securing device (e.g., ischial strap)	1	
Applies the distal securing device (e.g., ankle hitch)	1	
Applies mechanical traction	1	
Positions/secures the support straps	1	
Re-evaluates the proximal/distal securing devices	1	
Reassesses motor, sensory and circulatory function in the injured extremity	1	
Note: The examiner acknowledges "motor, sensory and circulatory function are present and normal"		
Note: The examiner must ask the candidate how he/she would prepare the patient for transportation		
Verbalizes securing the torso to the long board to immobilize the hip	1	
Verbalizes securing the splint to the long board to prevent movement of the splint	1	
Total:	**14**	

Critical Criteria

____ Loss of traction at any point after it was applied

____ Did not reassess motor, sensory and circulatory function in the injured extremity before and after splinting

____ The foot was excessively rotated or extended after splint was applied

____ Did not secure the ischial strap before taking traction

____ Final immobilization failed to support the femur or prevent rotation of the injured leg

____ Secured the leg to the splint before applying mechanical traction

Note: If the Sagar splint or the Kendricks Traction Device is used without elevating the patient's leg, application of manual traction is not necessary. The candidate should be awarded one (1) point as if manual traction were applied.

Note: If the leg is elevated at all, manual traction must be applied before elevating the leg. The ankle hitch may be applied before elevating the leg and used to provide manual traction.

BLEEDING CONTROL/SHOCK MANAGEMENT

Start Time: _____

Stop Time: _____ Date: _____

Candidate's Name: _____

Evaluator's Name: _____

	Points Possible	Points Awarded
Takes, or verbalizes, body substance isolation precautions	1	
Applies direct pressure to the wound	1	
Elevates the extremity	1	
Note: The examiner must now inform the candidate that the wound continues to bleed.		
Applies an additional dressing to the wound	1	
Note: The examiner must now inform the candidate that the wound still continues to bleed. The second dressing does not control the bleeding.		
Locates and applies pressure to appropriate arterial pressure point	1	
Note: The examiner must now inform the candidate that the bleeding is controlled.		
Bandages the wound	1	
Note: The examiner must now inform the candidate that the patient is now showing signs and symptoms indicative of hypoperfusion.		
Properly positions the patient	1	
Applies high concentration oxygen	1	
Initiates steps to prevent heat loss from the patient	1	
Indicates the need for immediate transportation	1	
Total:	**10**	

Critical Criteria

____ Did not take, or verbalize, body substance isolation precautions

____ Did not apply high concentration of oxygen

____ Applied a tourniquet before attempting other methods of bleeding control

____ Did not control hemorrhage in a timely manner

____ Did not indicate a need for immediate transportation

AIRWAY, OXYGEN, AND VENTILATION SKILLS
UPPER AIRWAY ADJUNCTS AND SUCTION

OROPHARYNGEAL AIRWAY

Start Time: _____ Date: _____
Stop Time: _____
Candidate's Name: _____
Evaluator's Name: _____

	Points Possible	Points Awarded
Takes, or verbalizes, body substance isolation precautions	1	
Selects appropriately sized airway	1	
Measures airway	1	
Inserts airway without pushing the tongue posteriorly	1	
Note: The examiner must advise the candidate that the patient is gagging and becoming conscious.		
Removes the oropharyngeal airway	1	

SUCTION

NOTE: The examiner must advise the candidate to suction the patient's airway.

	Points Possible	Points Awarded
Turns on/prepares suction device	1	
Assures presence of mechanical suction	1	
Inserts the suction tip without suction	1	
Applies suction to the oropharynx/nasopharynx	1	

NASOPHARYNGEAL AIRWAY

NOTE: The examiner must advise the candidate to insert a nasopharyngeal airway.

	Points Possible	Points Awarded
Selects appropriately sized airway	1	
Measures airway	1	
Verbalizes lubrication of the nasal airway	1	
Fully inserts the airway with the bevel facing toward the septum	1	
Total:	13	

Critical Criteria

___ Did not take, or verbalize, body substance isolation precautions
___ Did not obtain a patent airway with the oropharyngeal airway
___ Did not obtain a patent airway with the nasopharyngeal airway
___ Did not demonstrate an acceptable suction technique
___ Inserted any adjunct in a manner dangerous to the patient

MOUTH TO MASK WITH SUPPLEMENTAL OXYGEN

Start Time: _____ Date: _____
Stop Time: _____
Candidate's Name: _____
Evaluator's Name: _____

	Points Possible	Points Awarded
Takes, or verbalizes, body substance isolation precautions	1	
Connects one-way valve to mask	1	
Opens patient's airway or confirms patient's airway is open (manually or with adjunct)	1	
Establishes and maintains a proper mask to face seal	1	
Ventilates the patient at the proper volume and rate *(800–1200 ml per breath/10–20 breaths per minute)*	1	
Connects mask to high concentration of oxygen	1	
Adjusts flow rate to at least 15 liters per minute	1	
Continues ventilation of the patient at the proper volume and rate *(800–1200 ml per breath/10–20 breaths per minute)*	1	
Note: The examiner must witness ventilations for at least 30 seconds		
Total:	8	

Critical Criteria

___ Did not take, or verbalize, body substance isolation precautions
___ Did not adjust liter flow to at least 15 liters per minute
___ Did not provide proper volume per breath *(more than 2 ventilations per minute were below 800 ml)*
___ Did not ventilate the patient at a rate of 10–20 breaths per minute
___ Did not allow for complete exhalation

OXYGEN ADMINISTRATION

Start Time: _____
Stop Time: _____ Date: _____
Candidate's Name: _____
Evaluator's Name: _____

	Points Possible	Points Awarded
Takes, or verbalizes, body substance isolation precautions	1	
Assembles the regulator to the tank	1	
Opens the tank	1	
Checks for leaks	1	
Checks tank pressure	1	
Attaches non-rebreather mask to oxygen	1	
Prefills reservoir	1	
Adjusts liter flow to 12 liters per minute or greater	1	
Applies and adjusts the mask to the patient's face	1	
Note: The examiner must advise the candidate that the patient is not tolerating the nonre-breather mask. The medical director has ordered you to apply a nasal cannula to the patient.		
Attaches nasal cannula to oxygen	1	
Adjusts liter flow to six (6) liters per minute or less	1	
Applies nasal cannula to the patient	1	
Note: The examiner must advise the candidate to discontinue oxygen therapy		
Removes the nasal cannula from the patient	1	
Shuts off the regulator	1	
Relieves the pressure within the regulator	1	
Total:	**15**	

Critical Criteria

____ Did not take, or verbalize, body substance isolation precautions
____ Did not assemble the tank and regulator without leaks
____ Did not prefill the reservoir bag
____ Did not adjust the device to the correct liter flow for the non-rebreather mask (12 liters per minute or greater)
____ Did not adjust the device to the correct liter flow for the nasal cannula (6 liters per minute or less)

VENTILATORY MANAGEMENT
ENDOTRACHEAL INTUBATION

Start Time: _____
Stop Time: _____ Date: _____
Candidate's Name: _____
Evaluator's Name: _____

*Note: If a candidate elects to initially ventilate the patient with a BVM attached to a reservoir and oxygen, full credit must be awarded for steps denoted by "**" provided the first ventilation is delivered within the initial 30 seconds*

	Points Possible	Points Awarded
Takes or verbalizes body substance isolation precautions	1	
Opens the airway manually	1	
Elevates the patient's tongue and inserts a simple airway adjunct (oropharyngeal/nasopharyngeal airway)	1	
Note: The examiner must now inform the candidate "no gag reflex is present and the patient accepts the airway adjunct."		
**Ventilates the patient immediately using a BVM device unattached to oxygen	1	
**Hyperventilates the patient with room air	1	
Note: The examiner must now inform the candidate that ventilation is being properly performed without difficulty		
Attaches the oxygen reservoir to the BVM	1	
Attaches the BVM to high flow oxygen (15 liters per minute)	1	
Ventilates the patient at the proper volume and rate (800-1200 ml/breath and 10-20 breaths/minute)	1	
Note: After 30 seconds, the examiner must auscultate the patient's chest and inform the candidate that breath sounds are present and equal bilaterally and medical direction has ordered endotracheal intubation. The examiner must now take over ventilation of the patient.		
Directs assistant to hyper-oxygenate the patient	1	
Identifies/selects the proper equipment for endotracheal intubation	1	
Checks equipment — Checks for cuff leaks	1	
— Checks laryngoscope operation and bulb tightness	1	
Note: The examiner must remove the OPA and move out of the way when the candidate is prepared to intubate the patient.		
Positions the patient's head properly	1	
Inserts the laryngoscope blade into the patient's mouth while displacing the patient's tongue laterally	1	
Elevates the patient's mandible with the laryngoscope	1	
Introduces the endotracheal tube and advances the tube to the proper depth	1	
Inflates the cuff to the proper pressure	1	
Disconnects the syringe from the cuff inlet port	1	
Directs assistant to ventilate the patient	1	
Confirms proper placement of the endotracheal tube by auscultation bilaterally and over the epigastrium	1	
Note: The examiner must ask, "If you had proper placement, what would you expect to hear?"		
Secures the endotracheal tube (may be verbalized)	1	
Total:	**21**	

Critical Criteria

____ Did not take or verbalize body substance isolation precautions when necessary
____ Did not initiate ventilation within 30 seconds after applying gloves or interrupts ventilations for greater than 30 seconds at any time
____ Did not voice or provide high oxygen concentrations (15 liter/minute or greater)
____ Did not ventilate the patient at a rate of at least 10 breaths per minute
____ Did not provide adequate volume per breath (maximum of 2 errors per minute permissible)
____ Did not hyper-oxygenate the patient prior to intubation
____ Did not successfully intubate the patient within 3 attempts
____ Used the patient's teeth as a fulcrum
____ Did not assure proper tube placement by auscultation bilaterally over each lung **and** over the epigastrium
____ The stylette (if used) extended beyond the end of the endotracheal tube
____ Inserted any adjunct in a manner that was dangerous to the patient
____ Did not immediately disconnect the syringe from the inlet port after inflating the cuff

VENTILATORY MANAGEMENT
ESOPHAGEAL OBTURATOR AIRWAY INSERTION FOLLOWING AN UNSUCCESSFUL ENDOTRACHEAL INTUBATION ATTEMPT

Start Time: _____
Stop Time: _____ Date: _____
Candidate's Name: _____
Evaluator's Name: _____

	Points Possible	Points Awarded
Continues body substance isolation precautions	1	
Confirms the patient is being ventilated with high percentage oxygen	1	
Directs the assistant to hyper-oxygenate the patient	1	
Identifies/selects the proper equipment for insertion of EOA	1	
Assembles the EOA	1	
Tests the cuff for leaks	1	
Inflates the mask	1	
Lubricates the tube *(may be verbalized)*	1	
Note: The examiner should remove the OPA and move out of the way when the candidate is prepared to insert the device		
Positions the head properly with the neck in the neutral or slightly flexed position	1	
Grasps and elevates the patient's tongue and mandible	1	
Inserts the tube in the same direction as the curvature of the pharynx	1	
Advances the tube until the mask is sealed against the patient's face	1	
Ventilates the patient while maintaining a tight mask-to-face seal	1	
Directs confirmation of placement of EOA by observing for chest rise and auscultation over the epigastrium and bilaterally over each lung	1	
Note: The examiner must acknowledge adequate chest rise, bilateral breath sounds and absent sounds over the epigastrium		
Inflates the cuff to the proper pressure	1	
Disconnects the syringe from the inlet port	1	
Continues ventilation of the patient	1	
Total:	**17**	

Critical Criteria

____ Did not take or verbalize body substance isolation precautions
____ Did not initiate ventilations within 30 seconds
____ Interrupted ventilations for more than 30 seconds at a time
____ Did not direct hyper-oxygenation of the patient prior to placement of the EOA
____ Did not successfully place the EOA within 3 attempts
____ Did not ventilate at a rate of at least 10 breaths per minute
____ Did not provide adequate volume per breath (maximum 2 errors/minute permissible)
____ Did not assure proper tube placement by auscultation bilaterally and over the epigastrium
____ Did not remove the syringe after inflating the cuff
____ Did not successfully ventilate the patient
____ Do not provide high flow oxygen (15 liters per minute or greater)
____ Inserted any adjunct in a manner that was dangerous to the patient

VENTILATORY MANAGEMENT
DUAL LUMEN DEVICE INSERTION FOLLOWING AN UNSUCCESSFUL ENDOTRACHEAL INTUBATION ATTEMPT

Start Time: _____
Stop Time: _____ Date: _____
Candidate's Name: _____
Evaluator's Name: _____

	Points Possible	Points Awarded
Continues body substance isolation precautions	1	
Confirms the patient is being properly ventilated with high percentage oxygen	1	
Directs the assistant to hyper-oxygenate the patient	1	
Checks/prepares the airway device	1	
Lubricates the distal tip of the device *(may be verbalized)*	1	
Note: The examiner should remove the OPA and move out of the way when the candidate is prepared to insert the device		
Positions the patient's head properly	1	
Performs a tongue-jaw lift	1	

☐ USES COMBITUBE	☐ USES THE PTL
Inserts device in the mid-line and to the depth so that the printed ring is at the level of the teeth	Inserts the device in the mid-line until the bite block flange is at the level of the teeth

	Points Possible	Points Awarded
	1	
Inflates the pharyngeal cuff with the proper volume and removes the syringe	Secures the strap	1	
Inflates the distal cuff with the proper volume and removes the syringe	Blows into tube #1 to adequately inflate both cuffs	1	
Attaches/directs attachment of BVM to the first (esophageal placement) lumen and ventilates	1	
Confirms placement and ventilation through the correct lumen by observing chest rise, auscultation over the epigastrium and bilaterally over each lung	1	
Note: The examiner states, "You do not see rise and fall of the chest and hear sounds only over the epigastrium."		
Attaches/directs attachment of BVM to the second (endotracheal placement) lumen and ventilates	1	
Confirms placement and ventilation through the correct lumen by observing chest rise, auscultation over the epigastrium and bilaterally over each lung	1	
Note: The examiner states, "You see rise and fall of the chest, there are no sounds over the epigastrium and breath sounds are equal over each lung."		
Secures device or confirms that the device remains properly secured	1	
Total:	**15**	

Critical Criteria

____ Did not take or verbalize body substance isolation precautions
____ Did not initiate ventilations within 30 seconds
____ Interrupted ventilations for more than 30 seconds at any time
____ Did not hyper-oxygenate the patient prior to placement of the dual lumen airway device
____ Did not provide adequate volume per breath (maximum 2 errors/minute permissible)
____ Did not ventilate the patient at a rate of at least 10 breaths per minute
____ Did not insert the dual lumen airway device at a proper depth or at the proper place within 3 attempts
____ Did not inflate both cuffs properly
____ **Combitube** — Did not remove the syringe immediately following the inflation of each cuff
____ **PTL** — Did not secure the strap prior to cuff inflation
____ Did not conform, by observing chest rise and auscultation over the epigastrium and bilaterally over each lung, that the proper lumen of the device was being used to ventilate the patient
____ Inserted any adjunct in a manner that was dangerous to the patient

ANSWER KEY

Below are answers to the multiple-choice questions in each Chapter Review. Note that page numbers in parentheses refer to the textbook pages on which answers may be found or supported.

CHAPTER ONE

1. a (p. 3);   **2.** d (p. 3);   **3.** c (p. 8);
4. b (p. 9);   **5.** b (p. 9)

CHAPTER TWO

1. a (p. 16);   **2.** b (p. 17);   **3.** d (p. 19);
4. a (p. 21);   **5.** c (p. 23)

CHAPTER THREE

1. b (p. 37);   **2.** b (p. 37);   **3.** b (p. 38);
4. c (p. 41);   **5.** a (p. 41);   **6.** c (p. 43)

CHAPTER FOUR

1. b (p. 48);   **2.** b (p. 47);   **3.** c (p. 51);
4. b (p. 54);   **5.** a (p. 54)   **6.** c (p. 55)

CHAPTER FIVE

1. b (p. 59);   **2.** b (p. 60);   **3.** d (p. 61);
4. c (p. 61);   **5.** d (p. 68)

CHAPTER SIX

1. b (p. 79);   **2.** b (p. 79)   **3.** d (p. 84);
4. d (p. 88);   **5.** c (p. 87)   **6.** b (p. 91);
7. d (p. 91);   **8.** a (p. 94);   **9.** d (p. 95);
10. a (p. 96)

CHAPTER SEVEN

1. c (p. 105);   **2.** d (p. 112);   **3.** d (p. 113);
4. c (p. 116);   **5.** d (p. 116);   **6.** a (p. 117);
7. a (p. 117);   **8.** d (p. 118);   **9.** d (p. 121);
10. c (p. 122)

CHAPTER EIGHT

1. b (p. 128);   **2.** c (p. 130);   **3.** b (p. 137);
4. a (p. 130);   **5.** c (p. 137)

CHAPTER NINE

1. a (p. 144);   **2.** c (p. 144);   **3.** d (p. 145);
4. b (p. 149);   **5.** c (p. 144)

CHAPTER TEN

1. b (p. 157);   **2.** c (p. 160);   **3.** c (p. 160);
4. b (p. 162);   **5.** b (p. 162)

CHAPTER ELEVEN

1. b (p. 167);   **2.** a (p. 169);   **3.** d (p. 170);
4. d (p. 170);   **5.** d (p. 174)

CHAPTER TWELVE

1. d (p. 179);   **2.** a (p. 179);   **3.** b (p. 180);
4. a (p. 181);   **5.** b (p. 182)

CHAPTER THIRTEEN

1. b (p. 189);   **2.** c (p. 190);   **3.** c (p. 191);
4. a (p. 194);   **5.** d (p. 194)

CHAPTER FOURTEEN

1. c (p. 203);   **2.** b (p. 207);   **3.** b (p. 204);
4. b (p. 208);   **5.** c (p. 209)

CHAPTER FIFTEEN

1. b (p. 225);   **2.** c (p. 225);   **3.** c (p. 227);
4. d (p. 228);   **5.** a (p. 229)

CHAPTER SIXTEEN

1. d (p. 235);   **2.** a (p. 237);   **3.** d (p. 238);
4. a (p. 238);   **5.** c (p. 240)

CHAPTER SEVENTEEN

1. d (p. 247);   **2.** d (p. 247);   **3.** b (p. 249);
4. b (p. 249);   **5.** a (p. 252)

CHAPTER EIGHTEEN

1. a (p. 262);   **2.** c (p. 264);   **3.** a (p. 264);
4. a (p. 266);   **5.** a (p. 271)

CHAPTER NINETEEN

1. c (p. 275);   **2.** b (p. 276);   **3.** c (p. 278);
4. a (p. 280);   **5.** c (p. 280)

CHAPTER TWENTY

1. a (p. 289);   **2.** c (p. 291);   **3.** d (p. 294);
4. b (p. 294);   **5.** d (p. 296)

CHAPTER TWENTY-ONE

1. a (p. 304);   **2.** a (p. 305);   **3.** c (p. 307);
4. d (p. 309);   **5.** a (p. 310)

CHAPTER TWENTY-TWO

1. b (p. 318);   **2.** c (p. 321);   **3.** c (p. 322);
4. d (p. 323)   **5.** a (p. 327)

CHAPTER TWENTY-THREE

1. a (p. 342); **2.** d (p. 343); **3.** c (p. 345); **4.** a (p. 355); **5.** b (p. 355)

CHAPTER TWENTY-FOUR

1. c (p. 375); **2.** b (p. 376); **3.** c (p. 377); **4.** c (p. 378); **5.** a (p. 379)

CHAPTER TWENTY-FIVE

1. a (p. 414); **2.** a (p. 415); **3.** b (p. 415); **4.** a (p. 417); **5.** d (p. 418)

CHAPTER TWENTY-SIX

1. a (p. 427); **2.** d (p. 433); **3.** c (p. 440); **4.** c (p. 437); **5.** a (p. 442)

CHAPTER TWENTY-SEVEN

1. a (p. 447); **2.** b (p. 449); **3.** a (p. 447); **4.** b (p. 448) **5.** c (p. 453)

CHAPTER TWENTY-EIGHT

1. b (p. 463); **2.** a (p. 467); **3.** d (p. 468); **4.** b (p. 473); **5.** d (p. 475)

CHAPTER TWENTY-NINE

1. a (p. 486); **2.** c (p. 487); **3.** b (p. 496); **4.** d (p. 489); **5.** b (p. 489); **6.** b (p. 490); **7.** c (p. 496); **8.** a (p. 497); **9.** d (p. 486); **10.** a (p. 499)

GLOSSARY

abandonment leaving a patient after care has been initiated and before the patient has been transferred to someone with equal or greater medical training.

abdominal quadrants four divisions of the abdomen used to pinpoint the location of a pain or injury: the right upper quadrant, the left upper quadrant, the right lower quadrant, and the left lower quadrant.

abrasion (ab-RAY-zhun) a scratch or scrape.

abruptio placentae (ab-RUPT-si-o plah-SENT-ta) a condition in which the placenta separates from the uterine wall; a cause of prebirth bleeding.

absorbed poisons poisons that are taken into the body through unbroken skin.

acetabulum (AS-uh-TAB-yuh-lum) the pelvic socket into which the ball at the proximal end of the femur fits to form the hip joint.

acromioclavicular (ah-KRO-me-o-klav-IK-yuh-ler) **joint** the joint where the acromion and the clavicle meet.

acromion (ah-KRO-me-on) **process** the highest portion of the shoulder.

activated charcoal a powder, usually pre-mixed with water, that will adsorb some poisons and help prevent them from being absorbed by the body.

active rewarming application of an external heat source to rewarm the body of a hypothermic patient.

afterbirth the placenta, membranes of the amniotic sac, part of the umbilical cord, and some tissues from the lining of the uterus that are delivered after the birth of the baby.

air embolism gas bubble in the bloodstream. The plural is *air emboli*. The more accurate term is *arterial gas embolism (AGE)*.

airway the passageway by which air enters or leaves the body. The structures of the airway are the nose, mouth, pharynx, larynx, trachea, bronchi, and lungs.

allergen something that causes an allergic reaction.

allergic reaction an exaggerated immune response.

alveoli (al-VE-o-li) the microscopic sacs of the lungs where gas exchange with the bloodstream takes place.

amniotic (am-ne-OT-ik) **sac** the "bag of waters" that surrounds the developing fetus.

amputation (am-pyu-TAY-shun) the surgical removal or traumatic severing of a body part, usually an extremity.

anaphylaxis (an-ah-fi-LAK-sis) a severe or life-threatening allergic reaction in which the blood vessels dilate, causing a drop in blood pressure, and the tissues lining the respiratory system swell, interfering with the airway. Also called *anaphylactic shock*.

anatomical position the standard reference position for the body in the study of anatomy. The body is standing erect, facing the observer. The arms are down at the sides and the palms of the hands face forward.

anatomy the study of body structure.

angina pectoris (AN-ji-nah [or an-JI-nah] PEK-to-ris) pain in the chest, occurring when blood supply to the heart is reduced and a portion of the heart muscle is not receiving enough oxygen.

anterior the front of the body or body part. Opposite of *posterior.*

antidote a substance that will neutralize a poison or its effects.

aorta (ay-OR-tah) the largest artery in the body. It transports blood from the left ventricle to begin systemic circulation.

apnea (ap-ne-ah) absence of breathing.

arrhythmia (ah-RITH-me-ah) a disturbance in heart rate and rhythm.

arteriole (ar-TE-re-ol) the smallest kind of artery.

arteriosclerosis (ar-TE-re-o-skle-RO-sis) a condition in which artery walls become hard and stiff due to calcium deposits.

artery any blood vessel carrying blood away from the heart.

artificial ventilation forcing air or oxygen into the lungs when a patient has stopped breathing or has inadequate breathing.

asystole (ay-SIS-to-le) when the heart has ceased generating electrical impulses.

atria (AY-tree-ah) the two upper chambers of the heart. There is a right atrium (which receives unoxygenated blood returning from the body) and a left atrium (which receives oxygenated blood returning from the lungs).

auscultation (os-skul-TAY-shun) listening. A stethoscope is used to auscultate for characteristic body sounds.

auto-injector a syringe pre-loaded with medication that has a spring-loaded device that pushes the needle through the skin when the tip of the device is pressed firmly against the body.

autonomic (AW-to-NOM-ik) **nervous system** the division of the peripheral nervous system that controls involuntary motor functions.

AVPU a memory aid for *alert, verbal response, painful response, unresponsive* as a classification of a patient's level of responsiveness. See also *mental status.*

avulsion (ah-VUL-shun) the tearing away or tearing off of a piece or flap of skin or other soft tissue. This term also may be used for an eye pulled from its socket or a tooth dislodged from its socket.

bag-valve-mask (BVM) device a hand-held device with a face mask and self-refilling bag that can be squeezed to provide artificial ventilations to a patient. Can deliver air from the atmosphere or oxygen from a supplemental oxygen supply system.

bandage any material used to hold a dressing in place.

base station a two-way radio at a fixed site such as a hospital or dispatch center.

behavior the manner in which a person acts.

behavioral emergency when a patient's behavior is not typical for the situation; when the patient's behavior is unacceptable or intolerable to the patient, his family, or the community, or when the patient may harm himself or others.

bilateral on both sides.

blood pressure the force of blood against the walls of the blood vessels. Usually arterial blood pressure (the pressure in an artery) is measured. See also *diastolic blood pressure; systolic blood pressure.*

blunt trauma injury caused by a blow that does not penetrate through the skin or other body tissues.

body mechanics the proper use of the body to facilitate lifting and moving and prevent injury.

body substance isolation (BSI) a form of infection control based on the presumption that all body fluids are infectious. BSI calls for always using appropriate barriers to infection at the emergency scene, such as gloves, masks, gowns, and protective eyewear.

bones hard but flexible living structures that provide support for the body and protection to vital organs.

brachial (BRAY-ke-al) **artery** artery of the upper arm.

brachial pulse the pulse felt in the upper arm; the pulse checked during infant CPR.

bradycardia (BRAY-duh-KAR-de-uh) a slow heart rate; any pulse rate below 60 beats per minute.

breech presentation when the baby appears buttocks or both legs first during birth.

bronchi (BRONG-ki) the two large sets of branches that come off the trachea and enter the lungs. There are right and left bronchi. The singular is *bronchus.*

bronchoconstriction constriction, or blockage, of the bronchi that lead from the trachea to the lungs.

calcaneus (kal-KAY-ne-us) the heel bone.

capillary (KAP-i-lair-e) a thin-walled, microscopic blood vessel where oxygen/carbon dioxide and nutrient/waste exchange with the body's cells takes place.

cardiac compromise a blanket term for any heart problem.

cardiac muscle specialized involuntary muscle found only in the heart.

cardiovascular system the heart and the blood vessels; the circulatory system.

carina (kah-RI-nah) the fork at the lower end of the trachea where the two mainstem bronchi branch.

carotid (kah-ROT-id) **arteries** the large neck arteries, one on each side of the neck, that carry blood from the heart to the head.

carotid (kah-ROT-id) **pulse** the pulse felt along the large carotid artery on either side of the neck.

carpals (KAR-pulz) the wrist bones.

cartilage tough tissue that covers the joint ends of bones and helps to form certain body parts such as the ear.

cellular phone a phone that transmits through the air instead of over wires so that the phone can be transported and used over a wide area.

central nervous system (CNS) the brain and spinal cord.

central pulses the carotid and femoral pulses, which can be felt in the central part of the body.

cephalic (se-FAL-ik) **presentation** when the baby appears head first during birth. This is the normal presentation.

cerebrospinal (suh-RE-bro-SPI-nal) **fluid (CSF)** the fluid that surrounds the brain and spinal cord.

cerebrovascular (suh-RE-bro VAS-ku-ler) **accident (CVA)** see *stroke.*

cervix (SUR-viks) the neck of the uterus at the entrance to the birth canal.

chief complaint in emergency medicine, the reason EMS was called, usually in the patient's own words.

circulatory system see *cardiovascular system.*

clavicle (KLAV-i-kul) the collarbone.

closed extremity injury an injury to an extremity with no associated opening in the skin.

closed wound an internal injury with no open pathway from the outside.

cold zone area where the command post and support functions that are necessary to control a hazardous material incident are located.

compensated shock when the patient is developing shock but the body is still able to maintain perfusion. See *decompensated shock; shock.*

concussion mild closed head injury without detectable damage to the brain. Complete recovery is usually expected.

conduction the direct transfer of heat from one material to another through direct contact.

confidentiality the obligation not to reveal information obtained about a patient except to other health care professionals involved in the patient's care, or under subpoena, or in a court of law, or when the patient has signed a release of confidentiality.

congestive heart failure (CHF) the failure of the heart to pump efficiently, leading to excessive blood or fluids in the lungs, the body, or both.

consent permission from the patient for care or other action by the EMT-B. See also *expressed consent; implied consent.*

constrict (kon-STRIKT) get smaller.

contamination the introduction of dangerous chemicals, disease, or infectious materials. See also *decontamination.*

contraindications (KON-truh-in-duh-KAY-shunz) specific signs or circumstances under which it is not appropriate and may be harmful to administer a particular drug to a patient.

contusion (Kun-TU-zhun) a bruise; in brain injuries, a bruised brain caused when the force of a blow to the head is great enough to rupture blood vessels.

convection carrying away of heat by currents of air or water or other gases or liquids.

coronary (KOR-o-nar-e) **arteries** blood vessels that supply the muscle of the heart (myocardium).

cranium (KRAY-ne-um) the bony structure making up the forehead, top, back, and upper sides of the skull.

crepitation [krep-uh-TAY-shun] the grating sound or feeling of broken bones rubbing together; also called *crepitus*.

cricoid (KRIK-oid) **cartilage** the ring-shaped structure that circles the trachea at the lower edge of the larynx.

cricoid pressure pressure applied to the cricoid cartilage to suppress vomiting and bring the vocal cords into view. Also called *Sellick's maneuver*.

critical incident stress debriefing (CISD) a process in which teams of professional and peer counselors provide emotional and psychological support to EMS personnel who are or have been involved in a critical (highly stressful) incident.

crowning when part of the baby is visible through the vaginal opening.

crush injury an injury caused when force is transmitted from the body's exterior to its internal structures. Bones can be broken, muscles, nerves, and tissues damaged, and internal organs ruptured, causing internal bleeding.

cyanosis (SIGH-uh-NO-sis) a blue or gray color resulting from lack of oxygen in the body (see *hypoxia*).

danger zone the area around the wreckage of a vehicle collision or other accident within which special safety precautions should be taken.

DCAP-BTLS A memory aid to remember deformities, contusions, abrasions, punctures/penetrations, burns, tenderness, lacerations, and swelling—signs and symptoms of injury found by inspection or palpation during patient assessment.

decompensated shock occurs when the body can no longer compensate for low blood volume or lack of perfusion. Late signs such as decreasing blood pressure become evident. See *compensated shock; shock*.

decontamination the removal or cleansing of dangerous chemicals and other dangerous or infectious materials. See also *contamination*.

dermis (DER-mis) the inner (second) layer of skin found beneath the epidermis. It is rich in blood vessels and nerves.

designated agent an EMT-B or other person authorized by a medical director to give medications and provide emergency care. The transfer of such authorization to a designated agent is an extension of the medical director's license to practice medicine.

detailed physical exam an assessment of the head, neck, chest, abdomen, pelvis, extremities, and posterior of the body to detect signs and symptoms of injury. The examination of the head includes detailed examination of the face, ears, eyes, nose, and mouth. It is ususally done en route to the hospital after earlier on-scene assessments and interventions are completed.

diabetes mellitus (di-ah-BEE-tez MEL-i-tus) also called "sugar diabetes" or just "diabetes," the condition brought about by decreased insulin production. The person with this condition is a diabetic.

diaphragm (DI-uh-fram) the muscular structure that divides the chest cavity from the abdominal cavity. A major muscle of respiration.

diastolic (di-as-TOL-ik) **blood pressure** the pressure remaining in the arteries when the heart is relaxed and refilling.

dilate (DI-late) get larger.

dilution (di-LU-shun) thinning down or weakening by mixing with something else. Ingested poisons are sometimes diluted by drinking water or milk.

direct carry a method of transferring a patient from bed to stretcher in which two or more rescuers curl the patient to their chests, then reverse the process to lower the patient to the stretcher.

direct ground lift a method of lifting and carrying a patient from ground level to a stretcher in which two or more rescuers kneel, curl the patient to their chests, stand, then reverse the process to lower the patient to the stretcher.

disaster plan a predefined set of instructions that tells a community's various emergency responders what to do in specific emergencies.

dislocation the disruption or "coming apart" of a joint.

distal farther away from the torso. Opposite of *proximal*.

distention [dis-TEN-shun] a condition of being stretched, inflated, or larger than normal.

do not resuscitate (DNR) order a legal document, usually signed by the patient and his physician, which states that the patient has a terminal illness and does not wish to prolong life through resuscitative efforts.

dorsal referring to the back of the body or the back of the hand or foot. A synonym for *posterior*.

dorsalis pedis (dor-sal-is PEED-is) **artery** artery supplying the foot, lateral to the large tendon of the big toe.

draw sheet method a method of transferring a patient from bed to stretcher by grasping and pulling the loosened bottom sheet of the bed.

dressing any material (preferably sterile) used to cover a wound that will help control bleeding and help prevent additional contamination.

drowning death caused by changes in the lungs resulting from immersion in water. See also *near-drowning*.

duty to act an obligation to provide care to a patient.

dyspnea (DISP-ne-ah) shortness of breath; labored or difficult breathing.

eclampsia (e-KLAMP-se-ah) a severe complication of pregnancy that produces seizures and coma.

ectopic (ek-TOP-ik) **pregnancy** when implantation of the fertilized egg is not in the body of the uterus, occurring instead in the oviduct (fallopian tube), cervix, or abdominopelvic cavity.

edema (eh-DEEM-uh) swelling resulting from a buildup of fluid in the tissues.

embolism (EM-bo-lizm) a thrombus, or clot of blood and plaque, that has broken loose from the wall of an artery.

EMS Command the senior EMS person on the scene who establishes an EMS command post and oversees the medical aspects of a multiple-casualty incident.

endotracheal (EN-do-TRAY-ke-ul) **tube** a tube designed to be inserted into the trachea. Oxygen, medication, or a suction catheter can be directed into the trachea through an endotracheal tube.

epidermis (ep-i-DER-mis) the outer layer of skin.

epiglottis (EP-i-GLOT-is) a leaf-shaped structure that prevents food and foreign matter from entering the trachea.

epilepsy (EP-uh-lep-see) a medical condition that sometimes causes seizures.

epinephrine (EP-uh-NEF-rin) a hormone produced by the body. As a medication, it dilates respiratory passages and is used to relieve severe allergic reactions.

esophagus (eh-SOF-uh-gus) the tube that leads from the pharynx to the stomach.

evaporation the change from liquid to gas. When the body perspires or gets wet, evaporation of the perspiration or other liquid into the air has a cooling effect on the body.

evisceration (e-VIS-er-AY-shun) an intestine or other internal organ protruding through a wound in the abdomen.

exhalation (EX-huh-LAY-shun) a passive process in which the intercostal (rib) muscles and the diaphragm relax, causing the chest cavity to decrease in size and causing air to flow out of the lungs. Also called *expiration.*

expiration (EK-spuh-RAY-shun) See *exhalation.*

expressed consent consent given by adults who are of legal age and mentally competent to make a rational decision in regard to their medical well-being. See also *consent; implied consent.*

extremities (ex-TREM-i-teez) the portions of the skeleton that include the clavicles, scapulae, arms, wrists, and hands (upper extremities) and the pelvis, thighs, legs, ankles, and feet (lower extremities).

extremity lift a method of lifting and carrying a patient in which one rescuer slips hands under the patient's armpits and grasps the wrists, while another rescuer grasps the patient's knees.

femoral (FEM-or-al) **artery** the major artery supplying the thigh and leg.

femur (FEE-mer) the large bone of the thigh.

fetus (FE-tus) the baby as it develops in the womb.

fibula (FIB-yuh-luh) the lateral and smaller bone of the lower leg.

flow-restricted, oxygen-powered ventilation device (FROPVD) a device that uses oxygen under pressure to deliver artificial ventilations. Has automatic flow restriction to prevent over-delivery of oxygen to the patient.

flowmeter a valve that indicates the flow of oxygen in liters per minute.

focused history and physical exam the step of patient assessment that follows the initial assessment and includes the patient history, physical exam, and vital signs.

fracture (FRAK-cher) any break in a bone.

full thickness burn a burn in which all the layers of the skin are damaged. There are usually areas that are charred black or areas that are dry and white. Also called a third degree burn.

gag reflex vomiting or retching that results when something is placed in the back of the pharynx. This is tied to the swallow reflex.

glottic opening the opening to the trachea.

glucose (GLU-kos) a form of sugar, the body's basic source of energy.

golden hour the optimum limit of one hour between time of injury and surgery at the hospital.

hazardous material according to the U.S. Department of Transportation, "any substance or material in a form which poses an unreasonable risk to health, safety, and property when transported in commerce."

hazardous material incident the release of a harmful substance into the environment.

head-tilt chin-lift maneuver a means of correcting blockage of the airway by the tongue by tilting the head back and lifting the chin. Used when no trauma, or injury, is suspected. See also *jaw-thrust maneuver.*

hematoma (hem-ah-TO-mah) a swelling caused by the collection of blood under the skin or in damaged tissues as a result of an injured or broken blood vessel; in a head injury, a collection of blood within the skull or brain.

hemorrhage (HEM-o-rej) bleeding, especially severe bleeding.

hives red, itchy, possibly raised blotches on the skin that often result from allergic reactions.

hot zone area immediately surrounding a hazardous material incident which extends far enough to prevent adverse effects from the released hazardous material to personnel outside the zone.

humerus (HYU-mer-us) the bone of the upper arm, between the shoulder and the elbow.

humidifier a device connected to the flowmeter to add moisture to the dry oxygen coming from an oxygen cylinder.

hyperglycemia (HI-per-gli-SEE-me-ah) high blood sugar.

hyperthermia (HI-per-THURM-e-ah) an increase in body temperature above normal.

hyperventilate (HI-per-VEN-ti-late) to provide ventilations at a higher rate than normal.

hypoglycemia (HI-po-gli-SEE-me-ah) low blood sugar.

hypoperfusion (HI-po-per-FEW-zhun) inadequate perfusion of the cells and tissues of the body caused by insufficient flow of blood through the capillaries. Also called *shock.* See also *perfusion.*

hypopharynx (HI-po-FAIR-inks) the area directly above the openings of both the trachea and the esophagus.

hypothermia (HI-po-THURM-e-ah) a generalized cooling that reduces body temperature below normal.

hypovolemic (HI-po-vo-LE-mik) **shock** shock resulting from blood or fluid loss.

hypoxia (hi-POK-se-uh) an insufficiency of oxygen in the body's tissues.

ilium (IL-e-um) the superior and widest portion of the pelvis.

implied consent the consent it is presumed a patient or patient's parent or guardian would give if they could, for example an unconscious patient or a parent who cannot be contacted when care is needed. See also *consent; expressed consent.*

Incident Command the person or persons who assume overall direction of a large-scale incident.

Incident Command System (ICS) see *Incident Management System*

Incident Management System (IMS) a system used for the management of a multiple-casualty incident, involving assumption of responsibility for command and designation and coordination of such elements as triage, treatment, transport, and staging.

index of suspicion awareness, often based on the mechanism of injury, that a patient may have suffered injuries.

indications specific signs or circumstances under which it is appropriate to administer a drug to a patient.

induced abortion expulsion of a fetus as a result of deliberate actions taken to stop the pregnancy.

inferior away from the head; usually compared with another structure that is closer to the head (e.g., the lips are inferior to the nose). Opposite of *superior*.

ingested poisons poisons that are swallowed.

inhalation (IN-huh-LAY-shun) an active process in which the intercostal (rib) muscles and the diaphragm contract, expanding the size of the chest cavity and causing air to flow into the lungs. Also called *inspiration*.

inhaled poisons poisons that are breathed in.

inhaler a spray device with a mouthpiece that contains an aerosol form of a medication that a patient can spray into his airway.

initial assessment the first element in assessment of a patient; steps taken for the purpose of discovering and dealing with any life-threatening problems. The six parts of initial assessment are: forming a general impression, assessing mental status, assessing airway, assessing breathing, assessing circulation, and determining the priority of the patient for treatment and transport to the hospital.

injected poisons poisons that are inserted through the skin, for example by needle, snake fangs, or insect stinger.

inspiration (IN-spuh-RAY-shun) See *inhalation*.

insulin (IN-suh-lin) a hormone produced by the pancreas or taken as a medication by many diabetics.

interventions actions taken to correct a patient's problems.

intubation (IN-tu-BAY-shun) insertion of a tube. See also *endotracheal tube; nasogastric tube; orotracheal intubation*.

involuntary muscle muscle that responds automatically to brain signals but cannot be consciously controlled.

ischium (ISH-e-um) the lower, posterior portions of the pelvis.

jaw-thrust maneuver a means of correcting blockage of the airway by moving the jaw forward without tilting the head or neck. Used when trauma, or injury, is suspected to open the airway without causing further injury to the spinal cord in the neck. See also *head-tilt chin-lift maneuver*.

joints places where bones articulate, or meet.

jugular (JUG-yuh-ler) **vein distention (JVD)** bulging of the neck veins.

labor the stages of the delivery of a baby that begin with the contractions of the uterus and end with the expulsion of the placenta.

laceration (las-er-AY-shun) a cut.

laryngoscope (lair-ING-uh-skope) an illuminating instrument that is inserted into the pharynx to permit visualization of the pharynx and larynx.

larynx (LAIR-inks) the voice box.

lateral to the side, away from the midline of the body.

lateral recumbent (re-KUM-bunt) **position** lying on the side. See *recovery position*.

liability legal responsibility.

ligaments connective tissues that connect bone to bone.

limb presentation when an infant's limb protrudes from the vagina before the appearance of any other body part.

local cooling cooling or freezing of particular (local) parts of the body.

lungs the organs where exchange of atmospheric oxygen and waste carbon dioxide take place.

mainstem bronchi See *bronchi*.

malar (MAY-lar) the cheek bone, also called the *zygomatic bone*.

malleolus (mal-E-o-lus) protrusion on the side of the ankle. The *lateral malleolus*, at the lower end of the fibula, is seen on the outer ankle; the *medial malleolus*, at the lower end of the tibia, is seen on the inner ankle.

mandible (MAN-di-bl) the lower jaw bone.

manual traction the process of applying tension to straighten and realign a fractured limb before splinting. Also called *tension*.

manubrium (man-OO-bre-um) the superior portion of the sternum.

maxillae (mak-SIL-e) the two fused bones forming the upper jaw.

mechanism of injury a force or forces that may have caused injury.

meconium staining amniotic fluid that is greenish or brownish-yellow rather than clear as a result of fetal defecation; an indication of possible maternal or fetal distress during labor.

medial toward the midline of the body.

medical direction oversight of the patient care aspects of an EMS system by the medical director. *Off-line medical direction* consists of standing orders and protocols issued by the medical director that allow EMTs to give certain medications or perform certain procedures without speaking to the medical director or another physician. *On-line medical direction* consists of orders from the on-duty physician given directly to an EMT-B in the field by radio or telephone.

medical director a physician who assumes the ultimate responsibility for the patient care aspects of the EMS system.

mental status level of responsiveness. See also *AVPU*.

metacarpals (MET-uh-KAR-pulz) the hand bones.

metatarsals (MET-uh-TAR-sulz) the foot bones.

mid-axillary (mid-AX-uh-lair-e) **line** a line drawn vertically from the middle of the armpit to the ankle.

mid-clavicular (mid-clah-VIK-yuh-ler) **line** a vertical line through the center of each clavicle.

midline an imaginary line drawn down the center of the body, dividing it into right and left halves.

miscarriage see *spontaneous abortion.*

mobile radio a two-way radio that is used or affixed in a vehicle.

multiple birth when more than one baby is born during a single delivery.

multiple casualty incident (MCI) any medical or trauma incident involving multiple patients.

muscles tissues or fibers that cause movement of body parts and organs.

musculoskeletal (MUS-kyu-lo-SKEL-e-tal) **system** the system of bones and skeletal muscles that support and protect the body and permit movement.

myocardial infarction (MY-o-KARD-e-ul in-FARK-shun) the condition in which a portion of the myocardium dies as a result of oxygen starvation; a heart attack.

nasal (NAY-zul) **bones** the bones that form the upper third, or bridge, of the nose.

nasal cannula (NAY-zul KAN-yuh-luh) a device that delivers low concentrations of oxygen through two prongs that rest in the patient's nostrils.

nasogastric (NAY-zo-GAS-trik) **tube (NG tube)** a tube designed to be passed through the nose, nasopharynx, and esophagus. It is used to relieve distention of the stomach in an infant or child patient.

nasopharyngeal (NAY-zo-fah-RIN-jul) **airway** a flexible breathing tube inserted through the patient's nose into the pharynx to help maintain an open airway.

nasopharynx (NAY-zo-FAIR-inks) the area directly posterior to the nose.

nature of illness what is medically wrong with a patient.

near-drowning the condition of having begun to drown, but still able to be resuscitated.

negligence a finding of failure to act properly in a situation in which there was a duty to act, needed care as would reasonably be expected of the EMT-B was not provided, and harm was caused to the patient as a result.

nervous system the system of brain, spinal cord, and nerves that govern sensation, movement, and thought. See also *central nervous system; peripheral nervous system; autonomic nervous system.*

neurogenic shock hypoperfusion due to nerve paralysis (sometimes caused by spinal cord injuries) resulting in the dilation of blood vessels that increases the volume of the circulatory system beyond the point where it can be filled.

911 system a system for telephone access to report emergencies. A dispatcher takes the information, and alerts EMS or the fire or police departments as needed. *Enhanced 911* has the additional capability of automatically identifying the caller's phone number and location.

nitroglycerin a medication that dilates the blood vessels.

nonrebreather mask a face mask and reservoir bag device that delivers high concentrations of oxygen. The patient's exhaled air escapes through a valve and is not rebreathed.

occlusion (uh-KLU-zhun) blockage, as of an artery by fatty deposits.

occlusive dressing any dressing that forms an airtight seal.

ongoing assessment a procedure for detecting changes in a patient's condition. It involves: repeating the initial assessment, reestablishing patient priority, repeating and recording vital signs, repeating the focused assessment, and checking interventions.

open extremity injury an extremity injury in which the skin has been broken or torn through from the inside by an injured bone or from the outside by something that has caused a penetrating wound with associated injury to the bone.

open wound an injury in which the skin is interrupted, exposing the tissue beneath.

OPQRST a memory device for the questions asked to get a description of the present illness: Onset, Provokes, Quality, Radiation, Severity, Time.

oral glucose (GLU-kos) a form of glucose (a kind of sugar) given by mouth to treat an awake patient (who is able to swallow) with an altered mental status and a history of diabetes.

orbits the bony structures around the eyes; the eye sockets.

organ donor a person who has completed a legal document that allows for donation of organs and tissues in the event of death.

oropharyngeal (OR-o-fah-RIN-jul) **airway** a curved device inserted through the patient's mouth into the pharynx to help maintain an open airway.

oropharynx (OR-o-FAIR-inks) the area directly posterior to the mouth.

orotracheal (OR-o-TRAY-ke-ul) **intubation** placement of an endotracheal tube through the mouth and into the trachea. See also *endotracheal tube.*

oxygen a gas commonly found in the atmosphere. Pure oxygen is used as a drug to treat patients whose medical or traumatic condition may cause them to be hypoxic, or low in oxygen.

oxygen cylinder a cylinder filled with oxygen under pressure.

palmar referring to the palm of the hand.

palpation touching or feeling. A pulse or blood pressure may be palpated with the fingertips.

paradoxical [pair-uh-DOCK-si-kal] **motion** movement of a part of the chest in the opposite direction to the rest of the chest during respiration.

partial thickness burn a burn in which the epidermis (outer layer of skin) is burned through and the dermis (second layer) is damaged. Burns of this type cause reddening, blistering, and a mottled appearance. Also called a second degree burn.

passive rewarming covering a hypothermic patient and taking other steps to prevent further heat loss and help the body rewarm itself.

patella (pah-TEL-uh) the kneecap.

pathogens the organisms that cause infection, such as viruses and bacteria.

penetrating trauma injury caused by an object that passes through the skin or other body tissues.

perfusion the supply of oxygen to and removal of wastes from the cells and tissues of the body as a result of the flow of blood through the capillaries.

perineum (per-i-NE-um) the surface area between the vagina and anus.

peripheral nervous system (PNS) the nerves that enter and leave the spinal cord and that travel between the brain and organs without passing through the spinal cord.

peripheral pulses the radial, brachial, posterior tibial, and dorsalis pedis pulses, which can be felt at peripheral (outlying) points of the body.

personal protective equipment (PPE) equipment such as eyewear, mask, gloves, gown, or turnout gear or helmet that protect the EMS worker from infection and/or from exposure to hazardous materials and the dangers of rescue operations.

phalanges (fuh-LAN-jiz) the toe bones and finger bones.

pharmacology (FARM-uh-KOL-uh-je) the study of drugs, their sources, characteristics, and effects.

pharynx (FAIR-inks) the area directly posterior to the mouth and nose. It is made up of the oropharynx and the nasopharynx.

physiology the study of body function.

placenta (plah-SEN-tah) the organ of pregnancy where exchange of oxygen, foods, and wastes occurs between a mother and fetus.

placenta previa (plah-SEN-tah PRE-vi-ah) a condition in which the placenta is formed in an abnormal location (low in the uterus and close to or over the cervical opening) that will not allow for a normal delivery of the fetus; a cause of prebirth bleeding.

plane a flat surface formed when slicing through a solid object.

plantar referring to the sole of the foot.

plasma (PLAZ-mah) the fluid portion of the blood.

platelets components of the blood; membrane-enclosed fragments of specialized cells.

pocket face mask a device, usually with a one-way valve, to aid in artificial ventilation. A rescuer breathes through the valve when the mask is placed over the patient's face. Also acts as a barrier to prevent contact with a patient's breath or body fluids. Can be used with supplemental oxygen when fitted with an oxygen inlet.

poison any substance that can harm the body by altering cell structure or functions.

portable radio a hand-held two-way radio.

positive pressure ventilation see *artificial ventilation*.

posterior the back of the body or body part. Opposite of *anterior*.

posterior tibial (TIB-ee-ul) **artery** artery supplying the foot, behind the medial ankle.

power grip gripping with as much hand surface as possible in contact with object being lifted, all fingers bent at the same angle, hands at least 10 inches apart.

power lift also called the *squat lift position*. It is a lift from a squatting position with weight to be lifted close to the body, feet apart and flat on the ground, body weight on or just behind balls of feet, back locked in. The upper body is raised before the hips.

premature infant any newborn weighing less than 5½ pounds or born before the 37th week of pregnancy.

pressure dressing a bulky dressing held in position with a tightly wrapped bandage to apply pressure to help control bleeding.

pressure point a site where a main artery lies near the surface of the body and directly over a bone. Pressure on such a point can stop distal bleeding.

pressure regulator a device connected to an oxygen cylinder to reduce cylinder pressure to a safe pressure for delivery of oxygen to a patient.

priapism (PRY-ah-pizm) persistent erection of the penis that may result from spinal injury and some medical problems.

prolapsed umbilical cord when the umbilical cord presents first and is squeezed between the vaginal wall and the baby's head.

prone lying face down.

protocols lists of steps, such as assessment and interventions, to be taken in different situations. Protocols are developed by the medical director of an EMS system.

proximal closer to the torso. Opposite of *distal*.

pubis (PYOO-bis) the medial anterior portion of the pelvis.

pulmonary (PUL-mo-nar-e) **arteries** the vessels that carry blood from the right ventricle of the heart to the lungs.

pulmonary edema accumulation of fluid in the lungs.

pulmonary veins the vessels that carry oxygenated blood from the lungs to the left atrium of the heart.

pulse the rhythmic beats felt as the heart pumps blood through the arteries.

pulse quality the rhythm (regular or irregular) and force (strong or weak) of the pulse.

pulse rate the number of pulse beats per minute.

pulseless electrical activity (PEA) a condition in which the heart's electrical rhythm remains relatively normal, yet the mechanical pumping activity fails to follow the electrical activity, causing cardiac arrest.

puncture wound an open wound that tears through the skin and destroys underlying tissues. A *penetrating puncture wound* can be shallow or deep. A *perforating puncture wound* has both an entrance and an exit wound.

pupil the black center of the eye.

quality improvement a process of continuous self-review with the purpose of identifying and correcting aspects of the system that require improvement.

radial artery artery of the lower arm. It is felt when taking the pulse at the wrist.

radial pulse the pulse felt at the wrist.

radius (RAY-de-us) the lateral bone of the forearm.

rapid trauma assessment a rapid assessment of the head, neck, chest, abdomen, pelvis, extremities, and posterior of the body to detect signs and symptoms of injury.

reactivity (re-ak-TIV-uh-te) in the pupils of the eyes, reacting to light by changing size.

recovery position lying on the side. Also called *lateral recumbent position*.

red blood cells components of the blood. They carry oxygen to and carbon dioxide away from the cells.

respiration (RES-pir-AY-shun) breathing.

respiratory arrest when breathing completely stops.

respiratory failure the reduction of breathing to the point where oxygen intake is not sufficient to support life.

respiratory quality the normal or abnormal (shallow, labored, or noisy) character of breathing.

respiratory rate the number of breaths taken in one minute.

respiratory rhythm the regular or irregular spacing of breaths.

respiratory (RES-pir-uh-tor-e) **system** the system of nose, mouth, throat, lungs, and muscles that brings oxygen into the body and expels carbon dioxide.

rule of nines a method for estimating the extent of a burn. For an adult, each of the following areas represents 9% of the body surface: the head and neck, each upper extremity, the chest, the abdomen, the upper back, the lower back and buttocks, the front of each lower extremity, and the back of each lower extremity. The remaining 1% is assigned to the genital region. For an infant or child the percentages are modified so that 18% is assigned to the head, 14% to each lower extremity.

rule of palm a method for estimating the extent of a burn. The palm of the patient's hand, which equals about 1% of the body's surface area, is compared with the patient's burn to estimate its size.

SAMPLE history the present and past medical history of a patient, so called because the elements of the history begin with the letters of the word *sample*: signs/symptoms, allergies, medications, past medical history, last oral intake, events leading to the injury or illness.

scapula (SKAP-yuh-luh) the shoulder blade.

scene size-up steps taken by an ambulance crew when approaching the scene of an emergency call: checking scene safety, taking body substance isolation precautions, noting the mechanism of injury or nature of the patient's illness, determining the number of patients, and deciding what, if any, additional resources to call for.

scope of practice a set of regulations and ethical considerations that define the scope, or extent and limits, of the EMT-B's job.

seizure (SEE-zher) a sudden change in sensation, behavior, or movement. The most severe form of seizure produces violent muscle contractions called convulsions.

Sellick's maneuver see *cricoid pressure*.

shock See *hypoperfusion*. See also *compensated shock; decompensated shock; hypovolemic shock; neurogenic shock*.

side effect any action of a drug other than the desired action.

sign an indication of a patient's condition that is objective, or can be observed by another person; an indication that can be seen, heard, smelled, or felt by the EMT-B or others.

sphygmomanometer (SFIG-mo-mah-NOM-uh-ter) the cuff and gauge used to measure blood pressure.

spinous (SPI-nus) **process** the bony bump on a vertebra.

spontaneous abortion when the fetus and placenta deliver before the 28th week of pregnancy; commonly called a *miscarriage*.

sprain the stretching and tearing of ligaments.

staging officer the person responsible for overseeing and keeping track of ambulances and ambulance personnel at a multiple-casualty incident. The staging officer will direct ambulances to treatment areas at the request of the transportation officer.

staging sector the area where ambulances are parked and other resources are held until needed.

standing orders a policy or protocol that is issued by a medical director that authorizes EMT-Bs and others to perform particular skills in certain situations.

sternum (STER-num) the breastbone.

stoma [STO-mah] a permanent surgical opening in the neck through which the patient breathes.

strain muscle injury resulting from over-stretching or over-exertion of the muscle.

stroke a condition of altered function caused when an artery in the brain is blocked or ruptured, disrupting the supply of oxygenated blood or causing bleeding into the brain. Also called a *cerebrovascular accident (CVA)*.

stylet (STI-let) a long, thin, flexible metal probe.

subcutaneous (SUB-ku-TAY-ne-us) **layers** the layers of fat and soft tissues found below the dermis.

suctioning (SUK-shun-ing) use of a vacuum device to remove blood, vomitus, and other secretions or foreign materials from the airway.

superficial burn a burn that involves only the epidermis, the outer layer of the skin. It is characterized by reddening of the skin and perhaps some swelling. An example is a sunburn. Also called a first degree burn.

superior toward the head (e.g., the chest is superior to the abdomen). Opposite of *inferior*.

supine lying on the back.

symptom an indication of a patient's condition that cannot be observed by another person but rather is subjective, or felt and reported by the patient.

systolic (sis-TOL-ik) **blood pressure** the pressure created when the heart contracts and forces blood out into the arteries.

tachycardia (TAK-uh-KAR-de-uh) a rapid heart rate; any pulse rate above 100 beats per minute.

tarsals (TAR-sulz) the ankle bones.

temporal (TEM-po-ral) **bone** bone that forms part of the side of the skull and floor of the cranial cavity. There are a right and a left temporal bone.

temporomandibular (TEM-po-ro-mand-DIB-yuh-lar) **joint** the movable joint formed between the mandible and the temporal bone, also called the TM joint.

tendons tissues that connect muscle to bone.

thorax (THOR-ax) the chest.

tibia (TIB-e-uh) the medial and larger bone of the lower leg.

torso the trunk of the body; the body without the head and the extremities.

tourniquet (TURN-i-ket) a device used for bleeding control that constricts all blood flow to and from an extremity.

trachea (TRAY-ke-uh) the "windpipe"; the structure that connects the pharynx to the lungs.

traction splint a special splint that applies constant pull along the length of a lower extremity to help stabilize the fractured bone and to reduce muscle spasms in limb. Traction splints are used primarily on femoral shaft fractures.

transportation officer the person responsible for managing transportation of patients to hospitals from the scene of a multiple-casualty incident.

treatment officer the person responsible for overseeing treatment of patients who have been triaged at a multiple-casualty incident.

treatment sector the area in which patients are treated at a multiple-casualty incident.

trending the changes in a patient's condition over time, such as slowing respirations or rising pulse rate, that may show improvement or deterioration, and that can be shown by documenting repeated assessments.

triage the process of quickly assessing patients in a multiple-casualty incident and assigning each a priority for receiving treatment according to the severity of their illness or injuries. From a French word meaning "to sort."

triage officer the person responsible for overseeing triage at a multiple-casualty incident.

triage sector the area in which secondary triage takes place at a multiple casualty incident.

triage tag color coded tag indicating the priority group to which a patient has been assigned.

ulna (UL-nah) the medial bone of the forearm.

umbilical (um-BIL-i-kal) **cord** the fetal structure containing the blood vessels that carry blood to and from the placenta.

uterus (U-ter-us) the muscular abdominal organ where the fetus develops; the womb.

vagina (vah-JI-nah) the birth canal.

vallecula (val-EK-yuh-luh) a groove-like structure anterior to the epiglottis.

vein any blood vessel returning blood to the heart.

venae cavae (VE-ne KA-ve) the superior vena cava and the inferior vena cava. These two major veins return blood from the body to the right atrium. (*Venae cavae* is plural, *vena cava* singular.)

venom a toxin (poison) produced by certain animals such as snakes, spiders, and some marine life forms.

ventilation the breathing in of air or oxygen or providing breaths artificially. See also *artificial ventilation*.

ventral referring to the front of the body. A synonym for *anterior*.

ventricles (VEN-tri-kulz) the two lower chambers of the heart. There is a right ventricle (which sends oxygen-poor blood to the lungs) and a left ventricle (which sends oxygen-rich blood to the body).

ventricular fibrillation (ven-TRIK-u-ler fib-ri-LAY-shun) **(VF)** a condition in which the heart's electrical impulses are disorganized, preventing the heart muscle from contracting normally.

ventricular tachycardia (ven-TRIK-u-ler tak-i-KAR-de-uh) **(V-Tach)** a condition in which the heartbeat is quite rapid; if rapid enough, ventricular tachycardia will not allow the heart's chambers to fill with enough blood between beats to produce blood flow sufficient to meet the body's needs.

venule (VEN-yul) the smallest kind of vein.

vertebrae (VER-te-bray) the 33 bones of the spinal column (singular *vertebra*).

vital signs outward signs of what is going on inside the body, including respiration; pulse; skin color, temperature, and condition (plus capillary refill in infants and children); pupils; and blood pressure.

vocal cords two thin folds of tissue within the larynx that vibrate as air passes between them, producing sounds.

voluntary muscle muscle that can be consciously controlled.

warm zone area at a hazardous material incident where personnel and equipment decontamination and hot-zone support take place.

water chill chilling caused by conduction of heat from the body when the body or clothing is wet.

white blood cells components of the blood. They produce substances that help the body fight infection.

wind chill chilling caused by convection of heat from the body in the presence of air currents.

withdrawal referring to alcohol or drug withdrawal in which the patient's body reacts severely when deprived of the abused substance.

xiphoid (ZI-foid) **process** the inferior portion of the sternum.

zygomatic (ZI-go-MAT-ik) **bones** the cheekbones.

INDEX